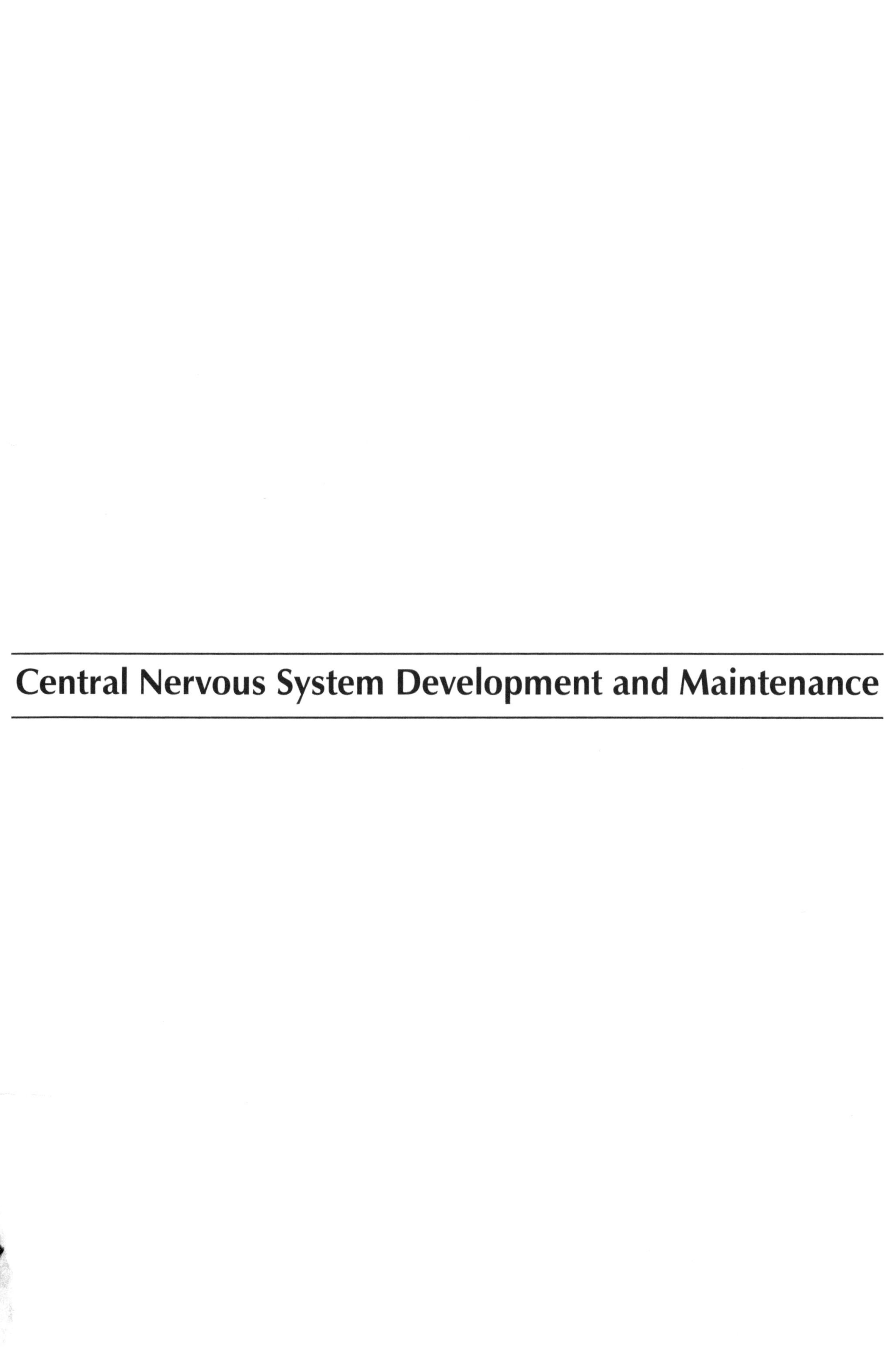

Central Nervous System Development and Maintenance

Central Nervous System Development and Maintenance

Editor: Scarlett Santos

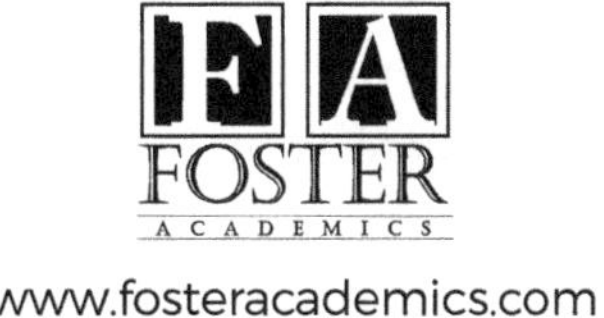

www.fosteracademics.com

www.fosteracademics.com

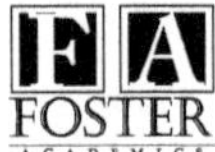

Cataloging-in-Publication Data

Central nervous system development and maintenance / edited by Scarlett Santos.
p. cm.
Includes bibliographical references and index.
ISBN 978-1-63242-724-3
1. Central nervous system. 2. Central nervous system--Diseases.
3. Nervous system--Diseases--Diagnosis. I. Santos, Scarlett.
RC280.N43 C45 2019
616.994 8--dc23

Foster Academics,
118-35 Queens Blvd., Suite 400,
Forest Hills, NY 11375, USA

ISBN 978-1-63242-724-3 (Hardback)

Contents

Preface

This book has been a concerted effort by a group of academicians, researchers and scientists, who have contributed their research works for the realization of the book. This book has materialized in the wake of emerging advancements and innovations in this field. Therefore, the need of the hour was to compile all the required researches and disseminate the knowledge to a broad spectrum of people comprising of students, researchers and specialists of the field.

The part of the nervous system which includes the brain and the spinal cord is known as central nervous system (CNS). It is a system responsible for integrating the received information, coordinating it, and influencing the activities of all body parts. In humans, the skull protects the brain, whereas the spinal cord is protected by the vertebrae. The brain and the spinal cord are enclosed in membranes, called meninges. The neuroglial cells are responsible for supporting the interneuronal space in the central nervous system. Neurological imaging of the brain is useful in diagnosing brain disorders. This book provides significant information about the central nervous system to help develop a good understanding of its development and maintenance. It aims to shed light on some of the unexplored aspects of central nervous system and the recent researches related to it. This book is a collective contribution of a renowned group of international experts.

At the end of the preface, I would like to thank the authors for their brilliant chapters and the publisher for guiding us all-through the making of the book till its final stage. Also, I would like to thank my family for providing the support and encouragement throughout my academic career and research projects.

Editor

1

Modeling immune functions of the mouse blood–cerebrospinal fluid barrier in vitro: primary rather than immortalized mouse choroid plexus epithelial cells are suited to study immune cell migration across this brain barrier

Ivana Lazarevic and Britta Engelhardt*

Abstract

Background: The blood–cerebrospinal fluid barrier (BCSFB) established by the choroid plexus (CP) epithelium has been recognized as a potential entry site of immune cells into the central nervous system during immunosurveillance and neuroinflammation. The location of the choroid plexus impedes in vivo analysis of immune cell trafficking across the BCSFB. Thus, research on cellular and molecular mechanisms of immune cell migration across the BCSFB is largely limited to in vitro models. In addition to forming contact-inhibited epithelial monolayers that express adhesion molecules, the optimal in vitro model must establish a tight permeability barrier as this influences immune cell diapedesis.

Methods: We compared cell line models of the mouse BCSFB derived from the Immortomouse® and the ECPC4 line to primary mouse choroid plexus epithelial cell (pmCPEC) cultures for their ability to establish differentiated and tight in vitro models of the BCSFB.

Results: We found that inducible cell line models established from the Immortomouse® or the ECPC4 tumor cell line did not express characteristic epithelial proteins such as cytokeratin and E-cadherin and failed to reproducibly establish contact-inhibited epithelial monolayers that formed a tight permeability barrier. In contrast, cultures of highly-purified pmCPECs expressed cytokeratin and displayed mature BCSFB characteristic junctional complexes as visualized by the junctional localization of E-cadherin, β-catenin and claudins-1, -2, -3 and -11. pmCPECs formed a tight barrier with low permeability and high electrical resistance. When grown in inverted filter cultures, pmCPECs were suitable to study T cell migration from the basolateral to the apical side of the BCSFB, thus correctly modelling in vivo migration of immune cells from the blood to the CSF.

Conclusions: Our study excludes inducible and tumor cell line mouse models as suitable to study immune functions of the BCSFB in vitro. Rather, we introduce here an in vitro inverted filter model of the primary mouse BCSFB suited to study the cellular and molecular mechanisms mediating immune cell migration across the BCSFB during immunosurveillance and neuroinflammation.

Keywords: Blood cerebrospinal fluid barrier, Choroid plexus, Immortomouse®, ECPC4

*Correspondence: bengel@tki.unibe.ch
Theodor Kocher Institute, University of Bern, Freiestrasse 1, 3012 Bern, Switzerland

Background

The choroid plexus (CP) is a highly-vascularized structure that folds from the ependymal lining of the lateral, third and fourth ventricles in a convoluted fashion into cerebrospinal fluid (CSF)-filled ventricular spaces. In contrast to brain microvessels at the blood–brain barrier (BBB), CP microvessels are fenestrated and allow for free diffusion of molecules from the blood into the CP stroma. Highly-polarized epithelial cells, which cover the entire surface of the CP, establish a barrier between the blood and the CSF, the blood–cerebrospinal fluid barrier (BCSFB). While preventing the free diffusion of blood components into CSF, the BCSFB regulates the transport of metabolites and is considered the major source of the CSF (reviewed in [1, 2]). Paracellular diffusion of molecules is prevented by unique tight junctions (TJs) constituted by the oligodendrocyte specific protein (OSP/claudin-11) that runs in parallel strands around the entire circumference of the CP epithelial cells [2, 3]. In addition to claudin-11, BCSFB TJs are composed of claudin-1, -2 and -3, occludin, and junctional adhesion molecules A and B (JAM-A and JAM-B), while the zonula occludens-1, 2, 3 (ZO1, 2, 3) scaffolding proteins connect BCSFB TJ proteins to the actin cytoskeleton (summarized in [4]). The adherens junctions (AJ) of the BCSFB are formed by homophilic interactions of the transmembrane epithelial cadherin (E-cadherin) that is linked to the actin cytoskeleton via α- and β-catenin [5, 6].

Over the last decades, evidence has accumulated for a potential role of the choroid plexus, and thus specifically the BCSFB, in controlling immune cell entry into the CNS. It has been shown that during experimental autoimmune encephalomyelitis (EAE), an animal model for multiple sclerosis (MS), functional expression of intercellular adhesion molecule (ICAM)-1 and vascular cell adhesion molecule (VCAM)-1 is upregulated on choroid plexus epithelial cells [3, 7, 8]. ICAM-1 and VCAM-1 mediate the migration of circulating autoaggressive T cells across the endothelial BBB in EAE (summarized in [9]) and have been suggested to also play a role in mediating immune cell trafficking across the BCSFB [10]. In addition, the recent observations that CCR6-deficient mice are resistant to EAE and that CCL20 is expressed by CP epithelial cells but not by the endothelial cells forming the BBB [11], support a role for the chemokine receptor CCR6 and its ligand CCL20 in mediating the migration of neuroantigen-specific CD4$^+$ Th17 cells into the CNS. Last but not least, the CP mediates neutrophil invasion into the CNS after traumatic brain injury [12] and in bacterial and viral infections [13].

Beyond these observations, our knowledge on the cellular and molecular mechanisms involved in immune cell migration across the BCSFB during immunosurveillance and neuroinflammation is sparse. Live cell imaging of single immune cells crossing the BCSFB in vivo is hindered by the poor accessibility of the CP within the brain ventricular spaces and its constant movement due to the CSF pulsations. Thus, reliable in vitro models of the BCSFB that preserve the differentiated characteristics of the choroid plexus epithelium are mandatory to study immune cell migration across the BCSFB. Primary cultures of bovine, porcine, sheep, rabbit and rat choroid plexus epithelial cells have been established and proven as reliable in vitro models of the BCSFB of the respective species [14–20]. In addition, a number of cell lines, notably the rat cell line Z310 [21–24] and human cell lines originating from either CP papillomas [25, 26] or carcinomas [27], have been used to model the BCSFB in vitro. A number of laboratories have previously established in vitro cultures of primary mouse CP epithelial cells [28–31]. However, there is a lack of a comprehensive characterization of these models regarding purity and growth as contact-inhibited monolayers, expression of CP epithelial cell markers, maturation of TJs and functional barrier characteristics [30]. Furthermore, an optimization of these in vitro models, which would allow for the study of immune functions of the mouse BCSFB including immune cell migration into the CNS, is still missing [8]. Given the availability of gene-targeted mice, an in vitro model of the mouse BCSFB would be advantageous to define the role of individual molecules for BCSFB immune functions.

The aim of the present study therefore, was to establish in vitro models of the mouse BCSFB specifically suited to study immune cell migration across the BCSFB in a two-chamber setup. To this end we first established the isolation and primary culture of mouse CP epithelial cells from different mouse strains. This included the Immortomouse®, which expresses the temperature sensitive Simian Virus 40 (tsSV40) large T Antigen under the MHC class I promoter and has proven a successful source for establishing conditionally immortalized epithelial cell lines from the intestine and other tissues [32, 33]. In addition, we analyzed the ECPC4 cell line, which was produced from CP carcinomas of transgenic mice expressing the SV40 large T antigen [34].

The three in vitro BCSFB models were analyzed for the development of epithelial contact-inhibited monolayers, expression of cytokeratin and transthyretin as markers for epithelial cell maturation, maturation of BCSFB specific junctional complexes, and the establishment of a tight barrier with low permeability to small molecular tracers with a high transepithelial electrical resistance (TEER). Our novel Immortomouse® derived lines and the ECPC4 cells did not fulfill these criteria as they lacked expression of cytokeratin and failed to grow into confluent monolayers with barrier characteristics. In contrast, highly-purified primary mouse choroid plexus epithelial cell (pmCPEC) cultures showed proper expression and distribution of CP epithelial markers including the junctional proteins and readily established a tight barrier. Inverted cultures, with pmCPECs grown on the lower side of a porous filter membrane, were found to be suitable in vitro models of the BCSFB to study the migration of encephalitogenic T cells across the BCSFB from the basolateral (blood facing) to the apical (CSF facing) side, which correctly models the in vivo situation.

Methods

Harvesting of choroid plexus tissues

Mice were sacrificed by CO_2 inhalation according to the approved animal protocol (approval number BE72/15 of the Cantonal Veterinary Office of the Canton Bern). Organ harvest was thus conducted strictly in compliance with the legal and ethical requirements demanded by the national guidelines and the legislations for animal experimentations. This implements Directive 2010/63/EU on the protection of animals used for scientific purposes and thus incorporates the principle of the Three Rs.

Primary mouse choroid plexus epithelial cell (pmCPECs) isolation and culture

Mouse choroid plexus epithelial cells (CPECs) were isolated by a modification of a protocol previously established for the isolation of rat CPECs [20]. In brief, sex-matched 6–10 week old C57BL/6 mice or Immortomice® (see below) were euthanized with CO_2, decapitated and the brain excised. For one preparation, CP was removed from 15 to 20 mice from the lateral and the 4th ventricles using a stereomicroscope. The CPs were collected, rinsed in Dulbecco's phosphate buffered saline (DPBS, Gibco, Paisley, UK) and digested with 0.1 mg/ml pronase (Roche, Mannheim, Germany) in DPBS for 30 min at 37 °C in a shaking water-bath. The digestion was ended by addition of 5 ml DPBS without pronase. The CP clumps were re-suspended and recovered by sedimentation controlled visually by eye. The supernatant, which contained mostly single non-epithelial cells and debris, was discarded. The sedimented CP clumps were further mechanically and enzymatically disaggregated by pipetting the clumps up and down for 10 to 20 s (depending on the size of the clumps) in 1 ml of 0.025 % Trypsin–EDTA (1×) (Gibco, Paisley, UK) containing 12.5 µg/ml DNAse I (Roche, Mannheim, Germany). This procedure was followed by a sedimentation step at RT for 1–2 min and ended based on visual control of the sedimentation. The supernatant, which is enriched for single CP epithelial cells and thus more turbid, was transferred to a new tube containing 5 ml of CPEC medium (DMEM/F12 1:1 (Gibco, Paisley, UK), FBS 10 % (Gibco, Paisley, UK), 2 mM glutamine (Gibco, Paisley, UK), 50 µg/ml gentamycine (Gibco, Paisley, UK). The procedure of mechanical/enzymatic disaggregation and sedimentation was repeated 5× as this was found to yield the highest number of CP epithelial cells. The single cell suspensions were pooled and pelleted by centrifugation at 800 g for 5 min at RT and the pellet was re-suspended in complete CPEC medium, which is CPEC medium supplemented with 5 µg/ml human insulin (Sigma Aldrich, St. Louis, MO, USA), 10 ng/ml hEGF (Peprotech, Rocky Hill, NJ, USA), 2 µg/ml hydrocortisone (Sigma, Buchs, Switzerland), 5 ng/ml bFGF (Sigma, Buchs, Switzerland) and 20 µM cytosine arabinoside (Ara-C) (Sigma, St. Louis, MO, USA). To allow for further enrichment of CP epithelial cells by differential attachment to plastic, cells were resuspended in 4 ml of complete CPEC growth medium and plated on 2 non-coated petri dishes (PD35), (Becton–Dickinson Biosciences (BD Biosciences), Franklin Lakes, NJ, USA). After 2–3 h of incubation at 37 °C and 7 % CO_2, adherent fibroblasts and macrophages, characterized by their extension of cellular processes, were visible under the microscope as described [20]. The supernatant was collected and pelleted for 5 min at 800 g. The single cell pellet was re-suspended in 0.5 ml complete CPEC growth medium and the cells were counted using a hemocytometer. 3×10^5 cells/cm^2 were plated either on permanox 8-well chamberslides (Thermo Fischer Scientific, Rochester, NY, USA) coated with 20 µg/ml laminin (Roche, Mannheim, Germany) for phase contrast microscopy, on laminin coated 0.33 cm^2 Transwell filters with 0.4 µm pore size (Corning, Kennebunk, ME, USA) for immunofluorescence stainings, or on laminin coated 5 µm pore size Transwell filters (Corning, Kennebunk, ME, USA) for transmigration assays. The cells were allowed to attach to the chamber slides or filter membranes at 37 °C and 7 % CO_2 for 48 h. On day 2 the cells were washed with DPBS and the medium was exchanged. The cells were grown to confluence for 1 week at 37 °C and 7 % CO_2 in complete growth medium, which was changed every other day. Continuous presence of the DNA synthesis inhibitor Ara-C specifically suppressed the growth of contaminating cells such as stromal fibroblasts. In contrast to CPECs, these cells express nucleoside transporters unable to distinguish ribose and arabinose residues and thus incorporate Ara-C into their genomic DNA, leading to the specific suppression of their growth [30, 35].

Establishment of inducible CP epithelial cell lines from the Immortomouse®

Immortomice® were obtained from Charles River Laboratories (Wilmington, MA, USA). Immortomice® are transgenic mice with a thermolabile Simian Virus 40 large T

Antigen (SV40 TAg) and limited expression of functional SV40 Tag in vivo, e.g. at 37 °C [36]. At the same time, expression of the thermolabile SV40 TAg under the control of the mouse major histocompatibility complex class I allows for further induction of expression by interferonγ (IFNγ). CPECs were isolated as described above and grown under non-permissive conditions (37 °C and in the absence of IFNγ). Upon reaching confluence, CPECs were passaged and shifted to permissive conditions (33 °C and 10 U/ml IFNγ (PeproTech, Rocky Hill, NJ, USA), allowing for increased expression of functional SV40 TAg. Confluent cell layers were split for up to 6 passages under permissive conditions accompanied by shifting aliquots of the cultures to non-permissive conditions at 37 or 39 °C and IFNγ withdrawal. The latter were tested for epithelial re-differentiation by evaluating their epithelial morphology and by immunostaining for epithelial-specific molecules. In order to establish conditionally immortalized cells, this standard procedure was modified several times at every step, as summarized in Table 1.

Culture of the ECPC4 cell line

The mouse carcinoma cell line ECPC4 [34] was purchased from the RIKEN BioResource Center (3-1-1 Koyadai, Tsukuba, Ibaraki 305-0074, Japan). ECPC4 cells were received at passage 37 and used for experiments until passage 41. ECPC4 cells were cultured at 37 °C and 7 % CO_2 in 5 ml growth medium (RPMI 1640 (Gibco, Paisley, UK)/10 % FBS (Gibco, Paisley, UK) in T25 flasks and split in a 1:4 ratio twice per week as described by the distributor.

Establishment of 'inverted' CPEC cultures

ECPC4 and pmCPECs were cultured on the lower ('inverted') side of filter inserts using a modification of a protocol previously established for porcine and human

Table 1 Culture options tested for the establishment of conditional immortoCPEC lines

Source (Immortomice®)			
Age	**Sex**	**Genotype**	**Number of mice per preparation**
2–12 weeks, 20 weeks	Female or male	tsSV40Tag heterozygous/homozygous	2 or 8–16

Primary culture (33 or 37 °C)					
Handling options				**Culture media supplements**	
Seeding density	**Laminin coated surface**	**Duration until passaging and/or temperature switch**	**Splitting ratio to passage 1**	**Fetal bovine serum (FBS)**	**Cytosine arabinoside (AraC)**
0.5×10^5–4.5×10^5 cells/cm^2 1×10^5 cells/filter limiting dilution cloning (1 cell/0.33 cm^2)	Petridishes 35 or 100 mm^2 8 well chamberslide 48 well plate 96 well plate	0–6 days 29/36 days (limited dilution)	1:2 1:3 1:5 Colony picking	2 % in the absence of fibroblast growth factor (FGF) 10 % (±FGF)	Days 0–4

De-differentiation under permissive conditions (33 °C + IFNγ)						
Handling options		**Culture media supplements**				
Temperature switch	**Splitting ratios**	**Conditioned medium**	**IFNγ**	**Fiborblast growth factor (FGF)**	**Fetal bovine serum**	**AraC**
With/without splitting of cells	1:2 1:3 1:4 1:5 1:8 limiting dilution cloning	±addition of supernatant from HIBCPPs (human choroid plexus papilloma *cell* line)	0 U/ml 5 U/ml 10 U/ml 30 U/ml 50 U/ml	± FGF	2 % 5 % 10 %	±AraC days 0–4

Re-differentiation under non-permissive conditions (37 or 39 °C)	
Handling options	**Culture media supplements**
Culture duration	**AraC**
7, 10, 14 days	day 0–4

in vitro models of the BCSFB [37]. In brief, CPECs were seeded in a volume of 100 µl on the lower side of laminin coated Transwell filters placed in inverted position in 12-well plates. The cells were seeded at the same density as on standard filter sides. After incubation for 24 and 48 h for ECPC4 and pmCPECs, respectively, the cells were washed twice with DPBS and the filters were flipped and placed into their original 24-well plate filled with 0.5 and 1 ml of growth medium per well in the upper and lower compartment, respectively.

Antibodies and buffers for immunofluorescence staining

The following primary antibodies were used for immunofluorescence staining: monoclonal mouse anti-pan Cytokeratin (mixture) antibody (1:100), (Sigma, C2562, St. Louis, MO, USA), monoclonal mouse anti-human E-cadherin (BD Biosciences, Franklin Lakes, NJ, USA, catalog number 610181, 10 µg/ml), monoclonal mouse anti-β-catenin (BD Biosciences, Franklin Lakes, NJ, USA, catalog number 610154, 10 µg/ml), polyclonal rabbit anti-human transthyretin (TTR) (Dako, Glostrup, Denmark, catalog number A0002, 4.5 µg/ml), polyclonal rabbit anti-claudin-1 (Cldn-1) (Invitrogen, Camarillo, CA, USA, catalog number 519000, 5 µg/ml), polyclonal rabbit anti-claudin-2, or -3 or -11 (Invitrogen, Camarillo, CA, USA, catalog numbers 516100, 341700, 364500, respectively, 10 µg/ml), polyclonal rabbit anti-zonula occludens 1 (ZO1) (Invitrogen, Camarillo, CA, USA, catalog number 617300, 5 µg/ml), and polyclonal goat anti-huVimentin (1:20, Chemicon International Inc. Temecula, CA, USA, catalog number AB1620). Rat anti-mouse ICAM-1 (25ZC7) and rat anti-mouse VCAM-1 (9DB3) were used as hybridoma culture supernatants.

The following 2nd stage antibodies were used: Cy3 donkey anti-mouse IgG (H + L) (Jackson ImmunoResearch, West Grove, PA, USA, catalog number 715-165-151, 2.5 µg/ml), Alexa488 goat anti-rabbit IgG (H + L) (Invitrogen, Eugene, OR, USA, catalog number A11034 10 µg/ml), and Cy3 donkey anti-goat IgG (H + L) (Jackson ImmunoResearch, West Grove, PA, USA, catalog number 705-165-147, 7 µg/ml), and Cy3 donkey anti-rat IgG (H + L) (Jackson ImmunoResearch, West Grove, PA, USA, catalog number 712-165-150, 2.5 µg/ml). The following buffers were made in house: 10 × TBS (50 mM Trizma Base (Sigma, St. Louis, MO, USA), 150 mM NaCl (Sigma, Buchs, Switzerland), 1 mM $CaCl_2 \cdot 2H_2O$ (Sigma St. Louis, MO, USA), adjusted to pH 7.4).

Immunofluorescence staining

Confluent cell layers grown on Transwell filters (Corning, Kennebunk, ME, USA) were gently washed with warm DPBS and subsequently fixed with either 1 % paraformaldehyde (PFA, MERCK, Darmstadt, Germany) in DPBS at RT for 10 min or with −20 °C methanol (for claudin and occludin staining) for 1 min. After fixation, the cells were washed 5× with DPBS. Blocking solution (5 % skimmed milk (Rapilait, Migros, Switzerland), 0.3 % Triton-X-100 (Schweizerhall, Basel, Switzerland Batch Nr. A11021), 0.04 % NaN_3 (Fluka Chemie, Buchs, Switzerland) in TBS pH 7.4) was incubated for 20 min at RT. Subsequently 35 µl of blocking buffer containing the 1st antibody was added for 1 h at RT. The primary antibody was removed from the cell layer by 5 washing steps with DPBS and 35 µl of blocking buffer containing the 2nd antibody was added to the filter inserts and incubated light protected for 45 min at RT. The cells were washed 5× with DPBS and incubated under light protection with 1 µg/ml 4′,6-diamidin-2-phenylindol (DAPI, AppliChem, Darmstadt, Germany) in DPBS for 2 min at RT. After washing 3× with DPBS, the cell carrying filters were cut out from the inserts, plated on glass-slides and mounted with embedding medium Mowiol (Sigma-Aldrich, Steinheim, Germany) prior to fluorescence microscopy. Immunostaining for cell surface ICAM-1 and VCAM-1 was performed on live cells. To this end live cells were incubated with the hybridoma culture supernatants for 20 min at RT. After washing with DPBS, the cells were fixed with 1 % formaldehyde in PBS for 5 min at RT, washed with DPBS for 10 min at RT and then incubated with the secondary antibody for 20 min at RT in the dark. After washing 3× with DPBS, the cell-carrying filters were cut out from the inserts, plated on glass-slides and mounted with embedding medium Mowiol prior to fluorescence microscopy.

Transepithelial electrical resistance

The transepithelial electrical resistance (TEER) across the CPEC monolayers was analyzed in triplicate by impedance spectroscopy employing the cellZscope R (Nanoanalytics, Muenster, Germany) according to the manufacturer's instructions. To this end cells were seeded on laminin coated 0.4 µm poresized filter inserts (Corning, Kennebunk, ME, USA or Greiner bio-one, Frickenhausen, Germany) in standard or inverted culture as described above. Upon complete pmCPECs attachment after 48 h, the filters were turned upside down and the medium was added to both compartments of the filter system allowing for further proliferation of the cells. The pmCPECs were transferred into the cellZscope and the TEER was measured over the last 72 h in culture to monitor the achievement of the resistance plateau. The ECPC4 cells were split in a 1:4 ratio as recommended by the distributor without counting the cells, and plated on standard and inverted sides of laminin coated Transwell filters. Upon attachment of ECPC4 cells to the porous membranes after 24 h, the filters were transferred into the cellZscope where they grew to confluence for further 3 days. One point TEER measurement of titrated and serum-depleted ECPC4 cells was performed every 24 h using the EndOhm-6 device (World Precision Instruments, Inc. Sarasota, FL, USA). Therefore, the filter inserts were transferred one by one into the chamber containing pre-warmed culture medium. In order to obtain accurate results, hydrostatic pressure on the membranes and air bubble formation were carefully avoided. The electrode was centered within the chamber and the TEER was measured using the Millicell Electrical Resistance System-2 epithelial volt-ohm meter (Millipore Corporation, Billerica, MA, USA). The displayed values were divided by the surface area of the filters, in order to yield the net resistances of the cell monolayers. Blank laminin coated inserts were used as empty filter references.

Transepithelial permeability

Prior to barrier investigations, the cells were seeded on laminin coated 0.33 cm^2 Transwell (Corning, Kennebunk, ME, USA) filters, pore diameter 0.4 µm, and the pmCPECs and ECPC4 cells were incubated for 48 and 24 h, respectively. Next, both compartments of the Transwell filter system were filled with fresh medium and the cells were cultured for further 5 days (pmCPECs) or 2–3 days (ECPC4). The paracellular permeability across the epithelial monolayers was measured in triplicate exactly as previously described [38, 39]. In brief, prior to experiments, 3 kDa dextran coupled with Alexa Fluor 680 (Molecular Probes, Eugene, OR, USA) was diluted, light protected, in assay medium (DMEM (Gibco, Paisley, UK), 5 % FCS (Gibco, Paisley, UK), 25 mM Hepes (Gibco, Paisley, UK), 2 % L-glutamine Gibco, Paisley, UK) to a final concentration of 10 µg/ml. 600 µl of the dextran free assay medium was added to the bottom of each well of an empty 24-Transwell plate (Corning, Kennebunk, ME, USA). Permeability assays were always performed on the same CPEC cultures previously analyzed for TEER. Filters were washed once with assay medium, and 100 µl of the dextran solution was added to the upper side of the filter inserts, which were subsequently placed into wells containing 600 µl of assay medium. The plate was incubated at 37 °C and the inserts were replaced into wells containing fresh assay medium, avoiding long exposure to light and room temperature every 10 min. 200 µl samples from all lower compartments were transferred to a 96-well plate. The dextran permeability was measured by scanning the 200 µl samples in the 96-well plate by infrared imaging (Odyssey Quantitative Fluorescence Imaging System, LI-COR, Bad Homburg, Germany). The epithelial permeability coefficient (Pe) was calculated using the clearance principle to obtain a concentration-independent transport parameter as previously described in detail [39]. A standard dilution curve (1 µg/ml–0.1 ng/ml) and empty filters were used to obtain the reference permeability of the empty filter inserts. The permeability coefficient for the in vitro BCSFB models was calculated as follows: the slope of the average tracer volume cleared was plotted versus time in order to obtain the linear regression designated as PSt. The slope of the tracer clearance curve of the coated empty filters was indicated as PSf. The permeability surface area product of the epithelial cell monolayer (PSe) was calculated from PSt and PSf: $1/PSe = 1/PSt - 1/PSf$. The PSe was divided by the filter surface area, in order to generate the epithelial Pe in cm/min.

The cell layer Pe for Lucifer Yellow (LY) (Sigma, St. Louis, MO, USA)—MW 457.3 g/mol diluted in assay medium—was determined as previously published in [40] according to the permeability assay for 3 kDa described above, with the assay medium being HBSS (1×) without phenol red (Gibco, Paisley, UK), supplemented with 5 % FCS and 25 mM Hepes, the LY solution of 50 µM and the LY standard dilution curve measured for 20–0.05 µM LY. The fluorescence detection was performed using the Tecan Infinite M1000 device and the Tecan i-control software (Tecan Trading AG, Männerdorf, Switzerland). Calculation of the Pe values by this methodology provides numbers to the 8th decimal. Entering these mathematically-correct numbers into the GraphPad Prism 6 Software for statistical analysis provides values to the 3rd decimal. These mathematically correct Pe values are shown in the "Results".

T cell migration across the BCSFB in vitro

In order to assure an unhindered passing of immune cells through the filter pores during the transmigration assay, the CPEC cells were seeded on laminin-coated inverted filters with 5 µm pore size. Inverted pmCPEC cultures were stimulated or not with TNFα (PromoCell GmbH, Heidelberg, Germany) (10 ng/ml) or IFNγ (100 U/ml) 16 h prior to the experiment. Encephalitogenic CD4$^+$ Th1 effector/memory proteolipid protein (PLP) peptide $aa_{139-153}$ specific T cells (line SJL/PLP7) were cultured as previously described [41]. On the day of the assay the CD4$^+$ T cells were collected in migrations-assay medium (MAM: DMEM (Gibco, Paisley, UK), 2 % L-Glutamine, 25 mM Hepes (Gibco, Paisley, UK), 5 % Calf Serum (CS) (Sigma, St. Louis, MO, USA)). pmCPEC inserts were washed with MAM twice before transferred into a new 24-well Costar plate well containing 600 µl of MAM. 100 µl of MAM containing 1×10^5 T cells was added per insert and T cells were allowed to transmigrate for 8 h at 37 °C. Additionally, a triplicate of input cell suspensions containing 1×10^5/600 µl of MAM were pipetted into 24-well plate wells. The number of transmigrated T cells, the number of the cells in input samples and their viabilities were assessed by the CASY Cell counter and analyzer (Schärfe System, Reutlingen, Germany) according to the manufacturer's instructions. The percentage of migrated T cells was calculated referring to the inputs as 100 %.

Statistical analysis

One-way ANOVA was performed followed by the Tukey multiple comparison test to compare three or more groups. For comparison of two groups, a Mann–Whitney test was performed. Results were expressed as mean ± SD and a P value <0.05 was considered significant. Statistical analysis was performed using the GraphPad Prism 6 software (GraphPad, San Diego, CA, USA).

Results

Isolation and culture of highly purified primary mouse choroid plexus epithelial cells (pmCPECs)

In order to provide a suitable in vitro model of the mouse BCSFB to investigate the cellular and molecular mechanisms mediating immune cell migration across the BCSFB, we established a procedure for the isolation and culture of highly purified primary mouse choroid plexus epithelial cells (pmCPECs) by adapting a previously-published protocol for the isolation and culture of rat choroid plexus epithelial cells [20]. CPECs were isolated by enzymatic digestion followed by a combined mechanical and enzymatic disaggregation of the choroid plexus from the lateral and 4th ventricles of sex and age matched mice. The preparations yielded 3.3–4.5 × 10^4 CPECs per mouse. The cells were plated on laminin-coated supports in a density of 3 × 10^5/cm^2. The pmCPECs formed islets of cuboidal shaped cells that within 5–7 days grew into confluent monolayers showing contact inhibition (Fig. 1). We did notice the occasional appearance of incompletely processed CP tissue particles (asterisk, Fig. 1a) and the formation of small dome-like epithelial structures after one week of culture (asterisk, Fig. 1b). The high purity of the CPEC culture was confirmed by positive immunofluorescence (IF) staining for cytokeratin in >95 % of cells within the monolayer. Junctional maturation was confirmed by the junctional localization of tight junction proteins, e.g. claudin-1 (e.g. Fig. 4b). Thus our protocol enabled the isolation and growth of highly pure mouse choroid plexus epithelial cells.

Conditionally immortalized Immortomouse® derived CPEC lines fail to re-differentiate into mature CPECs

Having established primary cultures of pmCPECs, we next aimed to establish conditionally immortalized CPEC lines which would produce proliferating cultures and thus reduce the number of mice needed for the in vitro model. The Immortomouse® that carries the thermolabile SV40 large T antigen under the control of an IFNγ inducible MHC class I promoter was used [36]. Previous studies have successfully used this mouse model to establish conditionally immortalized epithelial cell lines from other tissues [32].

When grown under non-permissive conditions (37 °C, no IFNγ) primary cultures of Immortomouse® CPECs were indistinguishable from CPECs of C57BL/6 mice (Fig. 2a). When placed under permissive conditions (33 °C, 10 U IFNγ) the CPECs started to proliferate and rapidly lost their typical cuboidal morphology starting in areas of lower cell density at the edges of the culture dishes while CPECs in the center of epithelial islets kept their cuboidal morphology (Fig. 2b). Immortalized CPECs also lost BCSFB specific expression of receptors and barrier functions as addition of the DNA synthesis inhibitor cytosine arabinoside (Ara-C) induced the cell

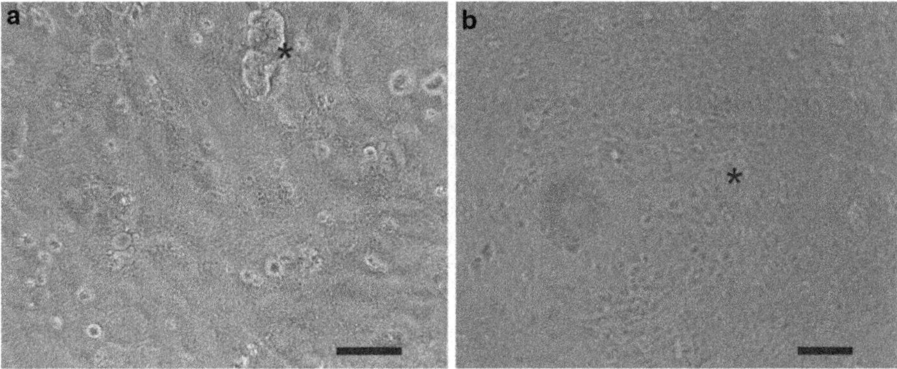

Fig. 1 Morphology of confluent primary mouse choroid plexus epithelial cells (pmCPECs). Representative phase contrast pictures of cells plated directly after choroid plexus dissection and cell disaggregation and cultured in complete growth medium for 8 days. The pmCPECs exhibit a predominant polygonal morphology with rare unprocessed tissue remnants (*asterisk*) visible in **a** and occasional dome like cell aggregates (*asterisk*) visible in **b**. The contrast of picture **a** was enhanced using Adobe Photoshop software. *Scale bar* in **a** = 50 μm and in **b** = 100 μm

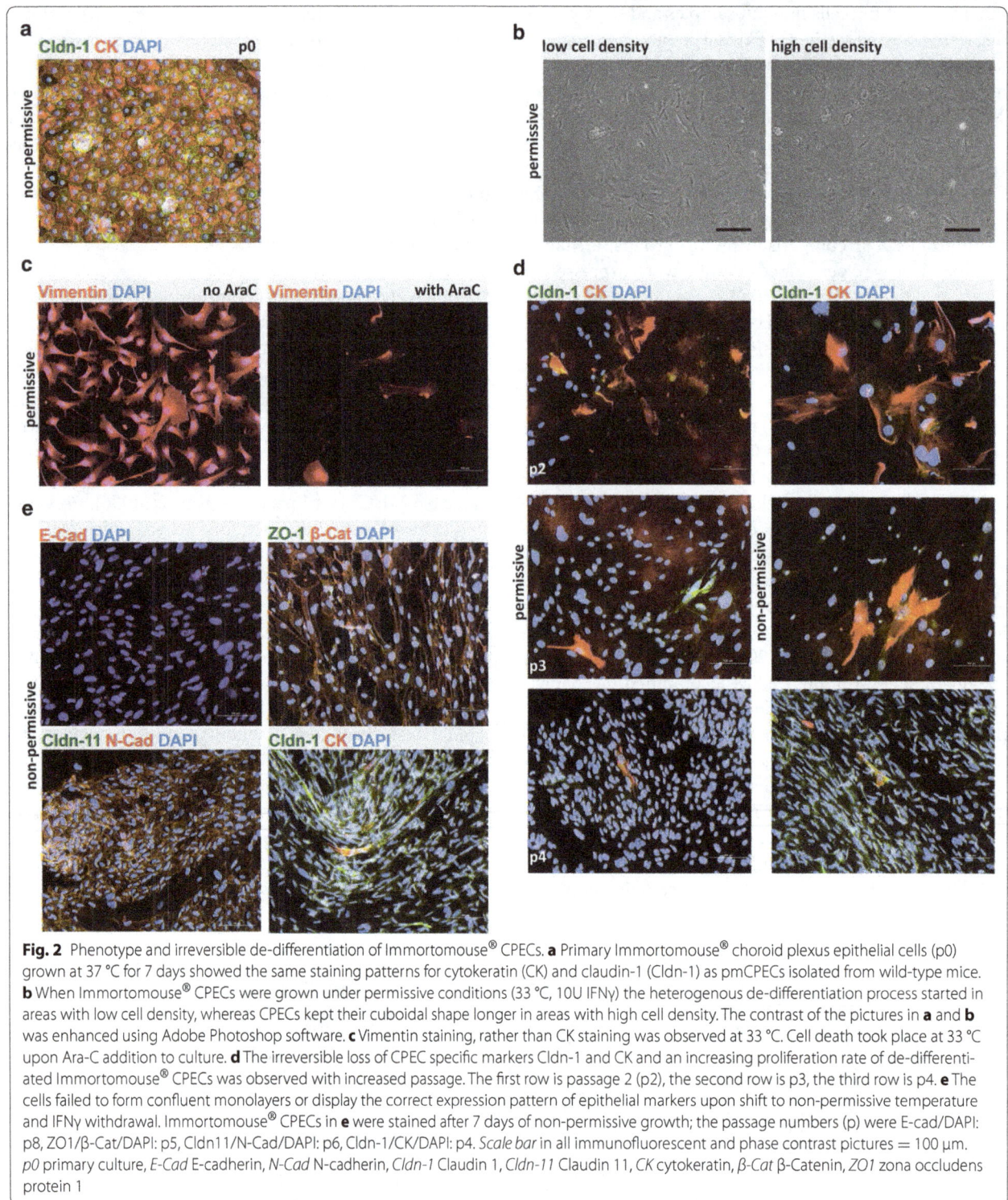

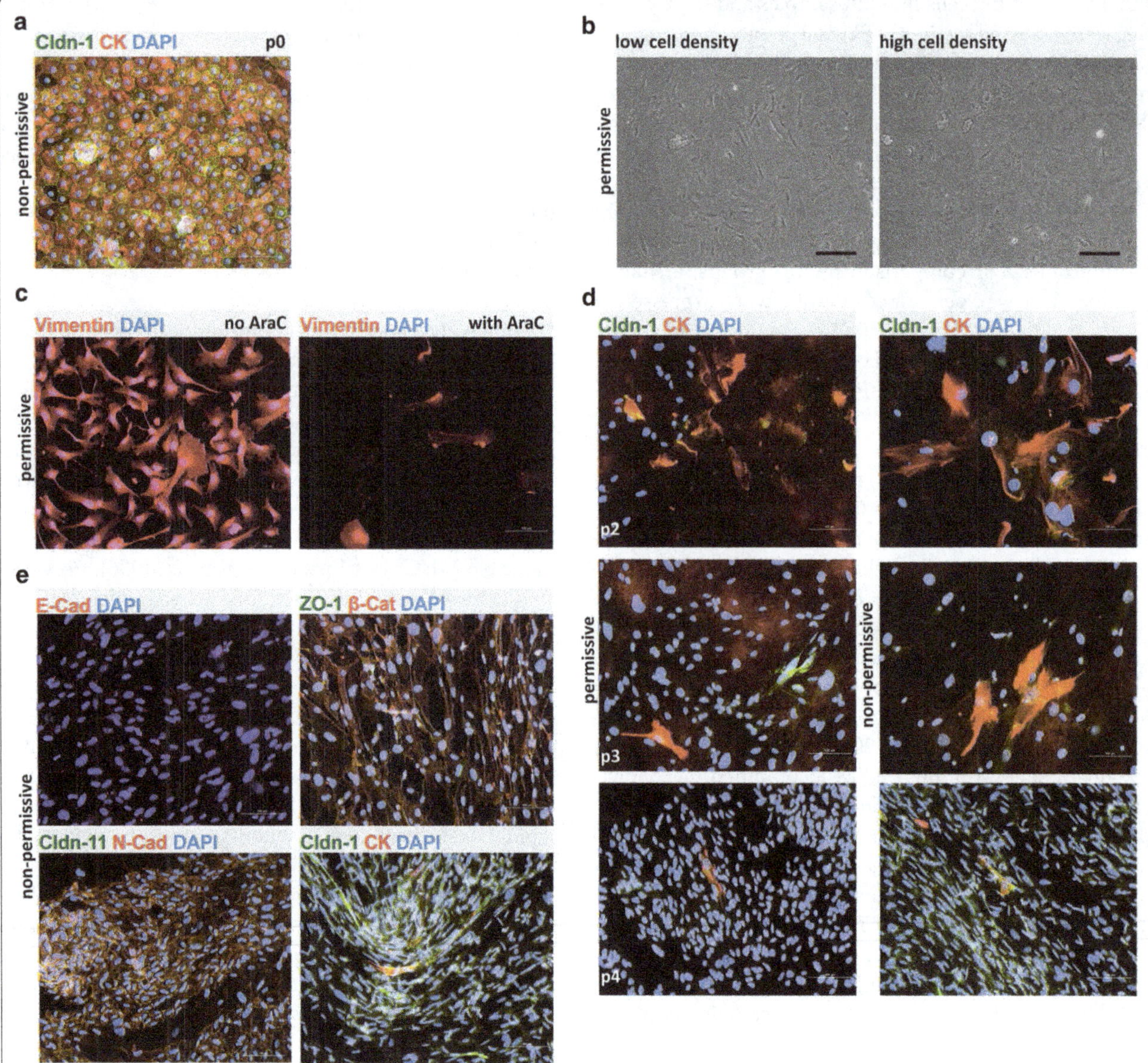

Fig. 2 Phenotype and irreversible de-differentiation of Immortomouse® CPECs. **a** Primary Immortomouse® choroid plexus epithelial cells (p0) grown at 37 °C for 7 days showed the same staining patterns for cytokeratin (CK) and claudin-1 (Cldn-1) as pmCPECs isolated from wild-type mice. **b** When Immortomouse® CPECs were grown under permissive conditions (33 °C, 10U IFNγ) the heterogenous de-differentiation process started in areas with low cell density, whereas CPECs kept their cuboidal shape longer in areas with high cell density. The contrast of the pictures in **a** and **b** was enhanced using Adobe Photoshop software. **c** Vimentin staining, rather than CK staining was observed at 33 °C. Cell death took place at 33 °C upon Ara-C addition to culture. **d** The irreversible loss of CPEC specific markers Cldn-1 and CK and an increasing proliferation rate of de-differentiated Immortomouse® CPECs was observed with increased passage. The first row is passage 2 (p2), the second row is p3, the third row is p4. **e** The cells failed to form confluent monolayers or display the correct expression pattern of epithelial markers upon shift to non-permissive temperature and IFNγ withdrawal. Immortomouse® CPECs in **e** were stained after 7 days of non-permissive growth; the passage numbers (p) were E-cad/DAPI: p8, ZO1/β-Cat/DAPI: p5, Cldn11/N-Cad/DAPI: p6, Cldn-1/CK/DAPI: p4. *Scale bar* in all immunofluorescent and phase contrast pictures = 100 μm. *p0* primary culture, *E-Cad* E-cadherin, *N-Cad* N-cadherin, *Cldn-1* Claudin 1, *Cldn-11* Claudin 11, *CK* cytokeratin, *β-Cat* β-Catenin, *ZO1* zona occludens protein 1

death of the immortalized CPECs. Furthermore, the cells showed expression of the mesenchymal intermediate filament vimentin (Fig. 2c). Loss of epithelial cell morphology and contact inhibition was accompanied by the continuous loss of expression of cytokeratin as well as loss of expression and junctional localization of E-cadherin and the choroid plexus specific claudins (claudin-1, -2, -3, -11) shown here over several passages (Fig. 2d).

Re-differentiation of the immortalized CPECs was attempted after passages 1–6 at 37 or 39 °C and withdrawal of IFNγ with re-differentiation at 39 °C found to be more effective. Evidence for re-differentiation of the immortalized CPECs into epithelial cells was documented by the re-expression of cytokeratin in a few epithelial cells and the partial reconstitution of AJs (detection of junctional localization of E/N-cadherin and β-catenin) and TJs (detection of junctional localization of ZO-1, claudin-1, claudin-11) (Fig. 2c, e and not shown). Unfortunately this process was limited to small, incoherent islands of epithelial cells and remained incomplete due to the continued expression of vimentin in the cultured cells and cytoplasmic detection of junctional molecules irrespective of passage number (Fig. 2e).

Interestingly, the addition of Ara-C to highly proliferating Immortomouse® CPECs at non-permissive conditions did not induce massive cell death during the re-differentiation time of 7–14 days. However, a selection for re-differentiated cuboidal epithelial cells could not be achieved (data not shown).

In a next step we compared a possible advantage of establishing CPEC lines from Immortomice® homozygous (T/T) or heterozygous (T/+) for the tsSV40Tag. Indeed we found that under permissive conditions Immortomouse® CPECs from mice homozygous for the tsSV40TAg (T/T) proliferated faster than those from heterozygous mice (T/+) (data not shown) but irrespective of their genotype they equally failed to re-differentiate into CP epithelial cells in different passages.

We further tested different concentrations of FBS and found that increasing concentrations of FBS in the CPEC cultures increased the proliferation rate of the immortalized cells, but reducing FBS concentrations under non-permissive conditions did not improve re-differentiation of the CPEC cell lines. Similarly, propagation of the CPEC lines also correlated with the concentration of IFN-γ. When propagating CPEC lines from Immortomice® at 33 °C in the absence or presence of increasing concentrations of IFN-γ we found that in the absence of IFN-γ, CPECs also lost their cuboidal morphology but died after passaging due to their poor proliferation ability. In contrast, increasing concentrations of IFN-γ up to 50 U/ml allowed us to propagate the CPECs over several passages. This supported the notion that the level of SV40Tag expression is critical for cell propagation. However, we did not observe improved re-differentiation of the CPEC lines when propagated in the absence or in the presence of higher concentrations of IFN-γ.

Thus, although we successfully established primary cultures of Immortomouse® CPECs and could readily propagate these cells, a total of 15 different trials applying different handling options and culture media (summarized in Table 1) failed to achieve successful re-differentiation of Immortomouse® CPECs. We therefore concluded that in contrast to other tissues the Immortomouse® is not a good source for establishing in vitro models of the mouse BCSFB.

Phenotypic characterization of the mouse choroid plexus carcinoma cell line ECPC4

Next we investigated the suitability of the commercially available mouse choroid plexus carcinoma cell line ECPC4 as an in vitro model to study immune function of the mouse BCSFB. ECPC4 cells were reported to be a useful model to study the BCSFB in vitro as they retain the characteristics of CPECs as shown by expression of BCSFB-specific proteins such as transthyretin and alpha2-macroglobulin [34]. When cultured according to the protocol of the manufacturer, ECPC4 cells grew with a high proliferation rate starting with a fibroblast like morphology (Fig. 3a) into confluent cell layers showing incomplete contact inhibition and thus partial overgrowth (Fig. 3b). In order to determine if exogenous addition of extracellular matrix proteins would improve monolayer formation by ECPC4, culture dishes were coated with laminin, rat-tail collagen, gelatin or poly-L-lysine on different glass and plastic surfaces. Irrespective of the condition chosen, we failed to observe any change in the proliferation rate or quality of monolayer formation of ECPC4 cells (data not shown).

To establish an in vitro model accessible from both sides and therefore suitable to study the migration of immune cells across the BSCFB, we cultured ECPC4 cells on porous membranes and tested their growth and viability. For our experiments we plated the ECPC4 cells directly on laminin coated filter inserts with a growth area of 0.33 cm^2 and let them grow to confluence.

To determine their CPEC specific characteristics we next performed immunofluorescence (IF) staining for CPEC specific molecules. We first confirmed expression of transthyretin (TTR), which is known to be highly expressed in the CP in vivo, in the cultured ECPC4 cells in a similar fashion as in Immortomouse® CPECs and pmCPECs (Fig. 3c). However, we could not detect the epithelial cell specific intermediate filament cytokeratin. Rather ECPC4 cells stained positive for the mesenchymal intermediate filament protein vimentin. Staining for the AJ molecules E-cadherin and β-catenin and the TJ proteins occludin, claudin-1, -2, -3 and -11 and ZO-1 showed interrupted junctional localization or no detectable expression, underscoring the immaturity of the junctional complexes between ECPC4 cells (Fig. 4a and data not shown). Thus although ECPC4 cells express CP characteristic proteins they fail to establish contact-inhibited monolayers with mature junctional complexes.

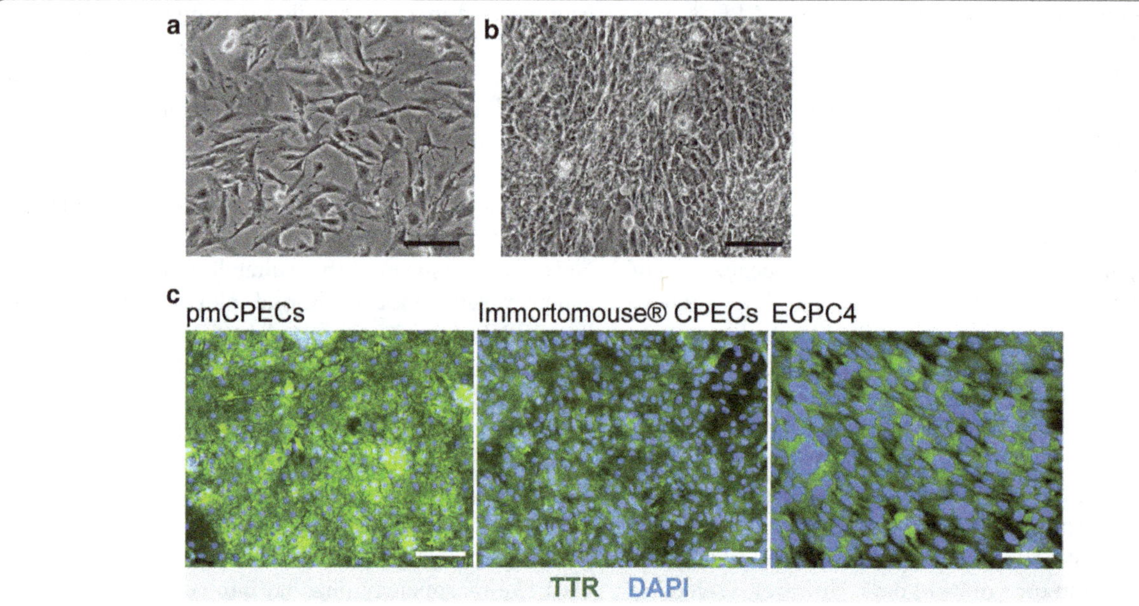

Fig. 3 Morphology, expression of transthyretin and propagation of ECPC4 cells. Representative phase contrast pictures of ECPC4 cells from passage 41 on d1 (**a**) and d4 (**b**) after sub-cultured in a 1:4 ratio as described by the distributer. The cells did not show typical epithelial morphology (**a**, **b**) and grew in overlapping layers (**b**). *Scale bars* 50 µm. **c** Immunofluorescence staining for the CPEC-specific marker transthyretin (TTR) is shown in pmCPECs, Immortomouse® CPECs from passage 6, grown for 7 days at non-permissive conditions and for the ECPC4 cells. *Scale bars* **a**, **b** and ECPC4 cells = 50 µm; pmCPECs and Immortomouse® CPECs = 100 µm

Phenotypic characterization of primary mouse choroid plexus epithelial cells (pmCPECs)

We next asked if pmCPECs grown on porous filter inserts will form monolayers with intact junctional complexes. We plated the freshly isolated choroid plexus single cell suspensions directly on laminin-coated filter inserts with a growth area of 0.33 cm^2 to avoid passaging and let the cells proliferate until they attained confluence. Immunofluorescence staining showed expression of TTR (data not shown) and the epithelial cell specific intermediate filament protein cytokeratin in >95 % of cells in the monolayer. In addition we observed continuous junctional staining for the AJ proteins E-cadherin and β-catenin and the TJ proteins claudin-1, -2, -3, -11, occudin and ZO-1 between the pmCPECs (Fig. 4b). Hence the immunostaining confirmed the high purity and the establishment of mature junctional complexes in pmCPEC cultures.

Comparison of barrier characteristics of ECPC4 and pmCPECs

To determine if the immunofluorescence staining of ECPC4 and pmCPECs correlated with their barrier characteristics we next established for both CPECs the 'inverted' culture as previously described for porcine CPECs [37]. To allow investigation of immune cell migration from the blood to the CSF side, CPECs were seeded on the lower surface of inverted filter inserts, which once the CPECs had attached, were turned around for performing the respective assays. Neither ECPC4 nor pmCPECs showed a difference in growth rate or differentiation when grown on the lower filter site compared to the upper filter site as confirmed by light microscopy and immunofluorescence staining for epithelial and junctional molecules exactly as described above (data not shown).

To determine the efficacy of the pmCPECs and the ECPC4 cell line to form a tight barrier with sealing junctional complexes between adjacent cells, we measured the TEER of the cultured cells over the last 72 h in culture to monitor the achievement of the resistance plateau by impedance spectroscopy. In parallel, the TEER was measured over empty laminin-coated filters as negative controls. After 7 days in culture, pmCPEC layers reached a TEER plateau between 100 and 200 Ω cm^2 (Fig. 5a), which is similar to TEER values previously measured across rat CPE monolayers, being 178 Ω cm^2 [20] and are slightly higher than those previously observed across mouse CPECs [8]. Interestingly, the inverted pmCPEC cultures displayed a significantly higher TEER than the standard cultures, shown by the calculated area under the curve (AUC) (Units: Ω cm^2 h) (Fig. 5a). However, the morphology of the pmCPECs growing on either side of the filter was indistinguishable (Fig. 5d).

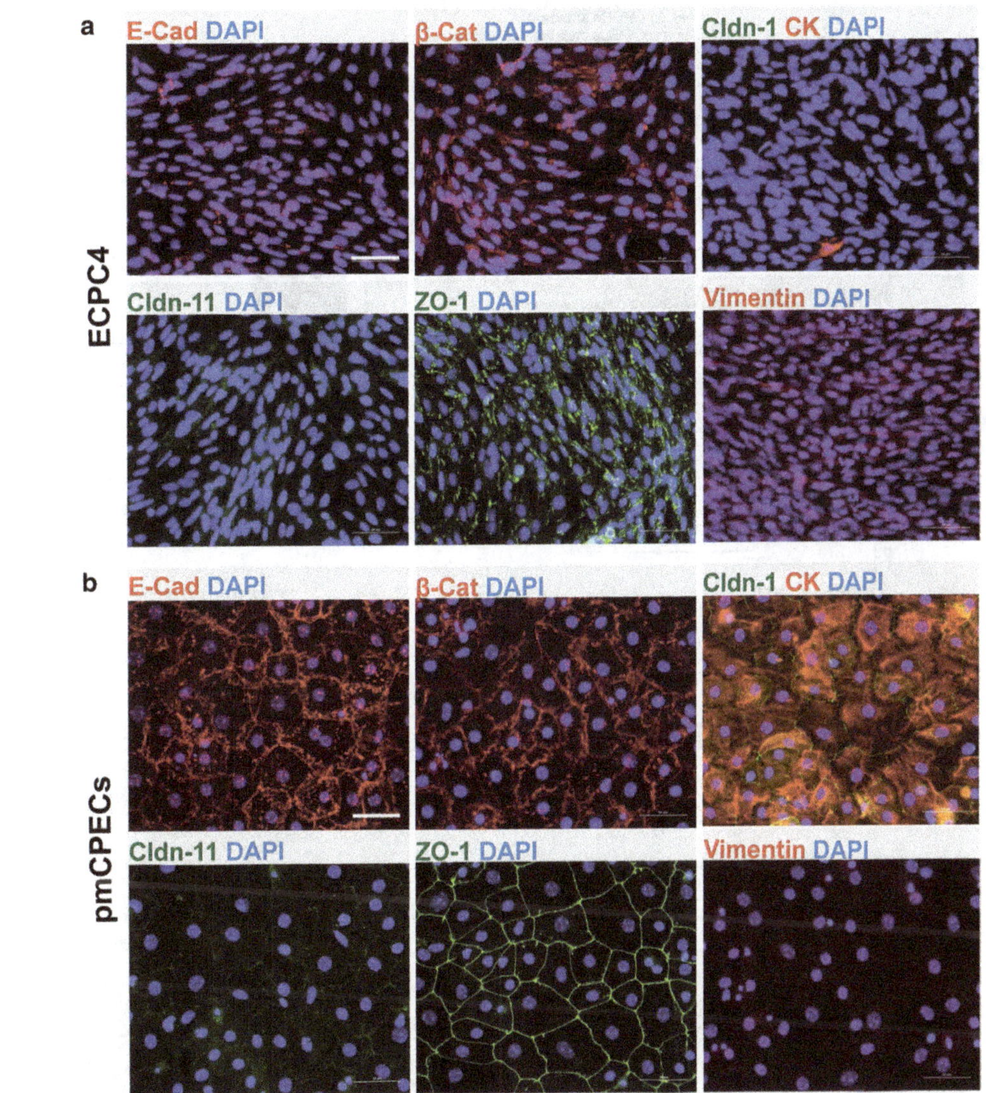

Fig. 4 Phenotype of ECPC4 cells and primary mouse choroid plexus epithelial cells (pmCPECs). Immunofluorescence staining for CPEC specific proteins is shown in ECPC4 cells (**a**) and pmCPECs (**b**). **a** There is weak staining for the adhesion junction (AJ) protein E-Cadherin (E-Cad) and its cytoskeleton linker β-catenin (β-Cat) of ECPC4 cells and their localization is not specifically at the plasma membrane. Staining for tight junctional (TJ) claudins-1 and -11 was absent or showed a weak cytosolic pattern, respectively. The scaffolding protein ZO1 staining was disrupted. Additionally, the cell line failed to stain for the early epithelial marker cytokeratin but rather was positive for the mesenchymal intermediate filament protein vimentin. ECPC4 cells from passage 41 were stained on d4 in culture. **b** In contrast, the staining of pmCPECs stained on d7 in culture, revealed a proper distribution of all epithelial markers. pmCPECs. All staining was performed at least 3 times. *Scale bars* 50 µm. *E-Cad* E-cadherin, *Cldn-1* Claudin 1, *Cldn-11* claudin 11, *CK* cytokeratin, *β-Cat* β-catenin, *ZO-1* zona occludens protein 1

Irrespective if grown in standard or inverted filters, the ECPC4 cells failed to establish a barrier with regard to TEER measurements. With 10 Ω cm^2 the TEER measured across ECPC4 monolayers remained close to the TEER values measured across laminin-coated empty filters (Fig. 5a).

The barrier characteristics of the CPEC monolayers were investigated by measuring the paracellular diffusion of the small water soluble tracers 3 kDa dextran and Lucifer Yellow (LY, MW 457 Da) across the epithelial monolayers for 40 min. Monolayers layers of pmCPEC established a tight barrier with permeability coefficients $Pe_{3kDa} = 0.024 \pm 0.021 \times 10^{-3}$ cm/min and $Pe_{3kDa} = 0.017 \pm 0.018 \times 10^{-3}$ cm/min for standard and inverted filter cultures, respectively (Fig. 5b). As expected, the permeability for the small tracer LY was higher than that observed for the larger 3 kDa dextran with $Pe_{LY} = 0.173 \pm 0.014 \times 10^{-3}$ cm/min and

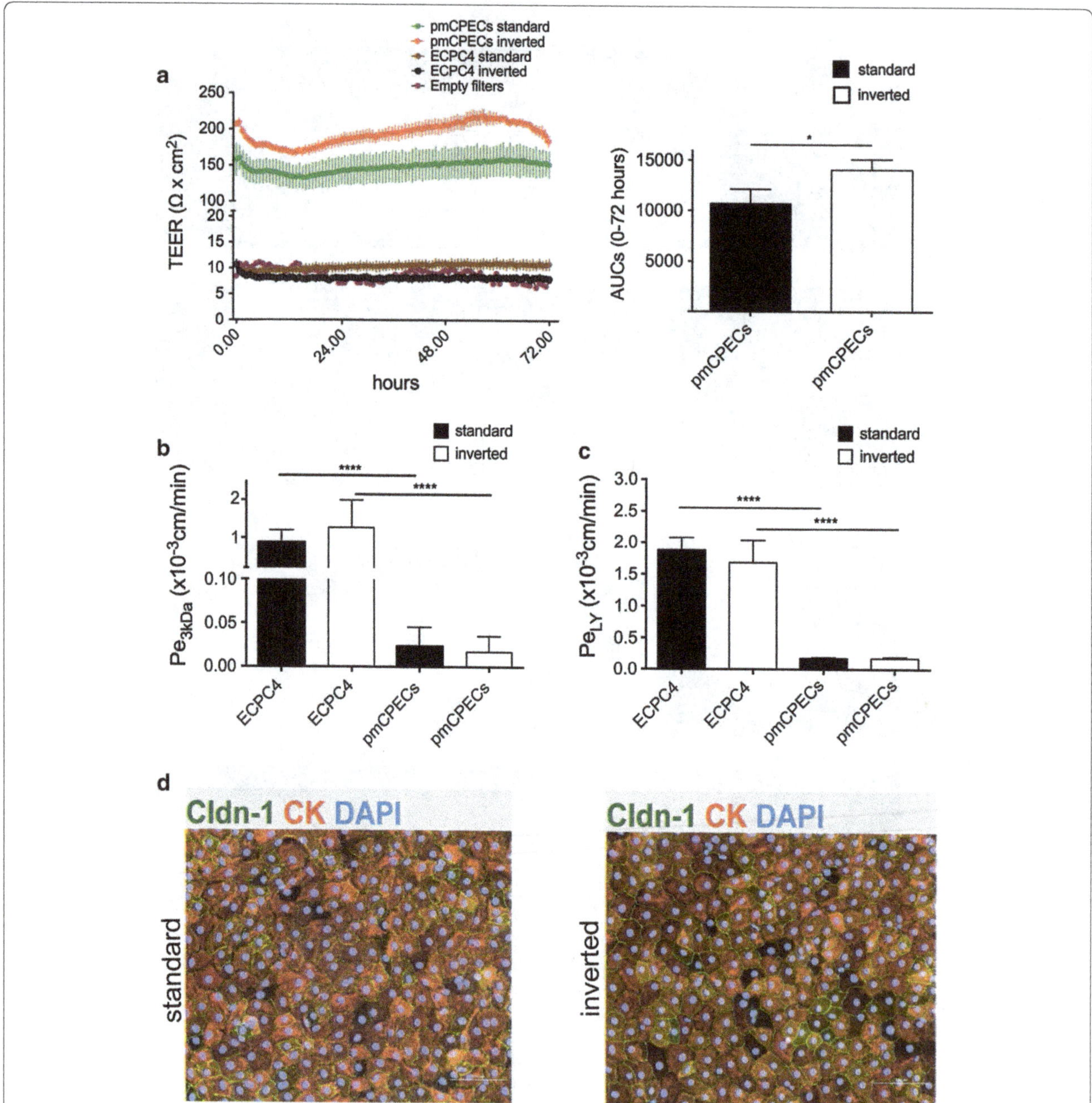

Fig. 5 Comparison of barrier characteristics of ECPC4 versus pmCPECs. **a** The time-dependent progression of the transepithelial electrical resistance (TEER) of ECPC4 cells and pmCPECs grown on standard (luminal) or inverted (abluminal) Transwell filter inserts was measured by impedance spectroscopy using the cellZscope device. The TEER of ECPE4 hardly differs from the TEER measured across laminin coated empty filters (EF). In contrast, pmCPECs reach a TEER of 150–200 Ω cm^2 on d7. The figure shows one representative experiment (of 4) of pmCPECs in comparison to ECPC4 over their last 72 h in culture with 3 filters per condition and 1 empty filter. The *colored lines* show the mean TEER values of triplicate measurements surrounded by *colored* areas, which represent the SD. The area under the *curve* (AUC) as a measure for the overall TEER across the cellular barriers over time (Unit: Ω cm^2 h) was assessed for a comparison of the overall resistance of the cell layers. *$p < 0.05$. **b, c** The permeability for Alexa Fluor 680-3 kDa dextran (Pe_{3kDa}) (**b**) was measured in 5 independent experiments with at least three filters per condition (ECPC4 standard: n = 3, ECPC4 inverted: n = 3, pmCPECs standard: n = 5, pmCPECs inverted n = 4) and the permeability for 457 Da Lucifer Yellow (Pe_{LY}) was measured once with at least 3 filters per condition (ECPC4 standard: n = 3, ECPC inverted: n = 3, pmCPECs standard: n = 5, pmCPECs inverted: n = 4) ****$p < 0.0001$ (**c**). **d** Immunofluorescence staining for claudin-1 (Cldn-1), cytokeratin (CK) and nuclei (DAPI) showed no differences between monolayers grown on the upper (standard) or lower (inverted) side of the filter. *Scale bar* 100 μm. *Bars* in **b, c** represent the mean permeability coefficients Pe ± SD

$Pe_{LY} = 0.173 \pm 0.021 \times 10^{-3}$ cm/min for standard and inverted filter pmCPEC cultures, respectively (Fig. 5c).

To compare pmCPEC barrier characteristics with those of ECPC4 monolayers, diffusion of 3 kDa dextran and LY was assessed in the same assays for the ECPC4 in parallel and found to be significantly higher than the Pe values measured for pmCPECs. Specifically, the permeability coefficient for 3 kDa dextran across ECPC4 was $Pe_{3kDa} = 0.889 \pm 0.311 \times 10^{-3}$ cm/min and $Pe_{3kDa} = 1.272 \pm 0.720 \times 10^{-3}$ cm/min for standard and inverted filter cultures, respectively (Fig. 5b). For LY, the permeability coefficients were $Pe_{LY} = 1.883 \pm 0.198 \times 10^{-3}$ cm/min and $Pe_{LY} = 1.687 \pm 0.351 \times 10^{-3}$ cm/min for standard and inverted filter cultures respectively (Fig. 5c). Thus, in contrast to pmCPECs ECPC4 failed to establish a tight barrier model in vitro.

Considering the different growth characteristics of ECPC4 versus pmCPECs we asked if optimizing the growth conditions of the ECPC4 cells on the filter inserts might improve their barrier characteristics. To this end we performed a titration of the ECPC4 cells on the laminin-coated filters to optimize their seeding concentration. ECPC4 cells were plated in two experiments at different concentrations (5×10^4, 1×10^5 and 5×10^5 cells per filter) and compared to the standard recommended by the distributor (ECPC4 split in a 1:4 ratio, concentration not known) and once at a lower concentration (1×10^4 cells per filter). The TEER of the ECPC4 cell layer was measured manually using the EndOhm device once per day on d3 and d4. The TEER of the cell layers with the maximum value being 22 Ω cm^2 was slightly higher than that of the empty filters with 12 Ω cm^2 (Fig. 6a). Next, we investigated the permeability of these titrated cells for 3 kDa dextran on day 4 in culture. Despite different seeding concentrations, the permeability coefficient for the ECPC4 cell layers was however similar, ranging from $Pe_{3kDa} = 1.220 \times 10^{-3}$ cm/min to $Pe_{3kDa} = 0.775 \times 10^{-3}$ cm/min (Fig. 6b). The ECPC4 plated at the lower concentration of 10^4 cells per filter showed an even higher $Pe_{kDa} = 3.340 \times 10^{-3}$ cm/min (data not shown). Immunofluorescence staining of the filters for ZO-1 and F-actin binding rhodamine phalloidin following the permeability measurements, confirmed closed monolayers without contact inhibition with higher and lower cell numbers (data not shown). Thus, changing the number of ECPE4 growing on filter inserts did not improve the barrier characteristics of these cells.

To change cell-substrate contacts as previously reported [42] we next investigated if ECPC4 grown on polyester (PET) instead of polycarbonate filter inserts have improved barrier properties and failed to find any improvement (data not shown). Finally, as serum withdrawal from the culture medium has been reported to result in improved barriers of porcine CPECs [15] we investigated if ECPC4 barrier properties improve after serum withdrawal from d2 to d4 after seeding. Serum withdrawal did not affect the monolayer integrity, however, it also failed to improve barrier characteristics of ECPC4 when compared to those continuously grown in 10 % FBS (data not shown). In summary, we conclude that in contrary to the commercially available ECPC4 cell line, the pmCPEC cultures form a tight cellular barrier when grown on filter inserts and are thus suited as in vitro model for the mouse BCSFB.

Comparison of barrier characteristics of pmCPECs on 0.4 and 5 µm pore sized filters

Having established a tight in vitro model of the mouse BCSFB we next adapted this model to the growth on

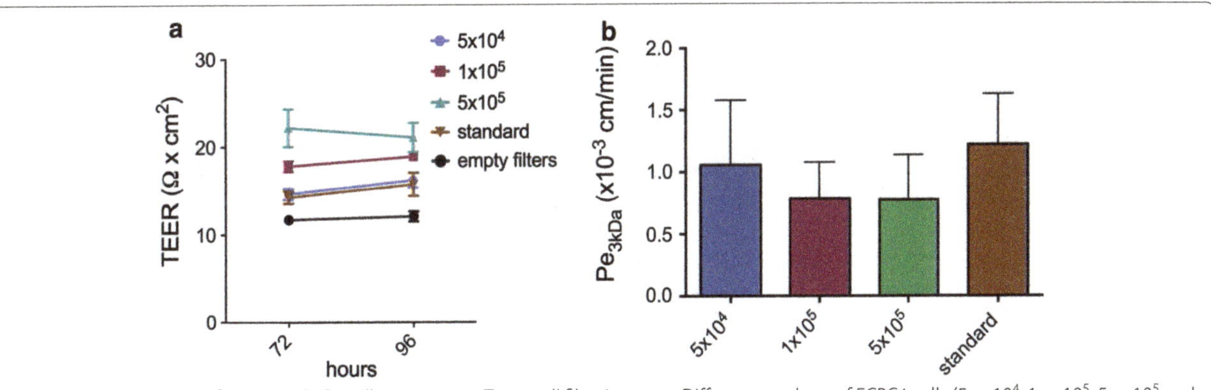

Fig. 6 Barrier properties of titrated ECPC4 cells growing on Transwell filter inserts. **a** Different numbers of ECPC4 cells (5×10^4, 1×10^5, 5×10^5 and standard) were plated on the inverted porous filter membranes in triplicate. Standard = ECPC4 continuously split in a ratio 1:4, according to the distributer's protocol (number of cells not counted). TEER was measured manually once per day on d3 and d4 in culture using the EndOhm device. The cells failed to build up a resistance irrespective of their seeding density. **b** The permeability coefficient (Pe) for Alexa Fluor 680–3 kDa dextran was assessed after the resistance measurement on d4. *Bars* represent the mean ± SD of all filters from two independent experiments, n = 6 for all groups

inverted filters with a larger pore size of 5 μm allowing immune cells to reach the pmCPEC monolayer from the upper filter compartment.

In order compare barrier integrities of pmCPECs grown to confluence on 5 μm pore versus 0.4 μm pore inverted filters, the time-dependent progression of the TEER was measured by impedance spectroscopy using cellZscope from d3 to d7 of culture (Fig. 7a). Monolayers of pmCPEC reached TEER values between 100 and 150 Ω cm^2 on day 7 of culture. Although the TEER of pmCPECs grown on 0.4 μm pore filters seemed apparently higher, this difference was not significant, as shown

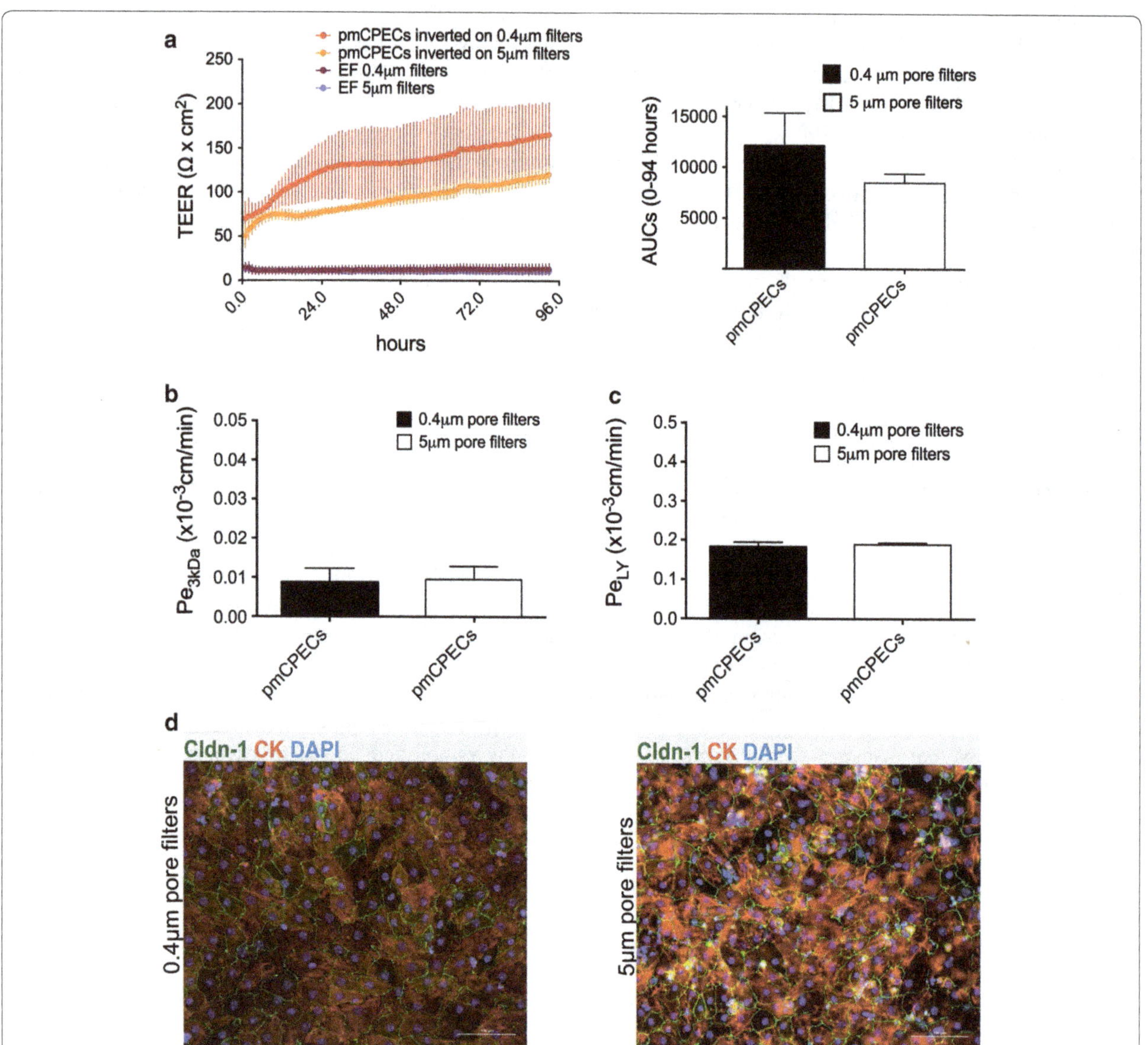

Fig. 7 Comparison of barrier characteristics of inverted cultures of pmCPECs on filters with 0.4 and 5 μm pores. **a** The time dependent progression of the transepithelial electrical resistance (TEER) of pmCPECs grown or inverted (abluminal) Transwell filter inserts with 0.4 and 5 μm pores was measured by impedance spectroscopy using the cellZscope device from d3 to d7 in culture. The pmCPECs on both kinds of filters reached a TEER of 100–150 Ω cm^2 on d7. The figure shows one experiment with 3 filters per condition and 3 empty filters per condition. The *colored lines* show the mean TEER values of triplicate measurements surrounded by *colored* areas, which represent the SD. The area under the curve (AUC; Units: Ω cm^2 h) was assessed for a comparison of the overall resistance of the cell layers over time with no significant difference detected. **b, c** The permeability of the pmCPEC grown on inverted Transwell filter inserts with 0.4 and 5 μm pores for two different small molecular tracers was determined following the TEER measurements in 1 experiment with n = 4 filters per condition. There was no difference for the permeability of Alexa Fluor 680–3 kDa dextran (Pe_{3kDa}) (**b**) or for 457 Da Lucifer Yellow (Pe_{LY}) (**c**) across the pmCPECs cultured on either type of filter. **d** Immunofluorescence staining for claudin-1 (Cldn-1), cytokeratin (CK) and nuclei (DAPI) on pmCPEC monolayers grown on the inverted sides of filter inserts with 0.4 and 5 μm pores. The difference in clarity between the pictures is due to different microscopic characteristics of the filters. *Scale bar* 100 μm. *Bars* represent the mean permeability coefficients Pe ± SD

by the calculated AUC of the TEER over time. Furthermore, the permeability of the pmCPEC grown on filter inserts with 0.4 and 5 μm pores for the Alexa Fluor 680–3 kDa dextran (Pe_{3kDa}) and 457 Da Lucifer Yellow (Pe_{LY}) (Fig. 7b, c) was comparable. The permeability coefficient for 3 kDa dextran was $Pe_{3kDa} = 0.009 \pm 0.003 \times 10^{-3}$ cm/min and $0.010 \pm 0.003 \times 10^{-3}$ cm/min for the pmCPECs grown on filters with 0.4 and 5 μm pores, respectively. The permeability coefficient for Lucifer Yellow (Pe_{LY}) was $Pe_{LY} = 0.183 \pm 0.011 \times 10^{-3}$ cm/min and $Pe = 0.189 \pm 0.004 \times 10^{-3}$ cm/min for the pmCPECs grown on filters with 0.4 and 5 μm pores, respectively. Finally, we confirmed comparable growth of contact inhibited monolayers of highly pure pmCPECs on the inverted sides of filter inserts with 5 and 0.4 μm pores by performing immunostainings for claudin-1 (Cldn-1) and cytokeratin (CK) (Fig. 7d). In summary, inverted filter cultures of pmCPEC could successfully be adapted to growth on 5 μm pore Transwell filters without impairing their barrier characteristics.

Encephalitogenic CD4^{+} T cells migrate across the BCSFB in vitro

Having ensured that barrier characteristics of the mouse BCSFB were maintained on 5 μm pore Transwell filters we next asked if encephalitogenic T cells could migrate from the blood to the CSF side across this pmCPEC monolayer. For this, the pmCPECs were stimulated or not with a combination of TNFα and IFNγ. Indeed we found that a small percentage of encephalitogenic T cells (3.8 %) could cross the non-inflamed pmCPEC monolayer by reaching the lower part of the chamber system after 8 h of incubation time. Stimulating the pmCPECs with a combination of TNFα and IFNγ to inflammation doubled T cell migration across the pmCPEC monolayers (8.1 %) within the same time (Fig. 8a). In contrast, spontaneous migration of encephalitogenic T cells across empty filters during that time amounted to almost 70 %. The viability of the transmigrated T cells was not impaired after crossing the pmCPEC monolayers (Fig. 8b). Similarly, the integrity of the pmCPECs monolayers was not affected by T cell diapedesis as confirmed by immunofluorescence staining for junctional molecules like ZO-1 and claudin-1 and cytokeratin after the 8 h co-incubation of T cells with the pmCPEC monolayers (Fig. 8c and data not shown). Stimulation of pmCPECs with a combination of TNFα/IFNγ induced increased expression of ICAM-1 and VCAM-1 at the protein level (Fig. 8d and not shown) suggesting a potential role of these molecules in the increased migration of T cells across the TNFα/IFNγ stimulated pmCPECs compared to non-stimulated pmCPECs. Thus, encephalitogenic T cells can migrate across our in vitro model of the BCSFB in the absence and presence of inflammatory stimuli. At the same time, this in vitro model of the mouse BCSFB provides a barrier for T cell migration and is thus suitable to study the mechanisms present at the BCSFB that limit immune cell entry into the CNS. Taken together, our in vitro model for the mouse BCSFB constituted of primary mouse CPECs in an inverted filter culture is highly suited to study the cellular and molecular mechanisms of T cell migration across this barrier.

Discussion

There is increasing evidence for an important role of the CP in CNS immunity. Comparative transcriptome analyses of choroid plexus tissue from healthy mice and mice suffering from neuroinflammatory conditions such as EAE showed the strongest upregulation of expression of genes encoding for adhesion molecules, chemokines and cytokines as well as T cell activation markers, supporting a function of the CP in mediating T cell migration into the CNS [43, 44]. To reach the CSF space at this site circulating T cells first have to cross the wall of the fenestrated CP microvessels allowing them to reach the CP stroma. In a next step they have to migrate across the BCSFB established by CP epithelial cells.

To delineate the cellular and molecular mechanisms mediating the migration of immune cells across the BCSFB from those involved at the BBB, suitable in vitro models established from CP epithelial cells are mandatory. Especially porcine and rat in vitro models of the BCSFB have been successfully established however only a few of these studies have specifically addressed the migration of leukocytes across the BCSFB (summarized in [45]).

In light of the fact that transgenic approaches enabling the specific manipulation of individual genes have advanced in mice and have become an irreplaceable tool to analyze gene function in development and pathology, mouse models of the BCSFB could significantly improve investigations on the potential immune functions of the CP. Although a number of laboratories has established in vitro models of the mouse BCSFB [28, 30, 31] these models have not been optimized for the in vitro study of the immune functions including immune cell migration from the periphery into the CNS [8].

Considering the small tissue size of the mouse CP, primary cultures of CPECs come with the obvious disadvantage of the necessity to sacrifice numbers of mice. In addition, primary cultures of CPECs have proven to have a limited life span of 1–2 weeks and have been reported upon passaging to show signs of dedifferentiation, death or fibroblast enrichment [14, 22, 29]. However, the low turnover rate of primary mouse CPECs can be overcome by the addition of growth factors like insulin-like growth

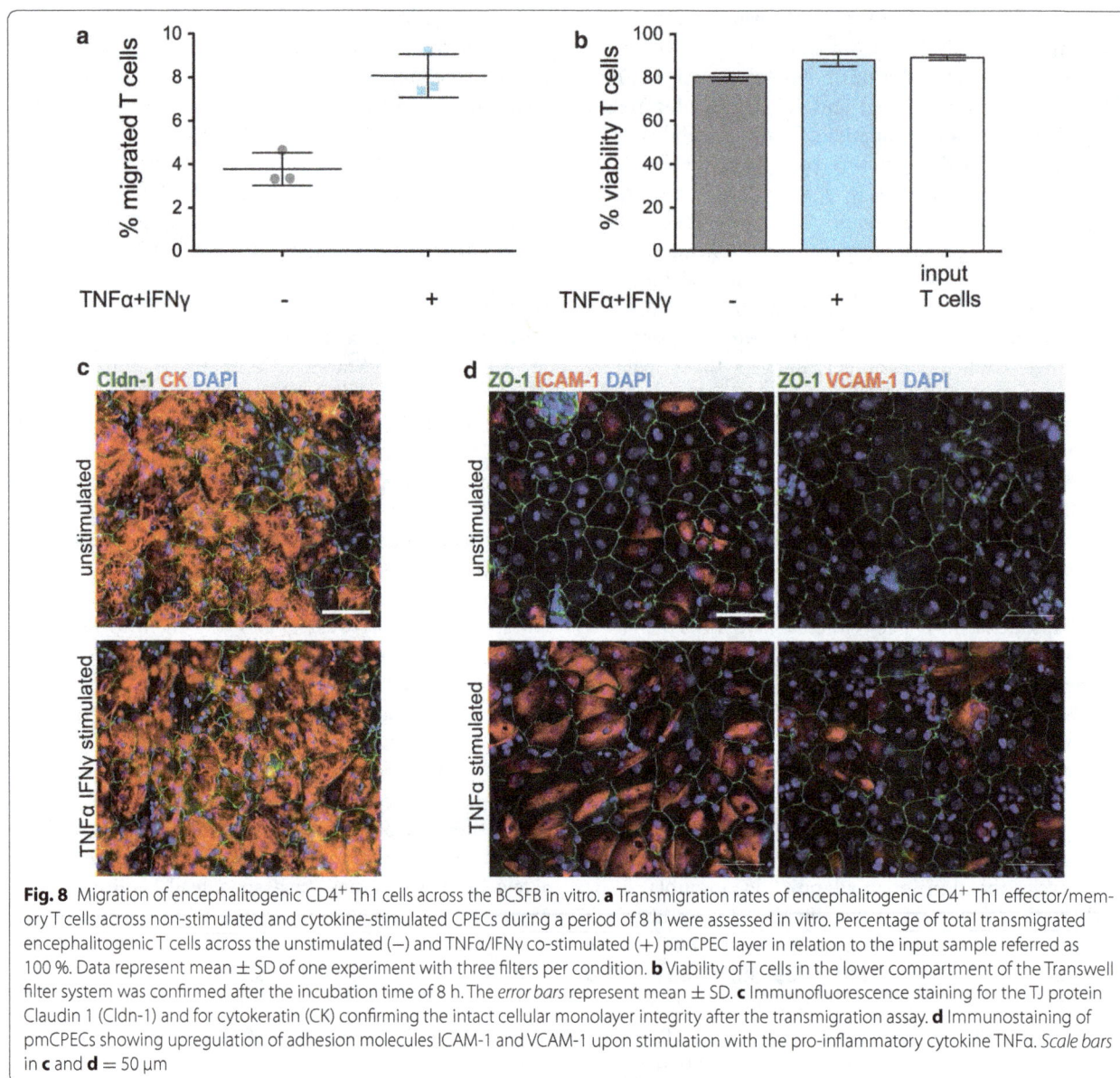

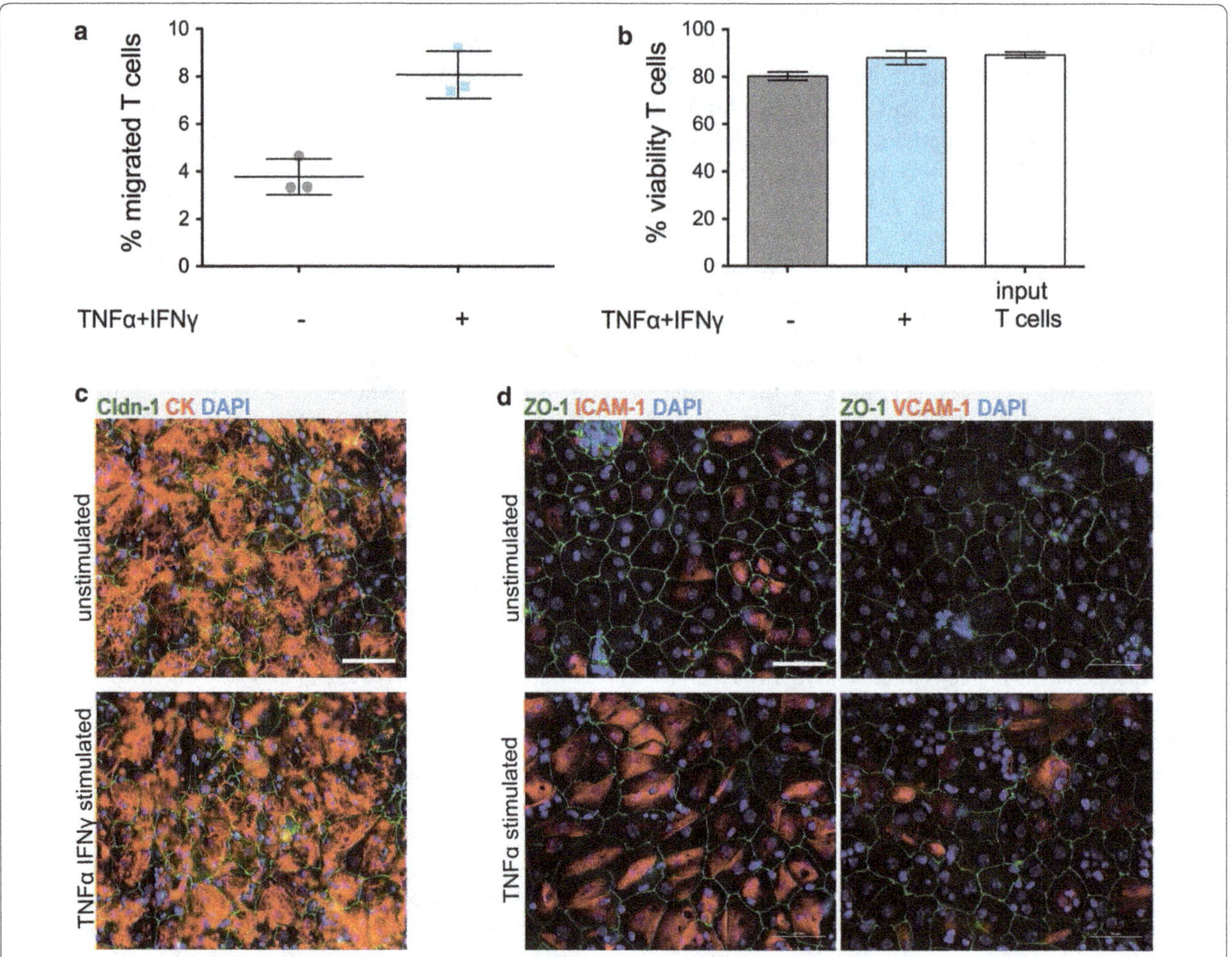

Fig. 8 Migration of encephalitogenic CD4$^+$ Th1 cells across the BCSFB in vitro. **a** Transmigration rates of encephalitogenic CD4$^+$ Th1 effector/memory T cells across non-stimulated and cytokine-stimulated CPECs during a period of 8 h were assessed in vitro. Percentage of total transmigrated encephalitogenic T cells across the unstimulated (−) and TNFα/IFNγ co-stimulated (+) pmCPEC layer in relation to the input sample referred as 100 %. Data represent mean ± SD of one experiment with three filters per condition. **b** Viability of T cells in the lower compartment of the Transwell filter system was confirmed after the incubation time of 8 h. The *error bars* represent mean ± SD. **c** Immunofluorescence staining for the TJ protein Claudin 1 (Cldn-1) and for cytokeratin (CK) confirming the intact cellular monolayer integrity after the transmigration assay. **d** Immunostaining of pmCPECs showing upregulation of adhesion molecules ICAM-1 and VCAM-1 upon stimulation with the pro-inflammatory cytokine TNFα. *Scale bars* in **c** and **d** = 50 μm

factor 1 (IGF-1) and epidermal growth factor (EGF) to the culture [31] implying that optimal culture conditions of these cells allow for appropriate expansion.

Nevertheless appropriate cell line models for the mouse BCSFB would be preferable. Cell lines in general bear the advantage of easy handling. They overcome the disadvantages of primary cell cultures such as repeated necessity to sacrifice significant numbers of mice and their short viability as well as their lack of suitability for high throughput experiments. Establishing cell lines from primary brain endothelial cells has been successfully achieved in the past by expression of the polyoma middle T oncogene [46] or a temperature-sensitive SV40 large T followed by expression of the catalytic subunit of telomerase [47]. In addition, CP tumors have been used to establish CPEC lines. Furthermore, the SV40 large T induced rat CPEC line Z310 establishes with a TEER of 150–200 Ω cm^2 barrier characteristics similar to those of primary rat CPECs [22]. At the same time, Z310 cells fail to express CPEC specific transporters and junctional proteins [48, 49] limiting its suitability for a number of research approaches. The slowly proliferating human CP papilloma cell line HIBCPP has proven a suitable in vitro model for the human BCSFB. If grown under optimized conditions, HIBCPP build a permeability barrier reaching a TEER of 200–500 Ω cm^2 and although they only show a partial contact inhibition, HIBCPP cells express the CPEC-specific junctional proteins including claudin-11 as observed in vivo [25, 50].

In the present study we have undertaken elaborate efforts to establish cell line and primary cell models for the mouse BCSFB from different mice that will allow study of the immune functions of this barrier including the molecular mechanisms mediating the migration of immune cells across the BCSFB. Having established primary cultures of mouse CPEC we chose to use the Immortomouse® as a cellular source for the establishment of CPEC lines. Immortomice® express a temperature- sensitive mutant of the SV40 large T antigen tsA58, which supports cell survival and growth by overcoming p53- and pRB-dependent cell cycle arrest, under the control of the MHC class I promoter. These mice have been successfully used to establish epithelial cell lines from the gastrointestinal tissues (summarized in [32]), the kidney [51] and the mammary gland [33] by expanding epithelial cultures under permissive culture conditions, namely at 33 °C and in the presence of IFNγ. Re-differentiation of epithelial cells was achieved by growing the cells under non-permissive conditions (37 or 39 °C and the absence of IFNγ). Taking this experimental approach using slight modifications of Whitehead et al. we successfully transformed Immortomouse® derived CPECs by growing the cells at 33 °C and the addition of IFNγ as reflected by their high proliferation rate over several passages which could not be observed under non-permissive conditions. However, irrespective of the passage tested subsequent withdrawal of IFNγ and culture of the Immorto®CPEC lines at 37° or 39° failed to induce epithelial re-differentiation of the cells. Rather, we observed in all our Immorto®CPEC lines continuous expression of the mesenchymal markers vimentin and N-cadherin accompanied by the lack of re-expression of cytokeratin and E-cadherin. This suggests that immortalization of the Immorto®CPECs induced irreversible and thus SV40 large T independent epithelial to mesenchymal transition (EMT). Spontaneous induction of temperature-sensitive growth phenotypes of mouse embryonal fibroblasts, independent of a temperature-sensitive immortalizing gene, have been observed before [52]. Taken together our observations suggest that the Immortomouse® is not well suited to establish CPEC lines that can be used to model the BCSFB in vitro.

We therefore next analyzed the mouse CP carcinoma cell line ECPC4, which was established from a CP carcinoma that had developed in transgenic mice expressing the SV40 large T antigen [34]. ECPC4 have been shown to exhibit a flattened, polygonal morphology and to maintain characteristics of CPECs such as expression of transthyretin (TTR) and α_2-macroglobulin when originally characterized in passages 13–15. ECPC4 cells have subsequently been used to study the activation of the kallikrein-kinin system or expression of inducible nitric oxide synthase (iNOS) in the CP in innate immunity responses [53, 54] using unknown passages of the cells. In the present study, we found that the commercially available ECPC4 from passage 37 and higher, despite continued expression of TTR, lacked contact inhibition and did not express CPEC specific molecules such as cytokeratin or E-cadherin. Rather, all ECPC4 cells stained positive for vimentin and failed to establish CPEC specific junctional complexes. These observations suggested a significant stage of de-differentiation of ECPC4, which was further supported by our observation that ECPC4 failed to establish barrier properties such as high TEER and low permeability for small soluble tracers. Thus, ECPC4 are not suitable as in vitro model for the mouse BCSFB to study immune functions including the migration of T cells across this barrier.

In depth characterization of the primary mouse CPEC cultures in the present study demonstrated this approach to be a valid in vitro model to study immune functions of the mouse BCSFB. Primary mouse CPECs were isolated and grown at high purity and formed contact-inhibited monolayers. CPECs maintained expression of CPEC specific molecules and developed mature junctional complexes. Primary mouse CPEC established a tight barrier with high trans-epithelial electrical resistance (TEER) values comparable to the TEER measured across primary CPEC cultures from different species [16, 18–20, 55, 56] and across the BCSFB in vivo in cats [57]. Barrier characteristics of our pmCPEC cultures were further confirmed by the establishment of a permeability barrier for small soluble tracers such as 3 kDa dextran and Lucifer Yellow reaching Pe values that are comparable to the Pe values measured for the small tracer [^{14}C]Sucrose across the BCSFB rat in vitro model [56, 58]. Furthermore, the permeability for 3 kDa dextran across the pmCPECs was more than fivefold lower than the permeability measured across the primary mouse brain microvascular endothelial cells pmBMECs assessed in our laboratory [38] and the permeability for Lucifer Yellow was more than twofold lower than across the pmBMECs [59] and threefold lower than across the novel human BBB model derived from hematopoietic stem cells [40].

Taken together cultured pmCPEC maintain important barrier characteristics of CPECs in vivo and are thus a suitable model for the mouse BCSFB in vitro.

To study T cell migration across the BCSFB in vitro, the pmCPEC cultures were adapted to grow on an inverted porous filter membranes as previously described in [37]. Interestingly, barrier characteristics of pmCPECs grown on the inverted side of the filter were significantly higher than those of pmCPECs grown on the upper side of the filter. As we failed to see any visible difference in morphology or in immunostaining of the pmCPEC monolayers, we cannot explain this difference at this time. We modelled the migration of encephalitogenic T cells across the non-stimulated and stimulated BCSFB in vitro and found that in the absence of inflammatory stimuli T cells migrated across the pmCPEC monolayer from the basolateral to the apical site. Addition of pro-inflammatory cytokines doubled the number of T cells crossing the pmCPEC monolayer in the same time—comparable to T cell diapedesis observed across a BBB in vitro model, respectively [60].

Taken together in the present study, we have successfully established an inverted in vitro filter model of the mouse BCSFB with barrier characteristics resembling that of the BCSFB in vivo. We provide proof of principle that this model is suited to study T cell migration from the blood to the CSF side across the BCSFB. This model of the mouse BCSFB can be used to investigate whether different immune cell subsets can cross the BCSFB and enable the cellular and molecular mechanism involved to be defined.

Conclusions

A suitable tool for reproducible high throughput investigations of the molecular and cellular mechanisms that mediate the migration of specific immune cells into the CNS via the mouse BCSFB is missing to date. Here we show that cell line models derived from the Immortomouse® and from the commercially available ECPC4 are not suited for this purpose. Rather pmCPECs growing on inverted Transwell filters were defined as a reliable in vitro model for experiments mimicking the T cell migration from the blood vessel side to the apical side facing the CSF. Moreover, our adapted 'inverted' BCSFB model is suitable for addressing not only the immune cell subset extravasation but also the passing of substances and pathogens, taking into account the correct orientation of the polarized cells as it occurs under physiological conditions within the brain.

Abbreviations

AJ: adherence junction; APC: antigen presenting cell; Ara-C: cytosine arabinoside; BBB: blood–brain barrier; BCSFB: blood–cerebrospinal fluid barrier; CAM: cell adhesion molecule; CD: cluster of differentiation; CK: cytokeratin; CNS: central nervous system; CSF: cerebrospinal fluid; CP: choroid plexus; CS: calf serum; CPEC: choroid plexus epithelial cell; Da: dalton; DC: dendritic cell; DMEM: Dulbecco's modified eagle medium; EAE: experimental autoimmune encephalomyelitis; E-Cad: epithelial cadherin; EGF: epidermal growth factor; EMT: epithelial to mesenchymal transition; F-actin: filamentous actin; FBS: fetal bovine serum; ICAM: intercellular adhesion molecule; IF: immunofluorescence; Ig: immunoglobulin; IGF: insulin like growth factor; INF-γ: interferon gamma; JAM: junctional adhesion molecule; LFA-1: leukocyte function associated antigen-1; LY: lucifer yellow; mAb: monoclonal antibody; MAdCAM: 1 mucosal vascular addressin cell adhesion molecule; MAM: migration assay medium; MCAM: melanoma cell adhesion molecule; MHC: major histocompatibility complex; MMP: matrix metalloprotease; MS: multiple sclerosis; OSP: oligodendrocyte specific protein; PBS: phosphate buffered saline; Pe: permeability coefficient; pmCPECs: primary mouse choroid plexus epithelial cells; PSGL-1: P-selectin glycoprotein ligand—1; SCI: spinal cord injury; SV: simian virus; TEER: transepithelial electrical resistance; TJ: tight junction; TNF-α: tumour necrosis factor alpha; ts: temperature sensitive; TTR: transthyretin; VCAM: vascular cell adhesion molecule; VLA-4: very late antigen-4; wt: wildtype; ZO: zonula occludens.

Authors' contributions

IL performed all experiments, analyzed the experimental data and wrote the manuscript. BE designed and supervised the study, provided help for data analysis and wrote the manuscript. Both authors read and approved the final manuscript.

Acknowledgements

We thank Dr. Henriette Rudolph for valuable advice regarding the optimization of the pmCPEC cultures on inverted filter membranes. Dr. Urban Deutsch and Prof. Dr. Sara Michie are both sincerely acknowledged for their critical review and the English editing of this manuscript.

Competing interests

The authors declare that they have no competing interests.

Funding Sources

This work was funded by the Swiss National Science Foundation (ProDoc Cell Migration Grant No. PDFMP3_137127), the Bangerter-Rhyner Foundation to BE and the Microscopy Imaging Center of the University of Bern. IL is enrolled in the Graduate School for Cellular and Biomedical Research of the University of Bern and the ProDoc Cell Migration funded by the SNSF grant ProDoc Cell Migration Grant No. PDAMP3_137087 and the Rector's Conference of Swiss Universities (CRUS).

References

1. Strazielle N, Ghersi-Egea JF. Choroid plexus in the central nervous system: biology and physiopathology. J Neuropathol Exp Neurol. 2000;59:561–74.
2. Wolburg H, Paulus W. Choroid plexus: biology and pathology. Acta Neuropathol. 2010;119:75–88.
3. Engelhardt B, Wolburg-Buchholz K, Wolburg H. Involvement of the choroid plexus in central nervous system inflammation. Microsc Res Tech. 2001;52:112–29.
4. Tietz S, Engelhardt B. Brain barriers: crosstalk between complex tight junctions and adherens junctions. J Cell Biol. 2015;209:493–506.
5. Vorbrodt AW, Dobrogowska DH. Molecular anatomy of intercellular junctions in brain endothelial and epithelial barriers: electron microscopist's view. Brain Res Brain Res Rev. 2003;42:221–42.
6. Lippoldt A, Jansson A, Kniesel U, Andbjer B, Andersson A, Wolburg H, et al. Phorbol ester induced changes in tight and adherens junctions in the choroid plexus epithelium and in the ependyma. Brain Res. 2000;854:197–206.
7. Steffen BJ, Breier G, Butcher EC, Schulz M, Engelhardt B. ICAM-1, VCAM-1, and MAdCAM-1 are expressed on choroid plexus epithelium but not endothelium and mediate binding of lymphocytes in vitro. Am J Pathol. 1996;148:1819–38.
8. Kunis G, Baruch K, Rosenzweig N, Kertser A, Miller O, Berkutzki T, et al. IFN-gamma-dependent activation of the brain's choroid plexus for CNS immune surveillance and repair. Brain. 2013;136:3427–40.
9. Engelhardt B, Ransohoff RM. Capture, crawl, cross: the T cell code to breach the blood–brain barriers. Trends Immunol. 2012;33:579–89.
10. Shechter R, Miller O, Yovel G, Rosenzweig N, London A, Ruckh J, et al. Recruitment of beneficial M2 macrophages to injured spinal cord is orchestrated by remote brain choroid plexus. Immunity. 2013;38:555–69.

11. Reboldi A, Coisne C, Baumjohann D, Benvenuto F, Bottinelli D, Lira S, et al. C-C chemokine receptor 6-regulated entry of TH-17 cells into the CNS through the choroid plexus is required for the initiation of EAE. Nat Immunol. 2009;10:514–23.
12. Szmydynger-Chodobska J, Strazielle N, Zink BJ, Ghersi-Egea JF, Chodobski A. The role of the choroid plexus in neutrophil invasion after traumatic brain injury. J Cereb Blood Flow Metab. 2009;29:1503–16.
13. Steinmann U, Borkowski J, Wolburg H, Schroppel B, Findeisen P, Weiss C, et al. Transmigration of polymorphnuclear neutrophils and monocytes through the human blood–cerebrospinal fluid barrier after bacterial infection in vitro. J Neuroinflammation. 2013;10:31.
14. Crook RB, Kasagami H, Prusiner SB. Culture and characterization of epithelial cells from bovine choroid plexus. J Neurochem. 1981;37:845–54.
15. Haselbach M, Wegener J, Decker S, Engelbertz C, Galla HJ. Porcine Choroid plexus epithelial cells in culture: regulation of barrier properties and transport processes. Microsc Res Tech. 2001;52:137–52.
16. Gath U, Hakvoort A, Wegener J, Decker S, Galla HJ. Porcine choroid plexus cells in culture: expression of polarized phenotype, maintenance of barrier properties and apical secretion of CSF-components. Eur J Cell Biol. 1997;74:68–78.
17. Holm NR, Hansen LB, Nilsson C, Gammeltoft S. Gene expression and secretion of insulin-like growth factor-II and insulin-like growth factor binding protein-2 from cultured sheep choroid plexus epithelial cells. Brain Res Mol Brain Res. 1994;21:67–74.
18. Ramanathan VK, Hui AC, Brett CM, Giacomini KM. Primary cell culture of the rabbit choroid plexus: an experimental system to investigate membrane transport. Pharm Res. 1996;13:952–6.
19. Zheng W, Zhao Q, Graziano JH. Primary culture of choroidal epithelial cells: characterization of an in vitro model of blood–CSF barrier. In Vitro Cell Dev Biol Anim. 1998;34:40–5.
20. Strazielle N, Ghersi-Egea JF. Demonstration of a coupled metabolism-efflux process at the choroid plexus as a mechanism of brain protection toward xenobiotics. J Neurosci. 1999;19:6275–89.
21. Kitazawa T, Hosoya K, Watanabe M, Takashima T, Ohtsuki S, Takanaga H, et al. Characterization of the amino acid transport of new immortalized choroid plexus epithelial cell lines: a novel in vitro system for investigating transport functions at the blood–cerebrospinal fluid barrier. Pharm Res. 2001;18:16–22.
22. Zheng W, Zhao Q. Establishment and characterization of an immortalized Z310 choroidal epithelial cell line from murine choroid plexus. Brain Res. 2002;958:371–80.
23. Shi LZ, Li GJ, Wang S, Zheng W. Use of Z310 cells as an in vitro blood–cerebrospinal fluid barrier model: tight junction proteins and transport properties. Toxicol In Vitro. 2008;22:190–9.
24. Monnot AD, Zheng W. Culture of choroid plexus epithelial cells and in vitro model of blood–CSF barrier. Methods Mol Biol. 2013;945:13–29.
25. Ishiwata I, Ishiwata C, Ishiwata E, Sato Y, Kiguchi K, Tachibana T, et al. Establishment and characterization of a human malignant choroids plexus papilloma cell line (HIBCPP). Hum Cell. 2005;18:67–72.
26. Nakashima N, Goto K, Tsukidate K, Sobue M, Toida M, Takeuchi J. Choroid plexus papilloma. Light and electron microscopic study. Virchows Arch A Pathol Anat Histopathol. 1983;400:201–11.
27. Takahashi K, Satoh F, Hara E, Murakami O, Kumabe T, Tominaga T, et al. Production and secretion of adrenomedullin by cultured choroid plexus carcinoma cells. J Neurochem. 1997;68:726–31.
28. Peraldi-Roux S, Dao BN-T, Hirn M, Gabrion J. Choroidal ependymocytes in culture: expression of markers of polarity and function. Int J Dev Neurosci. 1990;8:575–88.
29. Gabrion JB, Herbute S, Bouille C, Maurel D, Kuchler-Bopp S, Laabich A, et al. Ependymal and choroidal cells in culture: characterization and functional differentiation. Microsc Res Tech. 1998;41:124–57.
30. Menheniott TR, Charalambous M, Ward A. Derivation of primary choroid plexus epithelial cells from the mouse. Methods Mol Biol. 2010;633:207–20.
31. Barkho BZ, Monuki ES. Proliferation of cultured mouse choroid plexus epithelial cells. PLoS ONE. 2015;10:e0121738.
32. Whitehead RH, Robinson PS. Establishment of conditionally immortalized epithelial cell lines from the intestinal tissue of adult normal and transgenic mice. Am J Physiol Gastrointest Liver Physiol. 2009;296:G455–60.
33. Kohn EA, Du Z, Sato M, Van Schyndle CM, Welsh MA, Yang YA, et al. A novel approach for the generation of genetically modified mammary epithelial cell cultures yields new insights into TGFbeta signaling in the mammary gland. BCR. 2010;12:R83.
34. Enjoji M, Iwaki T, Hara H, Sakai H, Nawata H, Watanabe T. Establishment and characterization of choroid plexus carcinoma cell lines: connection between choroid plexus and immune systems. Jpn J Cancer Res. 1996;87:893–9.
35. Spector R. Pharmacokinetics and metabolism of cytosine arabinoside in the central nervous system. J Pharmacol Exp Ther. 1982;222:1–6.
36. Jat PS, Noble MD, Ataliotis P, Tanaka Y, Yannoutsos N, Larsen L, et al. Direct derivation of conditionally immortal cell lines from an H-2 Kb-tsA58 transgenic mouse. Proc Natl Acad Sci USA. 1991;88:5096–100.
37. Tenenbaum T, Papandreou T, Gellrich D, Friedrichs U, Seibt A, Adam R, et al. Polar bacterial invasion and translocation of *Streptococcus suis* across the blood–cerebrospinal fluid barrier in vitro. Cell Microbiol. 2009;11:323–36.
38. Steiner O, Coisne C, Cecchelli R, Boscacci R, Deutsch U, Engelhardt B, et al. Differential roles for endothelial ICAM-1, ICAM-2, and VCAM-1 in shear-resistant T cell arrest, polarization, and directed crawling on blood–brain barrier endothelium. J Immunol. 2010;185:4846–55.
39. Coisne C, Dehouck L, Faveeuw C, Delplace Y, Miller F, Landry C, et al. Mouse syngenic in vitro blood–brain barrier model: a new tool to examine inflammatory events in cerebral endothelium. Lab Invest. 2005;85:734–46.
40. Cecchelli R, Aday S, Sevin E, Almeida C, Culot M, Dehouck L, et al. A stable and reproducible human blood–brain barrier model derived from hematopoietic stem cells. PLoS ONE. 2014;9:e99733.
41. Abadier M, Haghayegh Jahromi N, Cardoso Alves L, Boscacci R, Vestweber D, Barnum S, et al. Cell surface levels of endothelial ICAM-1 influence the transcellular or paracellular T-cell diapedesis across the blood–brain barrier. Eur J Immunol. 2015;45:1043–58.
42. Lo CM, Keese CR, Giaever I. Cell-substrate contact: another factor may influence transepithelial electrical resistance of cell layers cultured on permeable filters. Exp Cell Res. 1999;250:576–80.
43. Murugesan N, Paul D, Lemire Y, Shrestha B, Ge S, Pachter JS. Active induction of experimental autoimmune encephalomyelitis by MOG35-55 peptide immunization is associated with differential responses in separate compartments of the choroid plexus. Fluids Barriers CNS. 2012;9:15.
44. Marques F, Mesquita SD, Sousa JC, Coppola G, Gao F, Geschwind DH, et al. Lipocalin 2 is present in the EAE brain and is modulated by natalizumab. Front Cell Neurosci. 2012;6:33.
45. Schwerk C, Tenenbaum T, Kim KS, Schroten H. The choroid plexus-a multi-role player during infectious diseases of the CNS. Front Cell Neurosci. 2015;9:80.
46. Wagner EF, Risau W. Oncogenes in the study of endothelial cell growth and differentiation. Semin Cancer Biol. 1994;5:137–45.
47. Weksler B, Romero IA, Couraud PO. The hCMEC/D3 cell line as a model of the human blood brain barrier. Fluids Barriers CNS. 2013;10:16.
48. Klas J, Wolburg H, Terasaki T, Fricker G, Reichel V. Characterization of immortalized choroid plexus epithelial cell lines for studies of transport processes across the blood–cerebrospinal fluid barrier. Cerebrospinal Fluid Res. 2010;7:11.
49. Szmydynger-Chodobska J, Pascale CL, Pfeffer AN, Coulter C, Chodobski A. Expression of junctional proteins in choroid plexus epithelial cell lines: a comparative study. Cerebrospinal Fluid Res. 2007;4:11.
50. Schwerk C, Papandreou T, Schuhmann D, Nickol L, Borkowski J, Steinmann U, et al. Polar invasion and translocation of Neisseria meningitidis and Streptococcus suis in a novel human model of the blood–cerebrospinal fluid barrier. PLoS ONE. 2012;7:e30069.
51. Resnick A. Chronic fluid flow is an environmental modifier of renal epithelial function. PLoS ONE. 2011;6:e27058.
52. May T, Wirth D, Hauser H, Mueller PP. Transcriptionally regulated immortalization overcomes side effects of temperature-sensitive SV40 large T antigen. Biochem Biophys Res Commun. 2005;327:734–41.
53. Takano M, Satoh C, Kunimatsu N, Otani M, Hamada-Kanazawa M, Miyake M, et al. Lipopolysaccharide activates the kallikrein-kinin system in mouse choroid plexus cell line ECPC4. Neurosci Lett. 2008;434:310–4.
54. Takano M, Ohkusa M, Otani M, Min KS, Kadoyama K, Minami K, et al. Lipid A-activated inducible nitric oxide synthase expression via nuclear factor-kappaB in mouse choroid plexus cells. Immunol Lett. 2015;167:57–62.
55. Southwell BR, Duan W, Alcorn D, Brack C, Richardson SJ, Kohrle J, et al. Thyroxine transport to the brain: role of protein synthesis by the choroid plexus. Endocrinology. 1993;133:2116–26.

56. Shu C, Shen H, Teuscher NS, Lorenzi PJ, Keep RF, Smith DE. Role of PEPT2 in peptide/mimetic trafficking at the blood–cerebrospinal fluid barrier: studies in rat choroid plexus epithelial cells in primary culture. J Pharmacol Exp Ther. 2002;301:820–9.
57. Welch K, Araki H. Features of the choroid plexus of the cat, studied in vitro. In: Cserr HR, Fenstermacher JD, editors. Fluid Environment of the Brain. New York: Academic Press Inc; 1975. p. 157–65.
58. Strazielle N, Belin MF, Ghersi-Egea JF. Choroid plexus controls brain availability of anti-HIV nucleoside analogs via pharmacologically inhibitable organic anion transporters. AIDS. 2003;17:1473–85.
59. Staat C, Coisne C, Dabrowski S, Stamatovic SM, Andjelkovic AV, Wolburg H, et al. Mode of action of claudin peptidomimetics in the transient opening of cellular tight junction barriers. Biomaterials. 2015;54:9–20.
60. Steiner O, Coisne C, Engelhardt B, Lyck R. Comparison of immortalized bEnd5 and primary mouse brain microvascular endothelial cells as in vitro blood–brain barrier models for the study of T cell extravasation. J Cereb Blood Flow Metab. 2011;31:315–27.

2

Dose escalation study of intravenous and intra-arterial *N*-acetylcysteine for the prevention of oto- and nephrotoxicity of cisplatin with a contrast-induced nephropathy model in patients with renal insufficiency

Edit Dósa[1], Krisztina Heltai[1], Tamás Radovits[1], Gabriella Molnár[1], Judit Kapocsi[2], Béla Merkely[1], Rongwei Fu[3], Nancy D. Doolittle[4], Gerda B. Tóth[4], Zachary Urdang[4] and Edward A. Neuwelt[4,5,6,7*]

Abstract

Background: Cisplatin neuro-, oto-, and nephrotoxicity are major problems in children with malignant tumors, including medulloblastoma, negatively impacting educational achievement, socioemotional development, and overall quality of life. The blood-labyrinth barrier is somewhat permeable to cisplatin, and sensory hair cells and cochlear supporting cells are highly sensitive to this toxic drug. Several chemoprotective agents such as *N*-acetylcysteine (NAC) were utilized experimentally to avoid these potentially serious and life-long side effects, although no clinical phase I trial was performed before. The purpose of this study was to establish the maximum tolerated dose (MTD) and pharmacokinetics of both intravenous (IV) and intra-arterial (IA) NAC in adults with chronic kidney disease to be used in further trials on oto- and nephroprotection in pediatric patients receiving platinum therapy.

Methods: Due to ethical considerations in pediatric tumor patients, we used a clinical population of adults with non-neoplastic disease. Subjects with stage three or worse renal failure who had any endovascular procedure were enrolled in a prospective, non-randomized, single center trial to determine the MTD for NAC. We initially aimed to evaluate three patients each at 150, 300, 600, 900, and 1200 mg/kg NAC. The MTD was defined as one dose level below the dose producing grade 3 or 4 toxicity. Serum NAC levels were assessed before, 5 and 15 min post NAC. Twenty-eight subjects (15 men; mean age 72.2 ± 6.8 years) received NAC IV (N = 13) or IA (N = 15).

Results: The first participant to experience grade 4 toxicity was at the 600 mg/kg IV dose, at which time the protocol was modified to add an additional dose level of 450 mg/kg NAC. Subsequently, no severe NAC-related toxicity arose and 450 mg/kg NAC was found to be the MTD in both IV and IA groups. Blood levels of NAC showed a linear dose response ($p < 0.01$). Five min after either IV or IA NAC MTD dose administration, serum NAC levels reached the 2–3 mM concentration which seemed to be nephroprotective in previous preclinical studies.

*Correspondence: neuwelte@ohsu.edu

[7] Blood–Brain Barrier and Neuro-Oncology Program, Oregon Health & Science University, 3181 S.W. Sam Jackson Park Road, L603, Portland, OR 97239, USA

Full list of author information is available at the end of the article

Conclusions: In adults with kidney impairment, NAC can be safely given both IV and IA at a dose of 450 mg/kg. Additional studies are needed to confirm oto- and nephroprotective properties in the setting of cisplatin treatment.

Keywords: Ototoxicity, Nephrotoxicity, Chemoprotection, Clinical trial, Cisplatin, *N*-Acetylcysteine

Background

Cisplatin is a common chemotherapeutic agent used to treat various types of malignant tumors. However, side effects such as neuro-, oto-, and nephrotoxicity limit the application of cisplatin. Cisplatin ototoxicity is of particular concern in children with malignant tumors where life-long hearing impairment can cause serious psychosocial deficits including social isolation, limited employment opportunities and associated earning potential, and an overall decrease in quality of life measures [1, 2]. The pathogenesis is not completely understood, but it is likely to be caused by depletion of intracellular glutathione (GSH) and generation of immune cell- and organ parenchymal-derived reactive oxygen species (ROS) and other free radicals [3]. Cisplatin is able to cross the blood-labyrinth barrier and enter the cochlea and sensory hair cells where it causes degeneration of the cochlear supporting cells, outer and inner hair cells and results in a progressive, irreversible hearing loss [4, 5]. For example, in medulloblastoma where the standard of care treatment includes cisplatin, ototoxicity occurs in approximately 80–90% of children treated with standard therapy [6]. Nephrotoxicity occurs in one-third of patients and can be potentially severe or life-threatening. Moreover, these toxicities utilize substantial healthcare resources and thus an inexpensive, effective, prophylactic protective strategy is of clear interest. Several oto- and nephroprotective approaches were developed (such as hydrating the patients during treatment, using less toxic cisplatin analogues) to avoid these reactions, including various chemoprotective agents used in experimental models (dimethylthiourea, melatonin, selenium, vitamin E, *N*-acetylcysteine [NAC], sodium thiosulfate) [5, 7–13].

N-Acetylcysteine is a sulfur-containing cysteine analog. It has been applied for decades as a mucolytic drug and as an antidote for acetaminophen overdose, as well as to prevent contrast-induced nephropathy (CIN) [14]. More recently, interest has been raised for the use of NAC in the prevention of cisplatin induced oto- and nephrotoxicity. Interestingly, CIN from iodine-based contrast agents and cisplatin share common mechanistic features including both intrinsic cellular- and inflammation-related ROS mediated cellular and stromal peroxidation damage [15–20]. The following properties of NAC are hypothesized to be paramount for the prevention of oto- and nephrotoxicity: (1) NAC is thought to act as a vasodilator through nitric oxide effects, thus improving blood flow, (2) NAC is a precursor to GSH, the body's endogenous ROS scavenger, (3) the antioxidant properties of NAC dampen inflammation caused by damage-associated molecular patterns that arise from biological macromolecule peroxidation by ROS and cellular necrosis, and (4) NAC prohibits apoptosis and promotes cell survival by the activation of an extracellular signal-regulated kinase pathway [14]. When NAC enters the systemic circulation it can only leave the blood vessels after N-deacetylation and subsequent carrier mediated active transport of L-cysteine by the alanine–serine–cysteine transporter (ASC-1) [21]. Once in the brain, L-cysteine may act as an antioxidant or can be converted to GSH. Our group and others have shown a low level delivery of radiolabeled NAC across the BBB [22–24]. We demonstrated that even at very high NAC concentration (1200 mg/kg) delivery was less than 0.5% of the administered dose per gram tissue after intravenous (IV) administration in rats, but was significantly enhanced by intra-arterial (IA) administration [24]. It is possible that NAC is a ligand for ASC-1 prior to deacetylation or that NAC is rapidly deacetylated in the blood and the observed radioactivity in the brain was due to radioactive cysteine. In the setting of inflammation, oxidative stress could impair the BBB to increase NAC leak [22, 23]. In case of a brain tumor, vessels supplying the tumor possess impaired barrier properties so both NAC and cisplatin can enter the tumor tissue to some degree.

A literature review revealed 38 trials evaluating NAC in the prevention of CIN, 15 with positive and 23 with negative outcomes, and 17 meta-analyses with conflicting conclusions [25]. There has been significant heterogeneity between studies due to various routes of administration and different dosages [25, 26]. Most trials followed Tepel's regimen of 600 mg of NAC orally twice a day for 48 h and 0.45% saline intravenously, before and after injection of the contrast agent, or placebo and saline as control [26].

Similarly to CIN, NAC has demonstrated mixed results in the literature as an otoprotectant in the context of cisplatin therapy [7, 14, 27–30]. Still, a handful of reports with positive results suggest otoprotective properties during cochlear insults through ROS mediated mechanisms. Dosing, route, and timing of NAC administration seem to be important variables in NAC medicated otoprotection. Whether or not NAC trafficking into the extravascular cochlear compartment occurs is an understudied question, and hence extravascular trafficking may not be required for otoprotective activity. NAC could potentially act by intravascular activity on ROS producing immune cells which can compromise blood-labyrinth barrier integrity and thus prevent enhanced cochlear uptake of cisplatin.

Preclinical ototoxicity studies demonstrated that IV or IA administration of NAC is required to achieve high blood concentration necessary for otoprotection [7, 8, 28, 31]. As Stenstrom observed, oral NAC is cleared via the portal vein on the first pass through the liver, however 31 of 38 reviewed trials ignored this first pass clearance and gave very small doses [14]. We assume that either the oral route or the applied low IV doses were likely a large factor in the negative results seen in previous clinical trials. We hypothesized that NAC at high IV and IA (via the descending aorta) doses can be injected with an acceptable toxicity profile in children with malignant tumors. Our primary goal was to perform a dose escalation study in pediatric patients. Due to rejection of our pediatric toxicity trial by the Institutional Review Board this phase I study used an adult population of subjects with stage 3 or worse kidney failure undergoing a radiologic procedure requiring iodine-based contrast media. Patients with renal failure were chosen with the thought that this population would be particularly sensitive to adverse events and thus the observed maximum tolerated dose (MTD) would include a large margin of safety when translated to the pediatric population. Using this study design we were also able to not only examine the chemoprotective properties of NAC, but could confirm its protection against CIN. The MTD will be evaluated for efficacy in a future trial, specifically in pediatric populations.

Methods

Study protocol

This was a prospective, non-randomized, single center dose escalation trial of patients with stage 3 or worse chronic renal disease (glomerular filtration rate [GFR] < 60 mL/min/1.73 m^2) who underwent a digital subtraction angiography (DSA) and/or vascular intervention with an isotonic nonionic contrast material (Iodixanol) between the years 2012 and 2015. Indication for the procedures was established by a vascular team including vascular surgeons, interventional radiologists, and vascular physicians. Interventions were carried out according to international guidelines. Our primary objective was to establish the MTD of both IV and IA NAC. The secondary objective was to determine NAC pharmacology given IV or IA.

The study was approved by the Institutional Review Committee (12935-0/2011-EKL) and all subjects gave written informed consent.

Eligibility requirements

Patients between 18 and 85 years of age at risk for CIN were eligible to participate if they had stage 3 or worse kidney impairment (renal failure staging was determined by the following formula: Modification of Diet in Renal Disease, GFR ([mL/min/1.73 m^2] $= 175 \times$ [Serum creatinine]$^{-1.154} \times$ [Age]$^{-0.203} \times$ [0.742 if the subject was female]) with a life expectancy of 4 weeks from the date of registration [32].

Exclusion criteria

Subjects were excluded if they had acute kidney injury (e.g., significant change over 4 weeks), were on dialysis, had a systolic blood pressure of < 90 mmHg, had decompensated heart failure at the time of admission, had a history of severe reactive airway disease, were at high risk for general anesthesia, were pregnant, had a positive serum human chorionic gonadotropin or was lactating, or who had contraindications to NAC or the contrast agent.

Treatment plan

Dose escalation

A group of three subjects was aimed to be evaluated at each of the following fixed dose levels of NAC: dose level 1, 150 mg/kg/day; dose level 2, 300 mg/kg/day; dose level 3, 600 mg/kg/day; dose level 4, 900 mg/kg/day; and dose level 5, 1200 mg/kg/day. The first dose level was based on the standard of care treatment of acetaminophen overdose [33]. The dose escalation was evaluated by the rate of grade 3 or 4 toxicities. In case of a severe toxicity reaction an additional dose level was added. Toxicity was graded according to National Cancer Institute Common Terminology Criteria for Adverse Events version 3.0. [34]. The dosing algorithm can be seen in Fig. 1. The NAC MTD was defined as one dose level below the dose that produced grade 3 or 4 toxicity.

Assignment for IV versus IA NAC

Patients were assigned to IV or IA using the last digit of their hospital identification number. Those with even last digits received IV NAC and those with odd last digits received IA NAC. If the MTD was achieved for one group, all subsequent subjects were treated with the other regimen.

Premedication

Since it has been previously shown that NAC has dose dependent anaphylactoid reactions in 23–48%

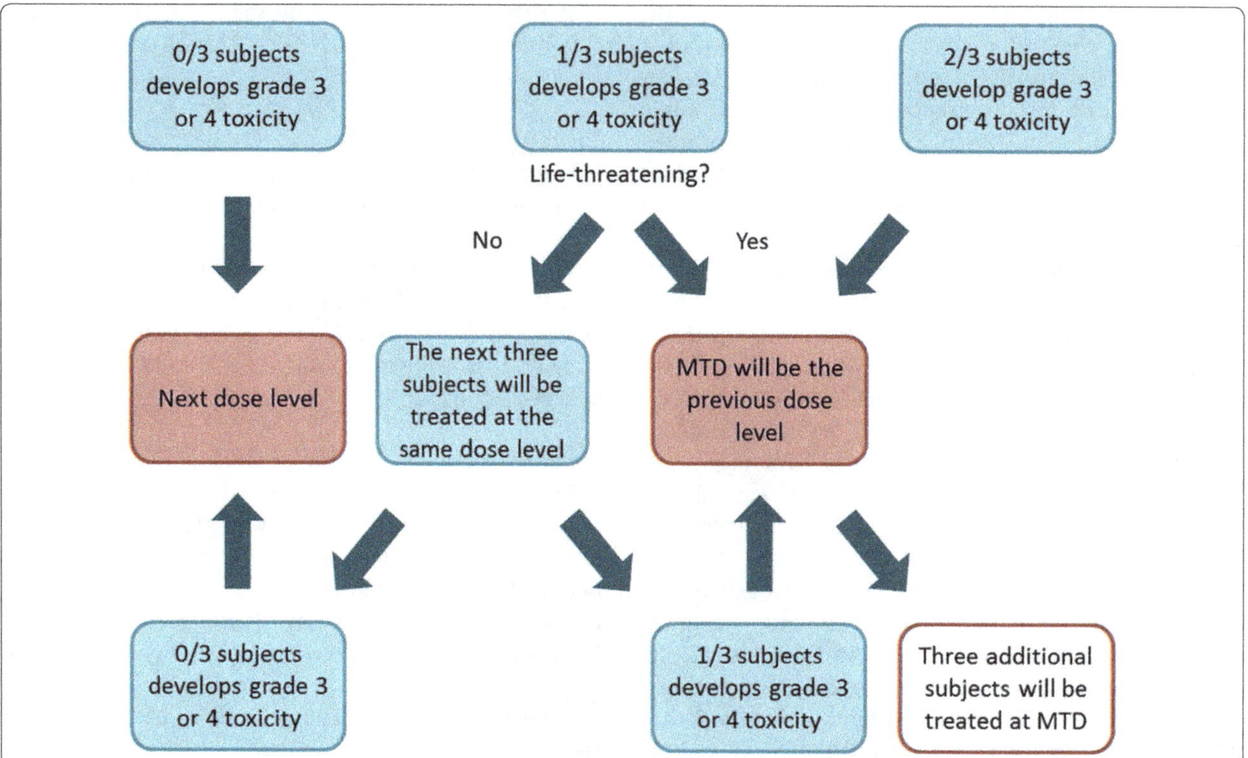

Fig. 1 Dosing algorithm for *N*-acetylcysteine to determine the maximum tolerated dose in adults with chronic kidney disease. The *N*-acetylcysteine maximum tolerated dose was defined as one dose level below the dose that produced grade 3 or 4 toxicity. *MTD* maximum tolerated dose

of patients, all participants received premedication prior to NAC administration [35]. Premedication regimen consisted of 100 mg IV methylprednisolone and 50 mg ranitidine 3 h prior to NAC, and 50 mg diphenhydramine 10 min prior to NAC. Additional doses of 25 mg diphenhydramine were given 10 min after the start of the NAC infusion and repeated as clinically indicated.

Administration of the study drug

The study drug (Acetylcysteine [Fluimucil Antidote]) is available as a 20% solution in 25 mL (200 mg/mL) single dose glass vials. The NAC was diluted to 150, 300, 450, and 600 mg/kg in 250 mL of diluent (5% dextrose in water [Isodex]). The 900 and 1200 mg/kg doses were designed to be diluted in 500 mL of diluent. Each of the above dilutions were given either IV through a peripheral vein using an infusion pump (Alaris GH) or IA down the descending aorta through a fluid injection system (Medrad Avanta) over a period of 25–55 min. In the case of IV injection, the flow rate was 1000 mL/h. For IA administration a pigtail catheter was used (the tip of the catheter was positioned at the level of the renal arteries) and a pulsed infusion of 16.5 mL volume at 16.5 mL/sec was performed and repeated for a total of 15 injections. In the event of grade 1 or 2 toxicities the infusion rate was reduced.

Subject monitoring

Vital signs (pulse and respiration rate), blood pressure, electrical activity of the heart, and oxygen saturation were recorded by a cardiologist at baseline, prior to NAC infusion, every 10 min during infusion, and for 30 min after completion of NAC infusion. The patient was closely monitored for anaphylactoid reaction throughout the endovascular procedure in the angiogram suite and in the recovery unit after the DSA and/or intervention. In the recovery unit, fluid intake and output were measured for 2–4 h until the subject was sent to the ward.

Laboratory analysis of the blood samples

Blood samples were taken at baseline, prior to NAC, then 5 and 15 min after the NAC administration, as well as 24, 48, and 72 h following the radiologic procedure. Study drug and GSH levels were assessed prior to, then 5 and 15 min after the completion of the study drug infusion. Serum NAC and GSH analyses were done in our Research Laboratory using a high-performance liquid chromatography assay. Details of this procedure have been described previously [28].

Statistical analysis

Statistical analysis was performed with SPSS 21.0 software (IBM Corp., Armonk, NY) and SAS 9.4 software (SAS Institute Inc., Cary, NC). Continuous variables were expressed as means and standard deviations and were compared between two groups using the Students' *t* test. A linear mixed-effects model was applied to evaluate dose response relationships and differences at various time points for pharmacological factors while accounting for correlations among the multiple observations within the same patient. All analyses were two-tailed, and values of $p \leq 0.05$ were considered statistically significant.

Results

Patient data

Twenty-eight subjects (13 women, 15 men; mean age: 72.2 ± 6.8 years) were enrolled. Fifteen subjects had DSA (lower or upper extremity angiography, N = 6; aortic arch and selective four-vessel cerebral angiography, N = 3; lower extremity plus aortic arch and selective four-vessel cerebral angiography, N = 3; renal angiography, N = 3) while 12 underwent percutaneous transluminal angioplasty with or without stent placement (internal carotid artery stenting, N = 4; renal artery stenting, N = 2; crural artery percutaneous transluminal angioplasty, N = 2; subclavian artery stenting, N = 1; common iliac artery stenting, N = 1; common iliac artery plus renal artery stenting, N = 1; superficial femoral artery stenting, N = 1). One patient (7_IV) did not have radiologic intervention due to NAC-related acute severe toxicity.

N-Acetylcysteine toxicity

The administered NAC volume and NAC infusion time did not differ significantly between the corresponding IV and IA groups (Table 1).

Maximum tolerated IV dose

Thirteen participants received IV NAC. Three patients completed dose level 1 and three completed dose level 2 without having grade 3 or 4 toxicity. The first subject (7_IV) enrolled to dose level 3 developed rashes, flushing, pruritus, and an intense bronchospasm immediately after completion of the study drug administration which

Table 1 *N*-Acetylcysteine and contrast agent volumes, *N*-acetylcysteine administration time, baseline serum creatinine levels, and 5-min *N*-acetylcysteine and glutathione concentrations

Parameter	NAC dose (mg/kg)	IV group (Mean ± SD)	IA group (Mean ± SD)	p value
NAC volume (mL)	150	63.25 ± 50.61	51.88 ± 6.6	0.31
	300	109.5 ± 6.89	132.5 ± 46.37	0.183
	600	294	NA	NA
	450	167.58 ± 44.63	166.13 ± 41.61	0.956
NAC administration time (min)	150	26.67 ± 2.89	31.67 ± 7.53	0.196
	300	31.67 ± 5.77	38.33 ± 2.89	0.173
	600	51	NA	NA
	450	40 ± 6.32	42.5 ± 8.22	0.569
CA volume (mL)	150	94.33 ± 69.89	109.17 ± 56.16	0.768
	300	80 ± 39.69	86.67 ± 64.29	0.887
	600	0	NA	NA
	450	89.5 ± 15.86	88.5 ± 25.81	0.937
Baseline serum creatinine (μmol/L)	150	201 ± 11.97	118.17 ± 15.53	0.402
	300	123.67 ± 33.23	160 ± 24.76	0.343
	600	157	NA	NA
	450	209.33 ± 54.4	171.5 ± 52.89	0.486
NAC concentration at 5 min (mM)	150	0.43 ± 0.1	1.66 ± 0.32	*< 0.001*
	300	1.04 ± 0.6	3.12 ± 0.77	*0.023*
	600	4.53	NA	NA
	450	2.03 ± 0.95	4.1 ± 1.22	*0.009*
GSH concentration at 5 min (mM)	150	0.13 ± 0.16	0.2 ± 0.04	0.514
	300	0.13 ± 0.03	0.96 ± 0.36	0.058
	600	0.21	NA	NA
	450	0.19 ± 0.04	0.89 ± 0.31	*0.003*

Italicized p-values indicate statistically significant values

IV intravenous, *IA* intra-arterial, *SD* standard deviation, *NAC* *N*-acetylcysteine, *NA* not applicable, *CA* contrast agent, *GSH* glutathione

rapidly progressed to respiratory and cardiac arrest. Successful cardiorespiratory resuscitation was performed according to the 2010 American Heart Association guidelines at which point the participant was transported to the intensive care unit where he was monitored for 3 days [36]. The patient left the hospital 6 days post NAC in good condition. Due to the serious toxicity in this subject, the protocol was modified and a new dose level of 450 mg/kg NAC was inserted between the 300 and 600 mg/kg doses. Participants 8_IV, 9_IV, and 10_IV received 450 mg/kg dose of NAC. None had grade 3 or 4 toxicity, therefore 450 mg/kg was considered to be the MTD and three additional patients were treated with the same dose in order to gain more data on NAC toxicity and pharmacokinetics (Fig. 2).

Maximum tolerated IA dose

Fifteen subjects received IA NAC. The first participant (1_IA) enrolled to the group developed an anaphylactic reaction with life-threatening symptoms. She was treated according to the 2011 World Allergy Organization anaphylaxis guidelines in the angiogram suite and was transported to the intensive care unit where she was monitored for 3 days [37]. The patient left the hospital 5 days post NAC infusion in good condition. The anaphylactic reaction occurred immediately after completion of the DSA. The time interval between the anaphylactic reaction and NAC infusion was 1 h. The case was discussed by a multidisciplinary team which considered the adverse reaction to be a consequence of the contrast agent rather than NAC based on the elapsed time from the study drug infusion to the time of the anaphylactic reaction. Also, the subject provided information after the adverse reaction that she developed hives on her chest 2 months previously after a cardiac catheterization. Furthermore, the cardiac catheterization was done in a different hospital, the hives were not mentioned in the final report, and the participant answered no for the question whether she had allergic reaction to anything in her life both prior to study enrollment and before the interventional procedure. Although two additional participants completed dose level 1 without having grade 3 or 4 toxicity, three more patients were treated with the same dose. Neither 300 nor 450 mg/kg dose produced severe toxicity. The 450 mg/kg

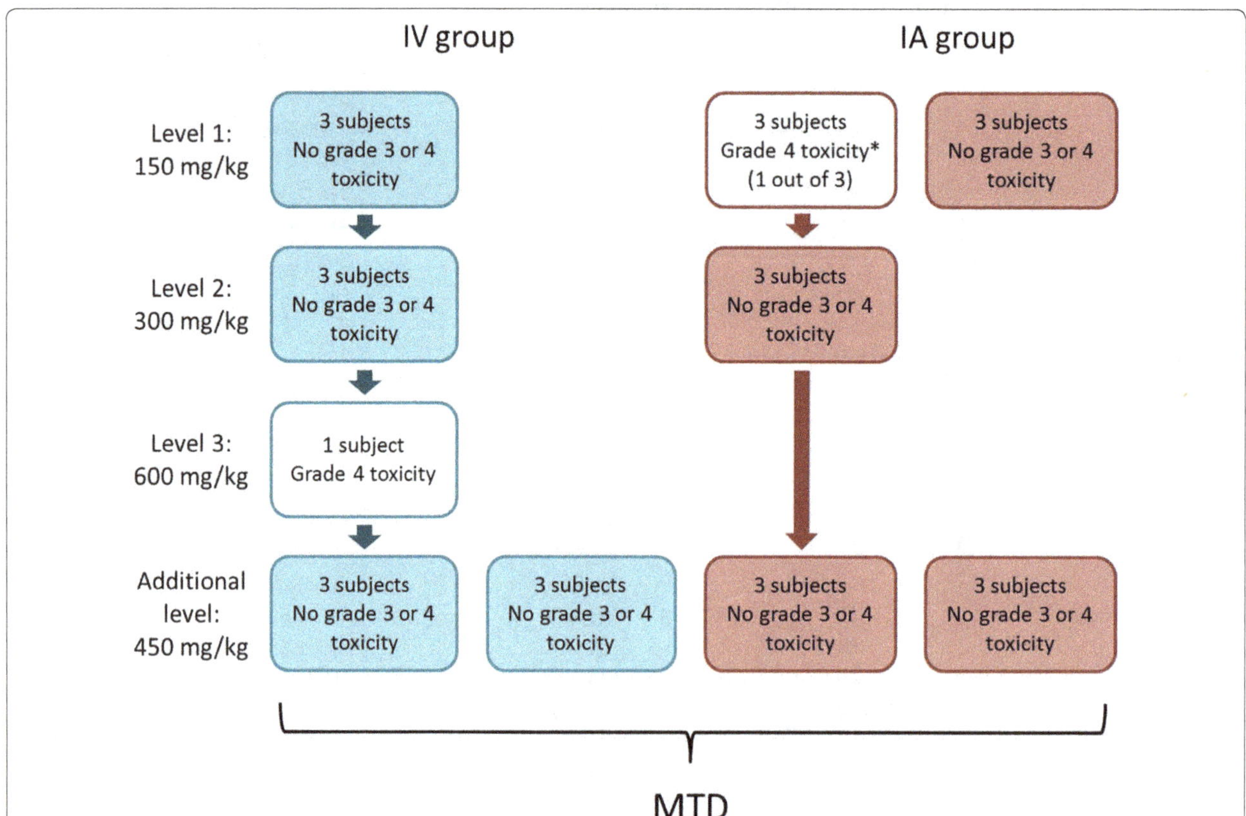

Fig. 2 Establishment of the maximum tolerated dose for *N*-acetylcysteine in adults with chronic kidney disease. Four hundred and fifty mg/kg *N*-acetylcysteine was found to be the maximum tolerated dose in both intravenous and intra-arterial groups. Asterisk: Adverse reaction to contrast agent rather than to *N*-acetylcysteine. *IV* intravenous, *IA* intra-arterial, *MTD* maximum tolerated dose

dose was considered to be the MTD and three additional subjects received that dose (Fig. 2).

Minor toxicities

Grade 1 or 2 toxicities were seen in six participants (21.4%). Two-thirds of the minor toxicities occurred at a dose of 450 mg/kg NAC. All of them resolved either spontaneously or by giving appropriate treatment over 30 min to 12 h following the toxicity (Table 2).

N-Acetylcysteine pharmacokinetics

Results of the high-performance liquid chromatography analysis are summarized in Fig. 3.

Serum NAC levels

At baseline, NAC and GSH were not detected in the serum samples. Blood levels of NAC showed a significant linear dose response both 5 min (slope, 1.07 mM increase for every 150 mg/kg rise in NAC dose; p = 0.001) and

Table 2 Toxicities attributed to *N*-acetylcysteine

Group	Patient number	Weight (kg)	NAC dose (mg/kg)	NAC volume (mL)	NAC toxicity
IV	4_IV	84	300	126	Grade 1, facial erythema
	7_IV	98	600	294	Grade 4, respiratory and cardiac arrest
	10_IV	96	450	216	Grade 2, pruritus and rash
	11_IV	103	450	231.75	Grade 1, coughing
IA	1_IA	55	150	41.25	Grade 4[a], anaphylaxis
	8_IA	101	300	151.5	Grade 1, nausea
	10_IA	95	450	213.75	Grade 1, coughing
	11_IA	80	450	180	Grade 1, facial erythema

NAC N-acetylcysteine, *IV* intravenous, *IA* intra-arterial

[a] Adverse reaction to contrast agent rather than to NAC

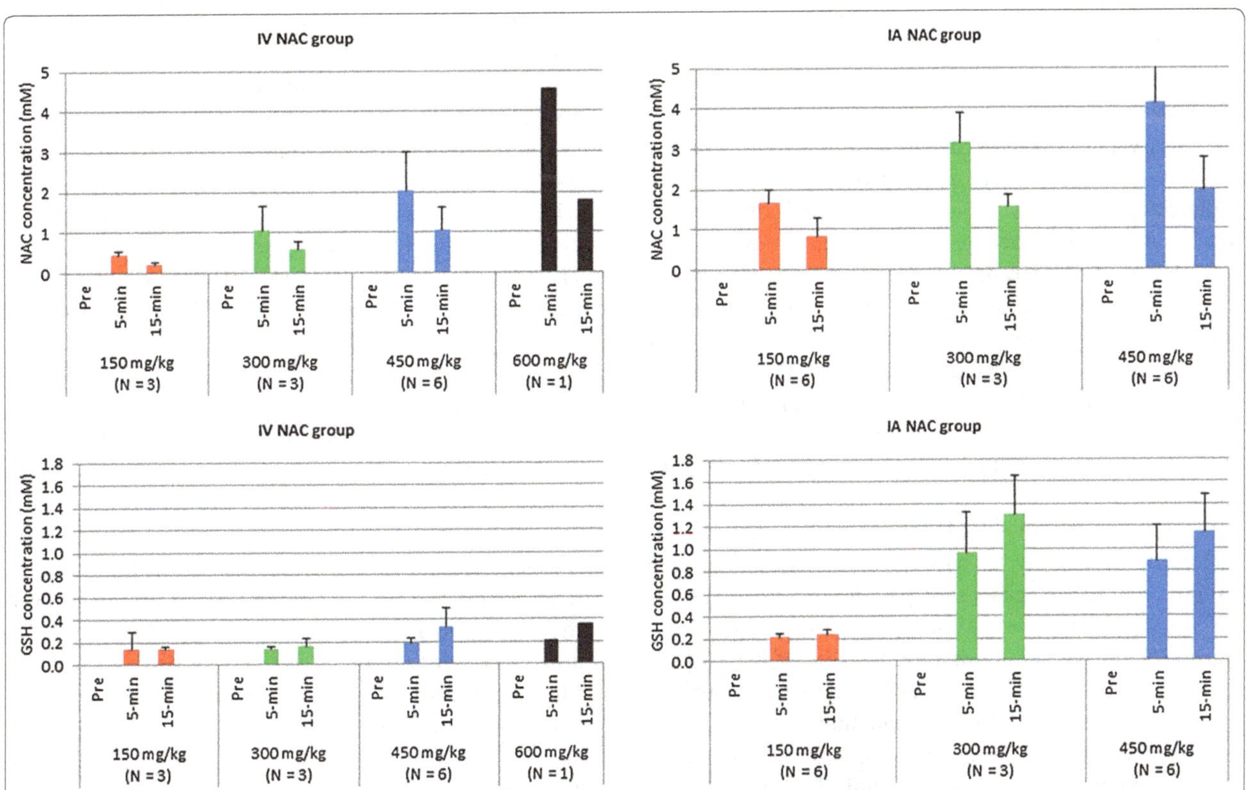

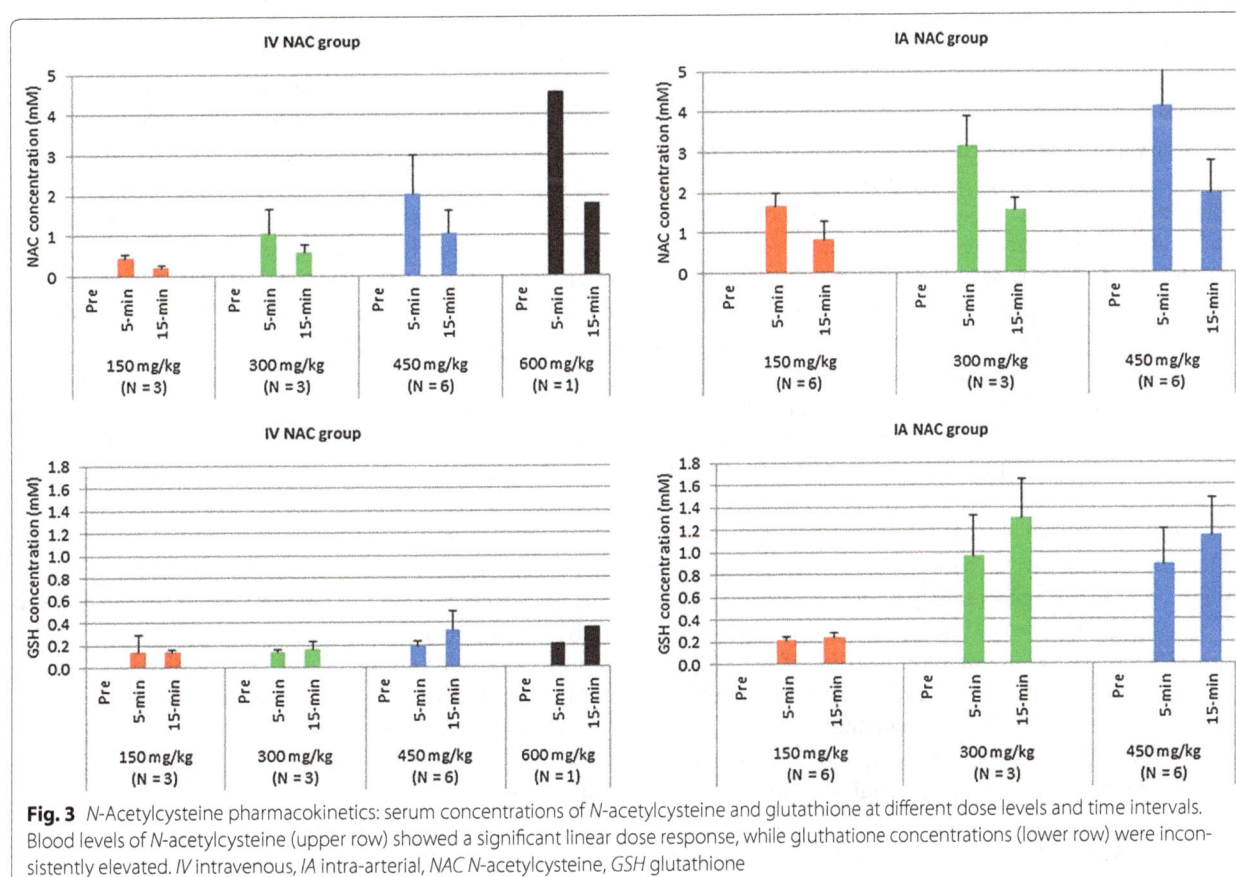

Fig. 3 *N*-Acetylcysteine pharmacokinetics: serum concentrations of *N*-acetylcysteine and glutathione at different dose levels and time intervals. Blood levels of *N*-acetylcysteine (upper row) showed a significant linear dose response, while gluthatione concentrations (lower row) were inconsistently elevated. *IV* intravenous, *IA* intra-arterial, *NAC N*-acetylcysteine, *GSH* glutathione

15 min after IV administration (slope, 0.48 mM increase for every 150 mg/kg rise in NAC dose; $p = 0.002$). Similar significant linear dose responses were observed after IA injection with a slope of 1.22 mM for every 150 mg/kg increase in NAC dose at 5 min ($p < 0.001$) and with a slope of 0.58 mM for every 150 mg/kg increase in NAC dose at 15 min ($p = 0.005$). In each group, NAC levels were nearly halved from 5 to 15 min post infusion. In particular, the overall mean NAC level was 1.63 mM (SE: 0.23) and 0.81 mM (SE: 0.21), respectively, 5 and 15 min after IV administration; and 2.93 mM (SE: 0.22) and 1.42 mM (SE: 0.15), respectively, 5 and 15 min after IA injection. At 5 min post infusion, NAC concentrations were significantly higher in the IA groups compared to the corresponding IV groups ($p < 0.001$; $p = 0.023$, $p = 0.009$, respectively) (Table 1, Fig. 3).

Serum GSH levels

A significant linear dose response relationship was noted for GSH concentrations in the IV group. Since the relationships were similar at 5 and 15 min, an overall dose response relationship was estimated to yield a 0.37 mM increase in GSH values for every 150 mg/kg rise in NAC dose ($p < 0.001$). In contrast to patients in the IV group, the overall dose response relationship was not significantly linear in the IA group ($p = 0.068$). The mean GSH concentrations were higher in the IA than in the IV group (Table 1, Fig. 3).

Discussion

Our goal was to provide the MTD of NAC as a correct scientific basis for future efficacy trials, particularly in pediatric populations. Four hundred and fifty mg/kg NAC was found to be the MTD in this study, and we have shown that it can be given with an acceptable toxicity both IV and IA in adults with impaired kidney function undergoing DSA with or without intervention. By determining the MTD we potentially gain the maximum concentration of NAC in the brain and cochlea to diminish the toxicity of agents like cisplatin, although the entry of NAC may be limited by the BBB and blood-labyrinth barrier.

A key factor in previous failed trials with NAC is that oral NAC is known to have 5–10% bioavailability in humans due to extensive first pass metabolism to GSH [38]. Oral NAC reaches a serum peak about an hour after ingestion and has an elimination half-life of 2.27 h [39]. Furthermore, there is no clear evidence that NAC effects are mediated indirectly by its metabolites.

The potential of oral NAC to be oto- and nephroprotective was examined in several preclinical studies. Dickey et al. determined in rats, that a single IV administration of 1500 mg/kg NAC is non-toxic, and three IV injections of 1200 mg/kg NAC, 4 h apart, are safe and well-tolerated [28]. In another study by Dickey et al. rats received NAC infusion at 100, 400 and 1200 mg/kg IV. Blood samples were taken 15 min post inoculation. Another group of rats was given NAC 1200 mg/kg orally, with blood samples collected after 15 and 60 min. Total NAC concentrations were analyzed and similarly to our findings, blood levels of NAC showed a rough linear dose response after IV administration of NAC. In contrast to the IV results, the group given NAC 1200 mg/kg by the oral route had very low levels of serum NAC [28]. In their third study, rats were treated with cisplatin 10 mg/kg intraperitoneally 30 min after NAC 400 mg/kg given by intraperitoneal, oral, or IV routes, compared with cisplatin alone. NAC was chemoprotective against the cisplatin nephrotoxicity, depending on the route of administration. Rats receiving NAC IV had very low blood urea nitrogen levels 3 days post treatment. In the case of oral or intraperitoneal NAC administration, the blood urea nitrogen concentrations were as high as in the group of rats who did not get NAC [28]. In their fourth study, rats were treated with cisplatin 10 mg/kg intraperitoneally 30 min after NAC 50 mg/kg infused IV or IA. The blood urea nitrogen levels were significantly lower in the IA group—the blood urea nitrogen levels were similar to those when NAC was injected IV at high dose (400 mg/kg)—indicating a significantly reduced rate of nephrotoxicity for the IA delivery [28]. Assuming that this rat chemoprotective model represents the effects of cisplatin as those of contrast agents in humans, these observations call into question if oral NAC or low dose IV NAC has any clinical impact on cisplatin induced oto- and nephrotoxicity.

Briguori et al. and Marenzi et al. were the only investigators who made dose comparisons in humans. Briguori et al. compared single dose NAC 600 mg orally twice a day for 48 h with double dose NAC 1200 mg (17.1 mg/kg for a 70 kg subject) orally twice a day for 48 h. Although these doses were not high and were given orally, the outcome was favorable for the double dose [40]. Marenzi et al. compared two IV doses (600 and 1200 mg total dose per patient) prior to the angioplasty and two oral doses (600 and 1200 mg twice a day for 48 h) after the procedure with placebo. A greater increase in serum creatinine was observed in the placebo group compared to patients treated with NAC and the higher NAC IV dose was even better than the lower dose, which implies that NAC actions may be dose dependent [41]. These observations are in line with the findings of the above mentioned rat studies and demonstrate the importance of this phase I trial.

It is also worth considering that the route of NAC administration markedly affects its biodistribution. In an animal study performed by our group, we found that when radiolabeled NAC was administered IA into the right carotid artery of the rat, high levels of radiolabel were found throughout the right cerebral hemisphere, regardless of whether or not the BBB was opened. Delivery was 0.41% of the injected dose, comparable to the levels found in the liver (0.57%) and kidney (0.70%). In contrast, the aortic infusion above the renal arteries prevented the brain delivery and changed the biodistribution of NAC. The change in tissue delivery with different modes of administration is likely due to NAC being deacetylated and the amino acid cysteine is rapidly bound by tissues via the amino acid transporters [24].

The limitations of our study include the special subject population: all patients were older than 50 years, had impaired kidney function, and atherosclerotic disease. Although serum creatinine values were measured both before and after contrast agent administration additional trials should be performed to determine whether either IV or IA 450 mg/kg NAC is protective against CIN or chemoprotective against cisplatin in pediatric subjects.

Conclusions

In conclusion, we found that NAC can be safely given both IV and IA at a dose of 450 mg/kg in adults with reduced renal function. Phase II and III studies are needed to determine whether high IV and IA doses can avoid oto- and nephrotoxicity of platinum-based chemotherapy, and if yes, whether a particular route of administration of NAC provides improved chemoprotection. A considerable hurdle with NAC is disentangling the mixed results from studies utilizing oral NAC administration; we advocate for careful analysis and comparison of oral route trials in humans with those of IV or IA. A phase I trial in children is currently underway with different doses of NAC after cisplatin to prevent ototoxicity (clinicaltrials.gov NCT02094625).

Abbreviations

ASC-1: alanine–serine–cysteine transporter; BBB: blood–brain barrier; CIN: contrast-induced nephropathy; DSA: digital subtraction angiography; GFR: glomerular filtration rate; GSH: glutathione; IA: intra-arterial; IV: intravenous; MTD: maximum tolerated dose; NAC: *N*-Acetylcysteine; ROS: reactive oxygen species.

Authors' contributions

Participated in research design: ED, NDD, EAN. Conducted experiments: ED, KH, TR, GM, JK, BM. Performed data analysis: ED, RF. Wrote or contributed to the writing of the manuscript: ED, RF, GBT, ZU. All authors read and approved the final manuscript.

Author details

[1] Heart and Vascular Center, Semmelweis University, 68 Városmajor Street, Budapest 1122, Hungary. [2] 1st Department of Internal Medicine, Semmelweis University, 26 Üllői Street, Budapest 1085, Hungary. [3] Public Health & Preventive Medicine, Oregon Health & Science University, 3184 S.W. Sam Jackson Park Rd, CB669, Portland, OR 97329, USA. [4] Department of Neurology, Oregon Health & Science University, 3184 S.W. Sam Jackson Park Rd, L603, Portland, OR 97329, USA. [5] Department of Neurosurgery, Oregon Health & Science University, 3184 S.W. Sam Jackson Park Rd, L603, Portland, OR 97329, USA. [6] Portland Veterans Affairs Medical Center, 3710 S.W. US Veterans Hospital Rd, Portland, OR 97239, USA. [7] Blood–Brain Barrier and Neuro-Oncology Program, Oregon Health & Science University, 3181 S.W. Sam Jackson Park Road, L603, Portland, OR 97239, USA.

Acknowledgements

We thank Leslie L. Muldoon and Emily Youngers for their expert editing of the manuscript.

Competing interests

The Portland Veterans Affairs Medical Center (PVAMC) and the Oregon Health & Science University (OHSU) Department of Veterans Affairs have a significant financial interest in Fennec, a company that may have a commercial interest in the results of this research and technology. Dr. Neuwelt, inventor of technology licensed to Fennec, has divested himself of all potential earnings. These potential conflicts of interest were reviewed and managed by the OHSU Integrity Program Oversight Council and the OHSU and PVAMC Conflict of interest in Research Committees.

Funding

This work was supported in part by a Veterans Affairs Merit Review Grant, the National Institutes of Health Grants R01 CA137488-22 and R01 CA199111-33 and by the Walter S. and Lucienne Driskill Foundation all to EAN.

References

1. Robinshaw HM. Early intervention for hearing impairment: differences in the timing of communicative and linguistic development. Br J Audiol. 1995;29:315–34.
2. Yoshinaga-Itano C, Sedey AL, Coulter DK, Mehl AL. Language of early- and later-identified children with hearing loss. Pediatrics. 1998;102:1161–71.
3. Rybak LP, Whitworth CA, Mukherjea D, Ramkumar V. Mechanisms of cisplatin-induced ototoxicity and prevention. Hear Res. 2007;226:157–67.
4. Assietti R, Olson JJ. Intra-arterial cisplatin in malignant brain tumors: incidence and severity of otic toxicity. J Neurooncol. 1996;27:251–8.
5. Neuwelt EA, Brummett RE, Remsen LG, Kroll RA, Pagel MA, McCormick CI, Guitjens S, Muldoon LL. In vitro and animal studies of sodium thiosulfate as a potential chemoprotectant against carboplatin-induced ototoxicity. Cancer Res. 1996;56:706–9.
6. Knight KR, Kraemer DF, Neuwelt EA. Ototoxicity in children receiving platinum chemotherapy: underestimating a commonly occurring toxicity that may influence academic and social development. J Clin Oncol. 2005;23:8588–96.
7. Dickey DT, Wu YJ, Muldoon LL, Neuwelt EA. Protection against cisplatin-induced toxicities by *N*-acetylcysteine and sodium thiosulfate as assessed at the molecular, cellular, and in vivo levels. J Pharmacol Exp Ther. 2005;314:1052–8.
8. Muldoon LL, Pagel MA, Kroll RA, Brummett RE, Doolittle ND, Zuhowski EG, Egorin MJ, Neuwelt EA. Delayed administration of sodium thiosulfate in animal models reduces platinum ototoxicity without reduction of antitumor activity. Clin Cancer Res. 2000;6:309–15.
9. Naziroglu M, Karaoglu A, Aksoy AO. Selenium and high dose vitamin E administration protects cisplatin-induced oxidative damage to renal, liver and lens tissues in rats. Toxicology. 2004;195:221–30.
10. Pace A, Savarese A, Picardo M, Maresca V, Pacetti U, Del Monte G, Biroccio A, Leonetti C, Jandolo B, Cognetti F, Bove L. Neuroprotective effect of vitamin E supplementation in patients treated with cisplatin chemotherapy. J Clin Oncol. 2003;21:927–31.
11. Sener G, Satiroglu H, Kabasakal L, Arbak S, Oner S, Ercan F, Keyer-Uysa M. The protective effect of melatonin on cisplatin nephrotoxicity. Fundam Clin Pharmacol. 2000;14:553–60.

12. Tsuruya K, Tokumoto M, Ninomiya T, Hirakawa M, Masutani K, Taniguchi M, Fukuda K, Kanai H, Hirakata H, Iida M. Antioxidant ameliorates cisplatin-induced renal tubular cell death through inhibition of death receptor-mediated pathways. Am J Physiol Renal Physiol. 2003;285:F208–18.
13. Wu YJ, Muldoon LL, Neuwelt EA. The chemoprotective agent *N*-acetylcysteine blocks cisplatin-induced apoptosis through caspase signaling pathway. J Pharmacol Exp Ther. 2005;312:424–31.
14. Stenstrom DA, Muldoon LL, Armijo-Medina H, Watnick S, Doolittle ND, Kaufman JA, Peterson DR, Bubalo J, Neuwelt EA. *N*-Acetylcysteine use to prevent contrast medium-induced nephropathy: premature phase III trials. J Vasc Interv Radiol. 2008;19:309–18.
15. Chu S, Hu L, Wang X, Sun S, Zhang T, Sun Z, Shen L, Jin S, He B. Xuezhikang ameliorates contrast media-induced nephropathy in rats via suppression of oxidative stress, inflammatory responses and apoptosis. Ren Fail. 2016;38:1717–25.
16. Gao L, Wu WF, Dong L, Ren GL, Li HD, Yang Q, Li XF, Xu T, Li Z, Wu BM, et al. Protocatechuic aldehyde attenuates cisplatin-induced acute kidney injury by suppressing nox-mediated oxidative stress and renal inflammation. Front Pharmacol. 2016;7:479.
17. He X, Li L, Tan H, Chen J, Zhou Y. Atorvastatin attenuates contrast-induced nephropathy by modulating inflammatory responses through the regulation of JNK/p38/Hsp27 expression. J Pharmacol Sci. 2016;131:18–27.
18. Kaur T, Borse V, Sheth S, Sheehan K, Ghosh S, Tupal S, Jajoo S, Mukherjea D, Rybak LP, Ramkumar V. Adenosine A1 receptor protects against cisplatin ototoxicity by suppressing the NOX3/STAT1 inflammatory pathway in the cochlea. J Neurosci. 2016;36:3962–77.
19. Li CZ, Jin HH, Sun HX, Zhang ZZ, Zheng JX, Li SH, Han SH. Eriodictyol attenuates cisplatin-induced kidney injury by inhibiting oxidative stress and inflammation. Eur J Pharmacol. 2016;772:124–30.
20. Onk D, Onk OA, Turkmen K, Erol HS, Ayazoglu TA, Keles ON, Halici M, Topal E. Melatonin attenuates contrast-induced nephropathy in diabetic rats: the role of interleukin-33 and oxidative stress. Mediators Inflamm. 2016;2016:9050828.
21. Helboe L, Egebjerg J, Moller M, Thomsen C. Distribution and pharmacology of alanine–serine–cysteine transporter 1 (asc-1) in rodent brain. Eur J Neurosci. 2003;18:2227–38.
22. Erickson MA, Hansen K, Banks WA. Inflammation-induced dysfunction of the low-density lipoprotein receptor-related protein-1 at the blood–brain barrier: protection by the antioxidant *N*-acetylcysteine. Brain Behav Immun. 2012;26:1085–94.
23. Farr SA, Poon HF, Dogrukol-Ak D, Drake J, Banks WA, Eyerman E, Butterfield DA, Morley JE. The antioxidants alpha-lipoic acid and *N*-acetylcysteine reverse memory impairment and brain oxidative stress in aged SAMP8 mice. J Neurochem. 2003;84:1173–83.
24. Neuwelt EA, Pagel MA, Hasler BP, Deloughery TG, Muldoon LL. Therapeutic efficacy of aortic administration of *N*-acetylcysteine as a chemoprotectant against bone marrow toxicity after intracarotid administration of alkylators, with or without glutathione depletion in a rat model. Cancer Res. 2001;61:7868–74.
25. Weisbord SD, Gallagher M, Kaufman J, Cass A, Parikh CR, Chertow GM, Shunk KA, McCullough PA, Fine MJ, Mor MK, et al. Prevention of contrast-induced AKI: a review of published trials and the design of the prevention of serious adverse events following angiography (PRESERVE) trial. Clin J Am Soc Nephrol. 2013;8:1618–31.
26. Tepel M, van der Giet M, Schwarzfeld C, Laufer U, Liermann D, Zidek W. Prevention of radiographic-contrast-agent-induced reductions in renal function by acetylcysteine. N Engl J Med. 2000;343:180–4.
27. Berglin CE, Pierre PV, Bramer T, Edsman K, Ehrsson H, Eksborg S, Laurell G. Prevention of cisplatin-induced hearing loss by administration of a thiosulfate-containing gel to the middle ear in a guinea pig model. Cancer Chemother Pharmacol. 2011;68:1547–56.
28. Dickey DT, Muldoon LL, Doolittle ND, Peterson DR, Kraemer DF, Neuwelt EA. Effect of *N*-acetylcysteine route of administration on chemoprotection against cisplatin-induced toxicity in rat models. Cancer Chemother Pharmacol. 2008;62:235–41.
29. Lorito G, Hatzopoulos S, Laurell G, Campbell KCM, Petruccelli J, Giordano P, Kochanek K, Sliwa L, Martini A, Skarzynski H. Dose-dependent protection on cisplatin-induced ototoxicity—an electrophysiological study on the effect of three antioxidants in the Sprague-Dawley rat animal model. Med Sci Monit. 2011;17:BR179–86.
30. Yoo J, Hamilton SJ, Angel D, Fung K, Franklin J, Parnes LS, Lewis D, Venkatesan V, Winquist E. Cisplatin otoprotection using transtympanic *L-N*-acetylcysteine: a pilot randomized study in head and neck cancer patients. Laryngoscope. 2014;124:E87–94.
31. Thomas Dickey D, Muldoon LL, Kraemer DF, Neuwelt EA. Protection against cisplatin-induced ototoxicity by *N*-acetylcysteine in a rat model. Hear Res. 2004;193:25–30.
32. Levey AS, Coresh J, Greene T, Stevens LA, Zhang YL, Hendriksen S, Kusek JW, Van Lente F. Using standardized serum creatinine values in the modification of diet in renal disease study equation for estimating glomerular filtration rate. Ann Intern Med. 2006;145:247–54.
33. Heard K, Dart R. Acetaminophen (paracetamol) poisoning in adults: Treatment. 8/30/2016 edition. http://www.uptodate.com: Wolters Kluwer; 2016.
34. Common terminology criteria for adverse events, version 3.0, DCTD, NCI, NIH, DHHS. [http://ctep.cancer.gov].
35. Sandilands EA, Bateman DN. Adverse reactions associated with acetylcysteine. Clin Toxicol (Phila). 2009;47:81–8.
36. Travers AH, Rea TD, Bobrow BJ, Edelson DP, Berg RA, Sayre MR, Berg MD, Chameides L, O'Connor RE, Swor RA. Part 4: CPR overview: 2010 American Heart association guidelines for cardiopulmonary resuscitation and emergency cardiovascular care. Circulation. 2010;122:S676–84.
37. Simons FE, Ardusso LR, Bilo MB, El-Gamal YM, Ledford DK, Ring J, Sanchez-Borges M, Senna GE, Sheikh A, Thong BY. World allergy organization guidelines for the assessment and management of anaphylaxis. World Allergy Organ J. 2011;4:13–37.
38. Fishbane S, Durham JH, Marzo K, Rudnick M. *N*-acetylcysteine in the prevention of radiocontrast-induced nephropathy. J Am Soc Nephrol. 2004;15:251–60.
39. Hultberg B, Andersson A, Masson P, Larson M, Tunek A. Plasma homocysteine and thiol compound fractions after oral administration of *N*-acetylcysteine. Scand J Clin Lab Invest. 1994;54:417–22.
40. Briguori C, Colombo A, Violante A, Balestrieri P, Manganelli F, Paolo Elia P, Golia B, Lepore S, Riviezzo G, Scarpato P, et al. Standard vs double dose of *N*-acetylcysteine to prevent contrast agent associated nephrotoxicity. Eur Heart J. 2004;25:206–11.
41. Marenzi G, Assanelli E, Marana I, Lauri G, Campodonico J, Grazi M, De Metrio M, Galli S, Fabbiocchi F, Montorsi P, et al. *N*-acetylcysteine and contrast-induced nephropathy in primary angioplasty. N Engl J Med. 2006;354:2773–82.

3

Misleading early blood volume changes obtained using ferumoxytol-based magnetic resonance imaging perfusion in high grade glial neoplasms treated with bevacizumab

Joao Prola Netto[1,2†], Daniel Schwartz[1,3†], Csanad Varallyay[1], Rongwei Fu[4,5], Bronwyn Hamilton[2] and Edward A. Neuwelt[1,6,7*]

Abstract

Background: Neovascularization, a distinguishing trait of high-grade glioma, is a target for anti-angiogenic treatment with bevacizumab (BEV). This study sought to use ferumoxytol-based dynamic susceptibility contrast magnetic resonance imaging (MRI) to clarify perfusion and relative blood volume (rCBV) changes in glioma treated with BEV and to determine potential impact on clinical management.

Methods: 16 high grade glioma patients who received BEV following post-chemoradiation radiographic or clinical progression were included. Ferumoxytol-based MRI perfusion measurements were taken before and after BEV. Lesions were defined at each timepoint by gadolinium-based contrast agent (GBCA)-enhancing area. Lesion volume and rCBV were compared pre and post-BEV in the lesion and rCBV "hot spot" (mean of the highest rCBV in a 1.08 cm^2 area in the enhancing volume), as well as hypoperfused and hyperperfused subvolumes within the GBCA-enhancing lesion.

Results: GBCA-enhancing lesion volumes decreased 39% ($P = 0.01$) after BEV. Mean rCBV in post-BEV GBCA-enhancing area did not decrease significantly ($P = 0.227$) but significantly decreased in the hot spot ($P = 0.046$). Mean and hot spot rCBV decreased ($P = 0.039$ and 0.007) when post-BEV rCBV was calculated over the pre-BEV GBCA-enhancing area. Hypoperfused pixel count increased from 24% to 38 ($P = 0.007$) and hyperperfused decreased from 39 to 28% ($P = 0.017$). Mean rCBV decreased in 7/16 (44%) patients from >1.75 to <1.75, the cutoff for pseudoprogression diagnosis.

Conclusions: Decreased perfusion after BEV significantly alters rCBV measurements when using ferumoxytol. BEV treatment response hinders efforts to differentiate true progression from pseudoprogression using blood volume measurements in malignant glioma, potentially impacting patient diagnosis and management.

Keywords: High grade glioma, Perfusion MRI, Ferumoxytol, Bevacizumab

Background

Treatment for newly diagnosed glioblastoma (GBM) consists of resection followed by radiotherapy with concomitant temozolomide (TMZ). Increased enhancement volume on T_1-weighted magnetic resonance imaging (MRI) using gadolinium-based contrast agent (GBCA) after chemoradiotherapy (CRT) in GBM patients can represent tumor progression or pseudoprogression. Diagnostic accuracy is critical in deciding appropriate therapy. Response assessment in neuro-oncology (RANO) suggests that differentiation of pseudoprogression from disease progression cannot be accomplished with a conventional MRI method in the first 12 weeks post-CRT [1].

Ferumoxytol, an iron oxide nanoparticle, is FDA-approved for iron replacement and used off-label for

*Correspondence: neuwelte@ohsu.edu
†Joao Prola Netto and Daniel Schwartz contributed equally to this work
[6] Department of Veterans Affairs Medical Center, 3710 SW U.S. Veterans Hospital Road, Portland, OR 97239, USA
Full list of author information is available at the end of the article

brain imaging, especially in patients with compromised renal function for whom GBCA is contraindicated [2]. Ferumoxytol as an MRI contrast agent for perfusion benefits from its intravascular property. Compared to GBCA, it may not require leakage correction or preload dosing [3]. Perfusion MRI has been used clinically as a biomarker to prospectively differentiate pseudoprogression from disease progression [4–7], and relative cerebral blood volume (rCBV) measurements using ferumoxytol as an MRI contrast agent can discriminate true progression from pseudoprogression in GBM using a mean rCBV threshold of 1.75 [3, 8]. The use of small paramagnetic iron oxides (SPIOs), such as ferumoxytol, was first published as an MR-based imaging agent for cancer in 1989, and has increased exponentially in the last decade. There were 728 publications on SPIOs and cancer between 1990 and 2010 and more than 864 in the last five years alone.

Bevacizumab (BEV) is an anti-vascular endothelial growth factor (VEGF) A antibody working as an angiogenesis inhibitor [9] that normalizes tumor vasculature [10], and decreases contrast-enhancing tumor volume and blood volume in lesions both in animal models [11, 12] and clinically [13–15]. No association has been found between tumor volume change after BEV and overall or progression-free survival [16]. After treatment with BEV, tumor perfusion decreases but tumor growth may only be temporarily inhibited [17, 18], leading to "pseudoresponse" and mismanaged therapy. Due to the likelihood of pseudoresponse and normalization of the blood–brain barrier, traditional methods to assess post-CRT tumor progression can be misleading in patients treated with BEV [1], and there is a concern that evaluating CBV for differentiating real progression from pseudoprogression as a result of CRT after treatment with BEV may produce false negative results. This study hypothesizes that perfusion decrease in high grade tumors after CRT and subsequent treatment with BEV can affect clinical management, and aimed to determine rCBV changes post-BEV using ferumoxytol-based dynamic susceptibility contrast (DSC) MR perfusion in patients with high grade glioma in a clinical setting.

Methods

Data collection

Sixteen patients (mean age in years [range]: 54 [39–63]; 6 males, 53 [44–62]; 10 females, 52 [43–61]) presenting with a total of 21 lesions (5 patients had two distinct and isolated lesions) were included in this retrospective study and provided written informed consent on one of four prospective Oregon Health & Science University HIPAA-compliant and IRB-approved MRI protocols (2753, 2864, 1562, and 813) using two contrast agents, GBCA and ferumoxytol, between 2009 and 2012. On average, pre-BEV MRI studies were performed 7 days (range: 0–21) before drug infusion, and post-treatment MRIs were performed 27 days after (range: 12–30).

Inclusion criteria were that patients have histological evidence of high grade glioma; evidence of increased or new enhancing tumor on clinical scan, which at time of scan could have represented tumor progression or treatment related changes; having received CRT and bevacizumab in the course of disease treatment; and an MRI study with gadoteridol and ferumoxytol DSC MRI less than 21 days before BEV and less than 30 days after. All patients received standard CRT with either 60 Gy in 30 fractions or 59.4 Gy in 33 fractions, with concomitant oral TMZ at a dose of 75 mg/m^2/day. After completion of CRT all patients continued on monthly TMZ (150–200 mg/m^2/day for 5 days in every 28 day cycle) for at least 6 months or until disease progression occurred [19].

Imaging

Patients underwent 3T MRI (Siemens Trio or Philips Achieva) with a multichannel head coil. All imaging protocols included anatomical and dynamic sequences in the axial plane. T_1-weighted scans (repetition time [TR]/echo time [TE] $\approx$ 900 ms/10 ms, field of view [FOV] = 240 mm^2, matrix = 256 × 256, ~44 2 mm slices with no gap) were acquired with a standard dose of 0.1 mmol/kg intravenous (IV) gadoteridol to assess contrast enhancing volume. DSC scans (90 measurements at 0.66 Hz, TR/TE/flip angle = 1500 ms/20 ms/45°, FOV = 192 mm^2, matrix 64 × 64, 27 3 mm slices with a 0.9 mm gap) were acquired, with a short IV bolus of 1 or 2 mg/kg (~5–10 ml) ferumoxytol injected at a flow rate of 3 ml/s followed by 20 ml of saline flush at the same rate. Approximately 20 measurements were obtained before the contrast reached the brain allowing an accurate baseline signal. Patients did not receive ferumoxytol directly after gadoteridol; in some cases, the two agents and their associated imaging acquisitions were separated by at least 12 min, and in some cases the acquisitions took place during sessions on consecutive days. However, recent work has shown that dual contrast sessions are feasible and yield reliable measurements of rCBV [20].

Image analysis

Tumor volume measurements were taken as the product of the extent of the GBCA-enhancing areas in three orthogonal axes as measured by a neuroradiologist with 8 years of experience (JPN). All DSC data were processed by JPN using NordicICE. CBV maps were generated by applying a tracer kinetic model to the first pass of the contrast bolus. Voxelwise CBV maps were coregistered to T_1-weighted images and then normalized by dividing by the mean of normal appearing white matter CBV in the same region in the contralateral hemisphere (rCBV), defined by JPN and chosen in the same axial slice as the lesion when possible, or if not possible, in the most proximal axial slice to the lesion.

One region of interest (ROI) was drawn on each GBCA-enhancing lesion (JPN) pre- (ROI_{pre}) and post-BEV (ROI_{post}) in each patient. The slice with the largest enhancing area was chosen based on the standard clinical evaluation for brain tumor assessment (RANO criteria) [1]. Care was taken to exclude blood vessels and areas of cystic change or necrosis, defined as abnormal areas with hyperintense signal on T_2-weighted and hypointense signal on T_1-weighted without discernible enhancement after GBCA injection.

Mean tumor rCBV, the voxelwise ferumoxytol-based DSC measurement, was calculated over each GBCA-enhancing ROI. Three means were calculated: (1) pre-BEV rCBV over ROI_{pre}, (2) post-BEV rCBV over ROI_{post}, and (3) post-BEV rCBV over ROI_{pre}. The third mean was calculated because BEV caused an expected reduction in the extent of GBCA enhancement, likely due to a reduction in vascular permeability secondary to vascular normalization; however, changes in local blood volume due to BEV likely occur beyond the extent of post-BEV GBCA enhancement.

The mean of "hot spot" (the mean of the highest rCBV in a 1.08 cm^2 area in the enhancing volume, the default size of a standard circular region of interest in Nordic ICE) rCBV values and pixel-wise rCBV histograms were obtained for each ROI. A standardized (% voxels in each bin/total voxels) histogram was determined using 40 bins 0.25 wide (range: 0–10). The proportion of voxels with rCBV > 1.75 was defined as hyperperfused subvolumes. This threshold value provides the optimal sensitivity and specificity for differentiating low grade from high grade glioma using rCBV [21]; it also has been used to differentiate treatment related changes and true progression using ferumoxytol or leakage-corrected GBCA perfusion MRI [3]. There is no established threshold for delineating hypoperfused subvolumes [15]. rCBV $\leq$ 0.75 was used, which represents perfusion at least 25% lower than normal appearing contralateral white matter.

A linear mixed effects model was used to compare differences in enhancing volume, mean and hot spot rCBVs, as well as hyperperfused and hypoperfused subvolumes before versus after BEV while taking into the account observations within the same patient. The Dunnett-Hsu method was used to adjust for multiple comparisons with the before BEV period as the control group. Least square (LS) mean $\pm$ standard error (SE) are reported. To assess the likelihood of BEV treatment to affect diagnostic criteria and clinical management, the proportion of patients with lesions that changed from high rCBV ($\geq$1.75) before BEV to low rCBV (<1.75) after BEV was also calculated. For patients with two lesions, if both lesions changed from high to low rCBV, or one lesion changed from high to low and the other lesion remained low before versus after BEV, it was counted as a change that would likely impact clinical management. If one lesion changed from high to low and the other lesion remained high, it was not counted as a change that would likely impact clinical management. All analyses were conducted using SAS 9.3 (SAS Institute Inc., Cary, NC, USA.).

Results

Fourteen patients were diagnosed with GBM, one with anaplastic astrocytoma, and one with anaplastic oligodendroglioma. Patients received BEV due to increasing enhancing lesion without clinical symptoms in 8 (50%) cases, increasing enhancing lesion with clinical symptoms in 7 (44%) cases, and clinical worsening but radiographically stable disease in 1 (6%) case.

After BEV treatment, 18 out of 21 (86%) GBCA-enhanced T_1-weighted tumor volumes decreased. The mean volume was significantly smaller post-BEV, decreasing approximately 39% (pre-BEV, 55,807 mm^3 $\pm$ 11,422; post-BEV 34,474 mm^3 $\pm$ 11,422; $P = 0.005$, Fig. 1, exemplified in patient in Fig. 2).

When examining perfusion measurements in each lesion after BEV treatment, there was no significant difference in mean rCBV values in ROI_{pre} vs. ROI_{post} (1.95 $\pm$ 0.35–1.65 $\pm$ 0.32, respectively, $P = 0.227$, Fig. 3a). However, mean "hot spot" rCBV decreased between pre- and post-BEV (4.04 $\pm$ 0.64–3.13 $\pm$ 0.52, respectively, $P = 0.046$, Fig. 3c). When post-BEV rCBV values averaged over ROI_{pre} were compared to pre-BEV mean rCBV values over ROI_{pre}, mean and "hot spot" values decreased to 1.51 $\pm$ 0.30 ($P = 0.039$, Fig. 3b), and 2.81 $\pm$ 0.52 ($P = 0.007$, Fig. 3d), respectively. The relationship between rCBV changes and timing of the scan with respect to BEV administration was tested with Pearson's r. There were no significant findings in hot spot or mean rCBV analyses (Fig. 4).

For the assessment of the likelihood of BEV treatment to affect diagnostic criteria and clinical management, 7/16 (44%) patients had lesions that changed from high rCBV ($\geq$1.75) to low rCBV (<1.75) when mean pre-BEV rCBV values over ROI_{pre} were compared to mean rCBV post-BEV over ROI_{post} (Fig. 3a: red lines). In addition, 2/16 (13%) patients had lesions that changed from low rCBV (<1.75) to high rCBV ($\geq$1.75). Similarly, when calculating post-BEV rCBV over ROI_{pre}, 7/16 (44%) changed from high to low rCBV (Fig. 3b: red lines), and one (6%) changed from low to high rCBV.

More detailed examination of rCBV changes was accomplished through distribution analysis. The average

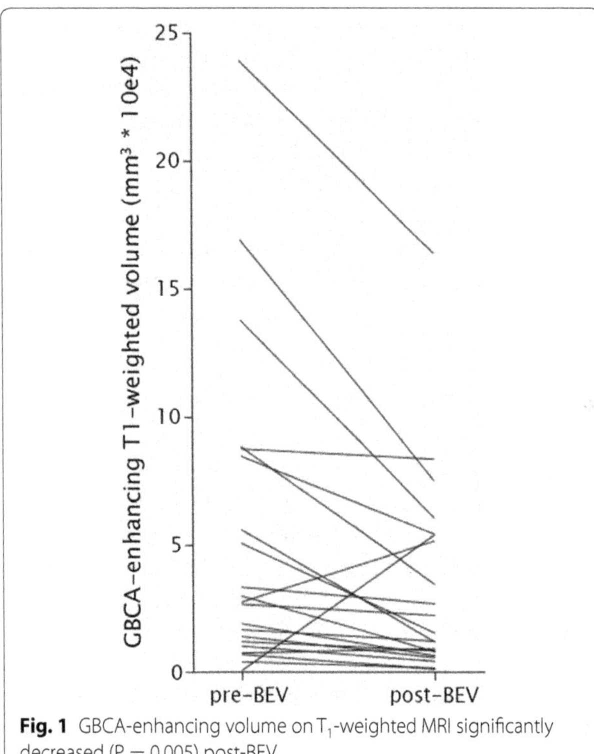

Fig. 1 GBCA-enhancing volume on T_1-weighted MRI significantly decreased ($P = 0.005$) post-BEV

histogram in ROI_{post} vs. ROI_{pre} demonstrated a significant increase in the mean proportion of hypoperfused voxels from 24% pre-BEV to 38% post-BEV ($P = 0.0007$), and a significant decrease in hyperperfused voxels from 39% pre-BEV to 28% post-BEV ($P = 0.017$, Fig. 5: gray vs. blue). Similarly, when the histogram of post-BEV rCBV was generated over ROI_{pre}, the mean proportion of hypoperfused voxels increased to 41% from pre-BEV ($P = 0.0001$), and the mean proportion of hyperperfused voxels decreased to 26% ($P = 0.006$) (Fig. 5: gray vs. red).

Discussion

This study used ferumoxytol to determine perfusion changes in patients with high grade glioma after treatment with bevacizumab. The results show that after treatment with anti-VEGF agent BEV there is a significant decrease in GBCA-enhancing volume, and a decrease in perfusion using ferumoxytol in the enhancing area of high grade gliomas after chemotherapy and radiation therapy but only when the pre-treatment enhancing regions of interest (ROI_{pre}) were used. The use of pre-treatment enhancing regions of interest (ROI_{pre}) over which to assess post-BEV perfusion maps increased sensitivity in all cases, suggesting that this method should be considered when quantifying blood volume changes after BEV. However, given the reduction in mass effect known to accompany BEV treatment it is possible that tissue shift could account for the difference. In the histogram analysis, it becomes clear that the decrease in the mean rCBV happens as expected due to BEV treatment, quantified by an increase in hypoperfused and a decrease in hyperperfused subvolumes. Nearly half of lesions changed from high rCBV before the BEV administration to low rCBV post-BEV. This is particularly important for cases in which perfusion MRI will be used to assess new or increasing enhanced areas for possible treatment.

Several publications describe the association between high CBV and tumor progression and low CBV and pseudoprogression and treatment related changes [8, 22, 23]. The ideal cutoff value has been under intense debate [4, 6, 24, 25]. We use 1.75 as a threshold rCBV value at our institution given significant indications that using this threshold for planning subsequent treatment is correlated well with overall survival [3]. Given that a significant percentage of lesions changed from high rCBV before the BEV administration to low rCBV after its infusion (44%), it is important to acquire perfusion MRI before the administration of BEV if rCBV will be used to determine whether a new or increased enhancing lesion represents true progression of disease or changes due to CRT. Other previously published threshold values range from 0.7 to 2.6; had they been utilized in this study, it is possible that the interpretation of the effects of bevacizumab on rCBV as it pertains to criteria for pseudoprogression, may have been different [6, 24, 25]. Extreme threshold values, high or low, would have less impact as the majority of cases having values under or above the threshold before and after bevacizumab administration would increase, respectively.

The RANO treatment response evaluation criteria are based on clinical symptoms and conventional MRI (T_1-weighted GBCA-based contrast volume enhancement) findings. Treatment related changes and the diagnostic challenge it represents are well known, including the impossibility of reliable evaluation with conventional MRI. A number of advanced imaging techniques have been studied including diffusion, spectroscopy, DCE and DSC perfusion MRI and nuclear medicine techniques, all with variable results. Our group has shown that cerebral blood volume measurements based on DSC perfusion, particularly in cases where a blood pool agent such as ferumoxytol is used, is a reliable method that can be used to differentiate between pseudoprogression and real tumor progression [3]. In 56% of the lesions, there was no significant change in the diagnosis and interpretation of the perfusion values. There are several possible alternatives for this finding. If baseline rCBV was very high before bevacizumab administration and decreased after treatment, it is possible that rCBV values did not go below the threshold, maybe related to aggressive tumor

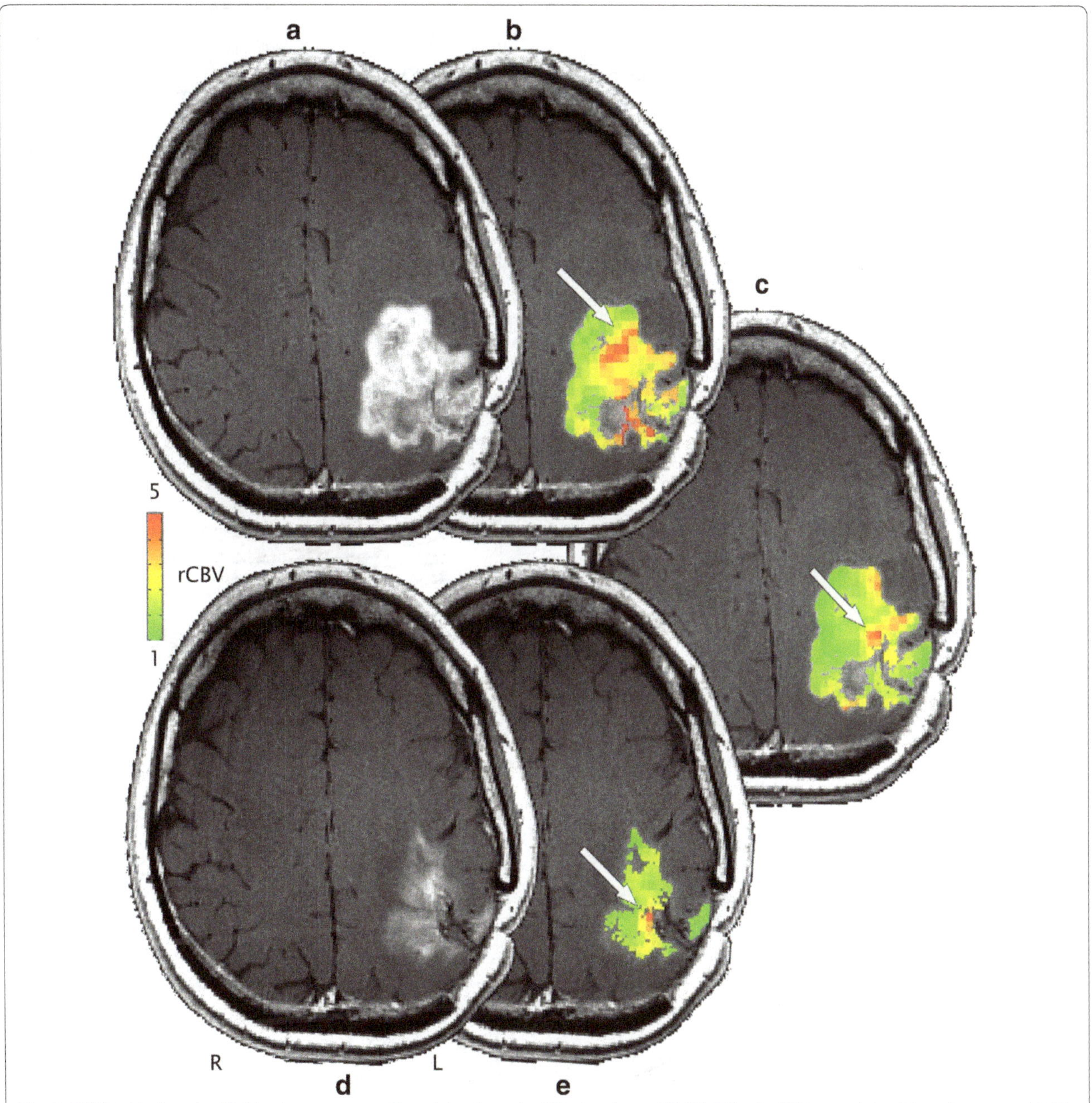

Fig. 2 GBM in 44 y/o male: GBCA enhancement on T_1-weighted pre- (**a**, ROI_{pre}) and post-BEV (**d**, ROI_{post}). rCBV maps derived from ferumoxytol DSC pre- (**b**) and post-BEV (**e**) overlaid on the enhancing volume. An overlay of the post-BEV rCBV map on ROI_{pre} can be found in **c**. "Hot spot" regions are indicated by *white arrows*; note the marked decrease in rCBV between **b** and **c**

progression with some resistance to the effect of bevacizumab. A floor effect is also possible in areas of tumors that are poorly perfused; if rCBV values were already very low before bevacizumab administration, an eventual decrease in perfusion values will not change the diagnosis of pseudoprogression.

Leakage correction is necessary for accurate quantification of perfusion MRI using GBCA; rCBV measurements using gadoteridol can adequately distinguish between patients with treatment related changes versus true progression only after leakage correction is applied [3]. The confounding effect of BEV and the infrequent use of leakage correction may be two critical factors contributing to the inconsistency in the literature of using rCBV to determine disease progression status [4, 26–28]. Finally, relative perfusion values from ferumoxytol-based DSC in GBM clearly match those in recent reports, without the need for leakage correction or preload dosing as is

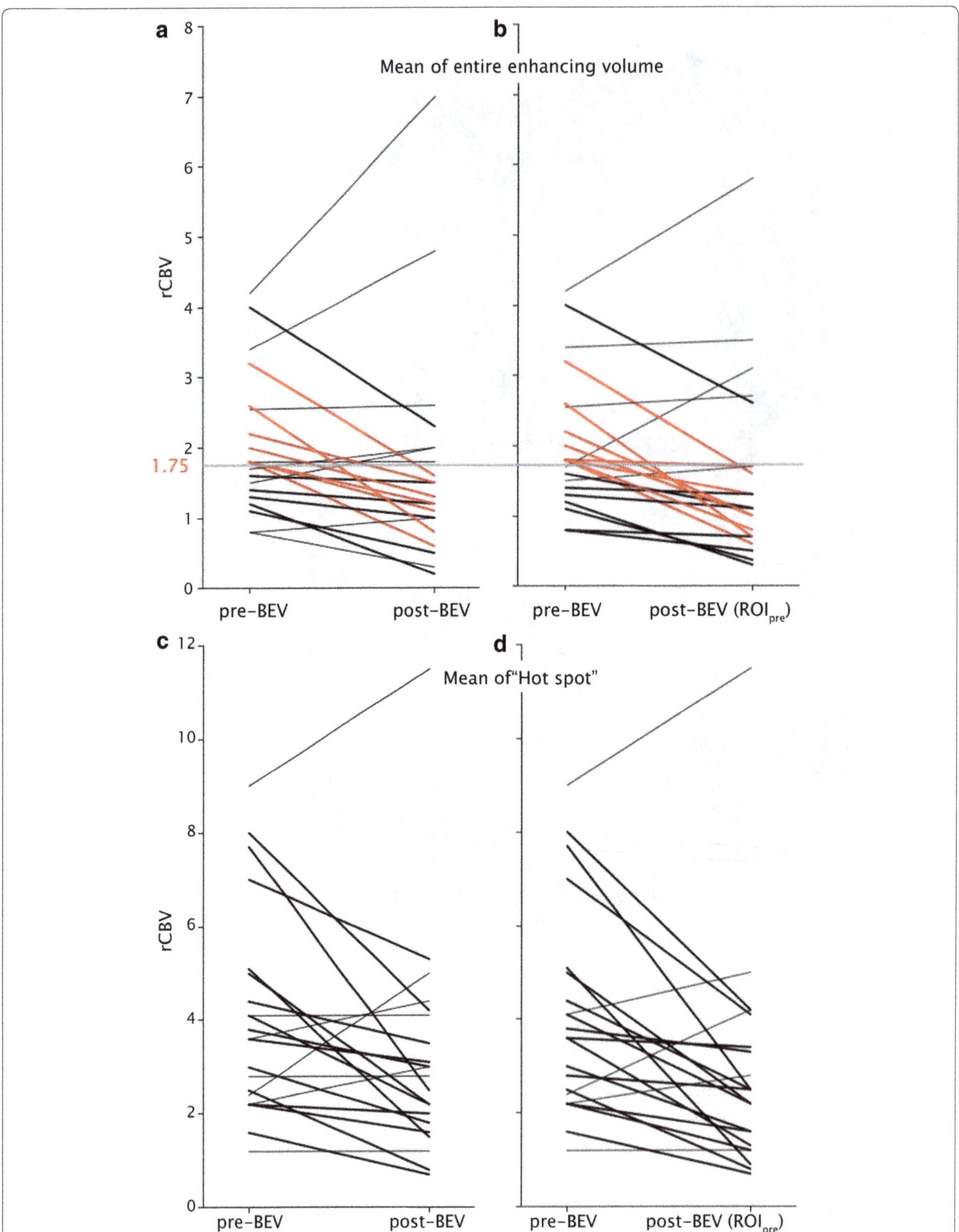

Fig. 3 Change in rCBV pre- and post-BEV for each of 21 lesions. A *black line* indicates a decrease in rCBV, *red* indicates a decrease in rCBV that passed the clinically relevant threshold of 1.75, and the remaining lesions are marked in *gray*. Values for the entire enhancing volume are shown in **a** and **b**. **c** and **d** depict hot spot changes. **a** and **c** depict the rCBV change between pre-BEV measured over ROI_{pre} and post-BEV rCBV measured over ROI_{post}. **b** and **d** depict the rCBV change between pre-BEV measured in ROI_{pre} and post-BEV rCBV in ROI_{pre}

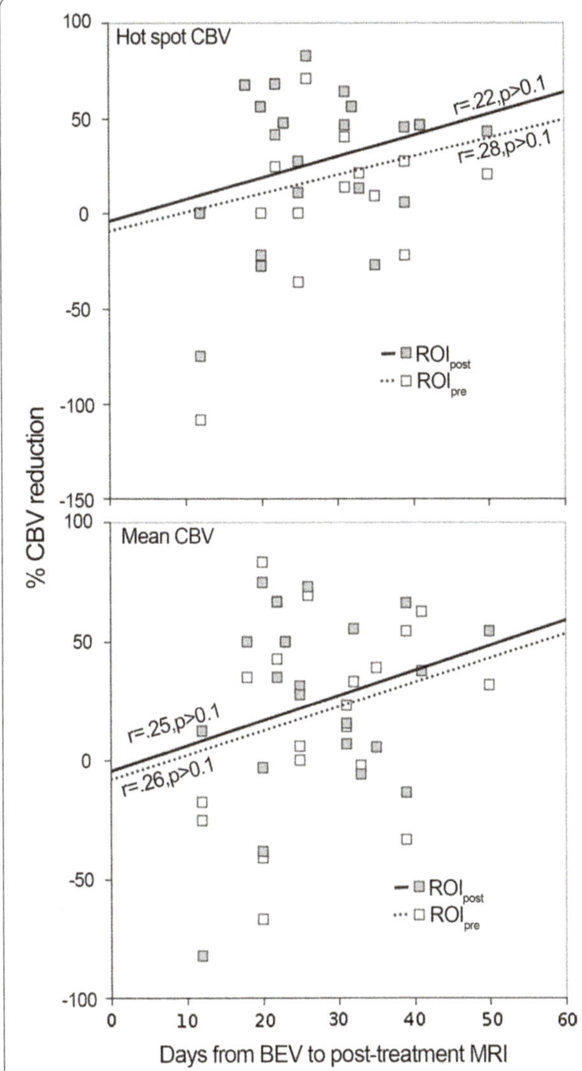

Fig. 4 Relationship between rCBV measurements and time interval to post-treatment MRI. *Top* hot spot rCBV measurements in ROIpost (*filled*) and ROIpre (*open*); *y axis* is % rCBV reduction, a negative value indicates rCBV increase. *Bottom* mean rCBV over the entire enhancing lesion. No significant relationships of rCBV with post-treatment MRI time intervals were found (all P > 0.1)

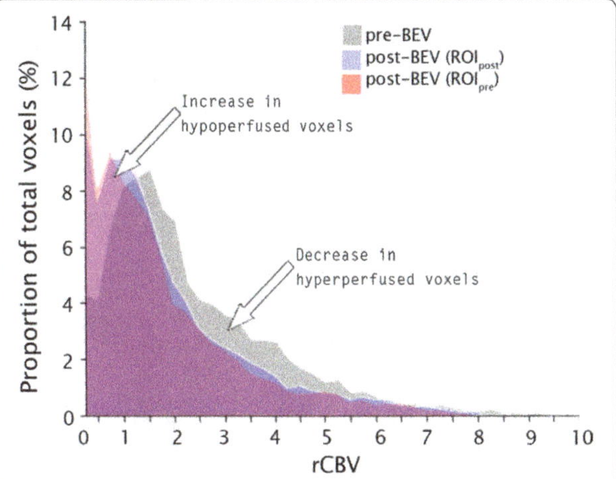

Fig. 5 Distribution of the averaged over all patients' rCBV voxel values before administration of BEV (pre-BEV, *gray*), after it using the pre-BEV volume of enhancement (*red*, ROI_{pre}) and post-BEV volume of enhancement (*blue*, ROI_{post}). There is a significant increase in the proportion of hypoperfused voxels (P = 0.008) and a significant decrease in hyperperfused voxels (P = 0.01) in both ROIs after BEV administration

currently necessary for accurate assessment of tumor perfusion with GBCA [11].

Lastly, recent reports have showed clear region-specific long term deposition of gadolinium in the brain [29]. While it is not yet clear whether there are any adverse health effects of gadolinium accumulation, these reports are serious enough to warrant a FDA safety announcement [30]. Ferumoxytol does not extravasate from the blood pool into brain parenchyma nearly as readily as do most GBCAs used in clinical practice today. While the incidence of serious anaphylaxis risk is approximately 10 times higher using ferumoxytol compared to most GBCAs, the absolute incidence of severe side effects remains small, approximately 1:10,000. Current evidence and experience indicates that ferumoxytol is a safe and available alternative for GBCA for assessment of tumor progression versus CRT-related changes.

Limitations of this report include the choice of a single slice method for pixel-wise histogram analyses. This technique is based on the RANO criteria for assessment of brain tumor in the clinical practice and for clinical trials, but it is possible that important information was missed by not using the entire tumor. It is unlikely that results would change based on the location of the slice or the use of the entire tumor, and single slice measurements are the norm in clinical practice. In addition, it is difficult to precisely control the relative timing of BEV, CRT, and MRI exams. While it is plain that the timing of these exams with respect to treatment phase can have profound effects on results, the cohort in this study was carefully chosen to have as narrow a window of timing variability as possible.

Conclusions

In conclusion, due to blood volume reduction caused by BEV, the threshold of rCBV > 1.75, used to differentiate high rCBV from low rCBV after CRT, may be confounded early after BEV administration and thwart true diagnoses of vascular progression, true response, or treatment related changes. Ideally, pre-BEV measurements should be used and extreme care taken with clinical interpretation of perfusion MRI results in any patients who have received BEV, even when using an intravascular agent such as ferumoxytol.

Abbreviations

BEV: bevacizumab; CRT: chemoradiotherapy; DSC: dynamic susceptibility-weighted contrast; GBCA: gadolinium based contrast agent; GBM: glioblastoma multiforme; FOV: field of view; IV: intravenous; JPN: author and experienced radiologist; MRI: magnetic resonance imaging; RANO: response assessment in neuro-oncology; rCBV: relative cerebral blood volume; ROI: region of interest; TE: echo time; TMZ: temozolomide; TR: repetition time; VEGF: vascular endothelial growth factor.

Authors' contributions

JPN and DS equally contributed to the conception, design, and interpretation of the data, as well as drafting and revising the manuscript. CV assisted in the interpretation and drafting of the manuscript. RF assisted in analyzing the data and drafting the manuscript. BH assisted in the interpretation and drafting of the manuscript. EAN contributed to the conception and design of the study, as well as critically revising the manuscript. All authors read and approved the final manuscript.

Author details

[1] Department of Neurology, Oregon Health & Science University, 3181 SW Sam Jackson Park Road, Portland, OR 97239, USA. [2] Department of Neuroradiology, Oregon Health & Science University, 3181 SW Sam Jackson Park Road, Portland, OR 97239, USA. [3] Advanced Imaging Research Center, Oregon Health & Science University, 3181 SW Sam Jackson Park Road, Portland, OR 97239, USA. [4] School of Public Health, Oregon Health & Science University, 3181 SW Sam Jackson Park Road, Portland, OR 97239, USA. [5] Emergency Medicine, Oregon Health & Science University, 3181 SW Sam Jackson Park Road, Portland, OR 97239, USA. [6] Department of Veterans Affairs Medical Center, 3710 SW U.S. Veterans Hospital Road, Portland, OR 97239, USA. [7] Department of Neurosurgery, Oregon Health & Science University, 3181 SW Sam Jackson Park Road, L603, Portland, OR 97239, USA.

Acknowledgements

The authors thank Emily Youngers for editorial support. Material presented in this paper was previously presented as an abstract at the 2013 American Society for Neuroradiology Annual Meeting.

Competing interests

The authors declare that they have no competing interests.

Funding

This work was supported in part by National Institute of Health Grants NS044687, and CA137488-15S1, in part with Federal funds from the National Cancer Institute, National Institutes of Health, under Contract No. HHSN261200800001E, and by the Walter S. and Lucienne Driskill Foundation, all to EAN.

References

1. Wen PY, Macdonald DR, Reardon DA, Cloughesy TF, Sorensen AG, Galanis E, Degroot J, Wick W, Gilbert MR, Lassman AB, Tsien C, Mikkelsen T, Wong ET, Chamberlain MC, Stupp R, Lamborn KR, Vogelbaum MA, van den Bent MJ, Chang SM. Updated response assessment criteria for high-grade gliomas: response assessment in neuro-oncology working group. J Clin Oncol. 2010;28:1963–72. doi:10.1200/JCO.2009.26.3541.
2. Grobner T. Gadolinium—a specific trigger for the development of nephrogenic fibrosing dermopathy and nephrogenic systemic fibrosis? Nephrol Dial Transplant. 2006;21:1104–8. doi:10.1093/ndt/gfk062.
3. Gahramanov S, Muldoon LL, Varallyay CG, Li X, Kraemer DF, Fu R, Hamilton BE, Rooney WD, Neuwelt EA. Pseudoprogression of glioblastoma after chemo- and radiation therapy: diagnosis by using dynamic susceptibility-weighted contrast-enhanced perfusion MR imaging with ferumoxytol versus gadoteridol and correlation with survival. Radiology. 2013;266:842–52. doi:10.1148/radiol.12111472.
4. Barajas RF Jr, Chang JS, Segal MR, Parsa AT, McDermott MW, Berger MS, Cha S. Differentiation of recurrent glioblastoma multiforme from radiation necrosis after external beam radiation therapy with dynamic susceptibility-weighted contrast-enhanced perfusion MR imaging. Radiology. 2009;253:486–96. doi:10.1148/radiol.2532090007.
5. Gerstner ER, Frosch MP, Batchelor TT. Diffusion magnetic resonance imaging detects pathologically confirmed, nonenhancing tumor progression in a patient with recurrent glioblastoma receiving bevacizumab. J Clin Oncol. 2010;28:e91–3. doi:10.1200/JCO.2009.25.0233.
6. Hu LS, Baxter LC, Smith KA, Feuerstein BG, Karis JP, Eschbacher JM, Coons SW, Nakaji P, Yeh RF, Debbins J, Heiserman JE. Relative cerebral blood volume values to differentiate high-grade glioma recurrence from post-treatment radiation effect: direct correlation between image-guided tissue histopathology and localized dynamic susceptibility-weighted contrast-enhanced perfusion MR imaging measurements. AJNR Am J Neuroradiol. 2009;30:552–8. doi:10.3174/ajnr.A1377.
7. Iv M, Telischak N, Feng D, Holdsworth SJ, Yeom KW, Daldrup-Link HE. Clinical applications of iron oxide nanoparticles for magnetic resonance imaging of brain tumors. Nanomedicine (Lond). 2015;10:993–1018. doi:10.2217/nnm.14.203.
8. Gahramanov S, Raslan AM, Muldoon LL, Hamilton BE, Rooney WD, Varallyay CG, Njus JM, Haluska M, Neuwelt EA. Potential for differentiation of pseudoprogression from true tumor progression with dynamic susceptibility-weighted contrast-enhanced magnetic resonance imaging using ferumoxytol vs. gadoteridol: a pilot study. Int J Radiat Oncol Biol Phys. 2011;79:514–23. doi:10.1016/j.ijrobp.2009.10.072.
9. Mukherji SK. Bevacizumab (Avastin). AJNR Am J Neuroradiol. 2010;31:235–6. doi:10.3174/ajnr.A1987.
10. Pope WB, Young JR, Ellingson BM. Advances in MRI assessment of gliomas and response to anti-VEGF therapy. Curr Neurol Neurosci Rep. 2011;11:336–44. doi:10.1007/s11910-011-0179-x.
11. Gahramanov S, Muldoon LL, Li X, Neuwelt EA. Improved perfusion MR imaging assessment of intracerebral tumor blood volume and antiangiogenic therapy efficacy in a rat model with ferumoxytol. Radiology. 2011;261:796–804. doi:10.1148/radiol.11103503.
12. Pishko GL, Muldoon LL, Pagel MA, Schwartz DL, Neuwelt EA. Vascular endothelial growth factor blockade alters magnetic resonance imaging biomarkers of vascular function and decreases barrier permeability in a rat model of lung cancer brain metastasis. Fluids Barriers CNS. 2015;12:5. doi:10.1186/2045-8118-12-5.
13. Stadlbauer A, Pichler P, Karl M, Brandner S, Lerch C, Renner B, Heinz G. Quantification of serial changes in cerebral blood volume and metabolism in patients with recurrent glioblastoma undergoing antiangiogenic therapy. Eur J Radiol. 2015;84:1128–36. doi:10.1016/j.ejrad.2015.02.025.
14. Sawlani RN, Raizer J, Horowitz SW, Shin W, Grimm SA, Chandler JP, Levy R, Getch C, Carroll TJ. Glioblastoma: a method for predicting response to antiangiogenic chemotherapy by using MR perfusion imaging—pilot study. Radiology. 2010;255:622–8. doi:10.1148/radiol.10091341.
15. Vidiri A, Pace A, Fabi A, Maschio M, Latagliata GM, Anelli V, Piludu F, Carapella CM, Giovinazzo G, Marzi S. Early perfusion changes in patients with recurrent high-grade brain tumor treated with Bevacizumab: preliminary results by a quantitative evaluation. J Exp Clin Cancer Res. 2012;31:33. doi:10.1186/1756-9966-31-33.
16. Ellingson BM, Cloughesy TF, Lai A, Nghiemphu PL, Mischel PS, Pope WB. Quantitative volumetric analysis of conventional MRI response in recurrent glioblastoma treated with bevacizumab. Neuro Oncol. 2011;13:401–9. doi:10.1093/neuonc/noq206.
17. Mautner VF, Nguyen R, Knecht R, Bokemeyer C. Radiographic regression of vestibular schwannomas induced by bevacizumab treatment: sustain under continuous drug application and rebound after drug discontinuation. Ann Oncol. 2010;21:2294–5. doi:10.1093/annonc/mdq566.

18. Keunen O, Johansson M, Oudin A, Sanzey M, Rahim SA, Fack F, Thorsen F, Taxt T, Bartos M, Jirik R, Miletic H, Wang J, Stieber D, Stuhr L, Moen I, Rygh CB, Bjerkvig R, Niclou SP. Anti-VEGF treatment reduces blood supply and increases tumor cell invasion in glioblastoma. Proc Natl Acad Sci USA. 2011;108:3749–54. doi:10.1073/pnas.1014480108.
19. Gahramanov S, Varallyay C, Tyson RM, Lacy C, Fu R, Netto JP, Nasseri M, White T, Woltjer RL, Gultekin SH, Neuwelt EA. Diagnosis of pseudoprogression using MRI perfusion in patients with glioblastoma multiforme may predict improved survival. CNS Oncol. 2014;3:389–400. doi:10.2217/cns.14.42.
20. Thompson EM, Guillaume DJ, Dosa E, Li X, Nazemi KJ, Gahramanov S, Hamilton BE, Neuwelt EA. Dual contrast perfusion MRI in a single imaging session for assessment of pediatric brain tumors. J Neurooncol. 2012;109:105–14. doi:10.1007/s11060-012-0872-x.
21. Law M, Yang S, Wang H, Babb JS, Johnson G, Cha S, Knopp EA, Zagzag D. Glioma grading: sensitivity, specificity, and predictive values of perfusion MR imaging and proton MR spectroscopic imaging compared with conventional MR imaging. AJNR Am J Neuroradiol. 2003;24:1989–98.
22. Young RJ, Gupta A, Shah AD, Graber JJ, Chan TA, Zhang Z, Shi W, Beal K, Omuro AM. MRI perfusion in determining pseudoprogression in patients with glioblastoma. Clin Imaging. 2013;37:41–9. doi:10.1016/j.clinimag.2012.02.016.
23. Fatterpekar GM, Galheigo D, Narayana A, Johnson G, Knopp E. Treatment-related change versus tumor recurrence in high-grade gliomas: a diagnostic conundrum—use of dynamic susceptibility contrast-enhanced (DSC) perfusion MRI. AJR Am J Roentgenol. 2012;198:19–26. doi:10.2214/AJR.11.7417.
24. Sugahara T, Korogi Y, Tomiguchi S, Shigematsu Y, Ikushima I, Kira T, Liang L, Ushio Y, Takahashi M. Posttherapeutic intraaxial brain tumor: the value of perfusion-sensitive contrast-enhanced MR imaging for differentiating tumor recurrence from nonneoplastic contrast-enhancing tissue. AJNR Am J Neuroradio. 2000;21:901–9.
25. Gasparetto EL, Pawlak MA, Patel SH, Huse J, Woo JH, Krejza J, Rosenfeld MR, O'Rourke DM, Lustig R, Melhem ER, Wolf RL. Posttreatment recurrence of malignant brain neoplasm: accuracy of relative cerebral blood volume fraction in discriminating low from high malignant histologic volume fraction. Radiology. 2009;250:887–96. doi:10.1148/radiol.2502071444.
26. Baek HJ, Kim HS, Kim N, Choi YJ, Kim YJ. Percent change of perfusion skewness and kurtosis: a potential imaging biomarker for early treatment response in patients with newly diagnosed glioblastomas. Radiology. 2012;264:834–43. doi:10.1148/radiol.12112120.
27. Kong DS, Kim ST, Kim EH, Lim DH, Kim WS, Suh YL, Lee JI, Park K, Kim JH, Nam DH. Diagnostic dilemma of pseudoprogression in the treatment of newly diagnosed glioblastomas: the role of assessing relative cerebral blood flow volume and oxygen-6-methylguanine-DNA methyltransferase promoter methylation status. AJNR Am J Neuroradiol. 2011;32:382–7. doi:10.3174/ajnr.A2286.
28. Mitsuya K, Nakasu Y, Horiguchi S, Harada H, Nishimura T, Bando E, Okawa H, Furukawa Y, Hirai T, Endo M. Perfusion weighted magnetic resonance imaging to distinguish the recurrence of metastatic brain tumors from radiation necrosis after stereotactic radiosurgery. J Neurooncol. 2010;99:81–8. doi:10.1007/s11060-009-0106-z.
29. McDonald RJ, McDonald JS, Kallmes DF, Jentoft ME, Murray DL, Thielen KR, Williamson EE, Eckel LJ. Intracranial gadolinium deposition after contrast-enhanced MR imaging. Radiology. 2015;275:772–82. doi:10.1148/radiol.15150025.
30. United States Food and Drug Administration. FDA drug safety communication: FDA evaluating the risk of brain deposits with repeated use of gadolinium-based contrast agents for magnetic resonance imaging (MRI); 2015. http://www.fda.gov/Drugs/DrugSafety/ucm455386.htm.

4

Cerebrospinal fluid Aβ42, t-tau, and p-tau levels in the differential diagnosis of idiopathic normal-pressure hydrocephalus: a systematic review and meta-analysis

Zhongyun Chen[1], Chunyan Liu[1], Jie Zhang[1], Norman Relkin[2], Yan Xing[1*] and Yanfeng Li[3*]

Abstract

Objectives: The purpose of this systematic review and meta-analysis was to evaluate the performance of cerebrospinal fluid (CSF) beta amyloid 42 (Aβ42), total tau (t-tau), and phosphorylated tau (p-tau) as potential diagnostic biomarkers for idiopathic normal-pressure hydrocephalus (iNPH) and to assess their utility indistinguishing patients with iNPH from those with Alzheimer disease (AD) and healthy normal controls.

Methods: Studies were identified by searching PubMed, Embase, the Cochrane Library, Web of Science, Chinese National Knowledge Infrastructure (CNKI), Wanfang Chinese Periodical Database, VIP Chinese database, and Chinese Bio-medicine Database (CBM) before August 2016. The standardized mean difference (SMD) and 95% confidence interval (CI), comparing CSF Aβ42, t-tau, and p-tau levels between iNPH, AD and healthy controls, were calculated using random-effects models. Subgroup analyses were created according to ethnicity (Caucasian or Asian) and CSF type (lumbar or ventricular), and the publication bias was estimated using Egger's test and the Begg's test.

Results: A total of 10 studies including 413 patients with iNPH, 186 patients with AD and 147 healthy controls were included in this systematic review and meta-analysis. The concentrations of CSF t-tau, and p-tau were significantly lower in iNPH patients compared to AD (SMD = −1.26, 95% CI −1.95 to −0.57, $P = 0.0004$; SMD = −1.54, 95% CI −2.34 to −0.74, $P = 0.0002$, respectively) and lower than healthy controls (SMD = −0.80, 95% CI −1.50 to −0.09, $P = 0.03$; SMD = −1.12, 95% CI −1.38 to −0.86, $P < 0.00001$, respectively). Patients with iNPH had significantly lower Aβ42 levels compared with controls (SMD = −1.14, 95% CI −1.74 to −0.55, $P = 0.0002$), and slightly higher Aβ42 levels compared with AD patients (SMD = 0.32, 95% CI 0.00–0.63, $P = 0.05$). Subgroup analyses showed that the outcomes may have been influenced by ethnicity and CSF source. Compared to AD, overall sensitivity in differentiating iNPH was 0.813 (95% CI 0.636–0.928) for Aβ42, 0.828 (95% CI 0.732–0.900) for t-tau, 0.943 (95% CI 0.871–0.981) for p-tau. Relative to AD, overall specificity in differentiating iNPH was 0.506 (95% CI 0.393–0.619) for Aβ42, 0.842 (95% CI 0.756–0.907) for t-tau, 0.851 (95% CI 0.767–0.914) for p-tau.

Conclusion: The results of our meta-analysis suggest that iNPH may be associated with significantly reduced levels of CSF Aβ42, t-tau and p-tau compared to the healthy normal state. Compared to AD, both t-tau and p-tau were significantly decreased in iNPH, but CSF Aβ42 was slightly increased. Prospective studies are needed to further assess

*Correspondence: drxingyan@163.com; doctorliyf@163.com
[1] Department of Neurology, Aviation General Hospital of China Medical University & Beijing Institute of Translational Medicine, Chinese Academy of Sciences, No. 3 Anwai Beiyuan Road, Chaoyang District, Beijing 100012, China
[3] Department of Neurology, Peking Union Medical College Hospital, Beijing, China
Full list of author information is available at the end of the article

the clinical utility of these and other CSF biomarkers in assisting in the diagnosis of iNPH and differentiating it from AD and other neurodegenerative disorders.

Keywords: CSF biomarkers, Idiopathic normal-pressure hydrocephalus, Alzheimer's disease, Meta-analysis, Systematic review

Background

Normal pressure hydrocephalus (NPH) was first described in 1965 by Hakim, Adams and colleagues [1] as a syndrome of cerebral ventricular enlargement occurring in adults without elevated cerebrospinal fluid (CSF) pressure or macroscopic obstruction to CSF flow. Early studies identified NPH as a progressive but treatable disorder that often presents with the classical symptom triad of gait disturbance, dementia, and urinary incontinence. This condition is considered idiopathic NPH (iNPH) when there is no identifiable antecedent cause and secondary NPH (sNPH) when events such as severe head trauma, subarachnoid hemorrhage or meningitis precede its onset.

Recent studies have reported prevalence rates of iNPH ranging from 0.51 to 5.9% in the elderly population that increase with advancing age. This suggests that iNPH is much more common than previously recognized [2–4]. It is extremely underdiagnosed throughout most of the world [5] and less than 10–20% of patients with iNPH get appropriate specialized treatment [6, 7]. This is particularly unfortunate because iNPH and sNPH can be effectively treated by neurosurgical placement of a shunt, which leads to improvement or stabilization of symptoms in upwards of 80% of accurately diagnosed patients [8].

An important factor in the under-diagnosis of iNPH is that early clinical features may be subtle and its manifestations can overlap those of other neurological disorders such as AD and normal brain aging. Therefore, finding sensitive and specific tools for early and accurate differential diagnosis is vital for improving the detection and care of patients with iNPH.

Analysis of CSF biomarkers is performed as part of many neurodegenerative research studies and is increasingly employed in the clinical diagnostic work-up when neurodegenerative disorders are suspected. Aβ42, t-tau, and p-tau have been widely validated as CSF biomarkers for AD diagnosis. In particular, a pattern of reduced CSF Aβ42 with elevated CSF p-tau and t-tau is strongly associated with AD [9]. The Aβ42 protein is closely linked to AD pathology as the central component of extracellular neuritic plaques [10]. Tau is an intracellular microtubule-associated protein and its total level in CSF is thought to reflect the extent of ongoing neuronal death. Hyperphosphorylated forms of tau (p-tau) are more closely associated with neurofibrillary tangle formation in AD and measurement of CSF p-tau therefore adds specificity for AD to the CSF biomarker profile [10, 11].

Comparably fewer CSF biomarker studies have been performed on iNPH patients and there has been only moderate consistency among those performed. Some studies have reported that patients with iNPH have low Aβ42 similar to those in AD, but without increased t-tau and p-tau levels. There has been speculation that this pattern might be useful for differentiating iNPH from AD [12, 13]. However, other studies did not reach the same conclusion [14, 15]. Considering these inconsistent results, we conducted a meta-analysis to evaluate whether CSF Aβ42, t-tau, and p-tau levels are of value in the differential diagnosis of iNPH from AD and healthy normal controls.

Methods

Literature search

We did asystematic review and meta-analysis according to the PRISMA guidelines [16]. Two authors searched PubMed, Embase, the Cochrane Library, Web of Science, Chinese National Knowledge Infrastructure (CNKI), Wanfang Chinese Periodical Database, VIP Chinese database, and Chinese Bio-medicine Database (CBM) for relevant articles published before August 2016 by using Medical Subject Heading (MeSH) terms and the following free text terms: "((normal pressure OR normotensive) AND hydrocephal*) OR Hydrocephalus, Normal Pressure [Mesh]" AND "((biological) AND markers) OR biomarker OR CSF OR cerebrospinal" AND "Aβ42 OR Abeta42 OR Abeta-42 OR Aβ1-42 OR t-tau OR p-tau OR tau OR phospho-tau OR phosphorylated tau".

The search was confined to human studies published in English and Chinese. The titles and abstracts of each article were scanned independently by two authors (ZYC and CYL) to exclude studies that were clearly irrelevant. The full text of the remaining studies were then retrieved and assessed for eligibility according to the inclusion criteria. Any disagreement was resolved by discussion with a third author (JZ).

Study selection

Studies were eligible for the analysis if they fulfill the following criteria: (1) case–control studies which compared the CSF levels of Aβ42 and/or t-tau and/or p-tau between iNPH patients and AD patients or healthy controls;

(2) clearly stated iNPH and AD diagnostic criteria (see Additional file 1: Table S1); (3) original articles containing independent data, and data were expressed as mean and standard deviation (SD) or median and interquartile range (IQR).

The exclusion criteria for the study were as follows: (1) abstracts, reviews, case reports, animal experiments, experts' opinions and commentaries; (2) duplicate publications of the same dataset; (3) papers not specifically focused on iNPH (i.e.: NPH or sNPH).

Data extraction

Two authors extracted data from the included articles, which included the following: the first author's name, year of publication, country, number of cases and controls, age (mean ± SD or median and interquartile range), the number of females and males, the CSF levels of Aβ42, t-tau and p-tau concentration (mean ± SD or median and interquartile range), analytical technology, and CSF source.

Quality evaluation

The Newcastle-Ottawa Quality Assessment Scale (NOS) was used to assess the quality of each included study, and was performed by two authors independently, with a third author consulted in case of discrepancy. Three major components were collected: (1) the selection (0–4 points); (2) the exposure (0–3 points); 3) the comparability (0–2 points). Higher scores represent better quality in methodology. All studies in this systematic review had scores greater than or equal to seven, indicating good qualities.

Statistical analysis

Statistical analyses were performed using Review Manager 5.1.2 (Cochrane Collaboration, Oxford, UK), Meta DiSc 1.4 version (Cochrane Collaboration, Oxford, UK) and Stata 12.0 (Stata Corp, College Station, Texas, USA). Data given as median and IQR were converted into mean ± SD in accordance with the protocol provided by Wan et al. [17]. In studies where patients with iNPH were divided into shunt responder and shunt non-responders, we combined the two datasets for the purpose of the current evaluation [18].

The standardized mean difference (SMD) and the corresponding 95% CI were used as the main effect measure. Heterogeneity across the studies was estimated by using the Chi square based Cochran Q and the I^2 test statistics [19]. The heterogeneity was considered statistically significant if $P < 0.1$ or $I^2 > 50\%$, a random-effects model (DerSimonian–Laird method) of analysis was used; otherwise, the fixed-effects model (Mantel–Haenszel method) was applied instead. Sub-groups were created according to ethnicity (Caucasian or Asian) and CSF source (lumbar or ventricular). Sensitivity analysis was performed by removing studies one by one to detect its influence on pooled ORs. The Egger's test and the Begg's test were used to estimate the severity of publication bias [20]. Where publication bias existed, we used the Trim and Fill method to correct it. The overall sensitivity, specificity, positive likelihood ratio (PLR), and negative likelihood ratio (NLR), as well as their corresponding 95% CIs, were pooled based on the random effects model. In addition, the area under the curve (AUC) and Q* index were calculated to evaluate the diagnostic test accuracy. All statistical tests were 2-sided, and statistical significance was defined as $P < 0.05$.

Results

Included studies

A total of 121 relevant articles were identified in the initial search. Seventy-four articles remained after removal of duplicate studies and 28 articles were excluded based on titles and abstracts. After systematically reviewing the remaining 46 full-text articles, 36 articles were excluded for not fulfilling our inclusion criteria. Finally, ten articles met stringent search criteria for data analysis and three articles were included in the diagnostic analysis. A detailed flow chart of the search and selection process is depicted in Fig. 1.

Study characteristics

The characteristics of the ten studies included in the meta-analysis are listed in Table 1. A total of 413 patients with iNPH, 186 patients with AD, and 147 healthy controls were included in this meta-analysis. 2 studies were performed in the United States [21, 22], 2 in Japan [23, 24], 2 in Sweden [12, 25], 1 in Greece [13], 1 in Finland [26], 1 in South Korea [27] and 1 in Italy [28]. These studies were published between 2007 and 2015. With respect to the assay method used to measure CSF Aβ42, t-tau, p-tau levels, 9 studies were performed using ELISA methodology and 1 was conducted using other methods.

Meta-analysis

Pooled analysis (Table 2)

Aβ42 in iNPH versus AD/healthy controls Seven studies, including 268 patients with iNPH and 186 patients with AD and 6 studies, including 193 patients with iNPH and 147 healthy controls were used in the meta-analysis, respectively. A random-effect model was used to calculate pooled SMD because of highly significant heterogeneity among those studies (iNPH versus AD, $P < 0.06$, $I^2 = 50\%$; iNPH versus healthy controls, $P = 0.0003$, $I^2 = 79\%$). Patients with iNPH showed significantly decreased Aβ42 levels compared with healthy controls (SMD = −1.14,

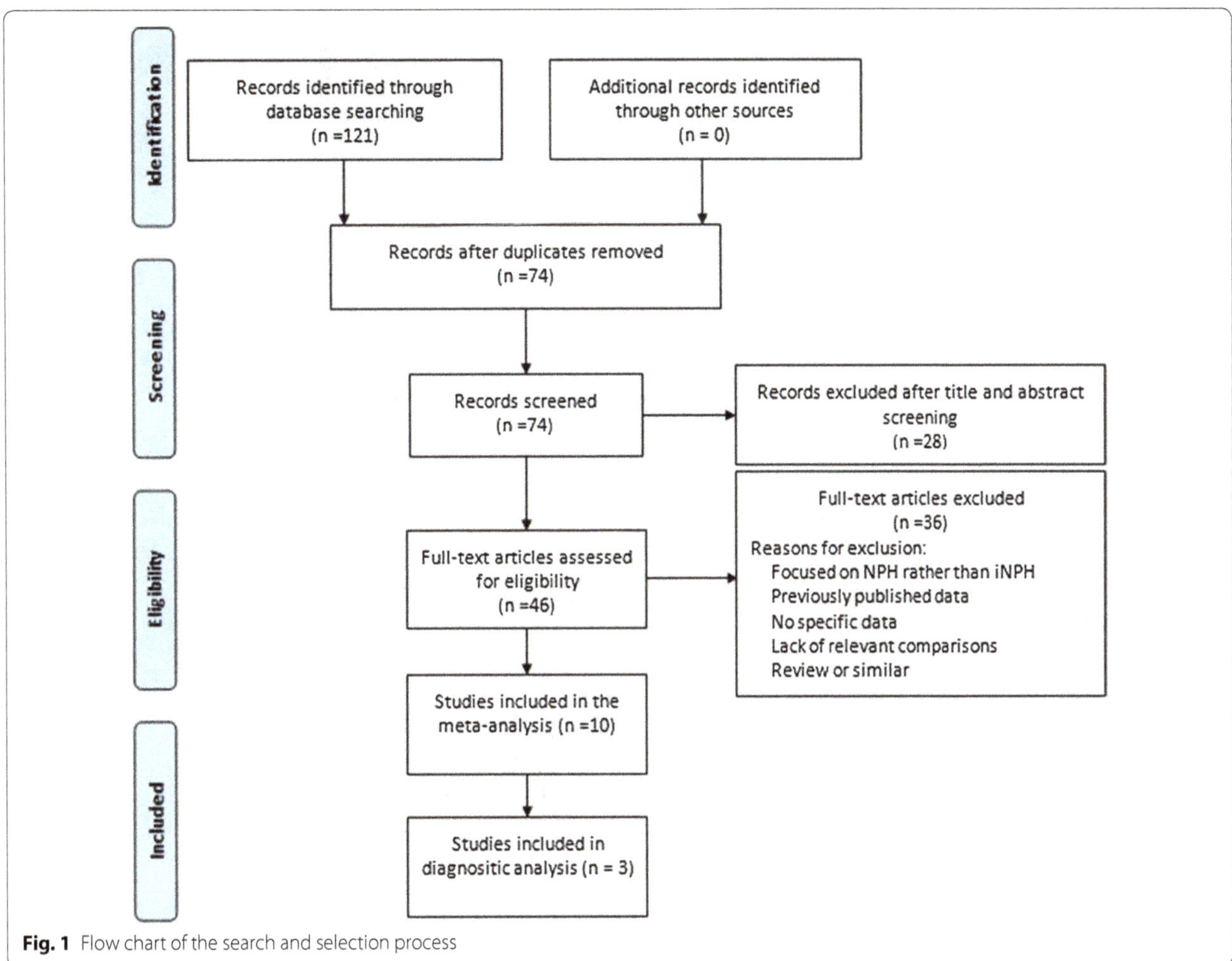

Fig. 1 Flow chart of the search and selection process

95% CI −1.74 to −0.55, $P = 0.0002$), and slightly increased Aβ42 levels compared with AD patients (SMD = 0.32, 95% CI 0.00–0.63, $P = 0.05$).

T-tau in iNPH versus AD/healthy controls Eight studies reported values for CSF t-tau in 323 iNPH patients and 206 AD patients and 6 studies reported values for CSFt-tau in 193 iNPH patients and 147 healthy controls. A significant heterogeneity across studies was found (iNPH versus AD, $P < 0.00001$, $I^2 = 90\%$; iNPH versus healthy controls, $P < 0.00001$, $I^2 = 86\%$), thus the random-effects model was used to calculate the pooled SMD. T-tau levels were significantly lower in iNPH patients than in AD (SMD = −1.26, 95% CI −1.95 to −0.57, $P = 0.0004$) and significantly lower than in healthy controls (SMD = −0.80, 95% CI −1.50 to −0.09, $P = 0.03$).

P-tau in iNPH versus AD/healthy controls Mean P-tau values of iNPH patients were compared with AD patients in 8 articles, including 323 iNPH patients and 206 AD patients. 6 studies reported CSF values for p-tau in 194 iNPH patients and 147 healthy controls. A significant heterogeneity across studies was found in iNPH versus AD ($P < 0.00001$, $I^2 = 92\%$), while no heterogeneity was found between iNPH and healthy controls ($P = 0.64$, $I^2 = 0\%$). P-tau levels were significantly lower in iNPH patients than in AD (SMD = −1.54, 95% CI −2.34 to −0.74, $P = 0.0002$) and significantly lower than in healthy controls (SMD = −1.12, 95% CI −1.38 to −0.86, $P < 0.00001$).

Subgroup analysis

A subgroup analysis was performed according to the categories of country (Asia or others) and CSF source (lumbar or ventricular) (see Table 2).

Of the ten studies included in this meta-analysis, 3 studies were performed in Asian populations, whereas 7 studies were performed in Caucasian groups. For Aβ42 levels in iNPH versus AD, the pooled SMD was 0.75 (95% CI 0.27–1.22, $P = 0.002$) in Asian groups and 0.17 (95% CI −0.07 to 0.40, $P = 0.16$) in Caucasian groups. For Aβ42 levels in iNPH versus healthy controls, the pooled SMD was −0.17 (95% CI −0.96 to 0.63, $P = 0.58$) in Asian

Table 1 Characteristics of studies included in the meta-analysis

Study	Country	Patients	N	Age	Male	Aβ42 (pg/ml)	t-tau (pg/ml)	p-tau (pg/ml)	Method	CSF type
Agren-Wilsson et al. [12]	Sweden	iNPH	62	72 (55–83)[d]	39/23	503 ± 103	171 ± 68	33 ± 10	ELISA	Lumbar
		Controls[a]	23	73 (59–88)[d]	10/13	716 ± 170	330 ± 179	58 ± 29		
Kapaki et al. [13]	Greece	iNPH	18	69 ± 14	11/7	400 ± 219	219 (118–280)[d]	34.8 (20–46.7)[d]	ELISA	Lumbar
		AD	67	66 ± 10	26/41	422 ± 149	571 (443–984)[d]	72 (60.4–100)[d]		
		Controls[a]	72	64 ± 11	41/31	721 ± 228	166 (117–233)[d]	45.1 (40–55.8)[d]		
Seppala et al. [26]	Finland	iNPH	101	NA	NA	399 ± 188	1261 ± 1354	78.1 ± 51.5	ELISA	Ventricular
		AD	51	75.4 ± 7.6	27/24	360 ± 202	1432 ± 1990	83.9 ± 50.1		
Jeppsson et al. [25]	Sweden	iNPH	28	69 ± 6.6	15/13	221 (156–325)[d]	39 (34–50)[d]	39 (33–50)[d]	ECL[e], xMAP	Lumbar
		Controls[a]	20	70 ± 3.6	11/9	498 (391–669)[d]	84 (64–107)[d]	59 (47–75)[d]		
Miyajima et al. [24]	Japan	iNPH	46	74.7 ± 6.9	27/19	314 ± 254	152 ± 98	24.2 ± 10.5	ELISA	Lumbar
		AD	10	78.4 ± 8.5	5/5	189 ± 116	536 ± 299	90.3 ± 32.2		
		Controls[a]	8	67.1 ± 6.7	2/6	255 ± 129	216 ± 138	31.6 ± 4.66		
Lim et al. [27]	South Korea	iNPH	25	73.3 ± 7.0	12/13	579.8 ± 182.3	131.9 ± 77.6	27.0 ± 9.6	ELISA	Lumbar
		AD	17	72.2 ± 10.0	10/7	409.2 ± 166.1	259.6 ± 161.5	51.3 ± 28.3		
		Controls[a]	10	63.0 ± 6.7	3/7	691.8 ± 212.7	196.9 ± 114.4	43.0 ± 28.5		
Pyykko et al. [21]	America	iNPH[b]	48	NA	27/26	476 ± 203	1210 ± 1186	77.1 ± 51.7	ELISA	Ventricular
		iNPH[c]	5	NA		428 ± 250	562 ± 443	50.4 ± 14.3		
		AD	16	78.3 (54.1–85.7)[d]	6/10	422 ± 259	1361 ± 1687	81.3 ± 51.2		
Tsai et al. [22]	America	iNPH	11	81.36 ± 2.58	2/9	251.17 ± 92.39	475.07 ± 335.23	47.35 ± 20.24	ELISA	Lumbar
		AD	11	61.46 ± 8.24	7/4	290.33 ± 146.74	651.53 ± 276.41	79.12 ± 30.00		
Schirinzi et al. [28]	Italy	iNPH	14	73.21 ± 4.63	8/6	477.50 ± 223.10	183.36 ± 99.81	25.36 ± 9.48	ELISA	Lumbar
		AD	14	69.85 ± 7.42	5/9	308.43 ± 91.38	662.79 ± 223.62	77.71 ± 21.65		
		Controls[a]	14	67.21 ± 7.67	8/6	862.86 ± 230.40	231.14 ± 78.42	40.50 ± 11.81		
Jingami et al. [23]	Japan	iNPH	55	76.4 (7.2)	NA	NA	297 (232–440)[d]	16.0 (11.3–23.7)[d]	ELISA	Lumbar
		AD	20	71.8 (12.8)	NA	NA	932 (716–1533)[d]	57.0 (32.1–102)[d]		

NA not available

[a] Healthy controls

[b] Shunt responder

[c] Shunt nonresponder

[d] Data are presented as median (Q1–Q3 range)

[e] Electrochemiluminescence

Table 2 Pooled analysis and subgroup analysis of CSF Aβ42, t-tau, and p-tau between iNPH and AD/healthy controls

	Stratification group	iNPH vs. AD							iNPH vs. healthy controls						
		Comparisons			SMD [95% CI]	Heterogeneity test			Comparisons			SMD [95% CI]	Heterogeneity test		
		Studies (N_{iNPH}/N_{AD})	Z	P		Q	P	I^2, %	Studies ($N_{iNPH}/N_{Control}$)	Z	P		Q	P	I^2, %
Aβ42	Total	7 (268/186)	1.98	0.05	0.32 (0.00, 0.63)	11.93	0.06	50	6 (193/147)	3.75	0.0002	−1.14 (−1.74, −0.55)	23.55	0.0003	79
	Study population														
	Caucasian	5 (197/159)	1.41	0.16	0.17 (−0.07, 0.40)	6.47	0.17	38	4 (122/129)	9.94	<0.00001	−1.60 (−1.91, −1.28)	0.67	0.88	0
	Asian	2 (71/27)	3.09	0.002	0.75 (0.27, 1.22)	0.79	0.37	0	2 (71/18)	0.41	0.68	−0.17 (−0.96, 0.63)	2.26	−0.13	56
	CSF source														
	Lumbar	5 (114/119)	1.49	0.14	0.39 (−0.12, 0.91)	11.41	0.02	65	6 (193/147)	3.75	0.0002	−1.14 (−1.74, −0.55)	23.55	0.0003	79
	Ventricular	2 (154/67)	1.41	0.16	0.21 (−0.08, 0.50)	0.00	0.95	5	–	–	–	–	–	–	–
t-tau	Total	8 (323/206)	3.57	0.0004	−1.26 (−1.95, −0.57)	70.50	<0.00001	90	6 (193/147)	2.22	0.03	−0.80 (−1.50, −0.09)	35.00	<0.00001	86
	Study population														
	Caucasian	5 (197/159)	2.30	0.02	−0.86 (−1.60, −0.13)	30.2	<0.00001	87	4 (122/129)	1.63	0.10	−0.87 (−1.91, 0.17)	34.81	<0.00001	91
	Asian	3 (126/47)	4.37	<0.00001	−1.88 (−2.72, −1.03)	8.69	0.01	77	2 (71/18)	2.41	0.02	−0.66 (−1.19, −0.12)	0.04	0.84	0
	CSF source														
	Lumbar	6 (169/139)	5.28	<0.00001	−1.66 (−2.28, −1.05)	21.18	0.0008	76	6 (193/147)	2.22	0.03	−0.80 (−1.50, −0.09)	35.00	<0.00001	86
	Ventricular	2 (154/67)	0.83	0.41	−0.12 (−0.41, 0.17)	0.03	0.87	0	–	–	–	–	–	–	–
p-tau	Total	8 (323/206)	3.78	0.0002	−1.54 (−2.34, −0.74)	89.64	<0.00001	92	6 (193/147)	8.36	<0.00001	−1.12 (−1.38, −0.86)	3.4	0.64	0
	Study population														
	Caucasian	5 (197/159)	2.49	0.01	−1.11 (−1.99, −0.24)	40.87	<0.00001	90	4 (122/129)	7.9	<0.00001	−1.21 (−1.51, −0.91)	1.82	0.61	0
	Asian	3 (126/47)	3.21	0.001	−2.23 (−3.59, −0.87)	20.55	<0.00001	90	2 (71/18)	2.99	0.003	−0.83 (−1.37, −0.29)	0.11	0.74	0
	CSF source														
	Lumbar	6 (169/139)	5.42	<0.00001	−2.03 (−2.77, −1.30)	27.56	<0.00001	82	6 (193/147)	8.36	<0.00001	−1.12 (−1.38, −0.86)	3.4	0.64	0
	Ventricular	2 (154/67)	0.80	0.42	−0.12 (−0.41, 0.17)	0.00	0.95	0	–	–	–	–	–	–	–

groups and −1.60 (95% CI −1.91 to −1.28, $P < 0.00001$) in Caucasian groups. For t-tau levels in iNPH versus AD, the pooled SMD was −1.88 (95% CI −2.72 to −1.03, $P < 0.00001$) in Asian groups and −0.86 (95% CI −1.60 to −0.13, $P = 0.02$) in Caucasian groups. For t-tau levels in iNPH versus healthy controls, the pooled SMD was −0.66 (95% CI −1.19 to −0.12, $P = 0.02$) in Asian groups and −0.87 (95% CI −1.91 to 0.17, $P = 0.10$) in Caucasian groups. For p-tau levels in iNPH versus AD, the pooled SMD was −2.23 (95% CI −3.59 to −0.87, $P = 0.001$) in Asian groups and −1.11 (95% CI −1.99 to −0.24, $P = 0.01$) in Caucasian groups. For p-tau levels in iNPH versus healthy controls, the pooled SMD was −0.83 (95% CI −1.37 to −0.29, $P = 0.003$) in Asian groups and −1.21 (95% CI −1.51 to −0.91, $P < 0.00001$) in Caucasian groups.

Of the ten studies included in this meta-analysis, 8 studies were performed using lumbar CSF while 2 studies were using ventricular CSF. For Aβ42 levels in iNPH versus AD, the pooled SMD was 0.39 (95% CI −0.12 to 0.91, $P = 0.14$) in lumbar CSF groups and 0.21 (95% CI −0.08 to 0.50, $P = 0.16$) in ventricular CSF groups. For t-tau levels in iNPH versus AD, the pooled SMD was −1.66 (95% CI −2.28 to −1.05, $P < 0.00001$) in lumbar CSF groups and −0.12 (95% CI −0.41 to 0.17, $P = 0.41$) in ventricular CSF groups. For p-tau levels in iNPH versus AD, the pooled SMD was −2.03 (95% CI −2.77 to −1.30, $P < 0.00001$) in lumbar CSF groups and −0.12 (95% CI −0.41 to 0.17, $P = 0.42$) in ventricular CSF groups.

Sensitivity analysis

Sensitivity analysis was performed by removing studies one by one and comparing the pooled estimate from the remaining studies with the pooled estimate from all studies. Sensitivity analysis of Aβ42 levels between iNPH and healthy controls, t-tau levels between iNPH and AD, and p-tau levels between iNPH and AD/healthy controls revealed that the direction and magnitude of pooled estimates did not change significantly, indicating that the results of the meta-analysis were relatively robust. In contrast, sensitivity analysis of Aβ42 levels in iNPH and AD, as well as t-tau levels in iNPH and healthy controls revealed that the pooled estimates were different when the leave-one-out approach was used. This suggests that results of those between-groups analyses were not stable and reliable (see Figs. 2, 3, 4, 5, 6, 7).

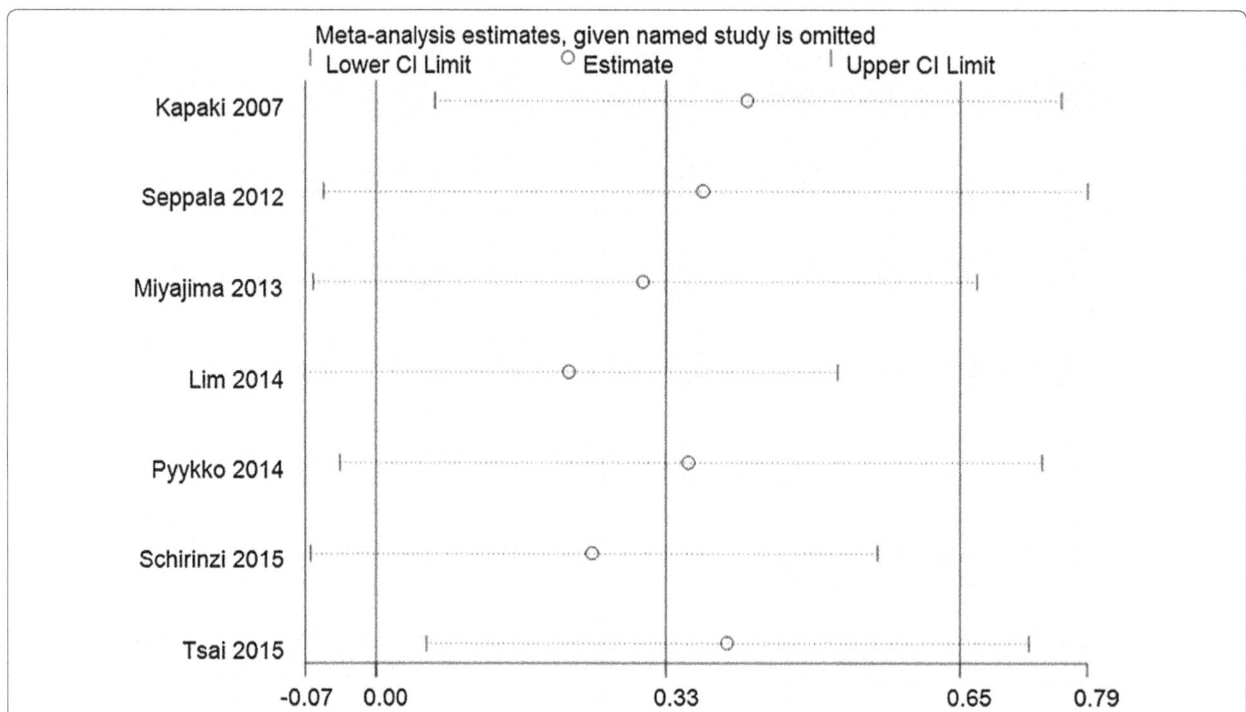

Fig. 2 Sensitivity analysis of CSF Aβ42 levels in iNPH compared to AD. Sensitivity analysis was performed by removing studies one by one and comparing the pooled estimate from the remaining studies with the pooled estimate from all studies. The *X axis* represents the pooled estimate and the *Y axis* represents the excluded studies. Analyses were conducted on the raw data and the pooled estimate was 0.33 (95% CI 0.00–0.65). The pooled estimate was different when the study of Seppala et al. [26], Miyajima et al. [24], Lim et al. [27], Pyykko et al. [21], Schirinzi et al. [28] were omitted separately. The pooled estimates (95% CI) were 0.37 (95% CI −0.05 to 0.79), 0.30 (95% CI −0.07 to 0.67), 0.22 (95% CI −0.07 to 0.51), 0.35 (95% CI −0.04 to 0.74), 0.25 (95% CI −0.07 to 0.56), respectively. This suggests that results of those between-groups analyses were not stable and reliable

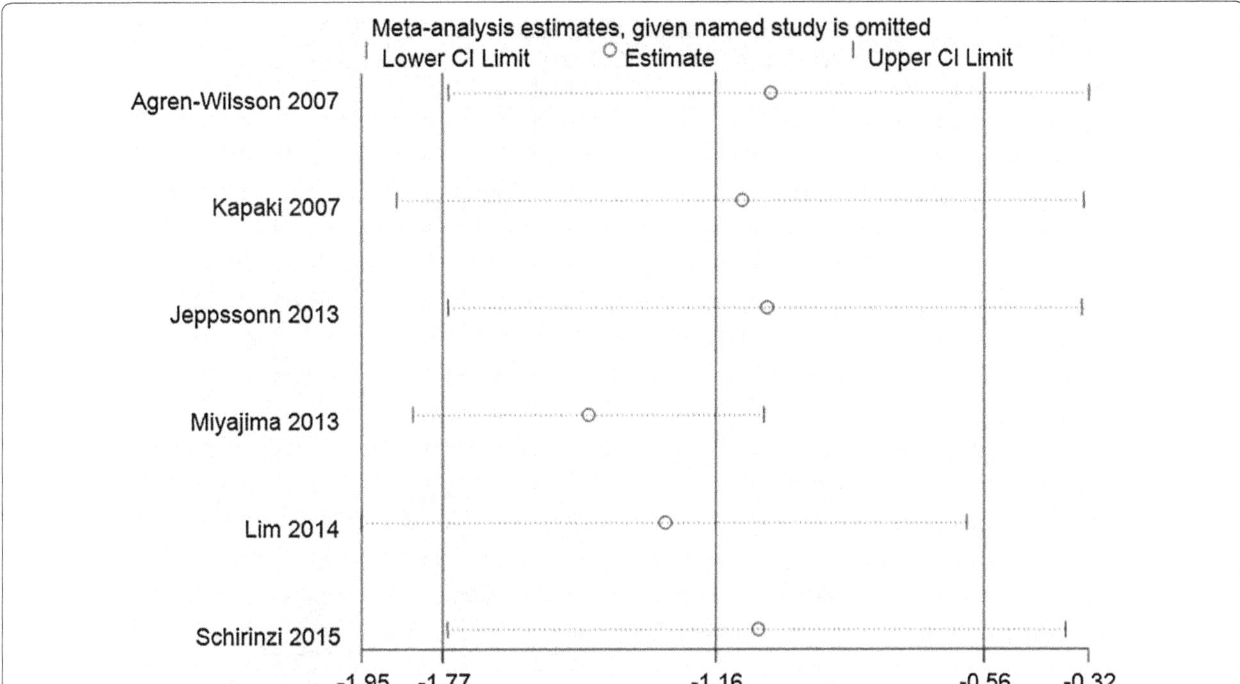

Fig. 3 Sensitivity analysis of CSF Aβ42 levels in iNPH compared to healthy controls. Analyses were conducted on the raw data and the pooled estimate was −1.16 (95% CI −1.77 to −0.56). The direction and magnitude of pooled estimates did not change significantly after removing studies one by one, indicating that the results of the meta-analysis were relatively robust

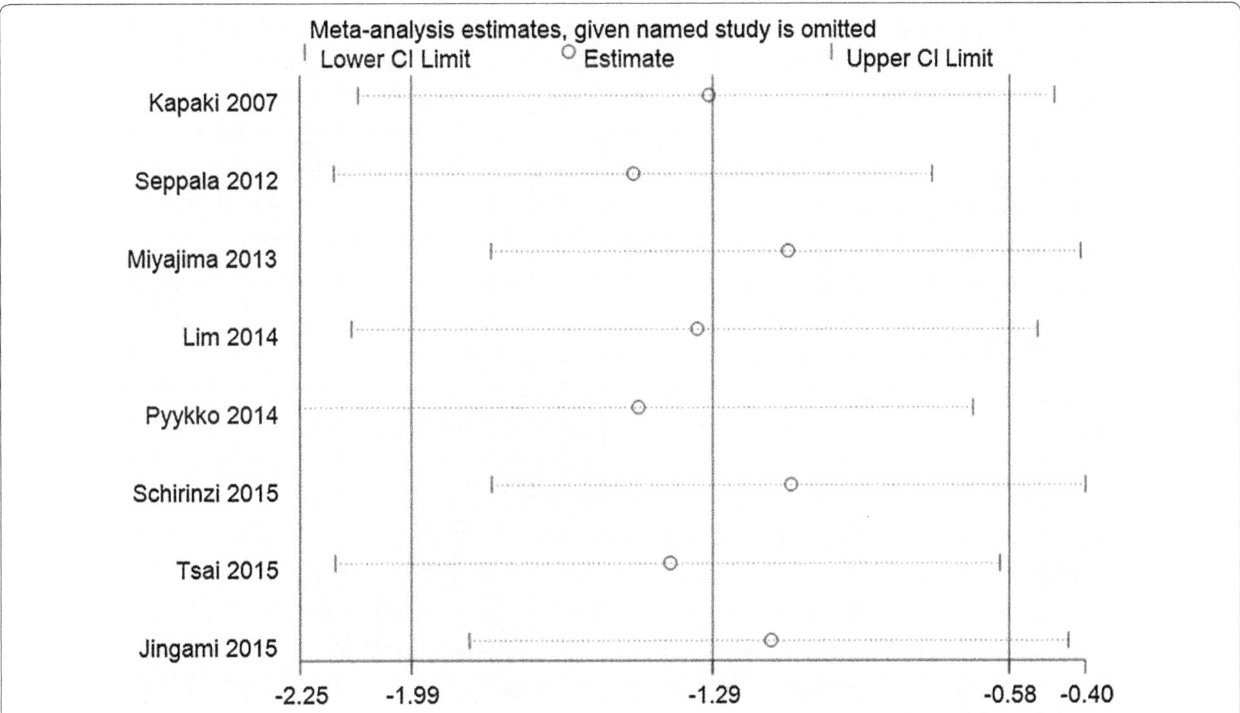

Fig. 4 Sensitivity analysis of CSF t-tau levels in iNPH compared to AD. Analyses were conducted on the raw data and the pooled estimate was −1.29 (95% CI −1.99 to −0.58). The direction and magnitude of pooled estimates did not change significantly after removing studies one by one, indicating that the results of the meta-analysis were relatively robust

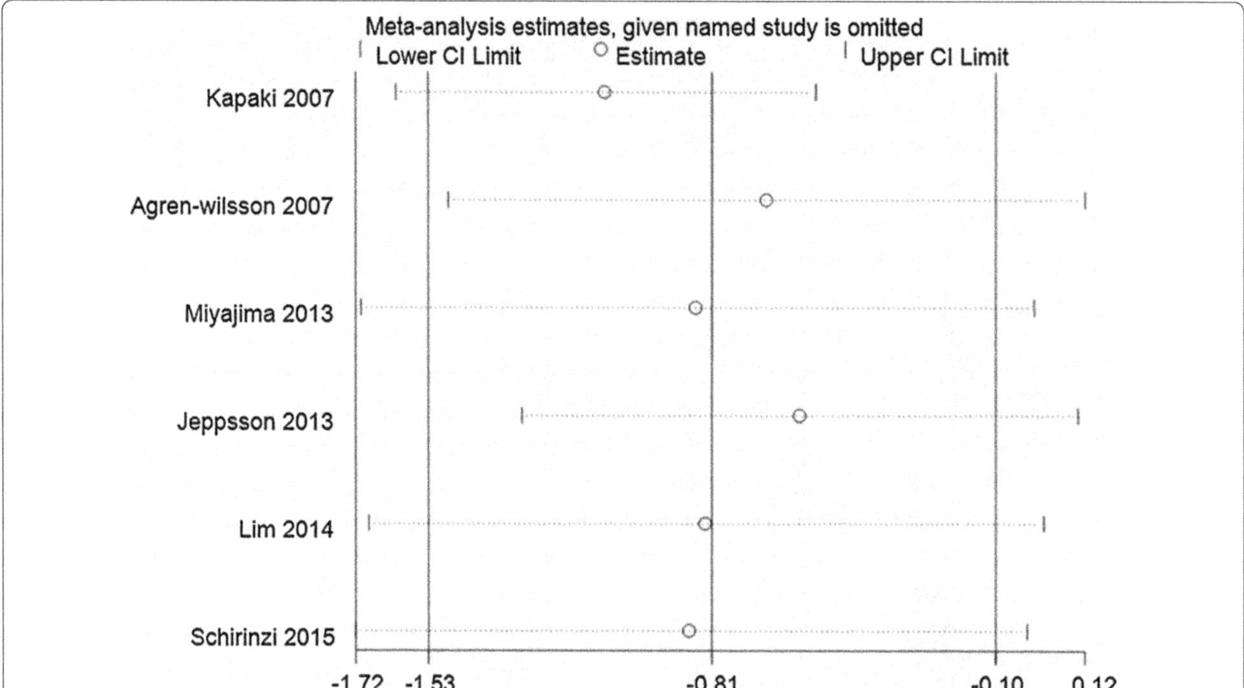

Fig. 5 Sensitivity analysis of CSF t-tau levels in iNPH compared to healthy controls. Analyses were conducted on the raw data and the pooled estimate was −0.81 (95% CI −1.53 to −0.10). The pooled estimate was different when the study of Agren-Wilsson et al. [12], Jeppsson et al. [25], Lim et al. [27] were omitted separately. The pooled estimates (95% CI) were −0.68 (95% CI −1.47 to 0.12), −0.59 (95% CI −1.29 to 0.11) and −0.83 (95% CI −1.68 to 0.21), respectively. This suggests that results of those between-groups analyses were not stable and reliable

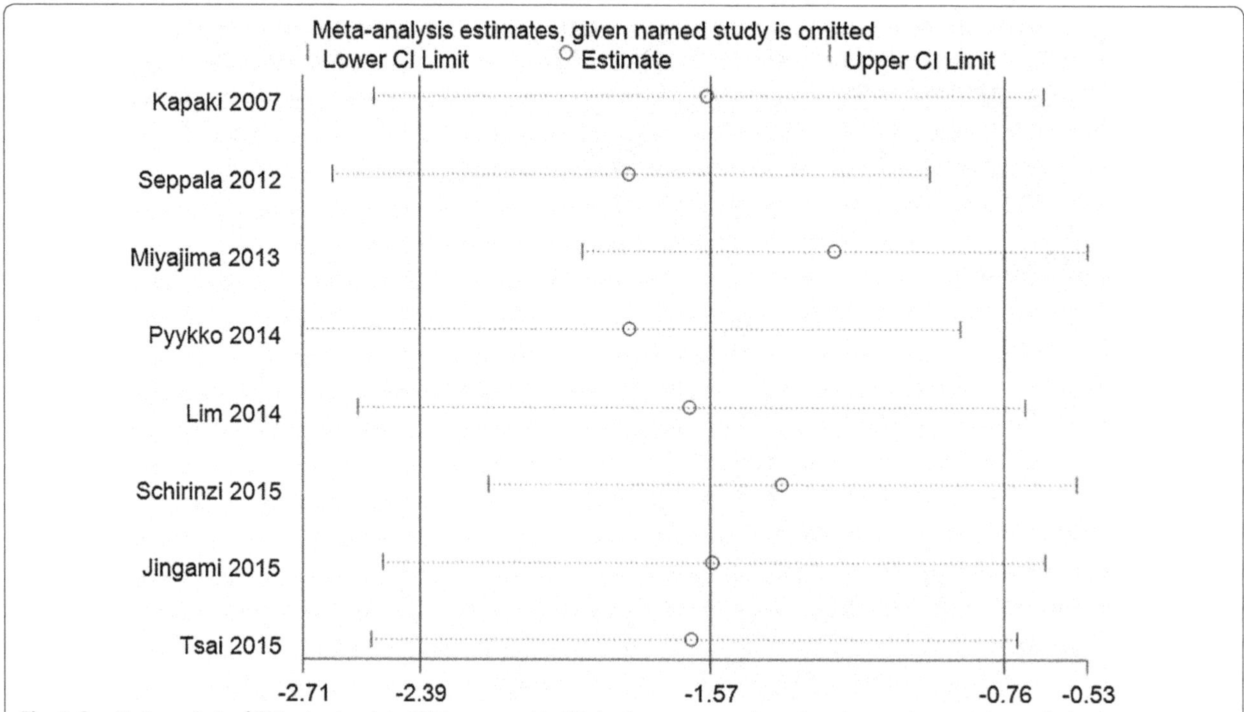

Fig. 6 Sensitivity analysis of CSF p-tau levels in iNPH compared to AD. Analyses were conducted on the raw data and the pooled estimate was −1.57 (95% CI −2.39 to −0.76). The direction and magnitude of pooled estimates did not change significantly after removing studies one by one, indicating that the results of the meta-analysis were relatively robust

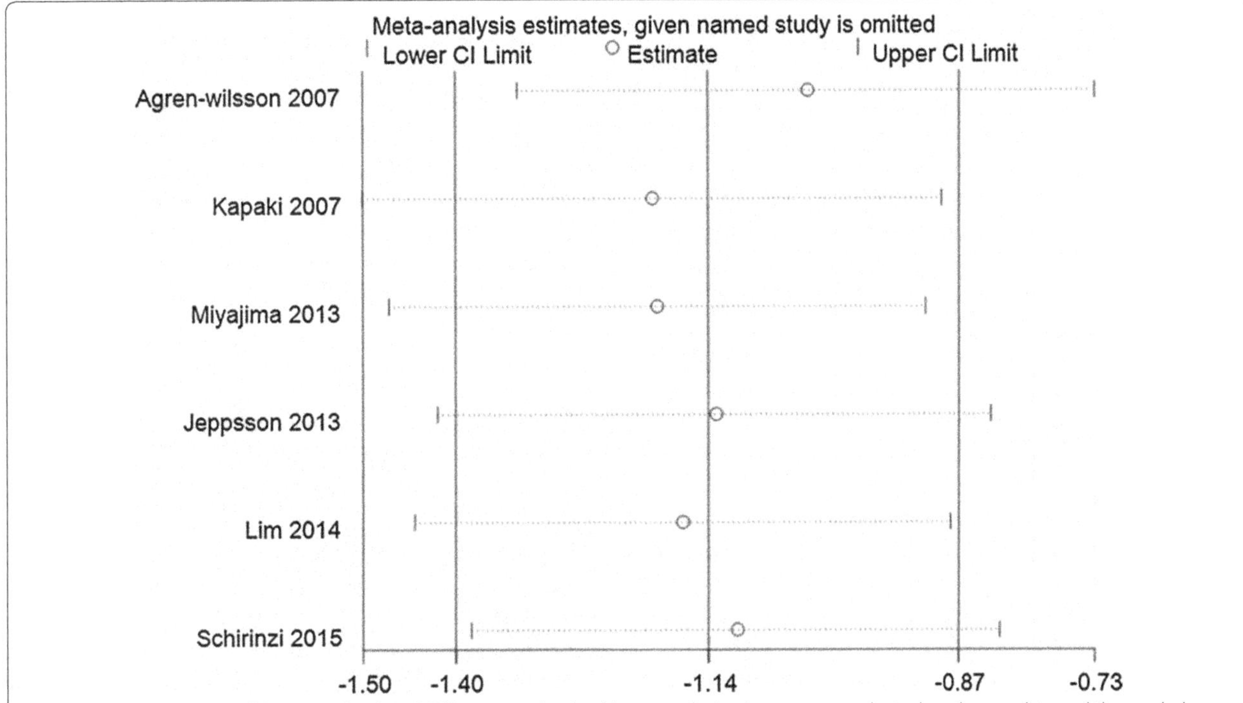

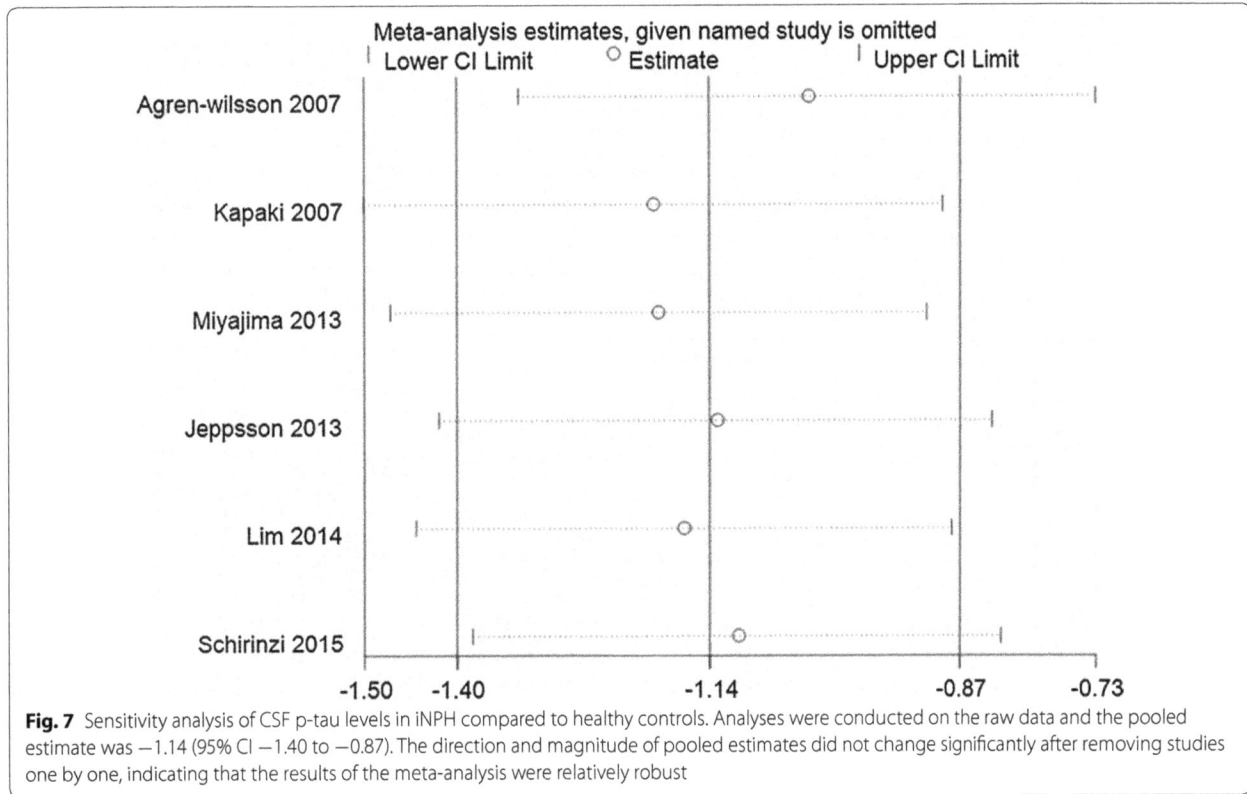

Fig. 7 Sensitivity analysis of CSF p-tau levels in iNPH compared to healthy controls. Analyses were conducted on the raw data and the pooled estimate was −1.14 (95% CI −1.40 to −0.87). The direction and magnitude of pooled estimates did not change significantly after removing studies one by one, indicating that the results of the meta-analysis were relatively robust

Publication bias

Begg and Egger tests were performed to assess for publication bias of the included studies and provide statistical evidence of publication funnel plot symmetry. Results showed that no significant publication bias was found in CSF Aβ42 levels between iNPH and AD (Begg's test: $Z = 0.60$, $P = 0.548$; Egger's test: $t = 0.73$, $P = 0.500$), Aβ42 levels between iNPH and healthy controls (Begg's test: $Z = 1.13$, $P = 0.260$; Egger's test: $t = 0.96$, $P = 0.390$), t-tau levels between iNPH and healthy controls (Begg's test: $Z = 0.00$, $P = 1.000$; Egger's test: $t = -0.44$, $P = 0.686$), p-tau levels between iNPH and healthy controls (Begg's test: $Z = 0.00$, $P = 1.000$; Egger's test: $t = 0.55$, $P = 0.609$). However evidence of publication bias was found in CSF t-tau levels between iNPH and AD (Begg's test: $Z = 0.87$, $P = 0.386$; Egger's test: $t = -2.77$, $P = 0.032$) and p-tau levels between iNPH and AD (Begg's test: $Z = 1.86$, $P = 0.063$; Egger's test: $t = -3.69$, $P = 0.010$). We therefore used the Trim and Fill method to correct it. There was no significant change in the results after using the trim and fill method, which suggested that the influence of publication bias on stability of results was weak.

Diagnostic results of included studies

Detailed data regarding the sensitivity, specificity and other diagnostic results were presented in Table 3. Compared to AD, higher Aβ42 concentrations differentiated iNPH with a sensitivity of 0.813 (95% CI 0.636–0.928) and a specificity of 0.506 (95% CI 0.393–0.619). The PLR and NLR of CSF Aβ42 concentrations in differentiating iNPH from AD were 2.032 (95% CI 0.918–4.498) and 0.324 (95% CI 0.156–0.673), respectively.

Relative to AD, the sensitivity and specificity of lower CSF t-tau concentrations in differentiating iNPH were

Table 3 Summary of the diagnostic results of the included studies

Study	Group compared	Cutoff value	Auc	Sensitivity	Specificity
Jingami et al. [23]	iNPH vs. AD				
	t-tau	766	0.9	75	98
	p-tau	24.4	0.91	95	74
Kapaki et al. [13]	iNPH vs. AD				
	Aβ42	268	0.58	90.9	44.4
	t-tau	294	0.84	92.5	77.8
	p-tau	47.4	0.83	88.7	86.7
Schirinzi et al. [28]	iNPH vs. AD				
	Aβ42	371	0.75	73.3	81.3
	t-tau	386	0.99	100	93.8
	p-tau	46	0.99	100	93.8

0.828 (95% CI 0.732–0.900) and 0.842 (95% CI 0.756–0.907), respectively. The PLR and NLR of CSF t-tau concentrations in differentiating iNPH were 8.199 (95% CI 1.738–38.678) and 0.112 (95% CI 0.018–0.699), respectively. The SROC AUC value was 0.963 ± 0.021, and the pooled diagnostic accuracy (Q*) was 0.909 ± 0.032.

Compared with AD, the sensitivity and specificity of lower CSF p-tau concentrations in distinguishing iNPH were 0.943 (95% CI 0.871–0.981) and 0.851 (95% CI 0.767–0.914), respectively. The PLR and NLR of CSF p-tau concentrations in distinguishing iNPH were 5.577 (95% CI 3.513–8.854) and 0.085 (95% CI 0.038–0.193), respectively. The SROC AUC value was 0.9453 ± 0.037, and the pooled diagnostic accuracy (Q*) was 0.884 ± 0.048.

Discussion

In this systematic review and meta-analysis, we explored whether concentrations of CSF Aβ42, t-tau, and p-tau are of potential value in differentiating iNPH from AD and from healthy normal controls. Our results suggest that concentrations of CSF t-tau and p-tau in iNPH patients are lower than in AD patients and lower than healthy controls. Concentrations of Aβ42 in iNPH patients are lower than in healthy controls but slightly higher than in AD patients. Lower CSF t-tau and p-tau levels appear to carry higher sensitivity and specificity in differentiating iNPH from AD.

The combined pattern of reduced CSF levels of Aβ42 and increased levels of CSF t-tau and p-tau is an established CSF biomarker for AD [9]. The low Aβ42 levels compared to healthy controls in AD are believed to result from sequestration of soluble beta amyloid in plaques, while the elevated concentrations of t-tau and p-tau are thought to reflect release from the intraneuronal compartment owing to nerve cell and neurite damage. Past studies have fairly consistently found iNPH patients have low CSF Aβ42 levels in a range that overlaps that of AD. In this meta-analysis, we found that high Aβ42 levels in CSF might be slightly helpful in differentiating iNPH from AD, whereas low CSF Aβ42 could potentially be useful as a marker for differentiating of iNPH from healthy normal elderly.

Various hypotheses have been proposed to explain the reduction of CSF Aβ42 levels in iNPH patients. One hypothesis is that delivery of Aβ42 to the CSF compartment is impaired as a consequence of reduced centripetal flow of extracellular fluid in the brain caused by the retrograde CSF flow dynamics in iNPH [14, 25]. Xie et al. [29] found that Aβ clearance from the extracellular fluid is increased during sleep, as the interstitial space increases 60% in size at this time. Hence, Graff-Radford et al. [14] hypothesized that reduced CSF Aβ42 levels in iNPH may be related to the smaller extracellular space and having less room for the convective flux of CSF and interstitial fluid during sleep. The increased CSF levels of many proteins obtained from lumbar CSF drainage in iNPH provides indirect support for this theory. However, Hladky and Barrand [30] raised doubts about this theory and proposed a hypothesis that the elimination of Abeta from the brain might be associated with the perivascular lymphatic drainage pathways. Another possible explanation is that hypometabolism in the periventricular zone, as sometime seen on PET and SPECT studies in iNPH patients, may play a role in lowering generation of CSF Aβ42 [25].

Contrary to the consistency of finding low Aβ42 level in iNPH, there is only moderate agreement regarding the concentrations of CSF t-tau and p-tau. In 2007, Kapaki et al. [13] found that t-tau was slightly increased in iNPH and obviously increased in AD compared to healthy controls, while p-tau levels were significantly increased only in AD. Therefore, the authors concluded that CSF p-tau alone or in combination with t-tau may be a useful marker in the differentiation of iNPH from AD. However, other studies found that both t-tau and p-tau concentrations were significantly reduced in iNPH patients compared to AD [23] and healthy controls [25]. Our results suggest that concentrations of CSF t-tau and p-tau in iNPH are lower than in AD and healthy controls and this difference might be used to differentiate iNPH from AD or healthy controls. Prior reports have found that the concentrations of t-tau and p-tau increased with age [31, 32]. Since the average ages of iNPH patients were older than the AD patients in this study, one might have expected to find higher t-tau and p-tau levels in the iNPH group. On the contrary, we found the opposite. Hence, the differences in the concentrations of t-tau and p-tau observed between iNPH and AD are more likely associated with the pathophysiology of iNPH than age differences [31]. Reduced clearance from extracellular fluid and decreased brain metabolism of periventricular zone in iNPH may contribute to this phenomenon of reduction in CSF t-tau and p-tau levels in iNPH [14].

Prior studies reported that the ventricular CSF t-tau and p-tau levels are higher than in lumbar CSF samples [26]. In the studies we analyzed, there was marked heterogeneity in CSF levels depending on the location from which the CSF was collected. Therefore we performed subgroup analysis taking into account the CSF sources (lumbar CSF vs. ventricular CSF). Results showed that the lumbar CSF t-tau and p-tau levels in iNPH were lower than in AD, while no differences were found in ventricular CSF samples. This finding may support the hypothesis that lower CSF levels of proteins in iNPH relate to the disturbed circulation of CSF to the lumbar region in this disorder. Other possible explanations for this discrepancy include insufficient sample size or methodologic differences such as neuronal injury associated with placing a ventricular catheter which may elevate ventricular CSF tau and p-tau levels [12]. A subgroup analysis was also performed according to the categories of country (Asia vs. Caucasian). Results showed that the CSF Aβ42 and t-tau levels were distinct in different races, which suggested that outcomes may have been influenced by ethnicity. However, insufficient sample size or methodologic differences may also explain this contrast.

Our systematic review and meta-analysis has some limitations that should be acknowledged. First, only a limited number of studies were eligible for inclusion, particularly in the diagnostic analyses, which reduced the power of our meta-analysis. Secondly, we observed marked heterogeneity suggesting that there was a significant difference among the included studies, which can be attributed to variation in sample size, age, ethnicity, CSF source, different metrics (means and medians), and methodologic differences in sample collection and the assays employed. Although random-effects and subgroup analyses were performed, these parameters could not completely explain the heterogeneity. Other factors can be identified that may have contributed to the heterogeneity across studies. We were unable to assess what stage of iNPH (mild, moderate, severe) was included in the respective studies, and this could introduce some of the variance in the CSF results. In addition, we assume that the reported cases were pure iNPH or pure AD, but it is known that these conditions can occur together in many cases. The possible coincident occurrence of iNPH with AD or complications due to other diseases, could not be evaluated because these factors were not reported in the included articles. This is likely to be an important contributing factor in the heterogeneity [15, 27, 33]. Thirdly, sensitivity analysis of Aβ42 levels between iNPH and AD, t-tau levels between iNPH and healthy controls indicated that the meta-analysis for these variables had poor reliability. Fourthly, we did not include unpublished and non-peer reviewed studies and our analysis was restricted to publications in English and Chinese, creating the possibility geographic source biases. Finally, a weak publication bias was found in relation to reports of CSF t-tau levels between iNPH and AD, and p-tau levels between iNPH and AD. However, there was no significant change in the results after using the Trim and Fill method, which suggests that the influence of publication bias on stability of results was weak.

Conclusion

Our study suggests that reduced CSF t-tau and p-tau maybe come useful markers for the differentiation of iNPH from AD or healthy controls. In addition, low Aβ42 levels contribute to distinguish iNPH and AD from healthy controls while Aβ42 levels are statistically slightly higher in iNPH compared to AD. Given the relative paucity of studies included and other limitations in this study, it is reasonable to assume our results should be interpreted with caution. In future, well-designed, large-scale prospective studies with well-controlled, standardization of experimental protocols for CSF biomarker measurements are warranted as a step towards improving the diagnosis and differential diagnosis of iNPH in clinical practice.

Authors' contributions

Conceived and designed the experiments: ZYC NR YX YFL. Analyzed the data: ZYC CYL. Contributed reagents/materials/analysis tools: JZ. Wrote the paper: ZYC NR YX. All authors read and approved the final manuscript.

Author details

[1] Department of Neurology, Aviation General Hospital of China Medical University & Beijing Institute of Translational Medicine, Chinese Academy of Sciences, No. 3 Anwai Beiyuan Road, Chaoyang District, Beijing 100012, China. [2] Department of Neurology and Neuroscience, Weill Medical College of Cornell University, Cornell Memory Disorders Program, 428 East 72 Street, Suite 500, New York, NY 10021, USA. [3] Department of Neurology, Peking Union Medical College Hospital, Beijing, China.

Competing interests

The authors declare that they have no competing interests.

References

1. Adams RD, Fisher CM, Hakim S, Ojemann RG, Sweet WH. Symptomatic occult hydrocephalus with "normal" cerebrospinal-fluid pressure. A treatable syndrome. N Engl J Med. 1965;273:117–26.
2. Akiguchi I, Shirakashi Y, Budka H, Watanabe Y, Watanabe T, Shiino A, et al. Disproportionate subarachnoid space hydrocephalus-outcome and perivascular space. Ann Clin Transl Neurol. 2014;1:562–9.
3. Jaraj D, Rabiei K, Marlow T, Jensen C, Skoog I, Wikkelso C. Prevalence of idiopathic normal-pressure hydrocephalus. Neurology. 2014;82:1449–54.
4. Tanaka N, Yamaguchi S, Ishikawa H, Ishii H, Meguro K. Prevalence of possible idiopathic normal-pressure hydrocephalus in Japan: the Osaki-Tajiri project. Neuroepidemiology. 2009;32:171–5.
5. Martin-Laez R, Caballero-Arzapalo H, Lopez-Menendez LA, Arango-Lasprilla JC, Vazquez-Barquero A. Epidemiology of idiopathic normal pressure hydrocephalus: a systematic review of the literature. World Neurosurg. 2015;84:2002–9.
6. Brean A, Eide PK. Prevalence of probable idiopathic normal pressure hydrocephalus in a Norwegian population. Acta Neurol Scand. 2008;118:48–53.
7. Marmarou A, Young HF, Aygok GA. Estimated incidence of normal pressure hydrocephalus and shunt outcome in patients residing in assisted-living and extended-care facilities. Neurosurg Focus. 2007;22:E1.
8. Klinge P, Hellstrom P, Tans J, Wikkelso C. One-year outcome in the European multicentre study on iNPH. Acta Neurol Scand. 2012;126:145–53.
9. Olsson B, Lautner R, Andreasson U, Ohrfelt A, Portelius E, Bjerke M, et al. CSF and blood biomarkers for the diagnosis of Alzheimer's disease: a systematic review and meta-analysis. Lancet Neurol. 2016;15:673–84.
10. Blennow K, de Leon MJ, Zetterberg H. Alzheimer's disease. Lancet. 2006;368:387–403.
11. Trojanowski JQ, Schuck T, Schmidt ML, Lee VM. Distribution of tau proteins in the normal human central and peripheral nervous system. J Histochem Cytochem. 1989;37:209–15.
12. Agren-Wilsson A, Lekman A, Sjoberg W, Rosengren L, Blennow K, Bergenheim AT, et al. CSF biomarkers in the evaluation of idiopathic normal pressure hydrocephalus. Acta Neurol Scand. 2007;116:333–9.

13. Kapaki EN, Paraskevas GP, Tzerakis NG, Sfagos C, Seretis A, Kararizou E, et al. Cerebrospinal fluid tau, phospho-tau181 and beta-amyloid1–42 in idiopathic normal pressure hydrocephalus: a discrimination from Alzheimer's disease. Eur J Neurol. 2007;14:168–73.
14. Graff-Radford NR. Alzheimer CSF biomarkers may be misleading in normal-pressure hydrocephalus. Neurology. 2014;83:1573–5.
15. Ray B, Reyes PF, Lahiri DK. Biochemical studies in normal pressure hydrocephalus (NPH) patients: change in CSF levels of amyloid precursor protein (APP), amyloid-beta (Aβ) peptide and phospho-tau. J Psychiatr Res. 2011;45:539–47.
16. Liberati A, Altman DG, Tetzlaff J, Mulrow C, Gotzsche PC, Ioannidis JP, Clarke M, et al. The PRISMA statement for reporting systematic reviews and meta-analyses of studies that evaluate healthcare interventions: explanation and elaboration. PLoS Med. 2009;6:e1000100.
17. Wan X, Wang W, Liu J, Tong T. Estimating the sample mean and standard deviation from the sample size, median, range and/or interquartile range. BMC Med Res Methodol. 2014;14:135.
18. Higgins J, Green S. Cochrane handbook for systematic reviews of interventions, Version 5.1.0 [updated March 2011], The Cochrane Collaboration; 2011.
19. Colditz GA, Burdick E, Mosteller F. Heterogeneity in meta-analysis of data from epidemiologic studies: a commentary. Am J Epidemiol. 1995;142:371–82.
20. Egger M, Davey Smith G, Schneider M, Minder C. Bias in meta-analysis detected by a simple, graphical test. BMJ. 1997;315:629–34.
21. Pyykko OT, Lumela M, Rummukainen J, Nerg O, Seppala TT, Herukka SK, et al. Cerebrospinal fluid biomarker and brain biopsy findings in idiopathic normal pressure hydrocephalus. PLoS ONE. 2014;9:e91974.
22. Tsai A, Malek-Ahmadi M, Kahlon V, Sabbagh MN. Differences in cerebrospinal fluid biomarkers between clinically diagnosed idiopathic normal pressure hydrocephalus and Alzheimer's disease. J Alzheimers Dis Parkinsonism. 2014;4(4). doi: 10.4172/2161-0460.1000150.
23. Jingami N, Asada-Utsugi M, Uemura K, Noto R, Takahashi M, Ozaki A, et al. Idiopathic normal pressure hydrocephalus has a different cerebrospinal fluid biomarker profile from Alzheimer's disease. J Alzheimers Dis. 2015;45:109–15.
24. Miyajima M, Nakajima M, Ogino I, Miyata H, Motoi Y, Arai H. Soluble amyloid precursor protein α in the cerebrospinal fluid as a diagnostic and prognostic biomarker for idiopathic normal pressure hydrocephalus. Eur J Neurol. 2013;20:236–42.
25. Jeppsson A, Zetterberg H, Blennow K, Wikkelso C. Idiopathic normal-pressure hydrocephalus: pathophysiology and diagnosis by CSF biomarkers. Neurology. 2013;80:1385–92.
26. Seppala TT, Nerg O, Koivisto AM, Rummukainen J, Puli L, Zetterberg H, et al. CSF biomarkers for Alzheimer disease correlate with cortical brain biopsy findings. Neurology. 2012;78:1568–75.
27. Lim TS, Choi JY, Park SA, Youn YC, Lee HY, Kim BG, et al. Evaluation of coexistence of Alzheimer's disease in idiopathic normal pressure hydrocephalus using ELISA analyses for CSF biomarkers. BMC Neurol. 2014;14:66.
28. Schirinzi T, Sancesario GM, Ialongo C, Imbriani P, Madeo G, Toniolo S, et al. A clinical and biochemical analysis in the differential diagnosis of idiopathic normal pressure hydrocephalus. Front Neurol. 2015;6:86.
29. Xie L, Kang H, Xu Q, Chen MJ, Liao Y, Thiyagarajan M, et al. Sleep drives metabolite clearance from the adult brain. Science. 2013;342:373–7.
30. Hladky SB, Barrand MA. Mechanisms of fluid movement into, through and out of the brain: evaluation of the evidence. Fluids Barriers CNS. 2014;11:26.
31. Paternico D, Galluzzi S, Drago V, Bocchio-Chiavetto L, Zanardini R, Pedrini L, et al. Cerebrospinal fluid markers for Alzheimer's disease in a cognitively healthy cohort of young and old adults. Alzheimers Dement. 2012;8:520–7.
32. Sjogren M, Vanderstichele H, Agren H, Zachrisson O, Edsbagge M, Wikkelso C, et al. Tau and Aβ42 in cerebrospinal fluid from healthy adults 21–93 years of age: establishment of reference values. Clin Chem. 2001;47:1776–81.
33. Kudo T, Mima T, Hashimoto R, Nakao K, Morihara T, Tanimukai H, et al. Tau protein is a potential biological marker for normal pressure hydrocephalus. Psychiatry Clin Neurosci. 2000;54:199–202.

5

Profiling of metalloprotease activities in cerebrospinal fluids of patients with neoplastic meningitis

Catharina Conrad[1,2], Kristina Dorzweiler[3], Miles A. Miller[4,5], Douglas A. Lauffenburger[4], Herwig Strik[1*] and Jörg W. Bartsch[3*]

Abstract

Background: Neoplastic invasion into leptomeninges and subarachnoid space, resulting in neoplastic meningitis (NM) is a fatal complication of advanced solid and hematological neoplasms. Identification of malignant involvement of the cerebrospinal fluid (CSF) early in the disease course has crucial prognostic and therapeutic implications, but remains challenging. As indicators of extracellular matrix (ECM) degradation and breakdown of the blood–brain-barrier, Matrix Metalloproteases (MMPs) and A Disintegrin and Metalloproteases (ADAMs) are potential analytes for cerebral pathophysiology and metastatic dissemination of tumor cells into the CSF.

Methods: We compared protease activities in CSF samples from patients with NM and control individuals using FRET-based metalloprotease substrates with distinct enzyme selectivity profiles in a real-time, multiplex approach termed "proteolytic activity matrix assay" (PrAMA). Protease activity dynamics can be tracked by fluorescence changes over time. By simultaneously monitoring a panel of 5 FRET-substrate cleavages, a proteolytic signature can be identified and analyzed to infer the activities of multiple specific proteases. Distinct patterns of substrate cleavage comparing disease vs. control samples allow rapid, reproducible and sensitive discrimination even in small volumes of CSF.

Results: Individual substrate cleavage rates were linked to distinct proteases, and PrAMA computational inference implied increased activities of MMP-9, ADAM8 and ADAM17 (4–5-fold on average) in CSF samples from NM patients that were inhibitable by the metalloprotease inhibitor batimastat (BB-94). The activities of these proteases correlated with blood–brain barrier impairment. Notably, CSF cell counts were not found to directly reflect the protease activities observed in CSF samples from NM patients; this may explain the frequent clinical observation of negative cytology in NM patients.

Conclusion: PrAMA analysis of CSF samples is a potential diagnostic method for sensitive detection of NM and may be suitable for the clinical routine.

Keywords: Neoplastic meningitis, Metalloproteases, CSF, Real-time protease activities, FRET-substrates

Background

Leptomeningeal metastasis (LM) resulting in Neoplastic Meningitis (NM) is a spread of malignant cells to the leptomeninges, the subarachnoid space and dissemination of tumor cells within the cerebrospinal fluid (CSF). NM is a complication of patients with progressive cancer (70%) and prognosis is poor once manifest NM with neurological deficits develops [1]. Patients with breast cancer, lung cancer, malignant melanoma and hematopoietic neoplasms are affected most frequently [1, 2].

Recently, the combination of neurological examination, radiographic imaging of the neuroaxis and CSF cytology are used to diagnose NM [3, 4]. However, all

*Correspondence: strik@med.uni-marburg.de; jbartsch@med.uni-marburg.de
[1] Department of Neurology, Philipps University Marburg, Baldingerstr, 35033 Marburg, Germany
[3] Department of Neurosurgery, Philipps University Marburg, Baldingerstr, 35033 Marburg, Germany
Full list of author information is available at the end of the article

these techniques suffer from limitations and may only detect NM at an advanced stage of malignant CSF invasion. CSF cytology has the highest specificity in diagnosis and detects tumor cells in the CSF in >95%, however the sensitivity of this method is generally less than 50% [3]. Depending on the quality of the cytospin preparation and the expertise of the clinical professional, the diagnostic accuracy of the CSF analysis is variable [2, 4]. Early diagnosis of NM as well as therapy monitoring is crucial for the patient outcome and an important prerequisite for disease control, since NM of solid tumors without therapy progresses to death within 4–6 weeks accompanied by severe neurological symptoms [5, 6]. To overcome the lack of sensitivity, research has focused on biomarkers and characterization of tumor cells in the CSF [7–10]. Proteomic approaches attempted to relate differential CSF protein profiles obtained from mass spectrometry-based studies to neoplastic diseases to identify potential biomarkers [11, 12]. Nevertheless, it is difficult to attribute disease identification and progression to a single protein. CSF profiling of the biological activity of multiple biomarkers may more accurately reflect the pathophysiological processes than one biomarker, increasing specificity and sensitivity [13].

The metastatic invasion of tumor cells and dissemination to secondary sites is promoted by deregulated activity of extracellular metalloproteases (MPs), such as matrix metalloproteases (MMPs) and A Disintegrin and Metalloproteases (ADAMs). Both classes of proteases are members the metzincin superfamily, meaning that they utilize a complexed zinc ion in their catalytic site to constitute proteolytic activity. Major roles for MMPs and ADAMs in cancer progression have been reported, in particular, tumor cell invasion, angiogenesis and metastasis [14, 15]. Cancer promoting protease function is part of a tightly regulated multidirectional network of numerous proteolytic enzymes and their physiological inhibitors, which is modulated context-dependent and involves proteolytic interactions of tumor, stromal and infiltrating immune cells [16]. The biological activities of MMPs and ADAMs in the context of neoplastic meningitis remain less clear but likely given the dissemination of tumor cells through the Virchow–Robin space into the CSF as outlined (Additional file 1: Fig. S1). The occurrence of extracellular proteases in the CSF has been reported under various pathological conditions of the brain including infection [17–21], inflammation [22–26], neurodegeneration [27–32], ischemia [33, 34] and neoplasm [35, 36]. Proteolytic enzymes involved in the disturbance of tissue integrity and the penetration of tumor cells into the subarachnoid space could serve as diagnostic markers for NM [37, 38]. Thus, the analysis of specific patterns of protease activation in the CSF may reflect whether a condition is benign or malignant, and may be a suitable approach for specific and sensitive detection of NM.

In order to obtain metalloprotease profiles for patients with NM in a pilot study, we utilized a multiplex approach for simultaneous detection of MMP and ADAM activities in the CSF of patients with NM compared to control individuals and tumor patients without NM. The Proteolytic Activity Matrix Analysis (PrAMA) is a combined experimental and mathematical method based on time-lapse fluorescence measurements of a panel of moderately specific FRET-based polypeptides in small volumes of biological samples. The observed cleavage patterns are compared to a standard table of catalytic efficiencies measured from purified mixtures of recombinant metalloproteinases and should reflect changes in specific enzyme activities [13, 39] in CSF samples from patients affected by NM.

Methods

Recruitment of patient cohorts and collection of cerebrospinal fluid (CSF)

This pilot study obtained ethical approval from the local Ethics Committee (Marburg University; File No. 101/15). Informed consent was provided from patients to use their biological specimens and clinicopathological data for research purposes. No selection criteria were applied, i.e. all available patients with suspected diagnosis of NM and with brain metastases undergoing routine lumbar puncture were recruited into the study. CSF samples in the control group were collected during therapeutic lumbar punctures from patients with normal pressure hydrocephalus (3/12) or idiopathic intracranial hypertension (9/12). Patients with normal CSF cytology and blood–brain-barrier (BBB) physiology without clinical evidence for neuro-infectious, neuro-inflammatory, neuro-degenerative or neoplastic brain pathologies were considered as controls. All CSF samples were collected at the Department of Neurology, Philipps University Marburg, Germany. Lumbar puncture to collect CSF was performed by medical staff according to clinical guidelines. Upon collection, CSF served primarily for diagnostic purposes, remaining CSF was placed on ice and centrifuged at 1000*g* to remove cells. Clarified CSF was aliquoted, snap-frozen in liquid nitrogen and stored at −80 °C for further analysis. Clinicopathological features were documented pseudonymized, patients were grouped in control individuals (crtl), patients with neoplastic meningitis (NM) and patients with brain metastases without neoplastic meningitis (w/o NM) according to neurological examination, contrast-enhanced MRI of the brain and neuroaxis and CSF cytology for clinical diagnosis.

Determination of MMP/ADAM activities in CSF

Cell-free cerebrospinal fluids were tested for MMP/ADAM activity by using the Proteolytic Activity Matrix Analysis (PrAMA) technique developed by Miller et al. using FRET-based polypeptide substrates PEPDab005, PEPDab010, PEPDab008, PEPDab013 and PEPDab014 (BioZyme Inc, Apex, NC), which vary in their specificities towards different ADAM family members and MMPs. PrAMA analysis was performed as described earlier [13, 39]. Briefly, for time-lapse fluorimetry, a final substrate concentration of 10 μM (diluted from 5 mM stock in DMSO) in 50 μl of activity buffer (1 μM $ZnCl_2$, 20 mM Tris–HCl pH 8.0, 10 mM $CaCl_2$, 150 mM NaCl, 6×10^{-4}% Brij-35) was incubated with 50 μl of CSF using 96-well microtiter white opaque plates, each sample was run in technical triplicates. Samples containing sufficient volumes were included for inhibitor studies and repetitive measurements. To some samples, the broad-range MMP/ADAM inhibitor batimastat (Tocris Bioscience, Bio-Techne, Wiesbaden, Germany) was added at a concentration of 1 μM dissolved in DMSO. Fluorescence units versus time were monitored with a Fluostar BMG Optima using excitation and emission wavelengths of 485 and 530 nM at 37 °C, respectively. A non-linear model was used for curve fitting as described previously [13], the signal of a negative control was subtracted (FRET-substrate only) and time-lapse fluorimetry data were normalized to a positive control (0.01% Trypsin). Specific protease activities were inferred with PrAMA by comparing the pattern of substrate cleavage rates for each sample to a matrix of known substrate specificities for ADAM8, ADAM17, MMP-2 and MMP-9 that was determined using purified enzymes [13]. All calculations and statistical evaluation of data was conducted using Matlab (2014b, MathWorks, Natick, MA).

Statistical analysis

The increase in fluorescence resulting from substrate proteolysis was tracked every 5 min for 4 h. For interpretation of time-lapse fluorimetry data, a non-linear curve-fitting model that accounted for substrate depletion and photobleaching decay served to determine cleavage rates. Cleavage rates are all presented in heat maps averaged over technical triplicates, clear outliers were excluded using Dixon's Q-Test with a 90% threshold. PrAMA inference was performed as described previously with 30% sampling error and threshold $\sigma_T = 1.4$ [13]. Based on normal distribution of values as tested by the David test at the significance level $p = 90\%$, statistical significance was determined using a two-tailed unpaired Student's *t test* to compare two sample groups. To compare more than two experimental groups, Analysis of Variance (ANOVA) was used. Values are denoted as not significant (ns, $p \geq 0.05$), significant * ($p \leq 0.05$), highly significant ** ($p \leq 0.01$), or very highly significant *** ($p \leq 0.001$).

To group the generated datasets, observed average cleavage rates were hierarchically biclustered mean-centered and variance-normalized by row, using Euclidean distance, average linkage and optimal leaf order. Clear patterns emerging from cluster analysis are indicated by dendrograms flanking the array.

To investigate the relationship between CSF cell count, blood–brain-barrier impairment and protease activities, Pearson's correlation coefficients (r) were calculated between these parameters, respectively. Statistical significance (p) was determined as described in the section above.

Results

Patient groups

According to the clinical diagnosis of medical professionals at the department of Neurology, patients were assigned to one of three groups: patients with neoplastic meningitis (NM, $n = 12$), patients with brain metastases but without leptomeningeal tumor spread (w/o NM, $n = 12$) or controls (ctrl, $n = 12$). CSF controls were characterized by normal CSF cytology, physiological protein concentrations, normal albumin and immunoglobulin quotients and absence of oligoclonal IgG bands, thus excluding inflammation, infection and impairment of the blood–brain-barrier. Comparison of baseline demographics for each group did not show significant differences. The mean age was 58.0 years (range 48–60 years) for patients with NM, 53.5 years (range 24–75 years) for patients with brain metastases w/o NM and 41.2 years (range 20–68 years) for controls. In our patient cohort, the NM cases were solely from female patients (gender male/female: NM 0/12) since NM is most prevalent in breast cancer patients. Accordingly, we recruited patients w/o NM and control group as far as possible from other female patients so that the proportion of female patients was higher than males (gender male/female: w/o NM 3/9 and crtl 1/11).

Protease activity is increased in the CSF of patients with neoplastic meningitis

Clinically obtained CSF samples from controls, patients with NM and patients with brain metastases but no leptomeningeal metastasis were subjected to time-lapse fluorimetry and analyzed for substrate cleavage rates of FRET peptides PEPDab 5, 8, 10, 13 and 14 in parallel (Fig. 1a; Additional file 1: Table S1). Distinct patterns of protease activity for disease and control samples were found. Overall, the observed reaction rates showed the strongest activity with PEPDab#10, which is most efficiently cleaved by ADAM17 [13]. Second strongest

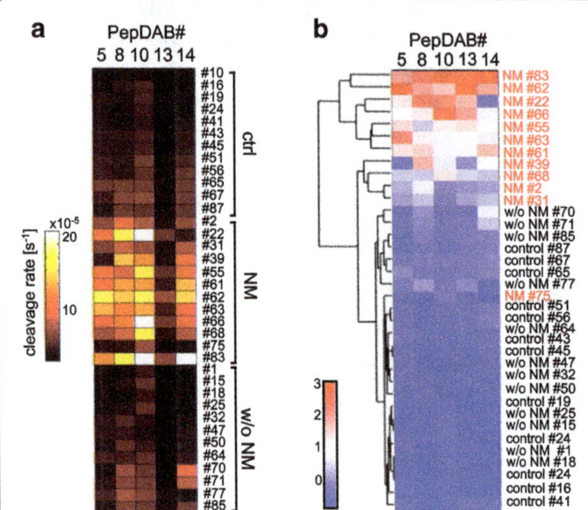

Fig. 1 Analysis of protease activities in the CSF of three patient cohorts. Cleavage signatures in CSF samples were analyzed from 12 control individuals (crtl), 12 patients with neoplastic meningitis (NM) and 12 patients with brain metastases of different primary tumors, but without neoplastic meningitis (w/o NM). Protease activities in real-time mode were determined using PEPDab substrates 5, 8, 10, 13 and 14 at final concentrations of 10 μM for 4 h. Heat map summarizing mean cleavage rates of 3 technical replicates for each clinical samples calculated from time-lapse fluorimetry **a**. Hierarchical bi-clustering result corresponding to (**a**), with data mean-centered and variance-normalized by row. CSF cleavage patterns of patients with NM (labeled *red*) cluster closely together, control individuals and patients with brain metastases w/o NM group together without forming main clusters for each condition (**b**)

substrate cleavage was detected for PEPDab#8, which is most selective for MMP-9. We discovered that enzymatic activity tracked by time-lapse fluorimetry increased in the CSF of patients with NM, whereas cleavage rates in the CSF of control individuals and patients with brain metastases w/o NM were similar and remained close to background fluorescence. Cleavage rates in the CSF were significantly different between ctrl and NM, as well as between NM and w/o NM for all PEPDab substrates analysed ($p = 0.01$ for PEPDab 5; $p = 4.2 \times 10^{-6}$ for PEPDab 8; $p = 0.00013$ for PEPDab 10; $p = 0.09$ for PEPDab 13; $p = 0.0009$ for PEPDab 14) whereas there were no significant changes detectable between crtl and patients with brain metastatic cancer w/o NM.

Resulting sample cleavage patterns were hierarchically bi-clustered, mean-centered and variance-standardized using Euclidean distance, average linkage and optimal leaf ordering (Fig. 1b). This type of cluster analysis groups 88% of the NM CSF samples in two main clusters as indicated by the dendrogram flanking the array; in contrast, substrate cleavage patterns in CSF samples of control individuals and patients with brain metastases w/o NM cluster closely together with no clear pattern. Of the NM CSF samples, sample#75 is the only one that does integrate into the group of neoplastic meningitis. These results suggest that disease samples can be clearly distinguished from control samples by their substrate cleavage signature.

Inference of protease identities in CSF samples revealed by the PrAMA method

Individual time-lapse measurement derived from relatively non-specific FRET-substrates can not generally be understood to relate to specific proteases. To address this issue, PrAMA inference uses panels of FRET-substrate cleavage measurements, coupled with known catalytic efficiencies previously determined with recombinant enzymes [13], Fig. 2a), to elucidate particular enzyme activities from cleavage signatures obtained in clinical samples containing multiple proteases. PrAMA inference is strengthened by comparison of reaction rates in the presence and absence of specific inhibitors [13]. We analyzed all CSF samples using a set of five PEPDab substrates along with the broad-spectrum MP inhibitor batimastat (BB-94). Addition of 1 μM BB-94 reduced the observed rates by at least 50% on average, supporting that although MMP and ADAM activities are the major components of the observed substrate cleavage, other non-MMP/ADAM protease activities are present in the samples (Fig. 2b). PrAMA inference of specific protease activities revealed significant differences between crtl and NM for MMP-9 (4.5-fold, $p = 9.9 \times 10^{-6}$), ADAM8 (4.7-fold, $p = 0.00054$) and ADAM17 (4.8 fold, $p = 0.00051$). Changes for MMP-2 were not significant, ADAM10 was not identified in the enzyme composition of the CSF samples by PrAMA. Of the proteases identified, PrAMA inference suggests the activities of MMP-9 and ADAM17 were the highest on average (Fig. 2c). To confirm that the observed peptide cleavage patterns are correlated with NM and not with a general presence of a malignancy, we included a patient cohort in our analyses with metastases but without leptomeningeal involvement.

Substrate cleavage patterns in CSF in follow-up lumbar CSF punctures

Following initial diagnosis of NM, patients are undergoing regular follow-up lumbar punctures in the clinical routine for intrathecal chemotherapeutic treatment and monitoring of disease progression. CSF samples obtained from patients who underwent 2-month follow-up lumbar punctures with cytologically proven stable diagnosis were subjected to PrAMA to demonstrate reproducibility of results. For all patient samples analyzed, substrate cleavage patterns in the CSF remained similar compared to baseline cleavage (Fig. 3a). Consistently, the inferred protease activities resembled baseline activities for ADAM8,

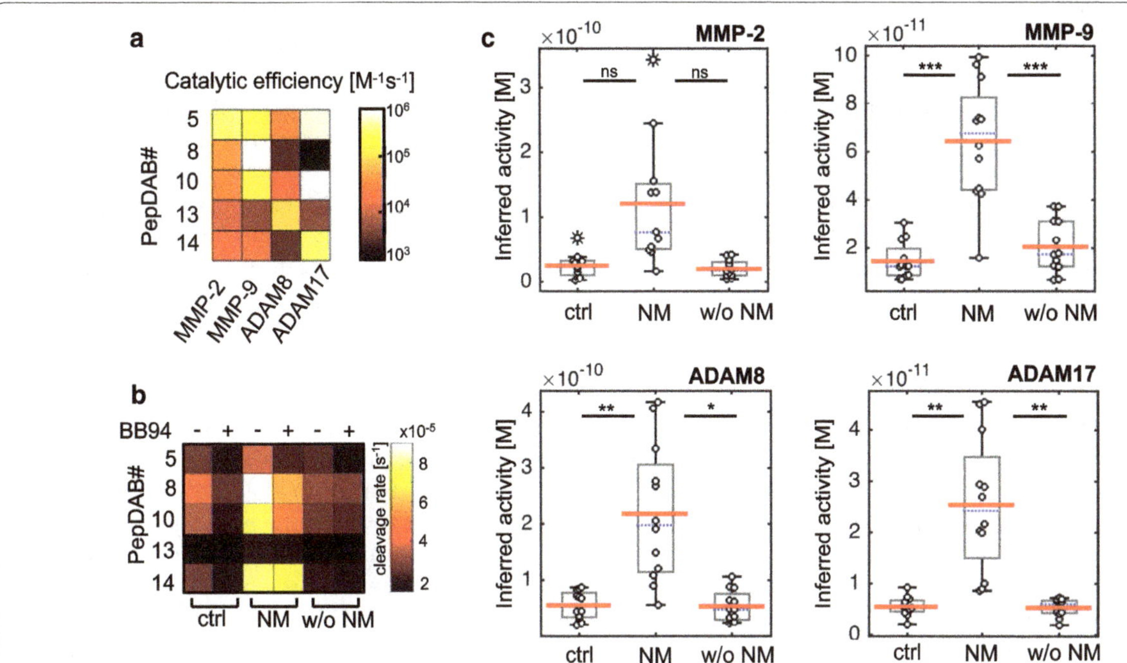

Fig. 2 Inferred protease activitity of MMP-9, ADAM8 and ADAM17 in CSF is increased in neoplastic meningitis. Catalytic efficiencies for FRET-based peptide substrates have been determined previously across a panel of purified recombinant enzymes [13]. Observed cleavage efficiencies for MMP-2, MMP-9, ADAM8 and ADAM17 for PEPDab Substrates 5, 8, 10, 13 and 14 (modified from [13] are shown **a**. Effects of broad-spectrum MMP-inhibitor batimastat (BB-94+) treatment on observed substrate cleavage in representative CSF samples. Combination of specific substrates and inhibitors allow to infer protease activities accurately (**b**). PrAMA inferred the cleavage signatures from (Fig. 1a), using parameters from (**a**). PrAMA inference results in CSF in patients with NM were compared to control individuals and patients with brain metastases w/o NM. The *box* indicates the interquartile range, *blue bar* indicates the median, *red bar* denote the mean values and *whiskers* indicate the 95% confidence interval. *Open dots* represent the individual samples (o), extreme values are marked with *asterisks*. Inferred differences were statistically significant for MMP-9, ADAM8 and ADAM17, stars indicate * p <0.01; ** p <0.005, *** p <0.001 (**c**)

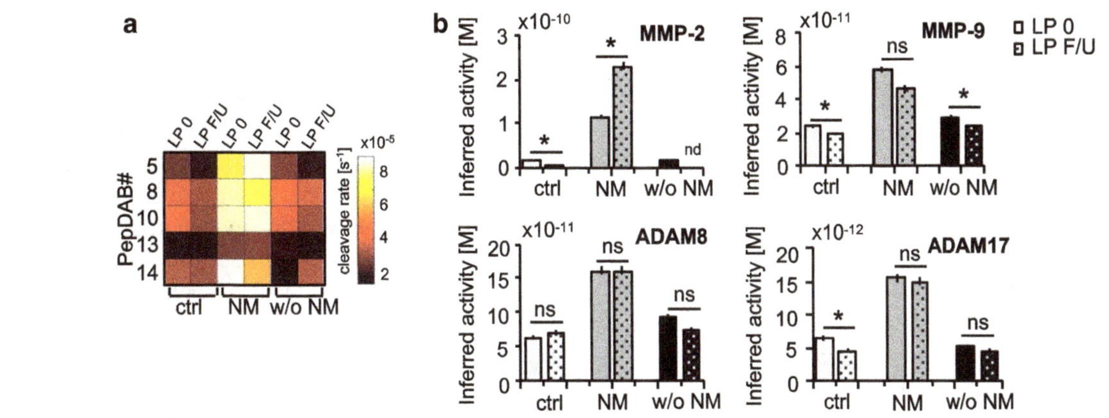

Fig. 3 PrAMA inference results are reproducible in follow-up lumbar punctures (LP). Substrate cleavage patterns in CSF samples obtained from same patients with unchanged clinical diagnosis within a time period of 2 months, baseline substrate cleavage in CSF is denoted as LP 0, cleavage rates in CSF of 2-month follow-up (F/U) lumbar punctures as LP F/U. Substrate cleavage is shown for controls (ctrl), patients with neoplastic meningitis (NM) and patients with brain metastases w/o NM in a heatmap (**a**). PrAMA inferred the cleavage signatures from (Fig. 2a), using parameters from (**a**). Calculated protease activities are presented as bar graph (*light grey*, control individuals; *grey*, NM; *black*, w/o NM), *error bars* indicate standard deviation of three technical replicates, *dotted columns* denote 2-months follow-up lumbar punctures, respectively (**b**). Note that both, cleavage patterns and PrAMA inference results, remain similiar for controls, NM and the patient with brain metastases w/o NM. Two-tailed, one-sample *t test* was used to compare initial protease activities with 2-month follow-up measurements, values were not significant (ns, $p \geq 0.05$) or significant * ($p \leq 0.05$)

ADAM17 and MMP-9 as observed in the respective CSF (Fig. 3b).

Correlation of protease activities with CSF cell counts and BBB disturbance

Conflicting results concerning the relationship of protease expression and CSF cell count have been reported for certain MMPs, and so far, only few studies have investigated the biological activity of proteases in CSF. For MMP-9, there were studies describing either a positive or a non-linear correlation of protein levels, CSF cell count and blood–brain-barrier impairment in various neurological diseases [21, 24, 27, 40].

To overcome this problem, we sought to use the PrAMA method that allows for sensitive detection of biochemical parameters reflecting the process of cellular invasion into the leptomeningeal space. Therefore we analyzed 16 patients presenting with pleocytosis in CSF cytology, including patients with neurological pathologies other than NM, to elucidate the relationship between substrate cleavage, cell count and CSF/serum albumin ratio, a routine parameter indicating blood–brain-barrier disturbance. Pearson's correlation statistics revealed a significant correlation of substrate cleavage rates and BBB impairment (expressed by the QAlb, albumin quotient) with a high to good correlation coefficient (r) depending on the inclusion of one patient (Additional file 1: Figs. S2 and S3). In contrast, cleavage rates and CSF cell count did not correlate, as no correlation coefficient was higher than 0.075 (Additional file 1: Fig. S3). The cellular source of the observed protease activity remains unclear; however, our results indicate that mere appearance of certain cell populations in the CSF does not reflect their biological activation. Notably, increased, uncontrolled MMP activation is implicated to play crucial roles in cerebral pathophysiology by mediating disruption of the blood–brain-barrier integrity and worsening the outcome [37, 38, 41]. In accordance, BBB disruption may be a result of increased protease activity in the CSF and vice versa.

Therapeutic progression monitoring of neoplastic meningitis by PrAMA

The key factor in the outcome of NM is early diagnosis, because even though clinically manifest NM is treated aggressively with a combination of radiation, systemic and intrathecal chemotherapy, therapy is palliative with the goal to extend survival and improve neurologic symptoms [6]. In order to evaluate whether PrAMA can be used to monitor therapy outcome, a case of a 62-year old breast cancer patient with leptomeningeal metastasis was assessed with collection of CSF samples before treatment and 3 months after intrathecal chemotherapy with liposomal cytarabine (cytosine arabinoside, araC, Fig. 4). Following treatment with araC for 3 months, substrate cleavage rates and inferred protease activities decreased by 2.3-, 2.4.- and fourfold for ADAM8, MMP-9 and ADAM17, respectively, after intrathecal treatment with araC, whereas the MMP-2 activity was not significantly changed. Coincidently the status of the patient appeared stable over 2 years together with continuously low protease activities. Thus, protease activity profiles may have clinical implementation to sensitively monitor treatment efficacy and disease progression (Fig. 4).

Discussion

Since abnormalities on MRI or in CSF require a substantial extent of disease in the case of leptomeningeal metastasis, it is likely that treatment delay due to the insensitivity of current methodologies contributes to the poor prognosis in NM. On the molecular level, CSF is a heterogeneous mixture of a low number of leukocytes, debris, small amounts of soluble protein, and tumor cells in the case of NM. The cellular components in the CSF are an important source of proteins determining the course of the disease relevance. Small molecules deriving from the brain or the blood reach the CSF compartment via diffusion. Conventional analytic approaches such as ELISA or Western Blot are often not suitable to detect low-abundance protein biomarkers in the CSF, which is characterized by a very low concentration of proteins. Compositional mass spectrometry-based proteomic studies of the CSF help to gain insight into dynamic disease-related changes, but generally are too complex for clinical routine [42]. Here we attempted to overcome this diagnostic constraint by providing a sensitive method of detecting increased proteolytic activities in small volumes of CSF samples only in NM patients with a reproducible and significant difference to samples from patients with brain metastasis and control patients.

MMP2, MMP-9, ADAM8, and ADAM17 are increased in CSF samples from NM patients. For a single case of a clinically stable patient, that is with no signs of impairment based on cytology, MRI and neurological examination, we observed almost similar activity values with the exception of MMP-2, which slightly increased in the follow-up sample. Moreover, in another patient treated intrathecally with the antimetabolite cytarabine, the increase of MMP-2 and all other proteases examined could be reverted, suggesting that the therapeutic progress is reflected by a decrease in MMP and ADAM activities as observed here.

Although we can clearly distinguish CSF samples from NM patients in contrast to control individuals and patients with brain metastases, the result of the PrAMA analysis has some limitations: firstly PrAMA inference suggests a major contribution of distinct proteases to the

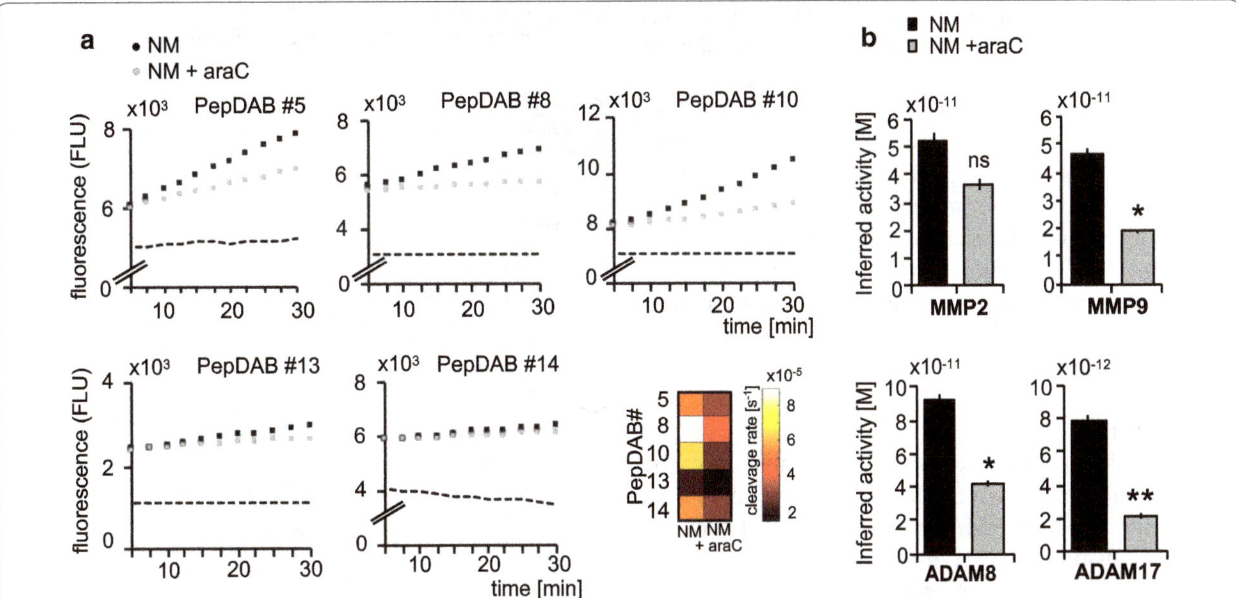

Fig. 4 Protease activity decreases following intrathecal treatment with liposomal cytarabin. In a 62-year old breast cancer patient with leptomeningeal metastasis, protease activities were analyzed prior and after intrathecal treatment with liposomal cytarabin. Time-lapse fluorimetry output of the same patient with neoplastic meningitis arising from breast cancer previous (NM, black dots) and following treatment of NM with Cytarabin (araC) (NM + AraC, grey dots) for 3 months. Substrate tracking (PEPDab 5, 8, 10, 13 and 14) for 30 min averaged over 3 technical replicates is shown, *dashed line* indicates the negative control. Cleavage rates were calculated as described previously using a non-linear kinetic model to fit the time-lapse data (**a**). PrAMA inference results for samples analysed in A, using significance threshold $\sigma_T = 1.4$. *Error bars* indicate standard deviation of technical triplicates (**b**). Two-tailed, one-sample *t test* was used to compare cleavage rates pre and post treatment with araC. Values were not significant (ns, $p \geq 0.05$), significant * ($p \leq 0.05$) or highly significant ** ($p \leq 0.01$)

observed metalloprotease activities, as they can be partially inhibited by BB-94 that works on MMP-2, MMP-9, ADAM8, ADAM17; secondly, based on activities not inhibited by BB-94, we postulate protease activities other than metalloproteases present in CSF samples.

With respect to the identity of the metalloproteases, we have attempted to confirm their presence by ELISA. Only in a very severe case of NM, a 53-year old patient with progressive breast cancer with severe neurologic deficits and diagnosis based on CSF cytology, we were able to detect MMP-9 and TNF-RI (as ADAM17 substrate) by ELISA (Additional file 1: Fig. S4). From this CSF sample, activities determined by PrAMA were up to 10-times higher than in all other NM cases. According to Dixon's Q-Test, this sample was defined as outlier and excluded from cluster analysis. Clusters of atypical, malignant cells dominated the cytogram and the blood–brain-barrier function was strongly impaired as determined by an albumin quotient of 80.4. Although multimodal treatment was initiated immediately, NM in this patient progressed to death within 3 months.

Although our results provide pilot data for the high impact of CSF profiling in disease at present, they underscore the value of multiplexing, i.e. with respect to a microfluidic platform [43] and to a series of other diseases related to CSF changes. Future studies in larger patient cohorts are required to validate our preliminary results. Mechanistically, invasion of malignant cells into the leptomeninges and the CSF is a multistep process that requires differential expression of migration- and invasion-related proteins. On a time scale, disease-related changes in the composition of the CSF are expected to precede transmigration of cells into the CSF. Most likely, the proteolytic activity in the CSF may increase before pathological signs can be detected by MRI or CSF cytology. The case of a 62 year-old patient with minimal CSF involvement from breast cancer surviving more than two years, which is described before, underlines the clinical experience that early detection and subsequent treatment of malignant cells in the CSF is crucial for long-term control of neoplastic meningitis. Very early detection of subclinical CSF invasion may therefore be crucial to improve the otherwise frustrating results of NM treatment.

Clinical data known to date implicate that conventional therapies are not sufficient to achieve long-term control or remission in cases of neoplastic meningitis (Strik, Proemmel 2010). Molecularly targeted therapies that aim at preventing tumor cells from invasion into the CSF space may offer more efficacy. At present, several pharmacological inhibitors of MPs are already available and ADAM-inhibitors are being developed. After a more detailed analysis of the pathophysiological mechanisms, pharmacological inhibition of MPs and ADAM proteins may be efficient tools to prevent or treat malignant CSF-invasion.

In this respect, our results from a multiplexed assay provide a novel perspective into MMP/ADAM contribution to the pathophysiology of NM. More importantly, the simple profiling of protease activities in CSF samples from patients with medical indications seems to reflect individual context-dependent protease function in invasive diseases and should be explored in a larger cohort of NM patients but also in other clinical applications including infectious diseases in the CNS.

Conclusion

Based on these pilot data we demonstrated that the simultaneous detection of metalloprotease activities in CSF samples by the PrAMA method could be of diagnostic value to distinguish NM from metastasis without NM and from controls with normal CSF. The observed cleavage profiles are consistently present in patients with a positive follow-up analysis and are modulated by successful treatment of NM. Moreover, we detected ADAM8, MMP-9, and ADAM17 activities in the CSF as major analytes in the CSF of patients with NM.

Abbreviations

ADAM: A Disintegrin And Metalloprotease; araC: cytarabin; BB-94: batimastat; BBB: blood-brain-barrier; Crtl: control; CSF: cerebrospinal fluid; ECM: extracellular matrix; ELISA: enzyme-linked immunosorbent assay; FRET: fluorescence resonance energy transfer; MMP: matrix-metallo-Protease; MP: metalloprotease; nd: not detectable; NM: neoplastic meningitis; ns: not significant; PrAMA: proteolytic activity matrix assay; QAlb: albumin quotient; w/o: without.

Authors' contributions

The study was conceived by CC, HS, and JWB, experiments were designed by CC and JWB, CC and KD performed the experiments, CC and MAM analyzed and interpreted the data, the final manuscript was prepared by CC, HS, MAM, DAL and JWB, the whole study was supervised by JWB. All authors read and approved the final manuscript.

Author details

[1] Department of Neurology, Philipps University Marburg, Baldingerstr, 35033 Marburg, Germany. [2] Department of Anesthesiology and Intensive Care Medicine, University Hospital, Albert-Schweitzer Campus 1, 48149 Münster, Germany. [3] Department of Neurosurgery, Philipps University Marburg, Baldingerstr, 35033 Marburg, Germany. [4] Department of Biological Engineering, Massachusetts Institute of Technology, Cambridge, MA 02139, USA. [5] Center for Systems Biology, Massachusetts General Hospital, Harvard Medical School, Boston, MA 02114, USA.

Acknowledgements

The authors wish to thank G. Engel, A. Hehenkamp, D. Blecker, S. Motzny, and M. Happel for help with CSF collection and patient documentation and S. Rakow for initial help with CSF analysis. We are grateful to M. Moss for helpful discussions.

Competing interests

The authors declare that they have no competing interests.

Funding

Work was generously supported by the P.E. Kempkes Foundation, Marburg, Germany.

References

1. Gleissner B, Chamberlain MC. Neoplastic meningitis. Lancet Neurol. 2006;5:443–52.
2. Strik H, Prömmel P. Diagnosis and individualized therapy of neoplastic meningitis. Expert Rev Anticancer Ther. 2010;10:1137–48.
3. Chamberlain MC, Glantz M, Groves MD, Wilson WH. Diagnostic tools for neoplastic meningitis: detecting disease, identifying patient risk, and determining benefit of treatment. Semin Oncol. 2009;36:S35–45.
4. Prömmel P, Pilgram-Pastor S, Sitter H, Buhk JH, Strik H. Neoplastic meningitis: How MRI and CSF cytology are influenced by CSF cell count and tumor type. Sci World J. 2013;2013:248072.
5. Grossman SA, Krabak MJ. Leptomeningeal carcinomatosis. Cancer Treat Rev. 1999;25:103–19.
6. DeAngelis LM, Boutros D. Leptomeningeal metastasis. Cancer Invest. 2005;23:145–54.
7. Weston CL, Glantz MJ, Connor JR. Detection of cancer cells in the cerebrospinal fluid: current methods and future directions. Fluids Barriers CNS. 2011;8:14.
8. Groves MD, Hess KR, Puduvalli VK, Colman H, Conrad CA, Gilbert MR, Weinberg J, Cristofanilli M, Yung WK, Liu TJ. Biomarkers of disease: cerebrospinal fluid vascular endothelial growth factor (VEGF) and stromal cell derived factor (SDF)-1 levels in patients with neoplastic meningitis (NM) due to breast cancer, lung cancer and melanoma. J Neurooncol. 2009;94:229–34.
9. Hegde U, Filie A, Little RF, Janik JE, Grant N, Steinberg SM, Dunleavy K, Jaffe ES, Abati A, Stetler-Stevenson M, Wilson WH. High incidence of occult leptomeningeal disease detected by flow cytometry in newly diagnosed aggressive B-cell lymphomas at risk for central nervous system involvement: the role of flow cytometry versus cytology. Blood. 2005;105:496–502.
10. Bromberg JE, Breems DA, Kraan J, Bikker G, van der Holt B, Smitt PS, van den Bent MJ, van't Veer M, Gratama JW. CSF flow cytometry greatly improves diagnostic accuracy in CNS hematologic malignancies. Neurology. 2007;68:1674–9.
11. Römpp A, Dekker L, Taban I, Jenster G, Boogerd W, Bonfrer H, Spengler B, Heeren R, Smitt PS, Luider TM. Identification of leptomeningeal metastasis-related proteins in cerebrospinal fluid of patients with breast cancer by a combination of MALDI-TOF, MALDI-FTICR and nanoLC-FTICR MS. Proteomics. 2007;7:474–81.
12. Roy S, Josephson SA, Fridlyand J, Karch J, Kadoch C, Karrim J, Damon L, Treseler P, Kunwar S, Shuman MA, Jones T, Becker CH, Schulman H, Rubenstein JL. Protein biomarker identification in the CSF of patients with CNS lymphoma. J Clin Oncol. 2008;26:96–105.
13. Miller MA, Barkal L, Jeng K, Herrlich A, Moss M, Griffith LG, Lauffenburger DA. Proteolytic Activity Matrix Analysis (PrAMA) for simultaneous determination of multiple protease activities. Integr Biol. 2011;3:422–38.
14. Mochizuki S, Okada Y. ADAMs in cancer cell proliferation and progression. Cancer Sci. 2007;98:621–8.
15. Kessenbrock K, Plaks V, Werb Z. Matrix metalloproteinases: regulators of the tumor microenvironment. Cell. 2010;141:52–67.
16. Mason SD, Joyce JA. Proteolytic networks in cancer. Trends Cell Biol. 2011;21:228–37.
17. Jones D, Alvarez E, Selva S, Gilden D, Nagel MA. Proinflammatory cytokines and matrix metalloproteinases in CSF of patients with VZV vasculopathy. Neurol Neuroimmunol Neuroinflamm. 2016;3:e246.
18. Patil T, Garg RK, Jain A, Goel MM, Malhotra HS, Verma R, Singh GP, Sharma PK. Serum and CSF cytokines and matrix metalloproteinases in spinal tuberculosis. Inflamm Res. 2015;64:97–106.
19. Perides G, Charness ME, Tanner LM, Péter O, Satz N, Steere AC, Klempner MS. Matrix metalloproteinases in the cerebrospinal fluid of patients with Lyme neuroborreliosis. J Infect Dis. 1998;177:401–8.

20. Kolb SA, Lahrtz F, Paul R, Leppert D, Nadal D, Pfister HW, Fontana A. Matrix metalloproteinases and tissue inhibitors of metalloproteinases in viral meningitis: upregulation of MMP-9 and TIMP-1 in cerebrospinal fluid. J Neuroimmunol. 1998;84:143–50.
21. Leppert D, Leib SL, Grygar C, Miller KM, Schaad UB, Holländer GA. Matrix metalloproteinase (MMP)-8 and MMP-9 in cerebrospinal fluid during bacterial meningitis: association with blood–brain barrier damage and neurological sequelae. Clin Infect Dis. 2000;31:80–4.
22. Uchida T, Mori M, Uzawa A, Masuda H, Muto M, Ohtani R, Kuwabara S. Increased cerebrospinal fluid metalloproteinase-2 and interleukin-6 are associated with albumin quotient in neuromyelitis optica: their possible role on blood–brain barrier disruption. Mult Scler J. 2016;23(8):1072–84.
23. Kieseier BC, Pischel H, Neuen-Jacob E, Tourtellotte WW, Hartung HP. ADAM-10 and ADAM-17 in the inflamed human CNS. Glia. 2003;42:398–405.
24. Leppert D, Ford J, Stabler G, Grygar C, Lienert C, Huber S, Miller KM, Hauser SL, Kappos L. Matrix metalloproteinase-9 (gelatinase B) is selectively elevated in CSF during relapses and stable phases of multiple sclerosis. Brain. 1998;121(Pt 12):2327–34.
25. Avolio C, Ruggieri M, Giuliani F, Liuzzi GM, Leante R, Riccio P, Livrea P, Trojano M. Serum MMP-2 and MMP-9 are elevated in different multiple sclerosis subtypes. J Neuroimmunol. 2003;136:46–53.
26. Light M, Minor KH, DeWitt P, Jasper KH, Davies SJ. Multiplex array proteomics detects increased MMP-8 in CSF after spinal cord injury. J Neuroinflamm. 2012;9:122.
27. Beuche W, Yushchenko M, Mäder M, Maliszewska M, Felgenhauer K, Weber F. Matrix metalloproteinase-9 is elevated in serum of patients with amyotrophic lateral sclerosis. Neuro Rep. 2000;11:3419–22.
28. Adair JC, Charlie J, Dencoff JE, Kaye JA, Quinn JF, Camicioli RM, Stetler-Stevenson WG, Rosenberg GA. Measurement of gelatinase B (MMP-9) in the cerebrospinal fluid of patients with vascular dementia and Alzheimer disease. Stroke. 2004;35:e159–62.
29. Stomrud E, Björkqvist M, Janciauskiene S, Minthon L, Hansson O. Alterations of matrix metalloproteinases in the healthy elderly with increased risk of prodromal Alzheimer's disease. Alzheimers Res Ther. 2010;2:20.
30. Lund TC, Stadem PS, Panoskaltsis-Mortari A, Raymond G, Miller WP, Tolar J, Orchard PJ. Elevated cerebral spinal fluid cytokine levels in boys with cerebral adrenoleukodystrophy correlates with MRI severity. PLoS ONE. 2012;7:e32218.
31. Mroczko B, Groblewska M, Zboch M, Kulczyńska A, Koper OM, Szmitkowski M, Kornhuber J, Lewczuk P. Concentrations of matrix metalloproteinases and their tissue inhibitors in the cerebrospinal fluid of patients with Alzheimer's disease. J Alzheimers Dis. 2014;40:351–7.
32. Jiang H, Hampel H, Prvulovic D, Wallin A, Blennow K, Li R, Shen Y. Elevated CSF levels of TACE activity and soluble TNF receptors in subjects with mild cognitive impairment and patients with Alzheimer's disease. Mol Neurodegener. 2011;6:69.
33. Zhang Y, Fan F, Zeng G, Zhou L, Zhang J, Jiao H, Zhang T, Su D, Yang C, Wang X, Xiao K, Li H, Zhong Z. Temporal analysis of blood-brain barrier disruption and cerebrospinal fluid matrix metalloproteinases in rhesus monkeys subjected to transient ischemic stroke. J Cereb Blood Flow Metab. 2016;37(8):2693–974.
34. Li YJ, Wang ZH, Zhang B, Zhe X, Wang MJ, Shi ST, Bai J, Lin T, Guo CJ, Zhang SJ, Kong XL, Zuo X, Zhao H. Disruption of the blood-brain barrier after generalized tonic-clonic seizures correlates with cerebrospinal fluid MMP-9 levels. J Neuroinflamm. 2013;10:80.
35. Friedberg MH, Glantz MJ, Klempner MS, Cole BF, Perides G. Specific matrix metalloproteinase profiles in the cerebrospinal fluid correlated with the presence of malignant astrocytomas, brain metastases, and carcinomatous meningitis. Cancer. 1998;82:923–30.
36. Si MY, Fan ZC, Li YZ, Chang XL, Xie QD, Jiao XY. The prognostic significance of serum and cerebrospinal fluid MMP-9, CCL2 and sVCAM-1 in leukemia CNS metastasis. J Neurooncol. 2015;122:229–44.
37. Brkic M, Balusu S, Van Wonterghem E, Gorlé N, Benilova I, Kremer A, Van Hove I, Moons L, De Strooper B, Kanazir S, Libert C, Vandenbroucke RE. Amyloid β oligomers disrupt blood-CSF barrier integrity by activating matrix metalloproteinases. J Neurosci. 2015;35:12766–78.
38. Feng S, Cen J, Huang Y, Shen H, Yao L, Wang Y, Chen Z. Matrix metalloproteinase-2 and -9 secreted by leukemic cells increase the permeability of blood-brain barrier by disrupting tight junction proteins. PLoS ONE. 2011;6:e20599.
39. Conrad C, Miller MA, Bartsch JW, Schlomann U, Lauffenburger DA. Simultaneous detection of metalloprotease activities in complex biological samples using the PrAMA (Proteolytic Activity Matrix Assay) method. Methods Mol Biol. 2017;1574:243–53.
40. Paemen L, Olsson T, Söderström M, van Damme J, Opdenakker G. Evaluation of gelatinases and IL-6 in the cerebrospinal fluid of patients with optic neuritis, multiple sclerosis and other inflammatory neurological diseases. Eur J Neurol. 1994;1:55–63.
41. Ong CW, Pabisiak PJ, Brilha S, Singh P, Roncaroli F, Elkington PT, Friedland JS. Complex regulation of neutrophil-derived MMP-9 secretion in central nervous system tuberculosis. J Neuroinflamm. 2017;14:31.
42. Dislich B, Wohlrab F, Bachhuber T, Müller SA, Kuhn PH, Hogl S, Meyer-Luehmann M, Lichtenthaler SF. Label-free quantitative proteomics of mouse Cerebrospinal fluid detects β-Site APP cleaving enzyme (BACE1) protease substrates in vivo. Mol Cell Proteom. 2015;14:2550–63.
43. Chen CH, Miller MA, Sarkar A, Beste MT, Isaacson KB, Lauffenburger DA, Griffith LG, Han J. Multiplexed protease activity assay for low-volume clinical samples using droplet-based microfluidics and its application to endometriosis. J Am Chem Soc. 2013;135:1645–8.

6

A comparison between the pathophysiology of multiple sclerosis and normal pressure hydrocephalus: is pulse wave encephalopathy a component of MS?

Grant A. Bateman[1,2*], Jeannette Lechner-Scott[2,3,4] and Rodney A. Lea[5]

Abstract

Background: It has been suggested there is a chronic neurodegenerative disorder, underlying the pathophysiology of multiple sclerosis (MS), which is distinct from the more obvious immune-mediated attack on the white matter. Limited data exists indicating there is an alteration in pulse wave propagation within the craniospinal cavity in MS, similar to the findings in normal pressure hydrocephalus (NPH). It is hypothesized MS may harbor pulse wave encephalopathy. The purpose of this study is to compare blood flow and pulse wave measurements in MS patients with a cohort of NPH patients and control subjects, to test this hypothesis.

Methods: Twenty patients with MS underwent magnetic resonance (MR) flow quantification techniques. Mean blood flow and stroke volume were measured in the arterial inflow and venous out flow from the sagittal (SSS) and straight sinus (ST). The arteriovenous delay (AVD) was defined. The results were compared with both age-matched controls and NPH patients.

Results: In MS there was a 35 % reduction in arteriovenous delay and a 5 % reduction in the percentage of the arterial inflow returning via the sagittal sinus compared to age matched controls. There was an alteration in pulse wave propagation, with a 26 % increase in arterial stroke volume but 30 % reduction in SSS and ST stroke volume. The AVD and blood flow changes were in the same direction to those of NPH patients.

Conclusions: There are blood flow and pulsation propagation changes in MS patients which are similar to those of NPH patients. The findings would be consistent with an underlying pulse wave encephalopathy component in MS.

Keywords: Multiple sclerosis, Normal pressure hydrocephalus, Cerebral blood flow, Pulse wave encephalopathy, Compliance, Cerebrospinal fluid

Background

Multiple sclerosis (MS) is considered to be an autoimmune inflammatory demyelinating disease of the central nervous system. The histopathology of MS shows inflammation to be most prominent in the white matter of the corpus callosum, subcortical white matter tracts, optic nerve and spinal tracts. There is T cell and macrophage-mediated damage leading to demyelination [1]. The immune-mediated aspects of MS dominate the research literature with all of the currently available therapies directed at modulating the immune response in this disease [2]. Despite the overwhelming dominance of the immune hypothesis in MS research, in a review of the literature, Juurlink noted that although the immune-modulating therapies reduce the number and severity of exacerbations, they do not prevent the long-term progression toward disability in MS [3]. If the amount of brain inflammation occurring during the disease process does not affect the degeneration, this suggests there

*Correspondence: grant.bateman@hnehealth.nsw.gov.au
[1] Department of Medical Imaging, John Hunter Hospital, Locked Bag 1, Newcastle Region Mail Center, Newcastle 2310, Australia
Full list of author information is available at the end of the article

may be some neurodegenerative process, other than the inflammation, mediating the slow decline. Although the autoimmune response of the body could secondarily elicit a neurodegenerative effect, in a major review Stys suggests that it was also possible that MS may be a degenerative disease that secondarily elicits an autoimmune response [4]. In the second scenario, the neurodegenerative disorder would perhaps lead to a breakdown of the blood–brain barrier and damage the myelin, thus leaving the myelin susceptible to immune attack in those individuals who were prone to such a response. Indeed, given that multiple sclerosis is characterized by simultaneous focal breakdown of the blood–brain barrier, the development of demyelinating lesions that are associated with immune-mediated inflammation and eventual axonal loss [3], it may be hard to discern which is the initiating event and which the secondary.

Multiple sclerosis has been noted to have some characteristics in common with normal pressure hydrocephalus (NPH). On the basis of decreased intracranial compliance [5], increased ventricular [6] and Virchow–Robin space size [7], the presence of Hakim's triad [8–10], increased pulsatility of the CSF through the aqueduct [11], reduced net flow of CSF through the same structure [12] together with decreased CSF pulsation at C2 level [13] (all of which are noted in NPH [3]), Juurlink suggested the possible initiating neurodegenerative process could be an underlying pulse wave encephalopathy [3]. Pulse wave encephalopathy was a concept originally developed by one of the current authors to describe how three of the causes of dementia (Alzheimer's disease, vascular dementia and normal pressure hydrocephalus) could be interrelated along a common pathophysiological spectrum [14]. The spectrum was suggested to be related to the strength of the pulse pressure waves induced in the craniospinal cavity by the arterial tree and the way the pulse waves interact with the compliance of the spinal canal and venous system [14]. It was hypothesized, increased arterial pulse pressure, if not damped sufficiently (either because it was too large or the available compliance of the spinal canal and/or veins too small), would lead to elevated capillary and venous pulse pressure and increased aqueduct pulsation (together with other pathological effects) [14]. However, the physiological evidence Juurlink has used to justify MS as being similar to NPH is tenuous at best. Firstly, Gorucu commented that the increase in stroke volume through the aqueduct in MS could be caused by hyperdynamic dilated ventricles secondary to the underlying atrophy [11]. Therefore, the increased aqueduct flow could be passive, rather than part of an active, pulsation driven process. Secondly, the estimation of net CSF flow through the aqueduct using MRI is currently under a cloud. Due to the very low flow rates being measured, the cumulative error in net aqueduct flow measurement is estimated to be up to 30 % [15]. Therefore, this may not be a valid metric. Finally, the reduced stroke volume through the spinal canal in MS was dismissed by the authors of the paper where it was originally described because there was also a reduction in the arterial blood flow in the MS patients. It was assumed there would have been an associated reduced arterial stroke volume and therefore less impetus to move the spinal canal CSF [13]. Therefore, much of the data is missing from the literature which would enable one to answer the question, "Is there an underlying pulse wave encephalopathy component in MS?" The required evidence includes an accurate measure of the total arterial pulsation stroke volume (which is the input into the system driven by pulse pressure), the intracranial compliance (which is the moderator of pulse pressure) and the stroke volume of the venous system (which is an output of the system). The purpose of the current study is to measure these variables utilizing a phase contrast MRI technique directed to the arterial input and venous output in a cohort of MS patients and compare them with normal controls and NPH patients.

Methods

Subjects

Patients with multiple sclerosis (MS) are regularly followed-up with routine MRI scans. As part of the standard protocol, MR flow quantification sequences were added to provide a surrogate marker of cerebral metabolism and brain volume. In the current study, twenty consecutive relapsing remitting MS patients had these sequences reviewed, all were female. The demographic details are summarized in Table 1. The mean age was 43 ± 12 year. The mean length of time from first symptoms to the MRI was 13 ± 8 year. The mean audio recorded cognitive screen score was 85 ± 12. The mean extended disability status scale for the patients was 2.5 ± 1.8. Seventeen patients were currently undergoing immunomodulation therapy at the time of the study; the other three had not received treatment for over a year. Twenty patients with NPH, who were previously studied with the same flow quantification technique (with the results being previously published in part [16]), were selected for comparison. This group comprised 12 males and 8 females. The NPH group was originally selected on the basis of the classical clinical triad of gait ataxia ± dementia ± incontinence together with ventriculomegaly. All 20 patients were confirmed to have NPH, having shown clinical improvement following CSF flow diversion (see [16] for more details). The controls were selected from a bank of spouses and volunteers recruited by advertisement and have been previously published [16, 17]. The controls were confirmed to be without structural brain pathology on standard

Table 1 Demographics and clinical information for multiple sclerosis patients

Patient number	Age (years)	Sex	Duration of disease (years)	Type	Treatment	ARCS	EDSS
1	21	F	9	RRMS	Natalizumab	79	1.5
2	38	F	2	RRMS	Interferon beta-1a	100	0
3	57	F	4	RRMS	Betaferon	73	1.5
4	36	F	11	RRMS	Natalizumab	78	5.5
5	46	F	21	RRMS	Natalizumab	81	6.0
6	62	F	17	RRMS	Nil	72	6.5
7	40	F	16	RRMS	Natalizumab	82	1.5
8	51	F	26	RRMS	Nil	90	2.5
9	40	F	13	RRMS	Natalizumab	77	3.5
10	31	F	9	RRMS	Natalizumab	71	3.0
11	50	F	28	RRMS	Nil	96	2.5
12	36	F	4	RRMS	Natalizumab	83	1.0
13	46	F	4	RRMS	Fingolimod	86	1.5
14	59	F	22	RRMS	Fingolimod	60	1.5
15	36	F	4	RRMS	Interferon beta-1a	95	1.5
16	62	F	25	RRMS	Glatiramer	93	1.5
17	47	F	14	RRMS	Betaferon	92	1.0
18	31	F	9	RRMS	Natalizumab	79	1.5
19	28	F	11	RRMS	Natalizumab	93	1.5
20	48	F	5	RRMS	Immunoglobulin	111	3.5

ARCS audio recorded cognitive screen; *EDSS* extended disability status scale; *F* female; *RRMS*,relapsing remitting multiple sclerosis

MRI and underwent Mini-Mental State examination and formal neuropsychological testing. The normal young were selected to match the MS patients and averaged 43 ± 16 year, all were females. The normal elderly averaged 74 ± 16 year and there were 6 women and 6 men.

MR and analysis

All patients were imaged on a 1.5 T superconducting magnet (Vario; Siemens, Erlangen Germany). In the brain, the patients were scanned with standard T1 and FLAIR sagittal images followed by T2 axial and diffusion-weighted axial images. A 3D T1 post contrast series was acquired. In the neck, post contrast T1 sagittal, inversion recovery sagittal and T2 axial images were performed. Two MR phase contrast flow quantification sequences were acquired with retrospective cardiac gating. The TR was 26.5 ms, TE 6.9 ms, flip angle 15°, slice thickness 5 mm, matrix 192 × 512, FOV 150 and a single excitation. The velocity encoding value was 75/s for the arterial acquisition and 40 cm/s for the venous. The arterial plane was selected to pass through the vertical segments of the carotid and basilar arteries at the skull base. The venous plane was selected to pass through the sagittal sinus above the torcular and then pass through the mid part of the straight sinus (Fig. 1C–E). The planar imaging, as well as the flow quantification raw data, was archived on DVD discs.

Regions of interest were placed around the carotid arteries, basilar artery, the sagittal sinus and the straight sinus in each patient. Care was taken to exclude aliasing by retrospectively manipulating the base lines of each resultant graph giving an effective arterial flow limit of 150 cm/s. Background subtraction was utilized to limit the effect of eddy currents. The addition of the flow from the three arteries gave the total arterial inflow. The sagittal sinus and straight sinus outflow was obtained from the regions of interest placed around these vessels. The percentage of the arterial inflow drained by each sinus was calculated for each patient.

The arteriovenous delay (AVD) is the time taken between the center of the primary arterial pulse and the center of the primary sagittal sinus outflow pulse. The arterial and venous waveforms were transected by a horizontal line representing the mean blood flow for each graph. The midpoint between the two sites where the mean flow crosses the flow curve is taken to be the midpoint of the pulse wave. Subtracting the arterial and sagittal venous midpoints gave the AVD. This is inversely proportional to the pulse wave velocity between these two points (Fig. 1F, G). The arterial pulse volume represents the degree to which the arterial tree expands in systole and is calculated from the graphs obtained from each carotid and basilar artery. The mean blood flow velocity for each artery for the entire heartbeat was subtracted from the mean blood flow

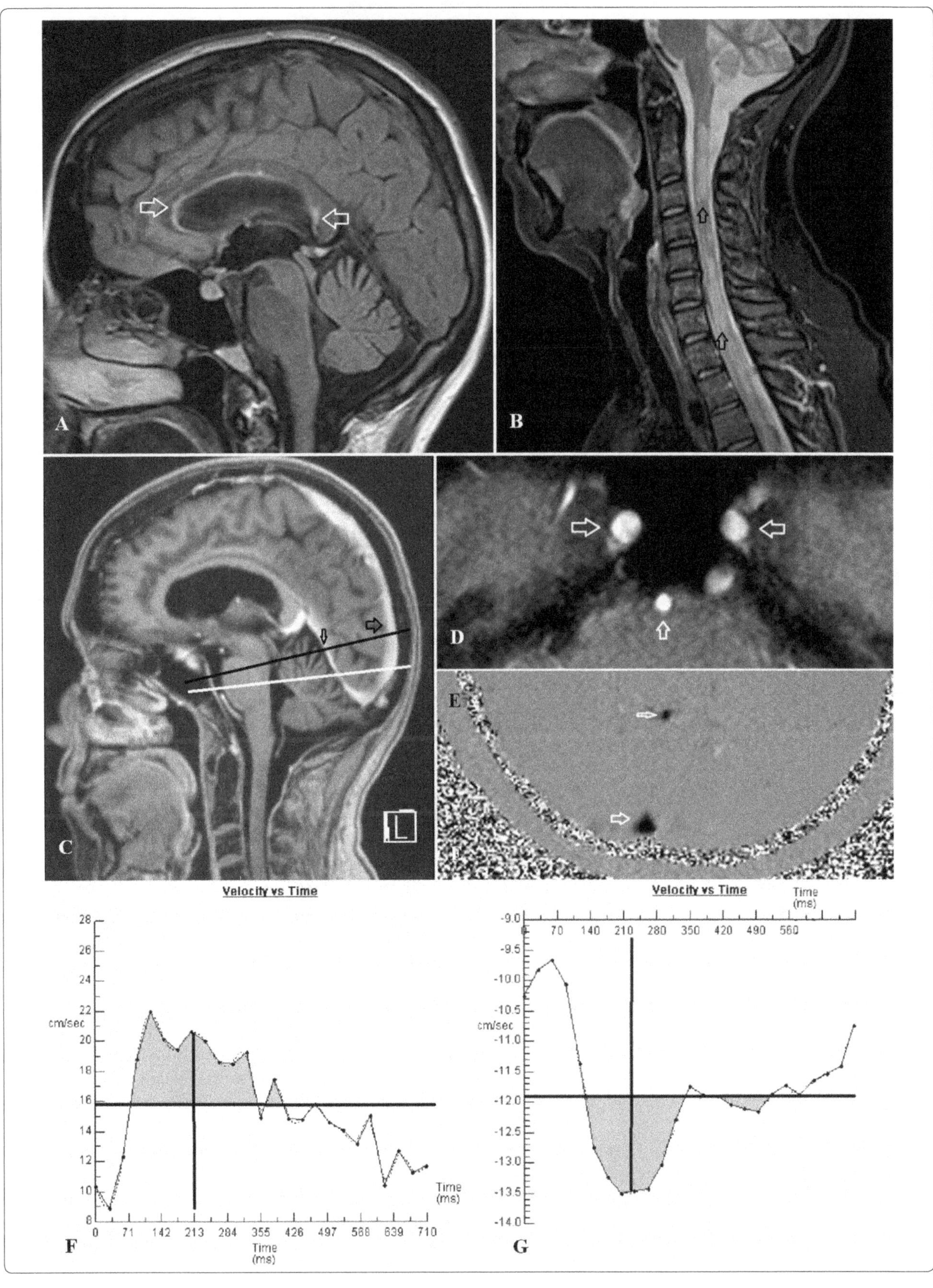
A
B
C
D
E
Velocity vs Time
cm/sec
Time (ms)
F
Velocity vs Time
cm/sec
Time (ms)
G

(See figure on previous page.)

Fig. 1 **A** A FLAIR sagittal image of a 48 year old female MS patient with *arrows* showing some plaques within the corpus callosum but no significant cerebral volume loss. **B** A T2 sagittal image of the cervical spine in the same patient with arrows showing extensive MS plaques. **C** A sagittal post contrast T1 image with the *black line* showing the position of the venous acquisition passing through the sagittal sinus (*large arrow*) and straight sinus (*small arrow*). The *white line* is the arterial acquisition passing through the skull base. **D** The localizer image from the arterial acquisition showing the carotid arteries just above foramen lacerum (*horizontal arrows*) and the mid basilar artery (*vertical arrow*). **E** The phase image from the venous acquisition showing the sagittal sinus (*large arrow*) and straight sinus (*small arrow*). **F** The arterial flow graph from the same patient. The *horizontal line* represents the mean flow velocity. Where the mean velocity transects the flow graph is the start and end of systole. The *grey area* above the *line* represents the arterial stroke volume which for the three arteries combined was 1184 μL. The *vertical line* represents the midpoint of the two transection points and is the midpoint of the primary arterial wave i.e. 213 mS. **G** The sagittal sinus flow graph from the same patient. The *horizontal line* is the mean flow velocity. The *grey area* is the sinus stroke volume which is 118 μL or 10 % of the arterial stroke volume. The *vertical line* is the midpoint of the two transection points and is the center of the primary pulse wave i.e. 223 mS giving an AVD of 10 mS in this patient which is less than 10 % of normal indicating very low compliance

velocity for the period of systole (systole was defined as the section of the graph between the transection points) for the same artery, giving the mean increase in flow velocity over systole for that vessel (Fig. 1F). This value when multiplied by the time taken for systole (the distance between transection points) to occur and the cross-sectional area of the vessel (region of interest) gives the volume of expansion of that vessel in systole. The addition of the value of vessel expansion obtained for both carotid and the basilar arteries gave the arterial stroke volume. The sagittal and straight sinus stroke volumes were obtained for each patient by a similar process to the arterial stroke volume except using the venous flow data (Fig. 1G). The percentage of the arterial stroke volume represented by each venous stroke volume was calculated.

Statistical analysis

Group means and standard deviations were obtained for each of the measurements. Comparison of mean differences between the study groups were tested using a general linear model–univariate analysis of variance (ANOVA). For each ANOVA, the measurement was entered as the dependent variable, with study group entered as a fixed factor and age entered as a covariate between study groups and relevant controls. All measurements were checked for normality using the one-sample Komogorov–Smirnov test and for equality of variance using the Levene's Test. A non-paired T test, with a p value of less than 0.05 was used to indicate statistical significance. All statistical analyses were performed using IBM® SPSS Statistics V22.

Results

The raw data supporting the findings of this study can be found in Additional file 1. The blood flow data is summarized in Table 2 with the compliance and pulsation data summarized in Table 3. The arterial inflow, SSS outflow, AVD and arterial stroke volume data for the normal elderly and NPH patients has been previously published [17]. The ST outflow and both venous sinus stroke volumes were not previously published and were calculated from the original raw data retrieved from the archive DVD discs. The MS and normal young data has not been previously published.

Blood flow

As expected, there was a non-significant reduction in arterial inflow with normal aging between the two control groups, with the reduction in blood flow being approximately 3 ml/min/year. The sagittal sinus showed a reduced outflow with aging in proportion to the inflow. There was no significant alteration in the percentage of the blood flow returned by each sinus compared to the arterial inflow. The multiple sclerosis patients were compared to the normal young. There was no significant difference in arterial inflow. There was a 13 % reduction in sagittal sinus outflow ($p = 0.01$), which gave a 5 % reduction in the percentage of the arterial inflow drained by this sinus ($p = 0.05$). The straight sinus flow and percentage return were not significantly different to the controls. The NPH patients were compared to the normal elderly. The arterial inflow, SSS and ST outflow volumes were significantly reduced by 20, 36 and 25 % respectively ($p = 0.02$, $p = 0.0005$, $p = 0.05$). The percentage of the arterial inflow returned by the SSS was reduced by 8 % ($p = 0.03$) but the ST as a percentage of the inflow was not significantly different from normal.

Craniospinal compliance and pulsation

There was no change in the AVD with aging. The arterial stroke volume was increased by 46 % in the normal elderly compared to the normal young ($p = 0.0006$). Despite the increase in arterial stroke volume, the two sinus stroke volumes were not significantly different between the control groups. However taken as a percentage of the arterial stroke volume both the venous stroke volumes were reduced with aging ($p = 0.02$ and $p = 0.02$ respectively). In MS the AVD was reduced by 35 % compared to the normal young ($p = 0.02$). There was an increase in arterial stroke volume of 26 % ($p = 0.02$) but

Table 2 Brain blood flow in normal, multiple sclerosis and normal pressure hydrocephalus patients

	Age (years)	Arterial inflow (ml/min)	SSS outflow (ml/min)	ST outflow (ml/min)	%SSS	%ST
Normal young n = 20						
Mean	43	792	356	108	46	14
SD	16	142	76	29	8	3
Normal elderly n = 12						
Mean	70	709	310	91	44	13
SD	5	110	65	30	9	4
p value NY vs NE	0.0001*	NS	0.03*	NS	NS	NS
Multiple sclerosis n = 20						
Mean	43	783	311	95	41	12
SD	12	160	44	28	7	4
p value MS vs NY	NS	NS	0.01*	NS	0.05*	NS
Normal pressure hydrocephalus n = 20						
Mean	74	567	197	68	36	13
SD	7	148	49	24	9	5
p value NPH vs NE	NS	0.02*	0.0005*	0.05*	0.03*	NS

SSS sagittal sinus sinus; *ST* straight sinus; *%SSS* percentage of arterial inflow drained by the SSS; *%ST* percentage of arterial inflow drained by ST; *SD* standard deviation; *t test *p* value <0.05; *MS* multiple sclerosis; *NS* not significant; *NPH* normal pressure hydrocephalus; *NY* normal young; *NE* normal elderly; *p* values are adjusted for age

Table 3 AVD and pulsation stroke volume

	AVD (ms)	Arterial SV (μL)	SSS SV (μL)	ST SV (μL)	%SSS SV	%ST SV
Normal young n = 20						
Mean	112	914	273	73	31	8.7
SD	67	264	96	30	9	3.9
Normal elderly n = 12						
Mean	111	1331	308	71	23	5.6
SD	50	374	124	20	7	1.8
p value NY vs NE	NS	0.0006*	NS	NS	0.02*	0.02*
Multiple sclerosis n = 20						
Mean	73	1152	188	50	16	4.4
SD	39	350	44	30	9	3.0
p value MS vs NY	0.02*	0.02*	0.007*	0.02*	0.0001*	0.0003*
Hydrocephalus n = 20						
Mean	47	963	170	42	19	4.4
SD	24	375	91	26	8	2.3
p value NPH vs NE	0.0002*	0.02*	0.0005*	0.002*	NS	NS

AVD arteriovenous delay; *ms* milliseconds; *SV* stroke volume; *SSS* superior sagittal sinus; *ST* straight sinus; *SD* standard deviation; *t test p value <0.05; *MS* multiple sclerosis; *NPH* normal pressure hydrocephalus; *NS* not significant; *NY* normal young; *NE* normal elderly; p values are adjusted for age

a decrease in SSS and ST stroke volumes of 31 and 32 % respectively ($p = 0.007$ and $p = 0.02$). Thus the percentages of the arterial stroke volume directed to the venous sinuses were greatly reduced ($p = 0.0001$ and $p = 0.0003$ respectively). In NPH the AVD was reduced by 58 % ($p = 0.0002$) compared to the normal elderly. The arterial stroke volume, SSS and ST stroke volumes were reduced by 28, 45 and 41 % ($p = 0.02$ $p = 0.0005$ and $p = 0.002$ respectively), however, as a percentage of the arterial stroke volume the venous stroke volumes were not significantly altered.

Discussion

There is a hydrodynamic spectrum underlying various forms of dementia. Vascular dementia is associated with increased arterial but normal venous stroke volume [17] with normal craniospinal compliance [18], Alzheimer's disease is associated with normal arterial and venous stroke volume [17] but reduced craniospinal compliance [16] and normal pressure hydrocephalus is associated with reduced arterial and venous stroke volume and a very low craniospinal compliance. The multiple sclerosis patients in the current study show increased arterial but reduced venous stroke volume together with reduced craniospinal compliance. Therefore, MS overlaps the other three forms of dementia but is most closely correlated with NPH.

The pulse pressure of the blood flowing from the arteries into the arterioles and then into the capillaries is normally damped as it proceeds. The pulse induces a change in volume of blood in the arteries over the cardiac cycle. However, there is non-pulsatile continuous flow proceeding into the capillaries [17]. The mechanism required to bring about the change in pulsation is known as the windkessel effect [19]. Arterial damping depends on expansion of the arteries in systole and contraction in diastole. This removes some energy from the flow in systole and returns it in diastole. The Monro–Kellie doctrine states that as the skull is rigid and the CSF incompressible, the volume of the arterial pulse stored in systole must be accommodated by the available compliance i.e. either the walls of the container (the dura mater) must be shifted to allow egress of CSF from the cranial to spinal cavities and/or the veins passing through the subarachnoid space must be compressed [20]. Thus the arterial tree can only be as compliant as the walls of the container allow. It is envisaged a breakdown in the windkessel effect will direct greater pulse pressure into the capillary beds of the neural structures leading to parenchymal derangement [18]. A larger CSF pulse pressure will also be transmitted through the thin walled veins as they traverse the subarachnoid space and increase the venous pulse pressure. For example, Alzheimer's disease (AD) is associated with a reduction in AVD of 36 % [16] which is almost identical to the MS patients in this study. The arterial pulse volume in AD is 1150 μL [17] which is also identical to MS. Is one neurodegenerative disease related to the other? It was suggested an increased capillary pulse pressure could account for the coiling and beading of the capillaries as well as the basement membrane disruption found in AD [18]. In the Framingham offspring study, higher central arterial pulse pressure was associated with lower brain volume, white matter hyperintensity and vascular and Alzheimer's type cognitive aging [21]. In another study, measurements of the arterial pulse and the invasively-measured CSF pulse pressure were strongly associated with temporal lobe and hippocampal volume loss [22], suggesting pulse waves may damage the brain. Finally, Chandra suggests a common mechanism for the neurodegeneration found within MS and AD due to increased amyloid precursor protein expression in the axons around MS plaques [23]. The purpose of the current study was to measure the arterial pulsation, the available compliance and the outflow venous pulsation to determine if there is a breakdown in the windkessel effect in multiple sclerosis, similar to NPH.

Blood flow changes

The arterial inflow to the brain reduces throughout life. In a cohort of normal controls of mean age 25 year previously studied by our group, the arterial inflow was 900 ml/min with the sagittal sinus returning 45 % of the arterial flow and the straight sinus 14 % [17]. In the current study, the normal young were mean age 43 year, the mean arterial inflow was 792 ml/min, the sagittal sinus returning 46 % and straight sinus 14 % of the flow. In the normal elderly of average age 70 year, the arterial inflow was 709 ml/min, the sagittal sinus returning 44 % and the straight sinus 13 % of the flow. Note the percentage of the arterial inflow returned by each sinus has not changed significantly over the 40 years spanned. The arterial inflow is noted to have reduced by 4.2 ml/min/year from 25 to 70 year which is similar to the findings of Stoquart–ElSankari et al. [24].

In normal pressure hydrocephalus there is a 23 % reduction in arterial inflow compared to the age matched controls. The reduction in sagittal sinus flow is somewhat larger at 36 % giving an 8 % reduction in the percentage of the inflow returning via this sinus. This is in comparison to the straight sinus where the percentage of the inflow is maintained. It has been previously noted in NPH that there is a 29 % reduction in sagittal sinus flow compared to controls with a 28 % increase in flow following CSF diversion [25]. Further investigation into this effect showed that the arterial inflow was unchanged. This indicates there must have been increased collateral flow bypassing the sinus before the shunt, which returns back to the normal venous pathway after the shunt. This suggests there is an elevation in sagittal sinus pressure but not straight sinus pressure in NPH which is reversible [26].

In MS, there was no significant difference in the arterial inflow between patients and controls. Some have suggested a reduction in total cerebral blood flow seen in some MS studies is due to small increases in venous pressure [27]. This would appear to be unlikely given the large perfusion pressure reserve available to the brain. However, increasing the sagittal sinus pressure by 1–2 mm Hg could affect the venous outflow by increasing collateral flow. Note that similar to NPH, the sagittal sinus returned 5 % less blood as a percentage compared to controls in MS. A previous study showed further evidence of increased SSS pressure in MS: strain-gauge plethysmography demonstrated a 63 % increase in the total venous resistance from the head in MS patients compared with healthy controls [28]. Given the pressure gradient from the sagittal sinus to the right heart is 2.5 mm Hg [29], this would give an increase in sinus pressure of 1.6 mm Hg if the blood flow was maintained. Indeed, direct measurement of the sinus pressure has shown an elevation of over 2 mm Hg in selected MS patients [30]. So it can be seen that there are similarities between the blood flow in NPH and MS patients.

Arterial stroke volume

The arterial stroke volume is the expansion of the arterial tree in systole, over and above the mean flow and this is the impetus for both displacement of CSF into the spinal canal and compression of the cortical veins [31]. Normal aging showed an increase in the stroke volume between the two control groups of 46 %. It has been previously suggested that aging is associated with reduced compliance in the walls of the central arteries and that the larger pulse pressure waves generated by aging would penetrate deeper into the microcirculation, microvascular disease would ensue, with the brain and kidney being most susceptible [32]. Note that in the present study the arterial stroke volume increased with aging despite the reduction in non-pulsatile blood flow (refuting the previously discussed assertion they are always linked [13]). In MS there was a 26 % increase in arterial stroke volume compared to the age-matched controls. Fjeldstat et al [33] found patients with MS have lower central arterial compliance than healthy controls, which preferentially affects the CNS vessels. The pulse wave velocity between the brachial and ankle arteries is significantly higher in MS patients compared to controls, indicating stiffer central arteries [34]. Both these findings place a larger pulse pressure wave within the carotid vessels which must be damped. Higher central arterial pulse pressure is also associated with worsening gait performance in MS but not controls, suggesting altered vascular compliance may contribute to the deterioration in physical function in MS [35]. In comparison, NPH is associated with a reduced arterial stroke volume compared to controls, indicating a point of difference between NPH and MS.

Arteriovenous delay

Compliance is defined as the ratio of the change in volume which occurs in a structure divided by the change in pressure which brings this about i.e. $C = \Delta V/\Delta P$ [19]. Aortic compliance is estimated by measuring the time the pulse wave takes to travel from the brachial to the ankle arteries [36] because the pulse wave velocity is inversely proportional to compliance. Thus, craniospinal compliance can be measured invasively (1) by injecting a volume of fluid into the subarachnoid space and measuring the change in pressure which occurs, or non-invasively (2) by measuring the time the pulse wave takes to traverse the available space. The AVD measures between the arteries at the skull base and the venous sinuses. It could be assumed that the pulse traversed the capillary bed, passed along the cortical veins to directly enter the sinuses but this was not so. Direct measurement of the pulse wave timing has shown that the peak pulse in the cortical veins lags behind the sinuses indicating that the pulse volume exits the arterial tree passes into the subarachnoid space and re-enters the cortical vessels just before their junction with the sinuses [37]. Therefore the pulse volume passes into the spinal canal with a minimal time lag [38] and then travels to the venous outflow with a time lag measured by the AVD. The time taken for the pulse to travel from the arteries to the sagittal sinus is thus a measure of the compliance of the arteries, subarachnoid space and veins between these two places. It is undefined how this would directly correlate with the other invasive techniques used to measure craniospinal compliance. From the present study, we note that the AVD does not change from the normal young to the normal elderly similar to a previous study [24] suggesting the compliance of the craniospinal system remains unchanged with normal aging. This is in comparison with the findings in NPH, in which the present study shows a 58 % reduction in AVD compared to age matched controls. Previously, in a smaller cohort, the compliance was estimated to be reduced by 50 % in NPH [25], Mase et al. [39] using another MRI technique confirmed a 64 % reduction in craniospinal compliance in NPH. The compliance as measured by the AVD was reduced in MS by 35 % compared to age match controls, indicating another similarity between the patient groups being currently studied: i.e. both NPH and MS have reduced compliance.

In a previously published control group of average age 33 year, the mean CSF pulse pressure at C1/C2 was 1.6 ± 0.6 mm Hg [40]. In one study, it has been noted the CSF pulse pressure in NPH is twice normal [41] and 2–3 times normal in another study [42]. Finally, NPH patients who responded to shunt had intracranial pulse pressures averaging over 4 mm Hg [43]. Note, that despite the arterial stroke volume in NPH being 28 % less than age-matched controls in this study, the pulse pressure in the subarachnoid space has been shown to be twice normal [41, 42]. This indicates very low compliance as discussed above. In MS the arterial stroke volume was increased by 26 % and the compliance as measured by the AVD was reduced by 35 % compared to the normal young, suggesting the possibility of an increased pulse pressure in the subarachnoid space in MS. The literature provides some evidence for this, the estimated peak-to-peak pulse pressure gradient in the spinal canal in MS patients was noted to be doubled compared to controls [44] and the pulse volumes were significantly increased in the epidural veins in the spine in adolescents with MS [45] suggesting an increase in spinal pulse pressure.

Local spinal canal compliance

Stivaros and Jackson noted, that displacement of CSF through the foramen magnum into the spinal subarachnoid space occurs due to the high compliance of the spinal arachnoid mater, accounting for at least 50 % of the pulse pressure volume displacement [46]. In a cohort of normal controls vs MS patients, the C2 stroke volume was reduced by 24 % [13]. The Monro–Kellie doctrine is essentially a restatement of the conservation of mass (if the arterial tree increases in volume then the CSF and venous volume must reduce by the same amount). If the spinal canal has the greater relative compliance than the veins then a larger percentage of the arterial stroke volume will be directed to the spine, if the veins are relatively more compliant than the spinal canal then their stroke volume will be greater as a percentage. In MS the arterial stroke volume was 26 % larger than controls but the percentage of the volume directed to the spinal canal was reduced by 24 % so we can conclude the spinal canal is much less compliant than normal in MS. One study found that there is no difference in the C2 stroke volume between normal elderly (at 71 year) and NPH [47]. In another study, the cervical stroke volume was reduced by 27 % compared to controls [48]. Given there is a 28 % reduction in arterial pulse volume in NPH compared to controls, the second study showing a 27 % reduction in cervical stroke volume would indicate an equal reduction in relative compliance between the spinal canal and the veins. The first study, where the spinal canal volumes were equal, would indicate the veins should be of somewhat lower relative compliance than the spinal canal. Thus, in both MS and NPH there is a reduction in spinal canal compliance.

Venous sinus compliance

In this study, the normal young, direct 31 % of the arterial stroke volume to the sagittal sinus and 8.7 % to the straight sinus. In MS this was much less i.e. 16 % of the arterial stroke volume was directed towards the sagittal sinus and 4.4 % to the straight sinus. Given the arterial stroke volume was larger in MS than in controls, this would tend to indicate that the compliance of the cortical veins leading to the sinuses is very low and thus resist compression in MS. In NPH the percentage of the arterial pulse directed to the sinuses was not significantly different to normal, suggesting as previously noted, that the reduction in compliance is probably equally shared between the spinal canal and veins.

A common pathophysiology of MS and NPH

There appears to be a common pathophysiological mechanism underlying MS and NPH. Both disorders generate collateral blood flow, bypassing the sagittal sinus, suggesting an increase in sinus pressure. Both disorders show a decrease in compliance compared to controls. Confounding the lower compliance in MS is the increased arterial stroke volume. Both conditions show a reduction in relative spinal canal and venous compliance but the relative changes between the spine and veins vary.

The arterial pulse pressure within the arteries of the neck represents a source of potential energy. In order for this energy to be removed from the arterial circulation before the capillary bed, it is necessary for the volume increase generated by the pulse pressure to be directed to the subarachnoid space and veins. If the compliance of the spine and veins is low, the pulse pressure damping is reduced and there is thought to be an increase in capillary pulse pressure, causing capillary disruption. In human hydrocephalus, the capillary wall shows blood–brain barrier dysfunction with increased vesicular and vacuolar transport, open inter-endothelial junctions, thin and fragmented basement membranes and discontinuous perivascular astrocytic end feet. The findings suggested an inter-endothelial route either for hydrocephalic oedema formation or resolution [49].

In addition to the capillary bed being affected, the breakdown in the windkessel mechanism may lead to an increased pulse pressure in the veins of the brain [17]. NPH is associated with a doubling in the subarachnoid space pulse pressure [41, 42] and the current data suggests an increase in subarachnoid pulse pressure may also occur in MS. The cortical veins and the vein of Galen are thin walled, so the pulse pressure within these structures will be identical to the CSF pulse pressure. Despite the suggested increase in cortical vein pulse pressure, there is a failure of the pulse pressure being converted into pulsatile flow in the veins in MS and in NPH [50]. The intracranial venous system is without valves so the pulse pressure is free to travel in both directions i.e. toward the sinuses and towards the smallest venules. In NPH there is thickening of the walls of the smallest venules which is termed perivenular collagenosis [51]. A similar process can be seen within the eyes of MS patients, which occur in the absence of demyelination (there is no myelin in the retina). Measurement of the retinal artery to retinal vein pulse delay (similar to the AVD) indicates the vessels are reduced in compliance by 25 % in MS compared to controls [52]. Reducing the compliance of the venules will make conversion of the pulse pressure to pulsatile flow ineffective. Therefore, the retinal veins will have a high pulse pressure. The retinal veins in MS are associated with a breakdown of the blood-retinal barrier with venous fluorescein leakage. Leaking venules are associated with a proteinaceous perivenous sheathing, which occurs especially at arterial/venous crossover points [53] where the venous pulse pressure would be at a maximum. All of these findings are analogous to those in NPH as already described.

If the pathophysiology between NPH and MS is so similar one might expect that there would be some overlap in presentation. The absolute compliance in NPH is much lower than MS and the intracranial pulse pressure is probably higher but there may be a few patients who present with both conditions. There have been a few isolated case reports of patients with MS who had shunt responsive hydrocephalus [54, 55]. It is likely that more patients exist but they may be misinterpreted as atrophy rather than NPH. Similarly, a theory has been put forward that syringomyelia secondary to Chiari I malformation develops in the cervical cord, due to an increase in local CSF pulse pressure secondary to reduced spinal canal compliance (pulse wave myelopathy) [56]. If this were true, then there should be a correlation between MS and syrinx formation in those whose spinal canal compliance dropped low enough. Firstly, as noted previously, the pulse volumes were significantly increased in the epidural veins in the spine in adolescents with MS [45], suggesting an increase in spinal pulse pressure and secondly, syringomyelia is noted in 4.5 % of patients with MS [57]. This suggests that the syrinx is more likely to be a consequence of the MS pathology rather than a coincidence [57].

Limitations of the method

There is no ideal plane to measure the arterial inflow with a single MR acquisition. A single arterial acquisition was required in this study to minimise the time the patient spent in the scanner, because the flow measurements were acquired after a full 40 min diagnostic MS study. Measured in the current plane, the carotid arteries were at the skull base and the extracranial carotid segments were excluded. However, the subarachnoid extent of the vertebral vessels extends from the upper surface of C1 so the subarachnoid vertebrals and the lower basilar artery were not measured. The effect was to miss some of the blood flow supplying the cerebellum, brainstem and spinal cord and also underestimate the arterial stroke volume contributed by the expansion of the posterior fossa vessels. Effectively, the current study measured the supratentorial blood flow and pulsation. The alternative would have been to place the arterial acquisition in the neck at C2 similar to Qvarlander et al. [48]. However, although all of the arterial flow would be measured, large segments of the extracranial carotid and vertebral arteries would have been added. The vessels within the subarachnoid space are constrained by the water bath of the CSF and the compliance of the walls of the container. The extracranial vessels are not so constrained so the neck positioning will significantly overestimate the arterial stroke volume (the normal elderly in Qvarlander et al. showed an arterial stroke volume of 1.6 times the current study, despite the mean flow being not significantly different). The positioning of the venous acquisition means the venous flow and pulsation were also being measured supratentorially, similar to the arterial measurement. The neck positioning of the venous acquisition would exclude the comparison between the straight and sagittal sinuses performed by this study and also vastly overestimate the venous stroke volume. The venous stroke volume in Qvarlander et al. was 6.3 times the sagittal sinus stroke volume for the normal controls. The AVD would also have been invalid if large sections of compliant extracranial vessels were added.

The venous stroke volume and flow as measured represent only a portion of the total. The sagittal sinus and straight sinus outflow being 60 % of the arterial inflow in the young controls. Other blood flow and pulsation leaves the brain via the basal sinuses, ophthalmic veins, emissary veins and direct connections to the transverse and sigmoid sinuses. This is the reason the percentage of the arterial stroke volume directed to the spinal canal, sagittal sinus and straight sinuses can all be reduced in MS because the extra is directed to the basal sinuses. Although the relative compliances of the spinal canal and the sinuses measured by the current study were reduced (and the total compliance reduced), if the basal sinuses were unchanged in compliance then a larger percentage of the pulse volume would be directed to them, or the Monro–Kellie doctrine would be violated. There is no way to measure the basal sinus components directly except by subtraction of the known stroke volumes. The acquisition planes as used were identical to the earlier studies [16, 17] and are therefore directly comparable.

The measurement of the AVD attempts to find the centre of each pulse wave, however, due to the waves not being perfect sine waves the centre based on the timing (as currently used) may not represent the centre of the volume of blood expansion but the error is expected to be small.

Conclusions

The pulsation pathophysiology of MS is similar to NPH suggesting that there may be an underlying pulse wave encephalopathy component to this disease which is being masked by the more obvious inflammatory overlay. It is uncertain if the neurodegenerative component is primary or secondary but the pulse wave encephalopathy which ensues could account for some of the chronic symptoms of MS and treatments aimed at altering the pulse wave propagation should be investigated.

Abbreviations
AVD: arteriovenous delay; AD: Alzheimer's disease; C2: cervical vertebra 2; MS: multiple sclerosis; NPH: normal pressure hydrocephalus; NY: normal young; NE: normal elderly; SSS: superior sagittal sinus; ST: straight sinus; SD: standard deviation.

Authors' contributions
GB conceived and designed the study, obtained and processed the MRI data and wrote the manuscript. JLS was involved in patient selection and clinical data acquisition. RL was involved in design and implementation of the statistical portion of the paper as well as interpretation of the data and writing the manuscript. All authors read and approved the final manuscript.

Author details
[1] Department of Medical Imaging, John Hunter Hospital, Locked Bag 1, Newcastle Region Mail Center, Newcastle 2310, Australia. [2] Newcastle University Faculty of Health, Callaghan Campus Newcastle, Newcastle, Australia. [3] Department of Neurology, John Hunter Hospital, Newcastle, Australia. [4] Hunter Medical Research Institute, Newcastle, Australia. [5] Institute of Health and Biomedical Innovation, Queensland University of Technology, Brisbane, Australia.

Competing interests
The authors declare that they have no competing interests.

References
1. Lassmann H. Multiple sclerosis pathology: evolution of pathogenic concepts. Brain Pathol. 2005;15:217–22.
2. Wingerchuk DM, Carter JL. Multiple sclerosis: current and emerging disease-modifying therapies and treatment strategies. Mayo Clin Proc. 2014;89:225–40.
3. Juurlink BH. Is there a pulse wave encephalopathy component to multiple sclerosis? Curr Neurovasc Res. 2015;12:199–209.
4. Stys PK. Pathoetiology of multiple sclerosis: are we barking up the wrong tree? F1000Prime. 2013. doi:10.12703/P5-20.
5. Lagana MM, Chaudhary A, Balagurunathan D, et al. Cerebrospinal fluid flow dynamics in multiple sclerosis patients through phase contrast magnetic resonance imaging. Curr Neurovasc Res. 2014;11:349–58.
6. Martola J, Stawiarz L, Fredrikson S, et al. Rate of ventricular enlargement in multiple sclerosis: a nine-year magnetic resonance imaging follow-up study. Acta Radiol. 2008;49:570–9.
7. Achiron A, Faibel M. Sandlike appearance of Virchow–Robin spaces in early multiple sclerosis: a novel neuroradiologic marker. Am J Neuroradiol. 2002;23:376–80.
8. Benedetti MG, Piperno R, Simoncini L, Bonato P, Tonini A, Giannini S. Gait abnormalities in minimally impaired multiple sclerosis patients. Multi Scler. 1999;5:363–8.
9. Gil Moreno MJ, Cerezo Garcia M, Marasescu R, Pinel Gonzales A, Lopez Alvarez L, Aladro Benito Y. Neuropsychological syndromes in multiple sclerosis. Psicothema. 2013;25:425–60.
10. Murphy AM, Bethoux F, Stough D, Goldman HB. Prevalence of stress urinary incontinence in women with multiple sclerosis. Int Neurourol J. 2012;16:86–90.
11. Gorucu Y, Albayram S, Balaci B, Hasiloglu ZI, Yenigul K, Yargic F, Keser Z, Kantarci F, Kiris A. Cerebrospinal fluid flow dynamics in patients with multiple sclerosis: a phase contrast magnetic resonance study. Funct Neurol. 2011;26:215–22.
12. Magnano C, Schirda C, Weinstock-Guttman B, et al. Cine cerebrospinal fluid imaging in multiple sclerosis. J Magn Reson Imaging. 2002;36:825–34.
13. ElSankari S, Baledent O, van Pesch V, Sindic C, de Broqueville Q, Duprez T. Concomitant analysis of arterial, venous and CSF flows using phase-contrast MRI: a quantitative comparison between MS patients and healthy controls. J Cereb Blood Flow Metab. 2013;33:1314–21.
14. Bateman GA. Pulse wave encephalopathy: a spectrum hypothesis incorporating Alzheimer's disease, vascular dementia and normal pressure hydrocephalus. Med Hypotheses. 2004;62:182–7.
15. Thomsen C, Stahlberg F, Stubgaard M, Nordell B. Fourier analysis of cerebrospinal fluid flow velocities: MR imaging study. The Scandinavian flow group. Radiology. 1990;177:659–65.
16. Bateman GA, Loiselle AM. Can MR measurement of intracranial hydrodynamics and compliance differentiate which patient with idiopathic normal pressure hydrocephalus will improve following shunt insertion? Acta Neurochir (Wein). 2007;149:455–62.
17. Bateman GA, Levi CR, Schofield P, Wang Y, Lovett EC. The venous manifestations of pulse wave encephalopathy: windkessel dysfunction in normal aging and senile dementia. Neuroradiology. 2007. doi:10.1007/s00234-008-0374-x.
18. Bateman GA, Levi CR, Schofield P, Wang Y, Lovett EC. Quantitative measurement of cerebral haemodynamics in early vascular dementia and Alzheimer's disease. J Clin Neurosci. 2006;13:563–8.
19. Wagshul ME, Eide PK, Madsen JR. The pulsating brain: a clinical review of experimental and clinical studies of intracranial pulsatility. Fluids Barriers CNS. 2011. doi:10.1186/2045-8118-8-5.
20. Wilson MH. Monro-Kellie 2.0: the dynamic vascular and venous pathophysiological components of intracranial pressure. J Cereb Blood Flow Metab. 2016;36:1338–50.
21. Tsao CW, Seshadri S, Beiser AS, et al. Relations of arterial stiffness and endothelial function to brain aging in the community. Neurology. 2013;81:984–91.
22. Wahlin A, Ambarki K, Birgander R, Malm J, Eklund A. Intracranial pulsatility is associated with regional brain volume in elderly individuals. Neurobiol Aging. 2014;35:365–72.
23. Chandra A. Role of amyloid from a multiple sclerosis perspective: a literature review. NeuroImmunoModulation. 2015;22:343–6.
24. Stoquart-ElSankari S, Baledent O, Gondry-Jouet C, Makki M, Godefroy O, Meyer ME. Aging effects on cerebral blood and cerebrospinal fluid flows. J Cereb Blood Flow Metab. 2007;27:1563–72.
25. Bateman GA. Vascular compliance in normal pressure hydrocephalus. Am J Neuroradiol. 2000;21:1574–85.
26. Bateman GA. The pathophysiology of idiopathic normal pressure hydrocephalus: cerebral ischemia or altered venous hemodynamics? Am J Neuroradiol. 2007. doi:10.3174/ajnr.A0739.
27. Beggs CB. Venous hemodynamics in neurological disorders: an analytical review with hydrodynamic analysis. BMC Med. 2013. doi:10.1186/1741-7015-11-142.
28. Beggs C, Shepherd S, Zamboni P. Cerebral venous outflow resistance and interpretation of cervical plethysmography data with respect to the diagnosis of chronic cerebrospinal venous insufficiency. Phlebology. 2014;29:191–9.
29. Bateman GA, Siddique SH. Cerebrospinal fluid absorption block at the vertex in chronic hydrocephalus: obstructed arachnoid granulations or elevated venous pressure? Fluids Barriers CNS. 2014. doi:10.1186/2045-8118-11-11.
30. Zamboni P, Galeotti R, Menegatti E, Malagoni AM, Gianesini S, Bartolomei I, Mascoli F, Salvi F. A prospective open-label study of endovascular treatment of chronic cerebrospinal venous insufficiency. J Vasc Surg. 2009;50:1348–58.
31. Bateman GA, Levi CR, Schofield P, et al. The pathophysiology of the aqueduct stroke volume in normal pressure hydrocephalus: can co-morbidity with other forms of dementia be excluded. Neuroradiology. 2005;47:741–8.
32. O'Rourke MF, Safar ME. Relationship between aortic stiffening and microvascular disease in brain and kidney: cause and logic of therapy. Hypertension. 2005;46:200–4.
33. Fjeldstad C, Frederiksen C, Fjedstad AS, Bemben M, Pardo G. Arterial compliance in multiple sclerosis: a pilot study. Angiology. 2010;61:31–6.

34. Talaat FM, Nassef SA, El-Fayomy NM, Abdelalim AM, El-Mazny AN, Fawzy MW. Arterial compliance and carotid artery changes in multiple sclerosis. Life Sci J. 2015;12:96–100.
35. Heffernan KS, Ranadive S, Weikert M, Lane A, Yan H, Fernhall B, Motl RW. Pulse pressure is associated with walking impairment in multiple sclerosis. J Neuro Sci. 2011;309:105–9.
36. Sagawara J, Hayashi K, Yokoi T, Cortez-Cooper MY, DeVan AE, Anton MA, Tanaka H. Brachial-ankle pulse wave velocity: an index of central artery stiffness? J Hum Hypertens. 2005;19:401–6.
37. Bateman GA. Pulse-wave encephalopathy: a comparative study of the hydrodynamics of leukoaraiosis and normal-pressure hydrocephalus. Neuroradiology. 2002;44:740–8.
38. Wagshul ME, Chen JD, Egnor MR, McCormak EJ, Roche PE. Amplitude and phase of cerebrospinal fluid pulsations: experimental studies and review of the literature. J Neurosurg. 2006;104:810–9.
39. Mase M, Miyati T, Yamada K, Kasai H, Hara M, Shibamoto Y. Non-invasive measurement of intracranial compliance using cine MRI in normal pressure hydrocephalus. Acta Neurochir Suppl. 2005;95:303–6.
40. Heiss JD, Snyder K, Peterson MM, et al. Pathophysiology of primary spinal syringomyelia. J Neurosurg Spine. 2012;17:367–80.
41. Eide PK, Brean A. Cerebrospinal fluid pulse pressure amplitude during lumbar infusion in idiopathic normal pressure hydrocephalus can predict response to shunting. Cerebrospinal Fluid. 2010. doi:10.1186/1743-8454-7-5.
42. Foltz EL. Hydrocephalus and CSF pulsatility: clinical and laboratory studies. In: Shapiro K, Marmarou A, Portnoy HD, editors. Hydrocephalus. New York: Raven Press; 1984. p. 337–62.
43. Eide PK, Sorteberg W. Diagnostic pressure monitoring and surgical management in idiopathic normal pressure hydrocephalus: a 6-year review or 214 patients. Neurosurgery. 2010;66:80–91.
44. Damadian RV, Chu D. The possible role of cranio-cervical trauma and abnormal CSF hydrodynamics in the genesis of multiple sclerosis. Physiol Chem Phys Med NMR. 2011;41:1–17.
45. Macgowan CK, Chan KY, Laughlin S, Marrie RA, Banwell B. Cerebral arterial and venous blood flow in adolescent multiple sclerosis patients and age-matched controls using phase contrast MRI. J Mag Res Imag. 2014;40:341–7.
46. Stivaros SM, Jackson A. Changing concepts of cerebrospinal fluid hydrodynamics: role of phase-contrast magnetic resonance imaging and implications for cerebral microvascular disease. Neurotherapeutics. 2007;4:511–22.
47. El Sankari S, Gondry-Jouet C, Fichten A, Godefroy O, Serot JM, Deramond H, Meyer ME, Baledent O. Cerebral fluid and blood flow in mild cognitive impairment and Alzheimer's disease: a differential diagnosis from idiopathic normal pressure hydrocephalus. Fluids Barriers CNS. 2011. doi:10.1186/2045-8118-8-12.
48. Qvarlander S, Ambarki K, Wahlin A, Jacobsson J, Birander R, Malm J, Eklund A. Cerebrospinal fluid and blood flow patterns in idiopathic normal pressure hydrocephalus. Acta Neurol Scand. 2016. doi:10.1111/ane.12636.
49. Castejon OJ. Submicroscopic pathology of human and experimental hydrocephalic cerebral cortex. Folia Neuropathol. 2010;48:159–74.
50. Bateman GA. The reversibility of reduced cortical vein compliance in normal-pressure hydrocephalus following shunt insertion. Neuroradiology. 2003;45:65–70.
51. Moody DM, Brown WR, Challa VR, Anderson RL. Periventricular collagenosis: association with leukoaraiosis. Radiology. 1995;194:469–76.
52. Kochkorov A, Gugleta K, Kavroulaki D, Katamay R, Weier K, Mehling M, Kappos L, Flammer J, Orgul S. Rigidity of retinal vessels in patients with multiple sclerosis. Klin Monbl Augenheilkd. 2009;226:276–9.
53. Birch MK, Barbosa S, Blumhardt LD, O'Brien C, Harding SP. Retinal venous sheathing and the blood-retinal barrier in multiple sclerosis. Arch Opthalmol. 1996;114:34–9.
54. O'Brien T, Paine M, Matotek K, Byrne E. Apparent hydrocephalus and chronic multiple sclerosis: a report of two cases. Clin Exp Neurol. 1993;30:137–43.
55. Algin O, Taskapilioglu O, Hakyemez B, Pariak M. Unusual patient with multiple sclerosis and shunt-responsive normal-pressure hydrocephalus. Clin Neuroradiol. 2012;22:101–4.
56. Bateman GA. Pulse wave myelopathy. An update of an hypothesis highlighting the similarities between syringomyelia and normal pressure hydrocephalus. Med Hypotheses. 2015;85:958–61.
57. Weier K, Naegelin Y, Thoeni A, Hirsch JG, Kappos L, Steinbrich W, Radue EW, Gass A. Non-communicating syringomyelia: a feature of spinal cord involvement in multiple sclerosis. Brain. 2008;131:1776–82.

7

Current research into brain barriers and the delivery of therapeutics for neurological diseases: a report on CNS barrier congress London, UK, 2017

John Greenwood[1], Margareta Hammarlund-Udenaes[2], Hazel C. Jones[3*], Alan W. Stitt[4], Roosmarijn E. Vandenbroucke[5,6], Ignacio A. Romero[7], Matthew Campbell[8], Gert Fricker[9], Birger Brodin[10], Heiko Manninga[11], Pieter J. Gaillard[12], Markus Schwaninger[13], Carl Webster[14], Krzysztof B. Wicher[15] and Michel Khrestchatisky[16,17]

Abstract

This is a report on the CNS barrier congress held in London, UK, March 22–23rd 2017 and sponsored by Kisaco Research Ltd. The two 1-day sessions were chaired by John Greenwood and Margareta Hammarlund-Udenaes, respectively, and each session ended with a discussion led by the chair. Speakers consisted of invited academic researchers studying the brain barriers in relation to neurological diseases and industry researchers studying new methods to deliver therapeutics to treat neurological diseases. We include here brief reports from the speakers.

Keywords: Blood–brain barrier, Blood–CSF barrier, Blood–retinal barrier, Neuroinflammation, Viral vectors, Drug delivery, Antibody therapy, MicroRNA, Liposomal technology, Protein capsules

Background

The blood–brain barrier (BBB), and the other blood–tissue barrier sites of the central nervous system (CNS), have been the subject of extensive research since their discovery over 100 years ago. Despite considerable advances in our understanding of the structural and functional interface of the BBB, there remain many gaps in our knowledge particularly regarding its role in disease and the challenges it presents to therapeutic intervention. In recent decades the classic concept of the BBB has also evolved such that it now cannot be considered in isolation from other cellular components of the CNS. Accordingly, the emergence of the concept of the neurovascular unit (NVU) has re-shaped our approach to studying the BBB. In addition, other blood–tissue interfaces, such as the blood–cerebrospinal fluid and blood–retinal barriers, are also providing additional insight into the communication between the blood and the CNS.

Our understanding of the normal structure and function of the blood–CNS barriers is well advanced but their roles in many diseases remains incomplete. Whereas blood–CNS dysfunction in some conditions is evident, such as in tumours, multiple sclerosis and stroke, in other diseases such as Alzheimer's disease, Parkinson's disease and epilepsy the involvement is less obvious. Indeed, gross changes, such as loss of structural integrity have clear pathological consequences, whereas subtle changes to function may be more difficult to ascertain and place within the overall pathogenesis of a disease. Whether cause or effect, therapeutic targeting of barrier dysfunction remains an attractive proposition and drives much of the translational research currently underway. However, various questions concerning barrier susceptibility to disease remain outstanding. These include the heterogeneity of the vasculature within the CNS and as a consequence its differential response. Indeed, it is known that

*Correspondence: hazelcjones@btinternet.com
[3] Gagle Brook House, Chesterton, Bicester OX26 1UF, UK
Full list of author information is available at the end of the article

in the normal BBB there is endothelial cell heterogeneity that is not only dependent on its position throughout the vascular bed (i.e. artery versus arteriole, versus capillary, versus venule, versus vein) but also within the same region of the vasculature. Moreover, the barrier within different structures of the CNS also differs and together such heterogeneity will undoubtedly impact on the variable response of the barrier to disease. For example, the microvascular pathology observed in diabetes is far more pronounced in the retina than in the brain, the response of white matter vessels and those in grey matter differ in multiple sclerosis, and in meningitis it is the meningeal vessels that are susceptible.

Aside from the direct relationship between barrier dysfunction and disease pathogenesis there is another longstanding and major challenge facing those working in the field. This relates to the problems posed by a structurally intact barrier that restricts the delivery of therapeutics to the brain. For almost 50 years this has proved to be largely insurmountable and only recently have advances been made that provide some optimism.

In this CNS barrier congress experts from various disciplines were brought together to collectively discuss the best ways to overcome these challenges, and pave the way for progress in the treatment of neurological disease. In recent years, our understanding of barriers has undergone re-evaluation and during the meeting various pressing questions were discussed. These included the role that non-endothelial cells in the NVU play in blood–brain barrier regulation, how much barrier dysfunction really occurs in different CNS diseases, why regional differences exist, and how do immune cells impact barrier function. Contrary to previous dogma, the CNS barriers are now recognised as complex, dynamic, interactive structures that contribute to disease on many levels. Recent advances in drug delivery technologies to the CNS were also presented and discussed at length. Pioneering groups have been perfecting new methods to ferry drugs across the CNS barriers, particularly the blood–brain barrier where access via other routes is problematic. Accordingly, the latest developments in liposome, peptide, antibody, and nanoparticle technology for therapeutic delivery were showcased and how far these technologies have to go before they can become widely available was discussed.

This CNS barrier congress allowed for the presentation of unpublished data, the exploration of new technologies, and provided a select platform for academic and industrial leaders in the field to form collaborations, exchange ideas and identify new strategies for development.

The specialised vascular barriers of the CNS and their influence on leukocyte migration

John Greenwood

The specialised vascular endothelial cells that line the vessels of the brain and retina form an impermeable but selective barrier between the blood and the neural parenchyma. Under normal physiological conditions this critical interface, termed the blood–brain/retinal barrier, strictly limits the passage of solutes and cells between these two compartments. During disease, however, the endothelial cells become activated resulting in a change of phenotype and an alteration in their regulatory function. Thus, in neuroinflammatory diseases such as multiple sclerosis and posterior uveitis, the function of these vascular barriers changes resulting in an enhanced influx of leukocytes. Accordingly, the endothelial cells of the CNS are recognised as playing a pro-active role in the propagation, maintenance and possibly resolution of CNS inflammatory lesions. Over the last few decades increasing evidence, from our laboratory and that of our collaborators, has shown that the endothelial cell responds to adherent leukocytes in variety of ways resulting in immediate facilitation of diapedesis to the longer-term regulation of gene expression. Many of these outside-in signaling cascades are generated through the engagement of endothelial immunoglobulin superfamily adhesion molecules such as ICAM-1, which act as signal transducers leading to the activation of the small GTPase rho, eNOS, phospholipase C, protein kinase C, src kinase and release of intracellular calcium [1]. In addition, we have reported more recently that downstream activation of MAP kinases, re-arrangements of the actin cytoskeleton and tyrosine phosphorylation of various cytoskeletal associated proteins results in the activation of divergent inflammatory outcomes [2]. Finally, we have established that the tightness of the endothelial cell junction and cell cytoskeletal stiffness dictates the route of leukocyte transmigration [3]. Deciphering the end-points of these signaling networks and identifying potential pharmacological targets, remains a major focus of the laboratory.

Non-VEGF mediated breakdown of the blood–retinal barrier: alternative strategies to treat diabetic macular oedema

Alan W. Stitt

Diabetic macular oedema (DMO) occurs as a symptom of diabetic retinopathy and often leads to significant vision-loss [4]. The condition is characterised by progressive breakdown of the blood retinal barrier (BRB) as a result of tissue ischaemia and/or inflammation which drive imbalances in vasoactive cytokines and growth factors causing compromise of normal neuroglial–vascular interactions and endothelial dysfunction [4]. Neutralisation of vascular endothelial growth factor (VEGF) using intravitreal injection of humanised antibodies has become a mainstream treatment for DMO. Unfortunately this is not effective for all DMO patients [5] and there is a need for additional therapeutic approaches which could be used instead of, or in conjunction with, current anti-VEGF drugs.

Our groups have recently focused on the permeability-inducing agent lysophosphatidylcholine (LPC) which is produced through activity of the enzyme lipoprotein-associated phospholipase A_2 (Lp-PLA_2). Using a range of in vitro and in vivo approaches, we have recently shown that inhibition of Lp-PLA_2 can prevent diabetes-induced compromise of the BRB in a manner that is comparable to intravitreal VEGF neutralisation [6]. Importantly, these protective effects were additive when both targets were inhibited simultaneously. Our mechanistic studies also demonstrated that LPC potently induced permeability, and that there was a coalescence of the LPC and VEGF pathways via a common VEGF-receptor-2 mediated mechanism [6, 7]. We have concluded that Lp-PLA_2 may be a useful therapeutic target for patients with DMO, perhaps in combination with currently administered anti-VEGF agents. Such studies demonstrate the utility of studying "real-world" clinical scenarios whereby new approaches can be evaluated alongside the current gold-standard therapies and offer hope for patients who are non-responsive to current treatment regimes.

The choroid plexus is an important player in the induction of neuroinflammation

Roosmarijn Vandenbroucke

The choroid plexus epithelium which forms the blood–CSF barrier is a unique single layer of epithelial cells situated at the interface between blood and cerebrospinal fluid (CSF). The choroid plexus epithelium has several different important functions: it forms a barrier to protect the brain from fluctuations in the blood, produces CSF and is responsible for the active removal of toxic molecules from the brain and thereby assures brain homeostasis. In recent years, the choroid plexus epithelium has gained increasing attention, especially its role in different pathologies. Indeed, subtle changes in the choroid plexus epithelial cells will result in changes in CSF composition, exerting wide-ranging effects on the brain and subsequently affecting disease progression. Therefore, understanding blood–CSF barrier functionality under physiological and pathophysiological conditions might open up new therapeutic strategies to treat inflammatory brain diseases.

Our research focusses on the effect of both systemic inflammation (sepsis) and neuroinflammation (the age-related disease Alzheimer's disease) on the blood–CSF barrier. More specifically, we study key molecules that play a role in the activation of detrimental processes at the blood–CSF barrier upon inflammation, focussing on barrier integrity and secretory activity. These studies might allow us to identify novel therapeutic strategies to prevent neuroinflammation.

To address the effect of sepsis, we used intraperitoneal lipopolysaccharide (LPS) injection and the caecal ligation and puncture (CLP) mouse model, while Alzheimer's disease was studied using the intracerebroventricular (icv) injection of soluble amyloid β oligomers (AβO) in mice. Our studies showed that both systemic [7] and central inflammation [8] induce increased blood–CSF barrier leakage. Interestingly, these effects could be attributed to matrix metalloproteinase (MMP) activity. Additionally, peripheral inflammatory triggers induced an increase in extracellular vesicle (EV) release by the choroid plexus epithelium into the CSF [9]. Detailed analysis by electron microscopy and inhibitor studies using the neutral sphingomyelinase 2 inhibitor GW4869, revealed that especially the biogenesis of exosomes is increased upon systemic inflammation. Strikingly, these choroid plexus-derived EVs are able to enter the brain parenchyma, are taken up by astrocytes and microglia and transfer a pro-inflammatory message to the brain [9]. Interestingly, we observed that the icv injection of AβO has similar effects on the extracellular vesicle production of the choroid plexus epithelial cells.

Clearly, our data show that both peripheral and central inflammatory triggers affect barrier and secretory activity of the choroid plexus epithelium and these results might open up new therapeutic strategies to treat neuroinflammatory diseases.

MicroRNAs and blood–brain barrier function in multiple sclerosis

Ignacio A. Romero

Blood–brain barrier dysfunction is a major hallmark of many CNS disorders such as multiple sclerosis. BBB breakdown is characterised by three main features: (1) increased permeability across the endothelium; (2) alteration in the expression of cell-surface receptors and/or transporters; and (3) activation of endothelial cells to support leukocyte extravasation into the CNS parenchyma. Many of these cerebrovascular pathophysiological effects are underpinned by overt acute or chronic changes in gene expression in cerebral endothelial cells and in other cells of the NVU.

MicroRNAs (miRs) are novel regulators of gene expression at the post-transcriptional level and may potentially play a key role in cerebrovascular pathophysiology. MiRs mainly suppress the expression of target genes either by blocking translation or by inducing mRNA degradation. We have first identified miRs whose levels in endothelial cells change following inflammatory stimuli. Inflammation induces upregulation of several key inflammatory miRs termed inflammiRs (miR-155 and miR-146) in brain endothelial cells. By contrast, there are other miRs termed brain endothelial housekeeping miRs (miR-125b and miR126) whose levels are elevated under quiescent conditions but are significantly reduced by pro-inflammatory cytokines [10–12]. These inflammation-induced changes in the finely-tuned balance of cerebral endothelial miR levels promote cerebrovascular dysfunction. For example, miR-155 contributes to BBB leakiness by reducing expression of tight junctional and focal adhesion components but it also promotes leukocyte firm adhesion to brain endothelium by indirectly increasing expression of cell adhesion molecules. Conversely, miR-146 inhibits leukocyte firm adhesion to brain endothelium by suppressing expression of key activators of the NF-κB pathway. Brain endothelial miRs could potentially be considered for targeted prophylaxis and therapies for BBB dysfunction.

However, we are still far from validating cerebrovascular miRs as potential therapeutic or prophylactic targets for neurovascular dysfunction in inflammatory and/or autoimmune disorders. First, there is the likelihood that several different miRs have combinatorial effects in specific CNS pathologies. Second, individual miRs likely have multiple gene targets and effects on other endothelial cellular pathways that contribute to the pathogenesis of inflammatory disease. In addition, non-specific delivery of miR modulators into other tissues or organs (e.g. liver, kidney) could cause unwanted side effects unless very specific delivery systems targeted at the cerebrovascular bed are available, Nevertheless, the potential for manipulating this novel class of regulators of gene expression for therapeutic purposes is huge and should be given considerable attention in the near future.

Dose dependent expression of claudin-5 is a modifying factor in neurological diseases

Matthew Campbell

Abnormalities in neuronal functioning in psychiatric conditions may derive in part from abnormalities in blood vessel–neuron interactions [13]. We have shown that the claudin-5 gene, a central component of the paracellular pathway of the BBB is associated with schizophrenia in individuals with the chromosomal disorder 22q11 deletion syndrome (22q11DS), a condition that confers a 30-fold increased lifetime risk of developing schizophrenia. A variant in this gene results in up to 50% less protein product and a targeted suppression of claudin-5 in distinct brain regions, or in an inducible "knockdown" mouse, identifies strong phenotypic correlations with schizophrenia. Additionally, post-mortem human schizophrenia donor brain tissues show evidence of BBB dysfunction, while some of the most common anti-psychotic drugs can directly regulate claudin-5 expression. Identifying the underlying cause of neuropsychiatric conditions at the level of the BBB suggests novel drug entities targeting the integrity of the BBB may have utility in treating these debilitating and socially isolating condition [14, 15]. All work involving animals was approved by the institutional ethics committee and all national licences were in place prior to commencement of work.

Impact of ABC transporters on blood–brain barrier function

Gert Fricker

The CNS requires a well-balanced homeostasis. Therefore, it is protected by the BBB, which is set up by endothelial cells of brain microvessels. These cells act as a dynamic regulator of ion balance, mediator of nutrient transport and barrier to harmful molecules. A central role accords to ATP-binding-cassette (ABC) export proteins, predominantly P-glycoprotein (P-gp, ABCB1), breast cancer resistance protein (BCRP, ABCG2) and multidrug resistance related proteins (MRPs, ABCCs). ABC transporters are predominantly expressed in microvessel endothelial cells, but are also located on other cell types, such as astrocytes, microglia, and neurons. In microvessel endothelial cells ABC transporters exhibit a polar distribution. P-gp is primarily found in luminal membranes, however, there is evidence that it also localizes to a certain amount to abluminal membranes as well as to pericytes and astrocytes. Studies using a fluorescent labeled construct of P-gp indicate that the export pump is not organized as a single molecule within membranes but forms clusters of several proteins close together [16]. BCRP appears to be predominantly located at the luminal surface of endothelial cells. Mrps are also expressed at the BBB, however, there is still considerable discussion about the extent of expression, involvement in drug transport and subcellular localization. Inhibition of ABC transporters significantly alters the brain disposition of transporter substrates as illustrated by studies in human: positron emission tomography (PET)-imaging revealed that cyclosporin A modulation of P-gp increased transfer of verapamil into the brain. In another PET-trial uptake of loperamide into the CNS was enhanced after inhibition of efflux pumps by tariquidar.

Various mechanisms control expression and function of ABC transporters. Regulation occurs either by ligand-activated transcription factors or by external stress signals which modulate ABC transporter function.

The nuclear receptors PXR (pregnane X receptor), AhR (arylhydroxycarbon-receptor), CAR (constitutive androstane receptor), VDR (vitamin D receptor) and PPAR-γ (peroxisome proliferator-activated receptor) and related signaling events are of particular interest, since they bind many xenobiotics and subsequently upregulate ABC-transporter expression. ABC transporters also contribute to various CNS diseases. For example, brain tissue from Alzheimer patients showed an inverse relationship between P-gp expression and disease progress and inhibition of P-gp in a rodent Alzheimer model increased amyloid-β levels in brain. Studies showed that St. John's Wort administration to mice resulted in significant reductions of parenchymal amyloid-β accumulation as well as in a moderate increase in cerebrovascular P-gp expression [17]. In summary, ABC-transporters are of outstanding relevance for the proper function of the blood–brain barrier. They are very sensitive to exogenous and endogenous stimuli and are involved in the progression of various CNS diseases.

In vitro models of the blood–brain barrier, pro's and con's

Birger Brodin

The brain capillary endothelium serves as a gateway for exchange of nutrients, hormones and metabolites between plasma and brain parenchyma, and acts as a barrier for CNS uptake of the majority of drug compounds. Mechanistic in vivo investigations of drug and nutrient transport, signalling and metabolism in the brain endothelium can be difficult to perform, since the brain endothelium is embedded within a complex structure, *the neurovascular unit*, itself within the multi-compartment brain and fluid system.

Cell isolation and culture protocols for growing brain endothelial cells in monolayers, either in monoculture or in co-culture with other cell types of the NVU, have been developed over the last 40 years. Although no ideal cell culture model of the blood–brain barrier is yet available, the in vitro models have evolved to become useful tools in the studies of barrier biology and drug delivery.

In vitro models based on primary cell cultures of animal origin (typically bovine, porcine or murine models) display endothelial cell morphology, expression of BBB tight junction proteins and high transendothelial electrical resistance, subject to astrocyte induction [18]. They display vectorial transport of efflux transporter substrates, indicative of luminal expression of ABC-type pumps [19]. The major drawback of these models may be downregulation of a number of solute carrier family proteins (SLC's) as compared to the expression in vivo. Alternatively, immortalized cell lines of mouse, rat and human origin, in general without astrocyte induction, tend to be considerably more leaky than the in vitro models based on primary cell cultures. Some immortalized cell lines do, however, show relatively higher expression of some BBB-specific SLC transporters than the models based on primary cell cultures and may serve as excellent tools for studies of uptake, receptor activation and some signal transduction systems. A recent approach, generation of in vitro models of the BBB using human stem cells, has resulted in cell monolayers with both high monolayer tightness and expression of BBB-specific marker proteins [20]. However, the stem cell cultures are not yet widely used, and have not been fully validated with respect to transport properties and functional transporter profiling.

In brief, established in vitro blood–brain barrier models all have their advantages and drawbacks. Primary cell lines of bovine, porcine and rodent origin generate tight monolayers whereas immortalized cell lines may have higher transporter expression levels but less tightness. Models derived from human stem cells shows great promise, but are not yet fully characterized.

Measuring blood–brain barrier transport of drugs—the hurdle in drug discovery and development

Margareta Hammarlund-Udenaes

Measurement of total drug levels in the brain has been a common but unhelpful practice for many years in drug discovery programs aiming at central drug effects. The paradigm has changed with the introduction of the pharmacologically more important unbound brain interstitial fluid to unbound blood concentration ratio, $K_{p,uu,brain}$, and with more high-throughput methods to estimate this parameter (the brain slice and the brain homogenate techniques).

By combining several of these measurements, the combinatory mapping approach (CMA) allows estimation of not only BBB transport, but also intracellular distribution of the pharmacologically active, unbound drug moiety [21]. CMA can also be used to assess possible lysosomal accumulation that may predict phospholipidosis as a serious side effect. The technique allows estimation of brain regional differences in BBB transport and binding, something that can influence effect/side effect patterns of drugs. In a study of six antipsychotic drugs, we found very different BBB and intracellular distribution patterns of the drugs [22]. There was a sixfold difference in regional BBB transport of risperidone (a P-glycoprotein substrate), with a more efficient efflux in cerebellum than in frontal cortex in rats, while other drugs such as quetiapine and clozapine showed very small differences in regional transport. In a separate study utilizing the CMA, we did not find any change in the BBB transport of five selected drugs in disease models of Alzheimer's disease

(ArcSwe) and Parkinson's disease (A30P) compared with wild-type mice, counteracting the view that the BBB is leaky in disease.

Microdialysis was used to study if liposomal delivery would improve the brain uptake of methotrexate [23]. With microdialysis it was possible to separate the liposomally-encapsulated drug from released drug in blood, and to measure the released compound in brain. While liposomes based on hydrogenated soy phosphatidylcholine did not change BBB uptake at all compared with administering the free drug, the egg-yolk phosphatidylcholine liposomes increased the uptake into the brain threefold, reaching concentrations that could be pharmacologically active also in humans.

In conclusion, there are three main conceptual parts of brain drug transport, the rate of transport, measured as the permeability surface area product, the extent of transport measured with $K_{p,uu,brain}$, and the nonspecific intra-brain binding, all contributing to different aspects of brain drug delivery. The extent of transport is considered clinically most relevant, as it measures the steady state relationship across the BBB, quantifying active efflux and influx processes.

NEUWAY pharma: qualified for CNS delivery

Heiko Manninga

NEUWAY Pharma GmbH, a German based biotech company, is focusing on the preclinical and clinical development of innovative therapeutics for treatment of brain diseases based on its proprietary CNS Drug Delivery Platform.

The presented platform is based on a protein derived from the JC-Virus, which naturally forms capsules, named Engineered Protein Capsules (EPCs). EPCs may be used as carrier to transport highly active drug substances—ranging from small molecules to large nucleic acid strands—across the intact BBB. NEUWAY has demonstrated that its EPC-based proprietary CNS drug delivery platform can deliver plasmids over the blood brain barrier into CNS cells leading to gene expression in the brain. In a proof of concept study it was shown that intravenous injection of EPCs loaded with DNA encoding for luciferase induced an activity of the resulting enzyme, which was detected by bioluminescent signals in the brain (Fig. 1). More accurate studies of the brains of such treated mice clearly showed that the signals from the brain cells are beyond the blood–brain barrier and not from other cells, e.g., blood vessels.

As EPCs can carry large nucleic acid strands, they may be useful for gene therapy of rare diseases. NEUWAYs current development focuses on lysosomal storage diseases, like metachromatic leucodystrophy. For this and other rare diseases, NEUWAY plans to run its own clinical development programs. NEUWAY is also open to partner its CNS drug delivery platform with

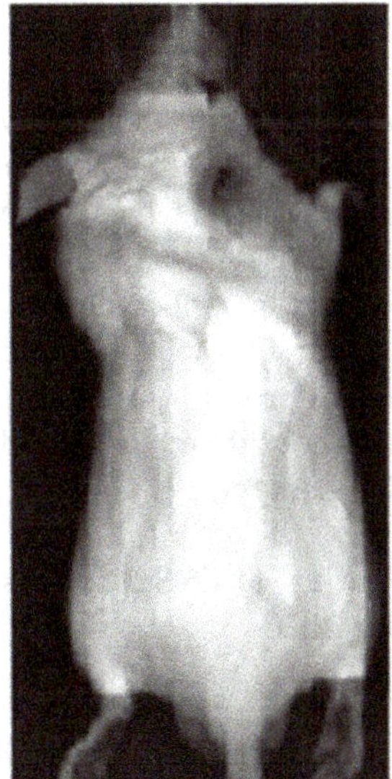
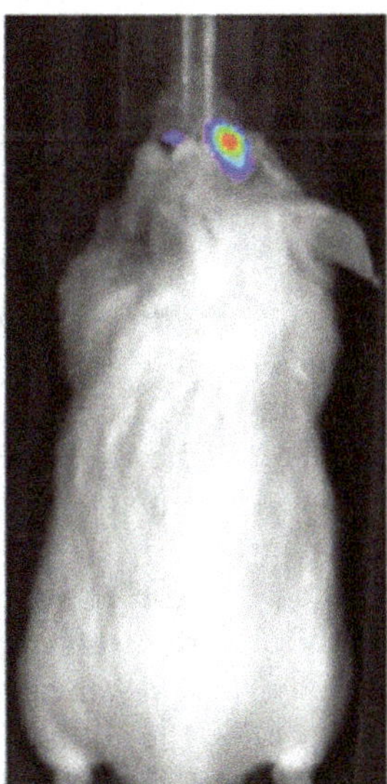
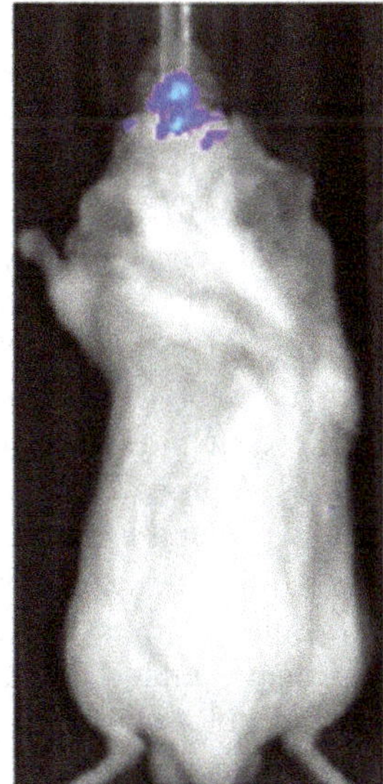

Fig. 1 The enzyme luciferase produces light when the conversion of luciferin occurs. If a plasmid coding for luciferase is administered intravenously, no light signal can be detected (left mouse). The enzyme was degraded in the bloodstream. If the luciferase plasmid packaged in Engineered Protein Capsules (EPCs) is applied directly into the brain (intracerebral, i.c., middle mouse), a luminous signal can be detected there after administration of luciferin. This is also observed when the luciferase plasmid is packaged in EPCs and injected intravenously (i.v., right mouse)

pharmaceutical or biotech companies preferably if large indications, like Alzheimer's disease, are addressed.

Investigations conformed to the Guide for the Care and Use of Laboratory Animals published by the US National Institutes of Health (NIH Publication No. 85-23, revised 1996).

All animal procedures were approved by the appropriate state agency (Protocol Number W17/11).

Liposomal technology and the blood–brain barrier

Pieter J. Gaillard

2-BBB is successfully harnessing liposomal technology to mediate safe targeting and enhanced drug delivery to the brain. The G-Technology® platform has been shown to enhance transport of therapeutics across the blood–brain barrier. Preclinical studies with the lead product, 2B3-101, containing doxorubicin, demonstrated significantly enhanced delivery and improved survival of mice in comparison to currently available compounds.

Phase I clinical trials with 2B3-101 have been completed, with Phase IIa set to determine preliminary antitumor efficacy at the maximum tolerated dose. The study population of this phase I/IIa trial consisted of patients who met all of the inclusion criteria and none of the exclusion criteria, and provided written informed consent. The protocol, any amendments and all other applicable study documents for the study were reviewed by the Independent Ethics Committees (IECs) of the following countries: NL: The "Nederlands Kanker Instituut Antoni van Leeuwenhoek Ziekenhuis"; BE: The "Association Hospitaliere de Bruxelles-Centre des Tumeurs de l'ULB"; USA: The "Office of Human Research Ethics of the University of North Carolina at Chapel Hill"; FR: The "Comite De Protection Des Personnes Ile De France III". Clinical trial identifier is NCT01386580.

2-BBB's second product in development, 2B3-201, containing methylprednisolone, is designed to treat patients with acute neuroinflammation. Superior efficacy, reduced side effects and enhanced plasma circulation half-life have been shown in rodent models, in comparison to competitive compounds. A phase I study in healthy volunteers was completed, addressing safety, tolerability and pharmacokinetics, and markers for pharmacological proof-of-concept. Collectively, preclinical and clinical evidence to date has demonstrated that G-Technology® offers a promising platform to safely enhance delivery of drugs to the brain. The study was approved by the Medical Ethics Committee of the BEBO Foundation (Assen, The Netherlands). Subjects provided written informed consent. Clinical trial identifier is NCT02048358.

The blood–brain barrier in gene therapy: hurdle or target?

Markus Schwaninger

Gene therapy provides attractive therapeutic options for the many diseases for which no treatment is still available. The adeno-associated virus (AAV) is a safe and efficient tool to transfer genes. However, conventional AAV-based vectors do not cross the BBB when administered systemically. This obstacle can be solved by administering vectors either intrathecally or using vectors based on AAV serotype 9 that cross the BBB to a limited extent. Still another approach is to target the BBB itself. In order to develop a brain endothelial selective vector, a novel strategy for in vivo screening of random ligand libraries displayed on viral capsids was used [24]. Several rounds of in vivo selection resulted in AAV-BR1, an AAV vector with unprecedented selectivity for brain endothelial cells after systemic intravenous administration. Due to its specific features, this vector allows for modulating and repairing the BBB. Its efficacy was tested in a mouse model of the hereditary disease incontinentia pigmenti [25], in which a deficiency of the Nemo gene leads to a loss of brain endothelial cells and breakdown of the BBB. Consequently, patients suffer from neurological disability and epileptic seizures. Intravenous injection of AAV-BR1 transferring the Nemo gene was able to largely reduce endothelial cell death and to ameliorate disruption of the BBB. Mice treated with AAV-BR1-Nemo showed less activation of astrocytes. Importantly, the occurrence of focal epileptic seizures was significantly reduced by the gene therapy [26]. Probably due to its high brain endothelial selectivity, the vector did not induce hepatocellular carcinoma or other adverse effects that have been observed in rodents during gene therapy with AAV vectors. Previous studies suggest that transduced brain endothelial cells may release enzymes that are missing in the CNS [27]. Thus, transducing brain endothelial cells with gene vectors offers the opportunity to overcome the BBB and to supply diverse proteins to the diseased brain (Fig. 2). The conceptual progress of this approach is that the BBB is no longer considered as a hurdle but as the target of a successful therapy.

Antibody therapeutics for CNS diseases and their delivery across the BBB

Carl Webster

The BBB protects and regulates the homeostasis of the brain. However, this barrier also limits the access of drugs, including large molecule therapeutics, to the brain and results in sub-therapeutic concentrations of drug reaching CNS targets. MedImmune have utilised their

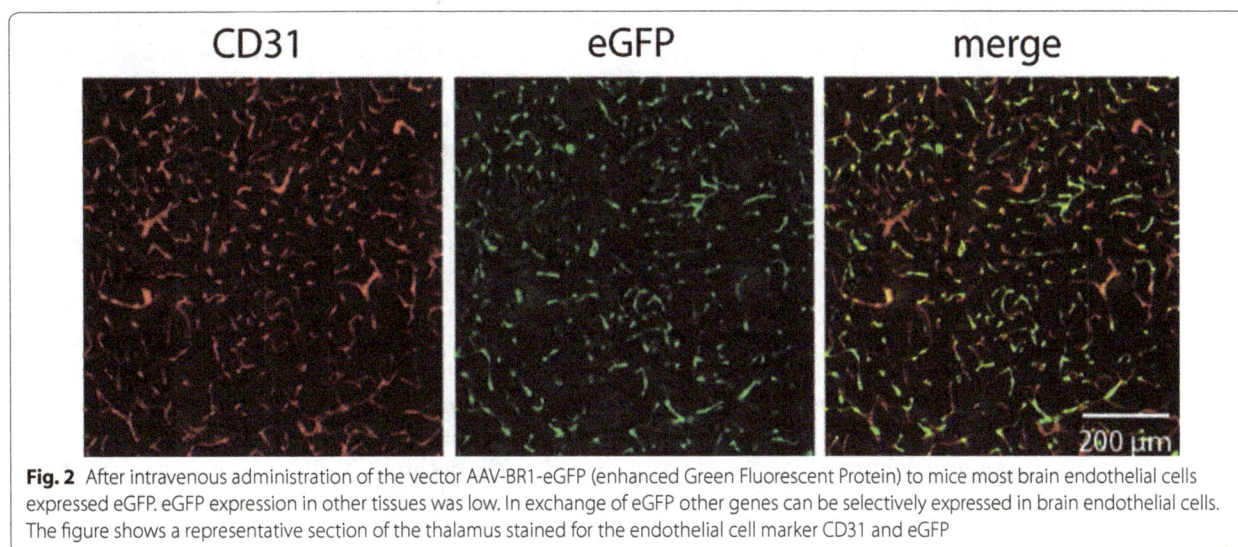

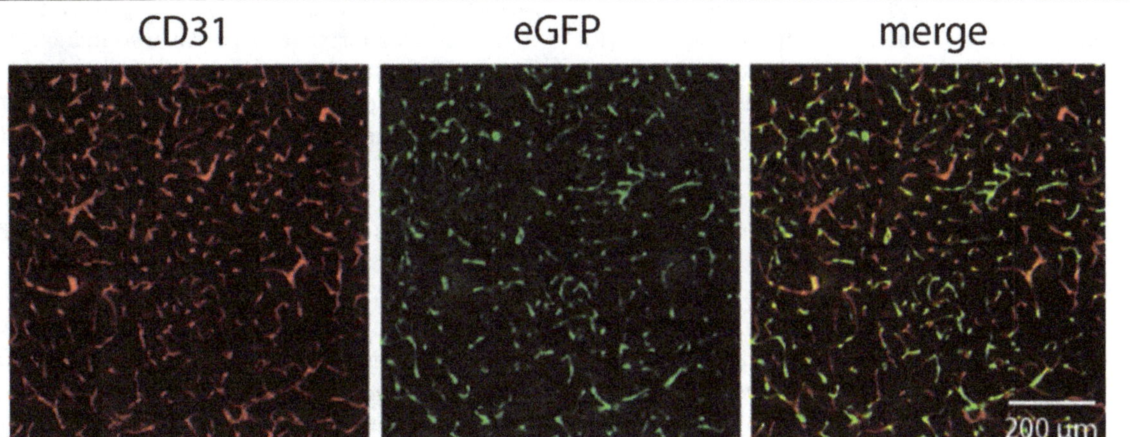

Fig. 2 After intravenous administration of the vector AAV-BR1-eGFP (enhanced Green Fluorescent Protein) to mice most brain endothelial cells expressed eGFP. eGFP expression in other tissues was low. In exchange of eGFP other genes can be selectively expressed in brain endothelial cells. The figure shows a representative section of the thalamus stained for the endothelial cell marker CD31 and eGFP

antibody engineering platform to develop a fully human monoclonal antibody that targets the blood brain barrier to deliver therapeutics to the CNS. The antibody was isolated from a phage display library by competitive elution using the known BBB transporting antibody FC5. A combination of pharmacodynamic (PD) and pharmacokinetic (PK) assays were used to confirm central penetration. In mice, the peripheral PK was in line with the expected half-life for a human antibody and showed no target mediated clearance at doses from 0.45 to 45 mg/kg. Brain penetration was around 3% of injected dose and persisted beyond 7 days. To confirm the antibody present in the CNS was able to access central targets, a fusion to interleukin-1 receptor antagonist (IL-1RA) was made. IL-1 is mediator of neuropathic pain and its antagonism is analgesic. Partial ligation of the sciatic nerve results in a neuropathic pain phenotype that manifests through increased sensitivity to mechanical pressure on the hind paw. Peripheral administration of the BBB-IL-1RA fusion resulted in dose dependent analgesia, confirming the ability of the BBB antibody to penetrate the CNS. However, the doses required were high and this fusion protein would not represent a commercially viable treatment for neuropathic pain. Other molecular targets represent better points of intervention in the pain signalling pathways and therefore an antibody against the ATP gated ion channel P2X4 was developed. P2X4 regulates the physiology and pathophysiology of spinal microglia and is implicated in pain signalling. Channel blocking antibodies against mouse P2X4 were obtained by immunising rats with recombinant mouse P2X4. Approximately 5000 hybridoma lines binding to P2X4 were identified of which 28 showed blocking activity. Lead antibodies were tested by intrathecal administration to mice where analgesia in the neuropathic pain model was demonstrated. Peripheral administration resulted in analgesia only when fused to the BBB antibody, confirming central exposure of the drug molecule was required. Doses as low as 3 mg/kg produce statistically significant analgesia, and this offers hope of a treatment to many people suffering from neuropathic pain.

All procedures described here were performed in accordance with the Animals (Scientific Procedures) Act 1986 and were approved by the MedImmune local ethics committee.

Harnessing bispecific antibodies to overcome the blood–brain barrier

Krzysztof B. Wicher

Penetration of the BBB remains a significant impediment in development of biologics for CNS-related diseases. To identify efficient brain-shuttles, we used shark single domain antibody phage libraries in a combined in vitro and in vivo selection process. To achieve the highest discovery rate of brain-penetrant clones, we employed next generation sequencing of phagemid DNA after subsequent rounds of selection. This way, we identified a panel of TfR1-specific shark antibodies, which are efficiently transported to mouse brain parenchyma. One of these antibodies (B2) fused to human IgG1 Fc showed more than 12-fold better brain uptake than the control, reaching therapeutic concentrations (5 nM) upon single intravenous injection of 25 nmol/kg (~ 1.9 mg/kg). Most of the brain-associated B2-hFc was found in brain parenchyma. Immunohistochemistry analyses showed the protein present both in the intestinal fluid and in the cells, including neurons. B2 antibody is safe upon administration of high doses in mice, as manifested by lack of significant acute adverse reactions or changes in blood morphology of injected animals. It binds to human TfR1 with comparable affinity as to mouse TfR1, but does not bind to TfR2. Moreover, in silico analysis indicates that B2 antibody would have relatively low immunogenic properties in humans.

We next constructed several different variants of bi-specific antibodies composed of B2 and rituximab, a well characterized anti human CD20 specific antibody used to treat peripheral B cell lymphomas. Many of these variants shuttle efficiently to brain and provide up to 14× better exposure than original antibody. The hybrid proteins retain their binding to both TfR1 and CD20 and at least some of them appear to mediate antibody-dependent cell cytotoxicity response on human $CD20^{+ve}$, but not on $CD20^{-ve}$, cells, similar to that of rituximab. Thus, they offer possible therapeutics for multiple sclerosis and cerebral B-cell lymphoma.

All research procedures/experiments described here were performed in accordance with Animals Scientific Procedures Act 1986 and European Directive 2010/63/EU. All studies performed were approved by the Royal Veterinary College Animal Welfare and Ethics Review Body and comply with the UK Home Office guidelines and codes of conduct.

Drug delivery across the blood–brain barrier using peptide conjugates

Michel Khrestchatisky

Drug delivery to the brain is hindered by the BBB. Receptor-mediated transport/transcytosis (RMT) can be used to shuttle therapeutics into the brain in a non-invasive manner. We developed peptide- and nanobody-based ligands that target specific receptors and that can be used as vector molecules to transport drugs or imaging agents across the BBB. Members of the low density lipoprotein receptor (LDLR) family appear relevant to deliver drugs into cells and organs and we report results on the development of peptide-vectors that target the rodent and human LDLR. Initial screening of complex peptide libraries followed by chemical optimization led to the development of a family of short cyclic peptides (eight natural or non-natural residues) with distinct properties in terms of affinity, stability and biodistribution.

Real time two-photon microscopy experiments on mice demonstrated the ability of a lead peptide-vector to transport a non-permeable agent such as RhoRedX across the BBB and the blood–spinal cord barrier. As a further proof of concept, following intravenous (iv) administration in mice, peptide-vectors efficiently transported to the brain molecules such as opiate peptides or neuropeptides, all known to poorly cross the BBB. In particular, a vector-neurotensin conjugate is under preclinical development for its potential to induce pharmacological hypothermia with neuroprotective effects in acute excitotoxic neurodegeneration.

Some tumors including glioblastoma are associated with high-level expression of receptors involved in cell metabolism such as the LDLR. Conjugating our peptide-vectors to ^{68}Gallium-NODAGA or -DOTA allowed PET imaging of glioblastoma in mouse brain. Others have shown that nanoparticles or liposomes functionalized with one of our lead peptide-vectors (peptide-22) permeate the BBB and exhibit higher glioma distribution than non-functionalized nanoparticles or liposomes; functionalized nanoparticles or liposomes loaded with paclitaxel and doxorubicin respectively elicit significantly prolonged life span of glioma-bearing mice [27, 28].

The lead peptide vectors also allowed uptake of vectorized protein cargos such as an antibody Fc fragment by brain endothelial cells and transport across an in vitro BBB model, and in vivo into the brain following iv administration in mice [29]. The peptide-vectors are currently assessed with industrial partners for their potential to transport therapeutic antibodies into the brain. In summary, we have developed a family of chemically optimized peptide-vectors that can be conjugated to a variety of different compounds such as small organic molecules, peptides, siRNAs and proteins including therapeutic antibodies. These peptide vectors bind the rodent and human LDLR and promote transport of cargos across the BBB and brain uptake in rodents. Such peptide-vectors appear promising for CNS delivery of different classes of drugs.

Conclusions

From the variety of talks, it was clear that significant progress is being made in understanding control processes at brain barrier interfaces and in novel drug delivery methods. Modification of the normal barrier processes occurs in inflammatory situations through signalling cascades which can be manipulated, barrier gene expression can be modified with micro RNAs and control can be exerted over barrier transporter functions. Techniques for enhancing delivery of therapeutics to the CNS involve cleverly-devised delivery vehicles such as drug-carrying liposomes, endothelial-specific viral vectors, peptide conjugates, engineered protein capsules, nanoparticles, bi-specific antibodies and human monoclonal antibodies. Methods to test the efficacy of therapeutic delivery were discussed using both in vitro and in vivo techniques. Overall this was a stimulating conference bringing together scientists from a number of different disciplines.

Authors' contributions
Authors contributed with an short report of their contribution to the conference. JG, HCJ and MH-U wrote the Abstract, Background and Conclusions. All authors read and approved the final manuscript.

Authors' information
HCJ is a Co-Editor of *Fluids and Barriers of the CNS*.

Author details
[1] Institute of Ophthalmology, University College London, London EC1V 9EL, UK. [2] Department of Pharmaceutical Biosciences, Uppsala University, 751 24 Uppsala, Sweden. [3] Gagle Brook House, Chesterton, Bicester OX26 1UF, UK. [4] Centre for Experimental Medicine, Queen's University Belfast, Belfast, Northern Ireland, UK. [5] Department of Biomedical Molecular Biology, Ghent University, Ghent, Belgium. [6] VIB-UGent Center for Inflammation Research, VIB, Ghent, Belgium. [7] School of Life, Health and Chemical Sciences, Open University, Milton Keynes, UK. [8] Smurfit Institute of Genetics, Lincoln Place Gate, Trinity College Dublin, Dublin 2, Ireland. [9] Institute of Pharmacy and Molecular Biotechnology, Ruprecht-Karls University, Heidelberg, Germany. [10] Department of Pharmacy, Faculty of Health and Medical Sciences, University of Copenhagen, Copenhagen, Denmark. [11] NEUWAY Pharma GmbH, Ludwig-Erhard-Allee 2, 53175 Bonn, Germany. [12] 2-BBB Medicines BV, Leiden, Netherlands. [13] Institute of Experimental and Clinical Pharmacology and Toxicology, University of Lübeck, Lübeck, Germany. [14] Antibody Discovery and Protein Engineering, MedImmune, Cambridge, UK. [15] Ossianix Inc., Stevenage, UK. [16] CNRS, NICN, Aix Marseille Univ, Marseille, France. [17] Vect-Horus, Faculte de Medecine Nord, 51 Boulevard Pierre Dramard, Marseille, France.

Acknowledgements
MH-U: The contributions of Irena Loryan and Yang Hu are mush appreciated.

AWS: The collaboration of Patric Turowski (UCL Institute of Ophthalmology, London, UK) is gratefully acknowledged.

IAR: The collaboration of C Cerutti, MA Lopez-Ramirez, and D Wu (Open University, UK) is gratefully acknowledged.

HM: The author would like to thank staff at Fraunhofer Institute for Cell Therapy and Immunology (Department of Cell Therapy, Experimental Imaging) for performing the animal studies, particularly: Alexander Kranz and Franziska Werner.

MS: The collaboration of Jakob Körbelin (UKE, Hamburg, Germany) is gratefully acknowledged.

CW: The author would like to thank staff at MedImmune Cambridge who contributed to this work, particularly: George Thom, Jon Hatcher, Iain Chessell and Wendy Williams.

KBW: The collaboration of Paweł Stocki, Jarosław Szary and Mykhaylo Demydchuk (Ossianix Inc., Stevenage UK) and of Frank S. Walsh and J. Lynn Rutkowski (Ossianix Inc., Philadelphia, USA) is gratefully acknowledged.

MK: The collaboration of Marion David, Pascaline Lécorché, Cedric Malicet, Yves Molino, Maxime Masse, Guillaume Jacquot and Jamal Temsamani (Vect-Horus, Marseille, France) and Jonathan Nowak, Romy Cohen, Anne Bernard (Aix Marseille Université, CNRS, NICN, Marseille, France) is gratefully acknowledged.

Competing interests
JG, MH-U, HCJ, REV, IAR, MC, GF, BB, MS declares that they have no competing interests. AWS: Part of the work described was funded by GlaxoSmithKline plc. HM: All work described in this abstract was funded by NEUWAY Pharma GmbH. HM is employee and shareholder in NEUWAY Pharma GmbH, is named inventor on patent (applications) covering the described work, and therefore has a theoretical competing interests. PJG: All work described in this abstract was funded by to-BBB technologies BV, and is currently owned by 2-BBB Medicines BV. PJG was employee and shareholder into-BBB technologies BV and is currently shareholder in 2-BBB Medicines BV, is named inventor on patent (applications) covering the described work, and therefore has a theoretical competing interests. CW: All work described in this abstract was funded by MedImmune. All collaborators at the time of the work were employees of MedImmune and therefore have a theoretical competing interests. KBW: The author and collaborators were employed by Ossianix, Inc. at the time of completion of this work. MK is Research Director at the CNRS and Director of the NICN laboratory supported by the CNRS and Aix-Marseille Université, and also co-founder, shareholder and scientific counsel of the biotechnology company Vect-Horus.

Funding
The papers in this publication were presented at a conference organised by Kisaco Research held March 22–23rd London, UK http://www.kisacoresearch.com.

References

1. Greenwood J, Heasman SJ, Alvarez JI, Prat A, Lyck R, Engelhardt B. Review: leucocyte-endothelial cell crosstalk at the blood–brain barrier: a prerequisite for successful immune cell entry to the brain. Neuropathol Appl Neurobiol. 2011;37:24–39.
2. Dragoni S, Hudson N, Kenny BA, Burgoyne T, McKenzie JA, Gill Y, et al. Endothelial MAPKs direct ICAM-1 signaling to divergent inflammatory functions. J Immunol. 2017;198:4074–85.
3. Martinelli R, Zeiger AS, Whitfield M, Sciuto TE, Dvorak A, Van Vliet KJ, et al. Probing the biomechanical contribution of the endothelium to lymphocyte migration: diapedesis by the path of least resistance. J Cell Sci. 2014;127:3720–34.
4. Duh EJ, Sun JK, Stitt AW. Diabetic retinopathy: current understanding, mechanisms, and treatment strategies. JCI Insight. 2017;2:14.
5. Ford JA, Lois N, Royle P, Clar C, Shyangdan D, Waugh N. Current treatments in diabetic macular oedema: systematic review and meta-analysis. BMJ Open. 2013;3:3.
6. Canning P, Kenny BA, Prise V, Glenn J, Sarker MH, Hudson N, et al. Lipoprotein-associated phospholipase A2 (Lp-PLA2) as a therapeutic target to prevent retinal vasopermeability during diabetes. Proc Natl Acad Sci USA. 2016;113:7213–8.
7. Vandenbroucke RE, Dejonckheere E, Van Lint P, Demeestere D, Van Wonterghem E, Vanlaere I, et al. Matrix metalloprotease 8-dependent extracellular matrix cleavage at the blood–CSF barrier contributes to lethality during systemic inflammatory diseases. J Neurosci. 2012;32:9805–16.
8. Brkic M, Balusu S, Van Wonterghem E, Gorlé N, Benilova I, Kremer A, et al. Amyloid beta oligomers disrupt blood–CSF barrier integrity by activating matrix metalloproteinases. J Neurosci. 2015;35:12766–78.
9. Balusu S, Van Wonterghem E, De Rycke R, Raemdonck K, Stremersch S, Gevaert K, et al. Identification of a novel mechanism of blood–brain communication during peripheral inflammation via choroid plexus-derived extracellular vesicles. EMBO Mol Med. 2016;8:1162–83.
10. Reijerkerk A, Lopez-Ramirez MA, van Het Hof B, Drexhage JA, Kamphuis WW, Kooij G, et al. MicroRNAs regulate human brain endothelial cell-barrier function in inflammation: implications for multiple sclerosis. J Neurosci. 2013;33:6857–63.
11. Lopez-Ramirez MA, Wu D, Pryce G, Simpson JE, Reijerkerk A, King-Robson J, et al. MicroRNA-155 negatively affects blood–brain barrier function during neuroinflammation. FASEB J. 2014;28:2551–65.
12. Cerutti C, Edwards LJ, de Vries HE, Sharrack B, Male DK, Romero IA. MiR-126 and miR-126* regulate shear-resistant firm leukocyte adhesion to human brain endothelium. Sci Rep. 2017;7:45284.
13. Keaney J, Walsh DM, O'Malley T, Hudson N, Crosbie DE, Loftus T, et al. Autoregulated paracellular clearance of amyloid-beta across the blood–brain barrier. Sci Adv. 2015;1:e1500472.
14. Campbell M, Hanrahan F, Gobbo OL, Kelly ME, Kiang AS, Humphries MM, et al. Targeted suppression of claudin-5 decreases cerebral oedema and improves cognitive outcome following traumatic brain injury. Nat Commun. 2012;3:849.
15. Campbell M, Humphries MM, Kiang AS, Nguyen AT, Gobbo OL, Tam LC, et al. Systemic low-molecular weight drug delivery to pre-selected neuronal regions. EMBO Mol Med. 2011;3:235–45.
16. Huber O, Brunner A, Maier P, Kaufmann R, Couraud PO, Cremer C, et al. Localization microscopy (SPDM) reveals clustered formations of P-glycoprotein in a human blood–brain barrier model. PLoS ONE. 2012;7:e44776.
17. Brenn A, Grube M, Jedlitschky G, Fischer A, Strohmeier B, Eiden M, et al. St. John's Wort reduces beta-amyloid accumulation in a double transgenic Alzheimer's disease mouse model-role of P-glycoprotein. Brain Pathol. 2014;24:18–24.

18. Helms HC, Abbott NJ, Burek M, Cecchelli R, Couraud PO, Deli MA, et al. In vitro models of the blood–brain barrier: an overview of commonly used brain endothelial cell culture models and guidelines for their use. J Cereb Blood Flow Metab. 2016;36:862–90.
19. Helms HC, Hersom M, Kuhlmann LB, Badolo L, Nielsen CU, Brodin B. An electrically tight in vitro blood–brain barrier model displays net brain-to-blood efflux of substrates for the ABC transporters, P-gp, Bcrp and Mrp-1. AAPS J. 2014;16:1046–55.
20. Lippmann ES, Azarin SM, Kay JE, Nessler RA, Wilson HK, Al-Ahmad A, et al. Derivation of blood–brain barrier endothelial cells from human pluripotent stem cells. Nat Biotechnol. 2012;30:783–91.
21. Loryan I, Melander E, Svensson M, Payan M, Konig F, Jansson B, et al. In-depth neuropharmacokinetic analysis of antipsychotics based on a novel approach to estimate unbound target-site concentration in CNS regions: link to spatial receptor occupancy. Mol Psychiatry. 2016;21:1527–36.
22. Loryan I, Sinha V, Mackie C, Van Peer A, Drinkenburg W, Vermeulen A, et al. Mechanistic understanding of brain drug disposition to optimize the selection of potential neurotherapeutics in drug discovery. Pharm Res. 2014;31:2203–19.
23. Hu Y, Rip J, Gaillard PJ, de Lange ECM, Hammarlund-Udenaes M. The impact of liposomal formulations on the release and brain delivery of methotrexate: an in vivo microdialysis study. J Pharm Sci. 2017;106:2606–13.
24. Korbelin J, Dogbevia G, Michelfelder S, Ridder DA, Hunger A, Wenzel J, et al. A brain microvasculature endothelial cell-specific viral vector with the potential to treat neurovascular and neurological diseases. EMBO Mol Med. 2016;8:609–25.
25. Ridder DA, Wenzel J, Muller K, Tollner K, Tong XK, Assmann JC, et al. Brain endothelial TAK1 and NEMO safeguard the neurovascular unit. J Exp Med. 2015;212:1529–49.
26. Dogbevia GK, Tollner K, Korbelin J, Broer S, Ridder DA, Grasshoff H, et al. Gene therapy decreases seizures in a model of incontinentia pigmenti. Ann Neurol. 2017;82:93–104.
27. Chen YH, Chang M, Davidson BL. Molecular signatures of disease brain endothelia provide new sites for CNS-directed enzyme therapy. Nat Med. 2009;15:1215–8.
28. Zhang B, Sun X, Mei H, Wang Y, Liao Z, Chen J, et al. LDLR-mediated peptide-22-conjugated nanoparticles for dual-targeting therapy of brain glioma. Biomaterials. 2013;34:9171–82.
29. Molino Y, David M, Varini K, Jabes F, Gaudin N, Fortoul A, et al. Use of LDL receptor-targeting peptide vectors for in vitro and in vivo cargo transport across the blood–brain barrier. FASEB J. 2017;31:1807–27.

8

Blood–brain barrier and foetal-onset hydrocephalus, with a view on potential novel treatments beyond managing CSF flow

M. Guerra[1*], J. L. Blázquez[2] and E. M. Rodríguez[1]

Abstract

Despite decades of research, no compelling non-surgical therapies have been developed for foetal hydrocephalus. So far, most efforts have pointed to repairing disturbances in the cerebrospinal fluid (CSF) flow and to avoid further brain damage. There are no reports trying to prevent or diminish abnormalities in brain development which are inseparably associated with hydrocephalus. A key problem in the treatment of hydrocephalus is the blood–brain barrier that restricts the access to the brain for therapeutic compounds or systemically grafted cells. Recent investigations have started to open an avenue for the development of a cell therapy for foetal-onset hydrocephalus. Potential cells to be used for brain grafting include: (1) pluripotential neural stem cells; (2) mesenchymal stem cells; (3) genetically-engineered stem cells; (4) choroid plexus cells and (5) subcommissural organ cells. Expected outcomes are a proper microenvironment for the embryonic neurogenic niche and, consequent normal brain development.

Keywords: Foetal-onset hydrocephalus, Blood–brain barrier, Cerebrospinal fluid, Cell therapy

Background

Foetal-onset hydrocephalus is a heterogeneous condition. Genetic [1] and environmental factors, such as vitamin B or folic acid deficiency [2], viral infection of ependyma [3], and prematurity-related germinal matrix and intraventricular hemorrhage [4], contribute to its occurrence. Recent studies have begun to identify the cellular pathologies that accompany foetal-onset hydrocephalus. Studies on numerous mutant animal models indicate that a disruption of the ventricular zone (VZ) of the cerebral aqueduct, starting early in development, triggers aqueduct stenosis and hydrocephalus [5–7]. A similar phenomenon seems to take place in cases of human foetal-onset hydrocephalus [8, 9]. The process of VZ disruption, which first affects the cerebral aqueduct, but also reaches the telencephalon, results in two neuropathological events: the formation of subependymal grey matter heterotopia (also known as 'periventricular heterotopia'), resulting from a failure of neuroblast migration during development of the embryonic brain, and the translocation of neural stem cells/neural progenitor cells into the foetal cerebrospinal fluid (CSF) [7, 10, 11]. Cerebral abnormalities are irreversible inborn defects and they could explain some of the neurologic impairments (e.g. epilepsy) of children born with hydrocephalus.

Foetal-onset hydrocephalus affects 1–3 of 1000 live births and is characterized by abnormal CSF flow accompanied by ventricular dilatation [12]. Although surgical diversion of CSF with shunts does prevent further damage to the brain caused by hydrocephalus, it does not solve the essential brain maldevelopment and neurological outcome associated with hydrocephalus. Indeed, 80–90% of the neurologic impairment suffered by shunt-dependent neonates with foetal-onset hydrocephalus is not reversed by surgery [13, 14]. The treatment of neurologic disorders is challenging because of the brain barriers that make it difficult to effectively and persistently deliver therapeutic compounds. The tight endothelial barrier can be bypassed using endogenous

*Correspondence: monserratguerra@uach.cl
[1] Instituto de Anatomía, Histología y Patología, Facultad de Medicina, Universidad Austral de Chile, Valdivia, Chile
Full list of author information is available at the end of the article

blood–brain barrier (BBB) transporters allowing carrier-mediated transport or receptor-mediated transport [15–17] (Fig. 1).

Recent years have witnessed research progress in the development of cell therapies for brain diseases, including neurological impairment associated with the onset of hydrocephalus. Expected applications for cell therapy are the regeneration of the disrupted VZ and drug delivery to improve the brain microenvironment and neurological function. We discuss this evidence in the present review.

Ontogenetic development of the blood–brain barrier (BBB) in animals and humans

The idea of a blood–brain barrier (BBB) that segregates blood from brain was developed 100 years ago, following the demonstration that vital dyes injected intravenously stained most organs but not the brain and spinal

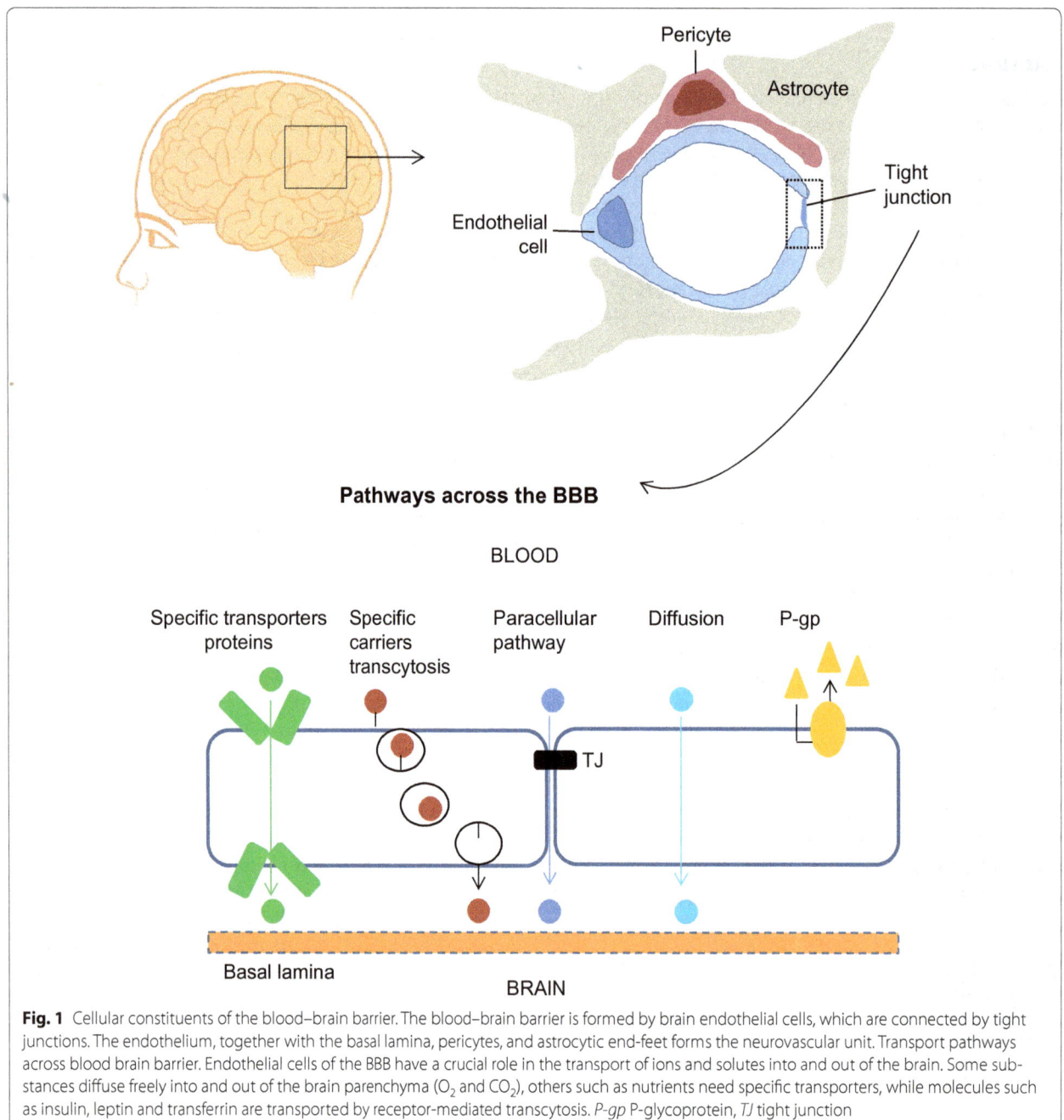

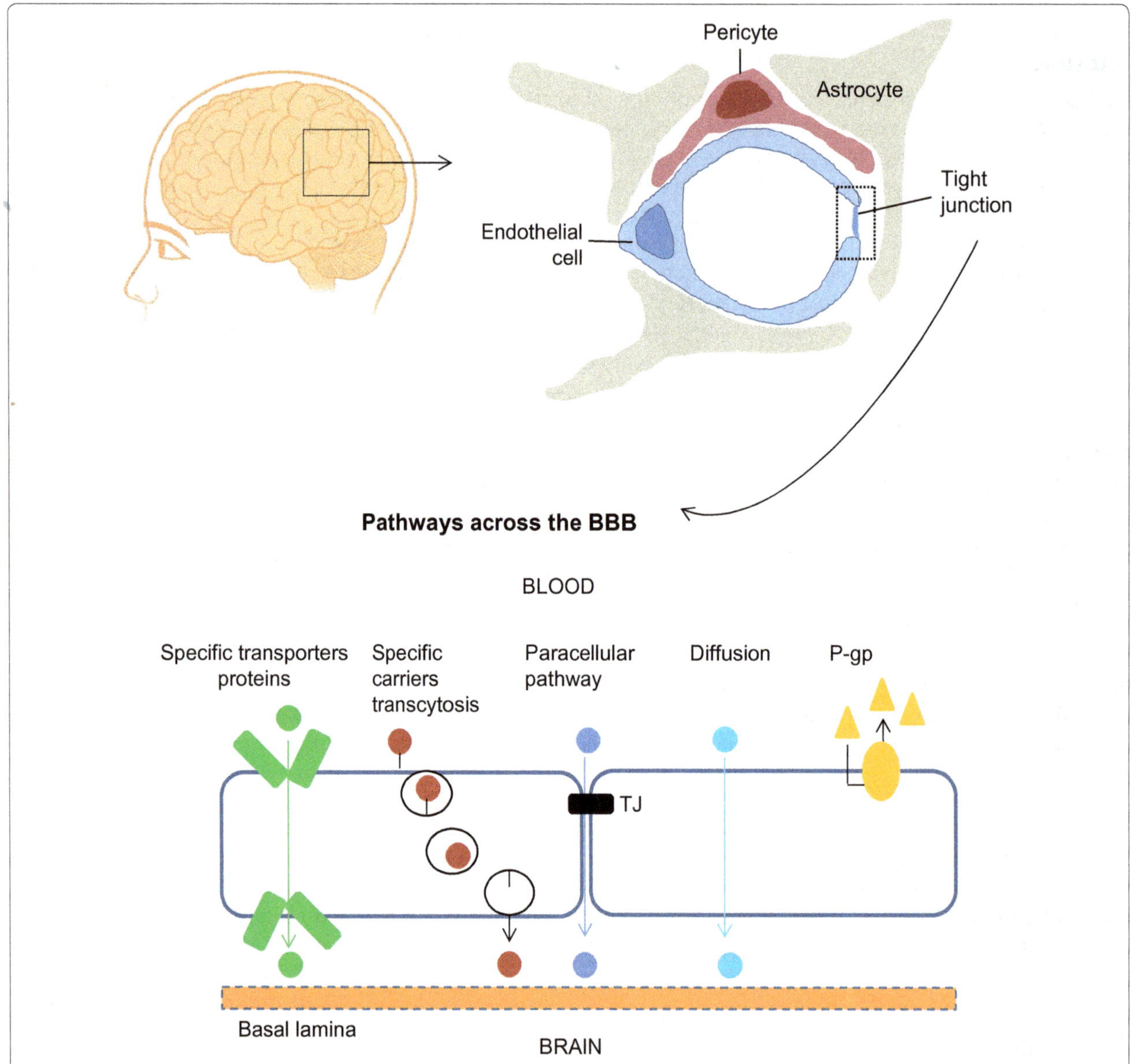

Fig. 1 Cellular constituents of the blood–brain barrier. The blood–brain barrier is formed by brain endothelial cells, which are connected by tight junctions. The endothelium, together with the basal lamina, pericytes, and astrocytic end-feet forms the neurovascular unit. Transport pathways across blood brain barrier. Endothelial cells of the BBB have a crucial role in the transport of ions and solutes into and out of the brain. Some substances diffuse freely into and out of the brain parenchyma (O_2 and CO_2), others such as nutrients need specific transporters, while molecules such as insulin, leptin and transferrin are transported by receptor-mediated transcytosis. *P-gp* P-glycoprotein, *TJ* tight junction

cord [18, 19]. The spatial organization of the barrier is complex, and although at its various locations (brain parenchyma, meninges, choroid plexus) it is formed by different cell types (endothelium, mesenchymal cells of meninges, choroidal cells), it behaves as a single, tight and fully efficient barrier [20, 21]. Adding further levels of complexity, there are discrete brain areas, known as circumventricular organs, in which the BBB is displaced from the endothelial site to the ependymal side, allowing small regions of the CNS to be directly exposed to blood without making the BBB generally leaky [20, 21].

The different cell organization of the barrier at its various brain locations allows it to display distinct barrier and permeability properties. Such innate barriers are dynamic and complex interfaces that strictly control the exchange between blood or CSF and brain compartments. Major barrier functions include: (1) maintenance of CNS homeostasis; (2) protection of the private neural environment from that of the blood; (3) provision of a constant supply of nutrients to the brain; (4) To convey inflammatory cells to specific sites in response to changes in the local environment [22, 23]. Several cell types contribute to the organization of the BBB, also known as the neurovascular unit, located at the capillaries in the brain parenchyma. Endothelial cells are at the heart of the BBB; pericytes control the expression of specific genes in endothelial cells; astrocytes convey molecules from and to the tight endothelium and contribute to the maintenance of the barrier postnatally [24–26]. Further, recent evidence has highlighted the role of neural activity in promoting the maturation of cerebrovascular networks during postnatal development [27].

The polarized nature of CNS endothelial cells is reflected in their four fundamental barrier properties that contribute to BBB function and integrity. First, tight junction (TJ) complexes between endothelial cells establish a high-resistance paracellular barrier to small hydrophilic molecules and ions. Second, in endothelial cells the transcellular vesicular trafficking of cargo molecules is limited to the receptor-mediated endocytosis/transcytosis. Third, the establishment of the restrictive paracellular and transcellular barriers allows CNS endothelial cells to use polarized cellular transporters to dynamically regulate the influx of nutrients and efflux of metabolic waste and toxins between the blood and brain parenchyma. Fourth, CNS endothelial cells lack the expression of leukocyte adhesion molecules (LAMs) such as E-selectin and Icam. The lack of these luminal surface molecules prevents the entry of immune cells from blood, resulting in a paucity of immune cells in the brain microenvironment [16]. BBB properties are not intrinsic to CNS endothelial cells but are induced and regulated by the neural environment [28].

The development of the BBB is a multistep process that begins with angiogenesis [29]. Barrier properties mature as nascent vessels come into close contact with pericytes and astroglia. This process includes elaboration of TJ, decreased transcytosis, downregulation of leukocyte adhesion molecules and increased transporter expression [30–33]. Full tightness of TJ is completed during maturation and needs to be maintained throughout life. If the barrier breaks down, there can be dramatic consequences, and neuroinflammation and neurodegeneration can occur [33–35]. Recently, neurovascular dysfunction, including BBB breakdown and cerebral blood flow dysregulation and reduction, has been recognized to contribute to Alzheimer's disease [35] and epilepsy [36].

The temporal profile of BBB development varies with species. In addition to tracer injections, the ultrastructure cellular properties of endothelial cells, the onset of specific BBB marker expression, and the presence of endogenous serum proteins in brain parenchyma have been used to study how barrier properties develop.

In humans, the vascularisation of the telencephalon begins at approximately the 8th week of gestation (GW). Post-mortem studies of preterm foetuses have shown that a barrier to trypan blue is present at the beginning of the second trimester of gestation [37]. By the 14th GW TJ proteins occludin and claudin-5 are expressed in the vessels of the germinal matrix, cortex and white matter [38]. The appearance of TJ proteins at this time appears sufficient to prevent endogenous albumin from entering the brain, providing evidence of early functionality of the barrier [38]. By the 18th week of gestation, TJ proteins demonstrate similar staining patterns to the TJ of the adult BBB [39]. Recruitment of pericytes to the developing capillary wall is critical for the formation and maintenance of the BBB. Astrocytes recruited at later stages further assist endothelium in acquiring BBB characteristics, barrier properties and CNS immune quiescence [23–26].

Some pathways have been implicated in the pericyte-mediated induction and regulation of the BBB. The best characterized genetic program is β-catenin signalling [40–42]. CNS-specific pathways (Wnt/β-catenin, Norrin/Frizzled4 and sonic hedgehog) [43] and genes (GPR124, Mfsd2a, apoE3) are also crucial in BBB differentiation and maturation [44, 45]. Loss-of-function of these genes results in CNS vasculature dysfunction.

In brief, methodological and technical achievements have allowed to establish that humans, rodents, and other animals (i.e. sheep, rabbits, chicken) [46–51] have a number of functional barrier mechanisms in place early in development. These include TJ proteins and several transporters. BBB develops in a caudal-rostral wave with the hindbrain BBB becoming functional first followed by the midbrain, and finally the forebrain [44]. Barrier transporting properties are induced very early. In contrast, barrier sealing properties are acquired gradually throughout development, first with the suppression of fenestrations, then the appearance of functional TJ and lastly with the suppression of transcytosis [30–33]. These findings are controversial because they support the view of a functional embryonic BBB protecting the developing brain and oppose the traditional perspective that "the vulnerable developing brain is only protected by the barrier properties of the placenta" [52] [for more comprehensive reviews see 53, 54].

The progressive maturation of the BBB components (i.e., expression of TJ proteins) should not be interpreted as a fully functionally operative barrier. When in development (pre- or postnatal) does the BBB starts to operate as a true, unique and fully tight barrier? This a key question from the physiological, pathological and therapeutic points of view. A functional BBB during the embryonic life implies that the nervous system develops in a defined and restricted environment; is this really the case? Does a functional embryonic BBB protect the embryonic brain from compounds (toxins or drugs) that escape the placental barrier? How does BBB dysfunction during embryogenesis impact brain development? Although BBB dysfunction has been associated with the initiation and persistence of various neurological disorders in the adult [33–36] and developing brain [55], it is unclear whether barrier dysfunction is a cause or a consequence of a particular neurological disorder. This is an area in which further research with modern technology is required [56]. On the other hand, a truly and fully functional BBB represents a challenge when targeting treatments towards the mother or foetus, or in the treatment of premature newborns.

Abnormalities of BBB in foetal-onset hydrocephalus: trigger or outcome?

All cells of the mammalian central nervous system are produced in two germinal zones associated with the ventricular walls, the ventricular zone (VZ) and the subventricular zone (SVZ) [57]. In the human, the SVZ has a massively expanded outer region that contributes to the large size and complexity of the brain cortex [58–61]. Although the bulk of neural proliferation and neuroblast migration occurs between 12 and 18 GW, it continues at a decreasing rate until about the 34th GW. As neurogenesis declines, ependymogenesis takes over (20–40 GW) by the progressive differentiation of neural stem cells (NSC) into multiciliated ependyma [57].

Over the years, based on our own and other investigators' evidence, we have progressively come to the view that a disruption of the VZ and SVZ, affecting equally NSC and ependymal cells, triggers the onset of foetal hydrocephalus and abnormal neurogenesis [7, 10, 11; Fig. 3a]. Disruption follows a program that has a temporal and spatial pattern, progressing as a "tsunami" wave running from the caudal to rostral regions of the developing ventricular system, leaving behind severe damage. In the hyh mice and HTx rat, animal models of foetal-onset hydrocephalus, the onset of VZ disruption is associated with the arrival of macrophages and lymphocytes to the zone that has just started to denude [6, 62], suggesting that an inflammatory/immune response could be associated with the progression and severity of hydrocephalus. Supporting this view, in the hyh mouse, the tumour necrosis factor alpha (TNFα) and its receptor TNFαR1 appear to be associated with the severity of the disease [63]. In human neonatal high pressure hydrocephalus, pro-inflammatory cytokines (IL-18 and IFNgamma) have been detected in the CSF [64].

At present, there is little information whether or not the BBB is affected in hydrocephalus. Recent studies have shown that at the neurovascular unit, endothelial cells, astrocytes, and pericytes synthesise and deposit different laminin isoforms into the basal lamina. Laminin α4 (endothelial laminin) regulates vascular integrity at embryonic/neonatal stage, while astrocyte laminin maintains vascular integrity in adulthood [65, 66]. The loss of pericyte laminin leads to hydrocephalus and BBB breakdown [67]. At variance, in the capillaries of the hydrocephalic HTx rat laminin immunoreactivity at the BBB is not different from that of control rats [68]. In HTx rats, tight junctions between endothelial cells of capillaries are apparently well formed and capillaries with partial defect of the basal membrane are occasionally found. However, the swelling of astrocytic end-feet around microvessels located in areas of injured white matter was interpreted as impairment of the BBB [68].

Other studies have focused on the role of aquaporins in the pathophysiology of hydrocephalus. Aquaporin-1 is highly expressed at the choroid plexus and is related to CSF production; aquaporin-4 is expressed at the ependyma, glia limitans, and at the perivascular end feet of astrocyte processes, facilitating the water movement across these tissue interfaces [69–71]. So far, the observations obtained from animal studies [72–75] and few cases in humans [74, 76] support an adaptive and protective role of aquaporins in hydrocephalus by decreasing CSF production and increasing edema clearance [77].

Although the evidence is poor, the possibility that an inflammatory process is somehow associated with the early stages of VZ disruption deserves to be explored. Pro-inflammatory interleukins have been detected in the CSF of hydrocephalic mutant rodents [63, 78], hydrocephalic patients [64, 76, 79]. It is well known that neuroinflammation is generally accompanied by impaired BBB function, which includes alterations in the junctional complexes [80–83]. Vascular endothelial growth factor (VEGF), which expression is significantly up-regulated during neuroinflammation, induces disruption of BBB, likely by down-regulating claudin-5 and occludin [84, 85]. Interestingly, VEGF is elevated in the CSF of patients with hydrocephalus and, when it is administered into the CSF of normal rats, it causes alterations of adherens junctions (AJ), ependyma disruption, and hydrocephalus [86]. Stable AJ are now considered to be required for the formation of TJ [87]. Surprisingly, the continuous crosstalk between components of AJ and TJ has been underestimated by researchers studying the BBB and hydrocephalus. The possibility that signals from the hydrocephalic CSF (cytokines, VEGF, others) may contribute to, or even trigger, the BBB disruption should be kept in mind.

Germinal matrix hemorrhage and the BBB

Germinal matrix (GM) haemorrhage and intraventricular haemorrhage (IVH) are the most common and most important events that cause neurological impairment in neonates born before 37 GW [88]. IVH occurs when a hemorrhage in the germinal matrix ruptures through the ependyma into the lateral ventricles, leading to hydrocephalus and other long-term sequelae. Prematurity associated with posthaemorrhagic hydrocephalus (PHH) results in high morbidity and mortality. Infants with a history of IVH/PHH have a higher incidence of seizures, neurodevelopmental delay, cerebral palsy, and death [88–90]. The pathogenesis of IVH is multifactorial and it has been primarily ascribed to a combination of intravascular, vascular, and extravascular factors, including: (1) disturbance in the cerebral blood flow; (2) inherent fragility of the GM-vasculature; (3) platelet and coagulation disorders [for comprehensive reviews see 91, 92]. It has been suggested that all or some of these conditions could lead to significant fluctuation in the cerebral blood flow or blood pressure inside the blood vessels, and may participate in the rupture of the microvasculature [93].

The morphology and functional properties of the GM-gliovascular interface have been studied in human embryos. The perivascular coverage by the end-feet of GFAP-reactive astrocytes increases consistently from 19 to 40 GW [94]. In a similar way, tight junction length, basal lamina area in the GM-vasculature and aquaporin-4 expression in astrocyte end-feet increase as a function of gestational age [94–97] (Fig. 2). It is worth ning that a lower degree of GFAP expression in astrocyte end-feet of the GM vasculature, as compared to that of the developing cortex and white matter, has been reported. It has been suggested that it may reflect cytoskeletal structural differences that would contribute to the fragility of the GM-vasculature and susceptibility to hemorrhage [94]. In addition, poorly developed TJs between endothelial cells, or immaturity of the basal lamina and/or pericytes have been also suggested as a risk factor for IVH [37, 94, 97].

Difficulties in the non-surgical treatment of hydrocephalus

Del Bigio and Di Curzio have recently written a critical review to summarize and evaluate research concerning pharmacological therapies for hydrocephalus [98]. Some approaches currently used to deliver therapeutic compounds to the brain include transcranial drug delivery, transnasal drug delivery, transient BBB opening, and small molecule lipidization [99–101]. Delivery of therapeutic compounds into the CSF is also emerging as an alternative. What has been the aim, so far, of all surgical and pharmacological attempts to treat hydrocephalus? (1) To repair disturbances in CSF flow/balance and (2) to prevent brain *damage* caused by hydrocephalus. Despite over five decades of research, no compelling non-derivative therapies have been developed for hydrocephalus. An alternative and promising task has recently been proposed: to prevent or diminish *abnormalities in brain development* which are inseparably associated with hydrocephalus.

Is there a real possibility to prevent/diminish brain abnormalities linked to foetal-onset hydrocephalus?

We believe that there is a hope. New medical technology could change the way to treat hydrocephalus and its outcomes, as a complement to CSF diversion by shunt surgery. Cell grafting therapy for brain diseases has been the subject of numerous publications. A few recent investigations have started to set the basis for a cell therapy for foetal-onset hydrocephalus. Potential cells to be used for brain grafting include: (1) pluripotential neural stem cells; (2) mesenchymal stem cells; (3) genetically engineered stem cells; (4) choroid plexus cells and (5) subcommissural organ cells. Expected outcomes are a proper microenvironment of the embryonic neurogenic niche and, consequently, normal brain development.

Neural stem cells

Based on the evidence that the common history of foetal-onset hydrocephalus and abnormal neurogenesis starts with the disruption of the VZ, neurospheres formed by normal neural stem cells/neural progenitor cells (NSC/NPC) have been grafted into the lateral ventricle of hydrocephalic HTx rats for regenerative purposes (for comprehensive reviews see 11, 102). After 48 h of transplantation, the grafted cells become selectively integrated into the

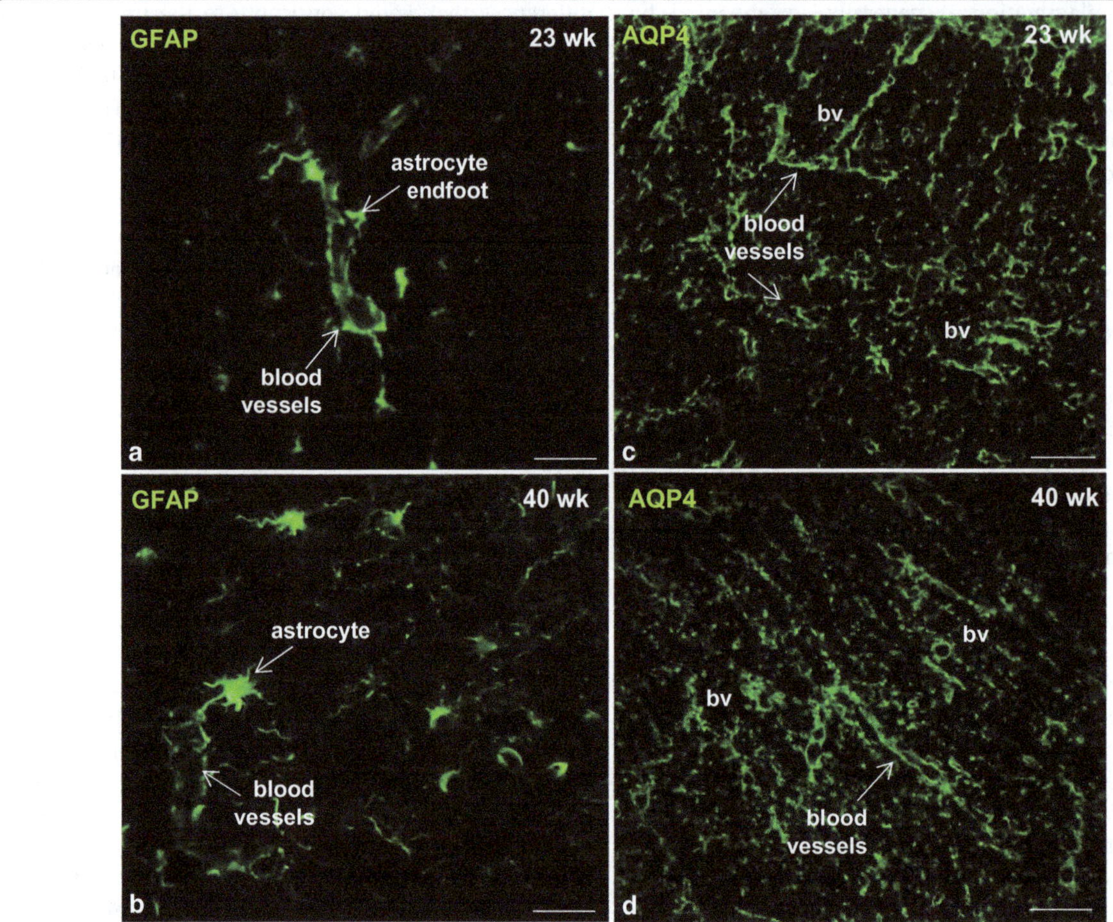

Fig. 2 Blood brain barrier in the developing human cerebral cortex. Telencephalon of premature newborns. Immunostaining shows the presence of GFAP (**a**, **b**) and aquaporin-4 (**c**, **d**) around brain microvessels as early as 23 weeks of gestation. *bv* blood vessels. *Scale bars* **a**, **b** 10 μm; **c**, **d** 30 μm

areas of VZ disruption [11]; Fig. 3b, c. Although the further fate of these cells is under investigation in our laboratory, the possibility to repopulate the disrupted VZ with neural stem cells (radial glia) and ependymal cells, avoiding the outcomes of VZ disruption (hydrocephalus and abnormal neurogenesis), may be in sight. Recently, the combination of endogenous NSC mobilization and lithium chloride treatment resulted in highly reduced incidence of hydrocephalus by inhibiting neuronal apoptosis in a rodent model of intraventricular haemorrhage [103].

The isolation and expansion of NSC of human origin are crucial for the successful development of cell therapy approaches in human brain diseases. A relevant step forward has been recently achieved in that an immortal foetal neural stem cell line [104] and a foetal striatum-derived neural stem cell line [105] has been obtained.

Mesenchymal stem cells

Mesenchymal stem cells (MSC) are versatile and multipotent adult stem cells. MSC are capable of differentiating into osteoblasts, chondroblasts, myocytes, and adipocytes [106, 107]. Furthermore, neuronal progenitor cells, as well as lung epithelial and renal tubular cells, can be derived from MSC [108]. MSC represent an alternative source of stem cells that can be harvested at low cost and isolated with minimal invasiveness. There are large MSC populations in umbilical cord blood, placental membranes and amniotic fluid [109, 110]. MSC are emerging as a replacement for NSC for therapeutic purposes, specifically for their plasticity, their reduced immunogenicity, and high anti-inflammatory potential [111]. It is now becoming clearer that they might be able to protect the nervous system through mechanisms other than cell replacement, such as the modulation of the immune system [111] and the release of neurotrophic factors [112, 113].

Mesenchymal stem cells have been used for the treatment of posthemorrhagic hydrocephalus. The intraventricular transplantation of MSC in an intraventricular haemorrhage model of newborn rats significantly

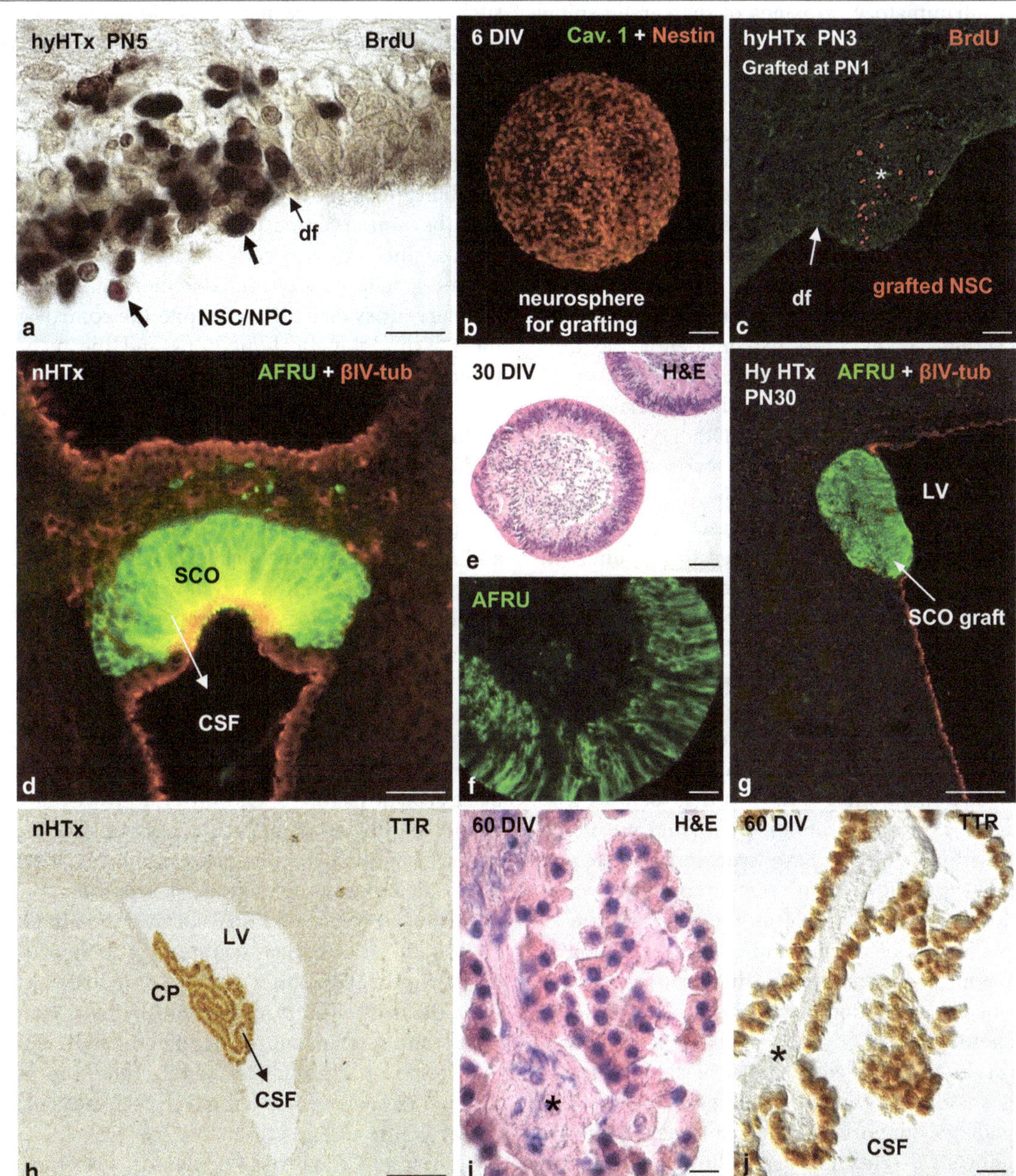

Fig. 3 **a** In the hydrocephalic HTx rat at postnatal day 5, ventricular zone disruption results in abnormal translocation of neural stem cells (NSC)/ neural precursor cells (NPC) into ventricular cerebrospinal fluid. Cells displaced to the ventricle and reaching the CSF retain proliferative capacity, as shown by injection of bromodeoxyuridine (BrdU) in living animals and tracking the BrdU-positive cells in tissue sections (*arrows*). *df* disruption front. **b**, **c** Neural stem cells (NSC) grafted into the cerebrospinal fluid (CSF) of a hydrocephalic HTx rat move selectively to the disrupted areas of the ventricular zone (VZ). Dispersed cells were grown in a neurosphere culture medium containing epidermal growth factor (EGF) and devoid of fetal bovine serum. Neurosphere immunostained for nestin after 6 days in vitro (DIV, **b**). Some of the grafted cells migrate through the subventricular zone; some of them move deeper into the brain tissue (*asterisk*, **c**). **d** Frontal section of the rat subcommissural organ (SCO) immunostained with antibodies against SCO-spondin (AFRU) and βIV-tubulin. *CSF* cerebrospinal fluid. **e**, **f** Organ culture of the bovine SCO. **e** After 30 DIV, SCO explants form spheres of secretory ependymocytes. Section of an SCO-explant stained with haematoxylin-eosin. **f** Section of a SCO-explant immunostained with AFRU. **g** Bovine SCO explant grafted into the lateral ventricle of a hydrocephalic HTx rat. The graft becomes integrated into the wall of the lateral ventricle (LV). SCO-spondin immunoreactive material is shown inside the cells. **h** Frontal section of a rat brain immunostained with antibodies against transthyretin (TTR).The choroid plexus (CP) is selectively immunoreactive. **i**, **j** Organ culture of the bovine choroid plexus. **i** Section of a CP-explant stained with haematoxylin-eosin. **j** Section of a CP-explant immunostained with anti-transthyretin. After 60 DIV, the choroid cells display a normal cytology and continue to express TTR. The vasculature and stroma of the villi were virtually missing (*asterisk*). *Scale bars* **a** 15 μm; **b**–**g** 50 μm; **h** 100 μm; **i**, **j** 12 μm. **a**–**c** were taken from Rodriguez et al. [11]. *Reprinted with permission of Pediatr Neurosurg*; **d** was taken from Ortloff et al. [151]. *Reprinted with permission of Cell Tissue Res*; **e**, **g** were taken from Guerra et al. [10]. *Reprinted with permission of JNEN*

attenuated inflammatory cytokines of the cerebrospinal fluid and brain tissue, and prevented the development of posthemorrhagic hydrocephalus [114]. The mechanism of protection seems to be related to the anti-inflammatory effects of these cells and the capacity of MSC to release the brain-derived neurotrophic factor [112, 113]. Substantial evidence has been obtained for the successful treatment of brain diseases, such as Parkinson's, using brain grafting of stem cells of various sources [115–117].

In brief, all these findings support that stem cells are promising therapeutic agents for brain regeneration and neuroprotection. A key point to consider is the time and opportunity when NSC should be transplanted. In normal human foetuses, neuronal proliferation and migration occur from the 12th to 30th GW, while in hydrocephalic foetuses VZ disruption starts at about the 16th GW and continues throughout the 2nd and 3rd trimester of pregnancy [118]. It seems reasonable to suggest that NSC grafting should be performed shortly after the disruption process of the VZ had been turned on. Foetal surgery to repair neural tube defects, such as spina bifida, is performed within a well-defined gestational period (19th–25th GW) according to the MOMS study [119]. This operation, that is becoming progressively standardized and safe, appears to be a good opportunity for NSC grafting into the brain ventricles of spina bifida foetuses. Worth mentioning is the fact that foetuses with spina bifida carry a VZ disruption [9, 10] and most children born with spina bifida have hydrocephalus. It may be hoped that grafting of stem cells into brain of hydrocephalic foetuses would result in the repopulation of the disrupted areas of the VZ and/or the generation of a protective microenvironment to diminish/prevent the outcomes of VZ disruption, namely, hydrocephalus and abnormal neurogenesis.

Warnings about unwanted outcomes of stem cell transplantation should be kept in mind permanently. The existing evidence supports that the short term application of stem cells is safe and feasible; however, concerns remain over the possibility of unwanted long-term effects [120–122]. In addition to unwelcome interactions of stem cells with the host immune system, there is evidence that they may promote tumorogenesis [123]. As animal models and first-in-man clinical studies have provided conflicting results, it is challenging to estimate the long-term risk for individual patients [124, 125]. Previous evidence has shown that the safety of stem cell therapies will depend on various factors including the differentiation status and proliferative capacity of the grafted cells, the timing and route of administration, and the long-term survival of the graft [126–130].

Human MSC have been also genetically engineered to release neuropeptides with neuroprotective potential such as brain-derived neurotrophic factor (BDNF), glial cell line-derived neurotrophic factor (GDNF) or insulin-like growth factor 1 (IGF-1) [131]. Glage et al. [132] grafted human MSC transfected to produce glucagon-like peptide-1 in the CSF of cats. This study showed that ventricular cell-based delivery of soluble factors has the capability to achieve concentrations in the CSF which may become pharmacologically active. Thus, genetically engineered stem cells should be also considered to deliver specific neuroprotective compounds to the central nervous system [131]. Despite the controversy about the pharmacokinetic limitations and the technical difficulties of ventricular drug delivery, the CSF pathway is a promising route of administration for soluble, highly biologically-effective neuropeptides [133, 134].

There are two brain glands, the choroid plexus (CP) and the subcommissural organ (SCO), that secrete proteins and peptides into the CSF, some of them with neurogenic and neuroprotective properties. These two glands play a key role in the secretion and flow of CSF, and participate in the physiopathology of hydrocephalus [135–138].

Choroid plexus

The choroid plexus (CP) cells are the main source of CSF, providing a full complement of proteins, peptides, nucleosides and growth factors such as the basic fibroblast growth factor (bFGF), insulin growth factor (IGF-II), nerve growth factor (NGF), and transforming growth factor (TGF), which influence a multitude of brain functions, including neurogenesis, neuroprotection, neurite extension as well as neuronal survival in vitro and in vivo [135, 139]. The marker secretory protein of the CP is transthyretin (Fig. 3h), a carrier of thyroxin throughout the CSF [140]. The transthyretin/thyroxin complex has a relevant role in neuronal differentiation and synaptogenesis in particular [140–142]. Thus, choroid plexus through its secretion into the CSF regulates nervous system structure and function [136, 142].

Grafting of CP has been explored for therapeutic purpose in some neurodegenerative disorders [for comprehensive reviews see 143, 144]. Surprisingly, CP grafting has not yet been considered in the treatment of hydrocephalus. The long-term survival of organ cultured CP (at least 2 months; ongoing experiments in our laboratory) and transplanted CP cells in vivo [145–147] provide a sound base to explore such a strategy. Worth noticing is that organ-cultured CP do not secrete CSF but they do secrete neurotrophic factors, such as transthyretin (ongoing experiments in our laboratory) (Fig. 3i, j).

Subcommissural organ

The subcommissural organ (SCO) is a distinctive ependymal secretory gland located at the entrance of the cerebral aqueduct. The SCO differentiates very early in ontogeny and remains fully active during the entire life span, secreting SCO-spondin to the CSF where it either assembles to form Reissner's fiber (RF) or remains soluble and circulates throughout the CSF compartments [148, 149]. The RF, extending through the Sylvius aqueduct (SA), fourth ventricle and central canal of the spinal cord, is indispensable for maintaining the patency of the SA and the normal flow of CSF [150–152]. An inborn defect of the SCO results in hydrocephalus [137, 138, 152].

In addition to SCO-spondin, the SCO secretes transthyretin, FGF, and the S100β protein, which support embryonic brain development [153, 154]. We have recently provided evidence to propose that these factors have similar roles in adult neurogenesis, regulating proliferation, migration and differentiation of neural stem cells and neural precursors in adult neurogenic niches [149].

The long-term survival of CP (Fig. 3h–j) and SCO explants (Fig. 3d–g) when they are cultured or transplanted into the ventricular CSF [146, 155, 156] provide a sound base to explore a CP/SCO cell-based therapy. When transplanted in the CSF, CP and SCO explants would allow a constant source and a homogenous distribution of neurotrophic and neuroprotective proteins, facilitating a uniform exposure of these compounds to the brain cells.

In order to translate cell therapies to humans, two strategies are envisaged. (1) To graft cells of human origin, mainly of human foetuses and (2) to graft cells of non-human origin. In such a case, a key question has to be solved: how to avoid the host versus graft immune reaction when the source of transplanted tissue is a non-human species.

Microencapsulation permits use of allo- and xeno-grafting without immunosuppression

Cell encapsulation technology represents an alternative approach to the delivery of biologically active compounds to the brain by overcoming the problem of graft rejection [157]. This strategy involves the use of untreated or genetically engineered cells that secrete proteins with therapeutic potential. Cells are immobilized within a polymeric semi-permeable membrane that permits the bidirectional diffusion of molecules such as the influx of oxygen, nutrients, growth factors, essentials for cell metabolism and the outward diffusion of waste products and therapeutic proteins. At the same time, the semi-permeable nature of the membrane prevents the grafted cells being exposed to host immune cells and antibodies, avoiding their destruction (Fig. 4) [158, 159]. Through the release of therapeutic proteins, the grafted encapsulated cells can modify a circumscribed brain microenvironment or the whole brain milieu when transplanted into the CSF, and provide clinical benefits [132, 160, 161].

The use of an appropriate material with the property of biocompatibility is a crucial factor that governs the long term efficiency of this technology. The ideal capsule should need to be implanted only once in a patient's lifetime; provide stable, predictable and reproducible function for a given period of time, and not burden the patient with immune suppressive regimens, discomfort, or other adverse effects. At present, alginates are regarded as the most suitable biomaterials for cell encapsulation due to their abundance and excellent biocompatibility properties [162, 163]. New polymers are being tested to be used as carriers and scaffolds for biomolecules and cell delivery in tissue engineering applications [159]. Encapsulation devices range from 'microscale' devices (100 nm–1 mm) to 'macroscale' (3–8 cm). Microcapsules, by virtue of their size, have a shorter diffusion distance for oxygen and other nutrients. However, they are mechanically and chemically fragile and cannot be retrieved once implanted within the brain parenchyma. Macrocapsules provide good cell viability and neurochemical diffusion, have good mechanical stability, and can be retrieved if needed or desired [159, 161].

Recent advances have increased the list of encapsulated cells that survive for a long-term in the brain and release therapeutic molecules ([161], Table 1); such neurotrophic factors do not cross the BBB.

Conclusions

Although many agents have therapeutic potential for hydrocephalus, few of these agents have been clinically used because of the brain barriers. Virtually there are no reports trying to prevent or diminish abnormalities in brain development which are inseparably associated with hydrocephalus. Cell therapies for brain diseases, by grating cells with regenerative properties (stem cells) or able to secrete therapeutic compounds for an efficient period of time when they are transplanted into the CSF (MSC, CP, SCO), should be strongly considered for developing new treatments for hydrocephalus. The development in new technologies, such as cell encapsulation, will allow the use of foreign cells for transplantation, overcoming the existing problem of xenografts. A carefully considered decision process is indispensable before cell grafting in order to avoid unwanted results. Detailed observation and follow-up of the graft hosts

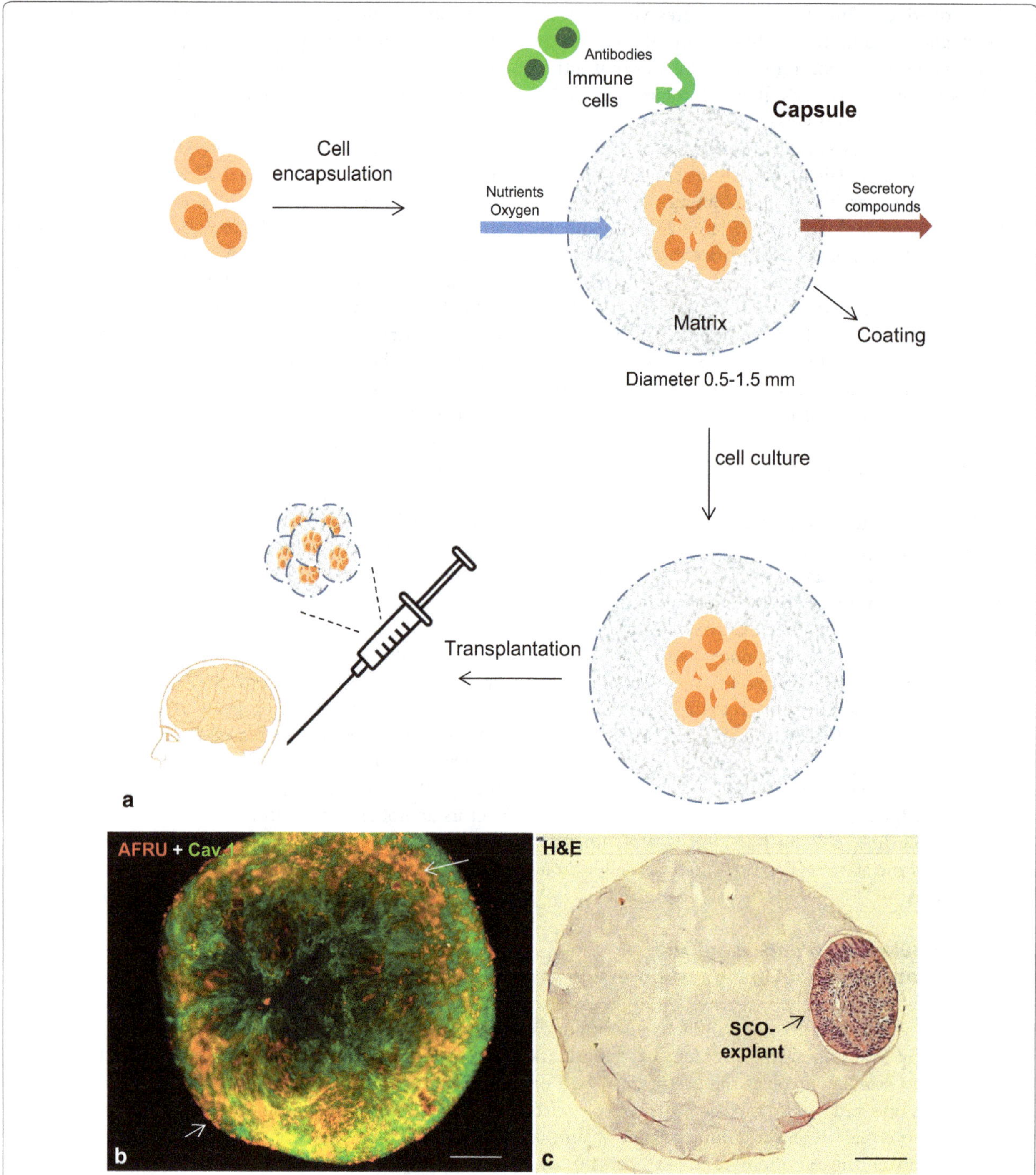

Fig. 4 **a** Therapeutic application of encapsulated cells. Encapsulated cells are protected by a membrane or capsular matrix that allows nutrients, waste, and therapeutic products to pass freely but also works as a barrier to immune cells. Capsules can be transplanted into the brain for the treatment of brain diseases. **b** Subcommissural organ (SCO) secretory explants stained in bloc with AFRU (*red*) and caveolin-1 (*green*) displaying extracellular material (*arrows*) on the surface of cells. **c** Secretory SCO-explants encapsulated within a microsphere. Haematoxylin and eosin stain. *Scale bars* **b** 30 µm; **c** 160 µm

Table 1 Examples of cell encapsulation for CNS and CNS-related diseases

Disease/model	Cells/experimental paradigm	Results and references
Alzheimer's disease	NGF in rats and primates	Neuroprotection [164]
Parkinson's disease	Neuropeptide Y in rats	Neuroprotection [165]
Huntington's disease	Choroid plexus in rats	Neuroprotection [143]
Epilepsy	GDNF, BDNF in rats	Neuroprotection, Decreased seizures [166, 167]
Stroke/ischaemia	Choroid plexus in rats	Neuroprotection [168]
Acute and chronic pain	Chromaffin cells (catecholamines, opioids) in rats	Reduced pain [169]

should be a key compromise. To achieve the stem cells transplantation goal for hydrocephalus/spina bifida patients will require a balanced and complementary basic-clinical working team.

Abbreviations

BBB: blood brain barrier; CP: choroid plexus; CSF: cerebrospinal fluid; GM: germinal matrix; IVH: intraventricular haemorrhage; MSC: mesenchymal stem cells; NPC: neural progenitor cells; NSC: neural stem cells; SCO: subcommissural organ; TJ: tight junction; VZ: ventricular zone.

Authors' contributions

All the authors contributed to the writing and editing of this manuscript. All authors read and approved the final manuscript.

Author details

[1] Instituto de Anatomía, Histología y Patología, Facultad de Medicina, Universidad Austral de Chile, Valdivia, Chile. [2] Departamento de Anatomía e Histología Humana, Facultad de Medicina, Universidad de Salamanca, Salamanca, Spain.

Acknowledgements

This work was supported by Grants from Fondef IdeA14I10236 to MG and Fondecyt (Chile) 1111018 to EMR. We apologize to authors whose work we could not cite because of the limit on the number of references and therefore in some instances we mostly cited the overview articles.

Competing interests

The authors declare that they have no competing interests.

References

1. Edwards JH. The syndrome of sex-linked hydrocephalus. Arch Dis Child. 1961;36:486–93.
2. Jellinger G. Anatomopathology of nontumoral aqueductal stenosis. J Neurosurg Sci. 1986;30:1–16.
3. Johnson RT, Johnson KP, Edmonds CJ. Virus-induced hydrocephalus: development of aqueductal stenosis in hamsters after mumps infection. Science. 1967;157:1066–7.
4. Boop FA. Posthemorrhagic hydrocephalus of prematurity. In: Cinalli C, Maixner WJ, Sainte-Rose C, editors. Pediatric hydrocephalus. Milan: Springer; 2004. p. 121–31.
5. Jiménez AJ, Tomé M, Páez P, Wagner C, Rodríguez S, Fernández-Llebrez P, Rodríguez EM, Pérez-Fígares JM. A programmed ependymal denudation precedes congenital hydrocephalus in the hyh mutant mouse. J Neuropathol Exp Neurol. 2001;60:1105–19.
6. Wagner C, Batiz LF, Rodríguez S, Jiménez AJ, Páez P, Tomé M, Pérez-Fígares JM, Rodríguez EM. Cellular mechanisms involved in the stenosis and obliteration of the cerebral aqueduct of hyh mutant mice developing congenital hydrocephalus. J Neuropathol Exp Neurol. 2003;62:1019–40.
7. Rodríguez EM, Guerra MM, Vío K, González C, Ortloff A, Bátiz LF, Rodríguez S, Jara MC, Muñoz RI, Ortega E, Jaque J, Guerra F, Sival DA, den Dunnen WF, Jiménez AJ, Domínguez-Pinos MD, Pérez-Fígares JM, McAllister JP, Johanson C. A cell junction pathology of neural stem cells leads to abnormal neurogenesis and hydrocephalus. Biol Res. 2012;45:231–42.
8. Domínguez-Pinos MD, Páez P, Jiménez AJ, Weil B, Arráez MA, Pérez-Fígares JM, Rodríguez EM. Ependymal denudation and alterations of the subventricular zone occur in human fetuses with a moderate communicating hydrocephalus. J Neuropathol Exp Neurol. 2005;64:595–604.
9. Sival DA, Guerra M, den Dunnen WF, Bátiz LF, Alvial G, Castañeyra-Perdomo A, Rodríguez EM. Neuroependymal denudation is in progress in full-term human foetal spina bifida aperta. Brain Pathol. 2011;21:163–79.
10. Guerra MM, Henzi R, Ortloff A, Lichtin N, Vío K, Jiménez AJ, Dominguez-Pinos MD, González C, Jara MC, Hinostroza F, Rodríguez S, Jara M, Ortega E, Guerra F, Sival DA, den Dunnen WF, Pérez-Fígares JM, McAllister JP, Johanson CE, Rodríguez EM. Cell junction pathology of neural stem cells is associated with ventricular zone disruption, hydrocephalus, and abnormal neurogenesis. J Neuropathol Exp Neurol. 2015;74:653–71.
11. Rodríguez EM, Guerra MM. Neural stem cells and fetal-onset hydrocephalus. Pediatr Neurosurg. 2017. doi:10.1159/000453074.
12. Rekate HL. A consensus on the classification of hydrocephalus: its utility in the assessment of abnormalities of cerebrospinal fluid dynamics. Childs Nerv Syst. 2011;27:1535–41.
13. Bourgeois M, Sainte-Rose C, Cinalli G, Maixner W, Malucci C, Zerah M, Pierre-Kahn A, Renier D, Hoppe-Hirsch E, Aicardi J. Epilepsy in children with shunted hydrocephalus. J Neurosurg. 1999;90:274–81.
14. Klepper J, Büsse M, Strassburg HM, Sörensen N. Epilepsy in shunt-treated hydrocephalus. Dev Med Child Neurol. 1998;40:731–6.
15. Obermeier B, Verma A, Ransohoff RM. The blood–brain barrier. Handb Clin Neurol. 2016;133:39–59.
16. Chow BW, Gu C. The molecular constituents of the blood–brain barrier. Trends Neurosci. 2015;38:598–608.
17. Abbott NJ, Patabendige AA, Dolman DE, Yusof SR, Begley DJ. Structure and function of the blood–brain barrier. Neurobiol Dis. 2010;37:13–25.
18. Ehrlich P. Das sauerstoff-bedürfnis des organismus. Eine Farbenanalytische Studie. Habilitation Thesis, Berlin; 1885.
19. Ehrlich P. Ueber die beziehungen von chemischer constitution, vertheilung, und pharmakologischen wirkung. Collected Studies on Immunity. Wiley. Berlin: Wiley; 1906. p. 404–42.
20. Ge S, Song L, Pachter JS. Where is the blood–brain barrier… really? J Neurosci Res. 2005;79:421–7.
21. Wilhelm I, Nyúl-Tóth Á, Suciu M, Hermenean A, Krizbai IA. Heterogeneity of the blood-brain barrier. Tissue Barriers. 2016;4(1):e1143544.
22. Nico B, Ribatti D. Morphofunctional aspects of the blood-brain barrier. Curr Drug Metab. 2012;13:50–60.
23. Begley DJ, Brightman MW. Structural and functional aspects of the blood-brain barrier. Prog Drug Res. 2003;61:39–78.

24. Sweeney MD, Ayyadurai S, Zlokovic BV. Pericytes of the neurovascular unit: key functions and signaling pathways. Nat Neurosci. 2016;19:771–83.
25. Armulik A, Genove G, Mae M, Nisancioglu MH, Wallgard E, Niaudet C, He L, Norlin J, Lindblom P, Strittmatter K, Johansson BR, Betsholtz C. Pericytes regulate the blood-brain barrier. Nature. 2010;468:557–61.
26. Abbott NJ, Ronnback L, Hansson E. Astrocyte–endothelial interactions at the blood-brain barrier. Nat Rev Neurosci. 2006;7:41–53.
27. Lacoste B, Gu C. Control of cerebrovascular patterning by neural activity during postnatal development. Mech Dev. 2015;138(Pt 1):43–9.
28. Obermeier B, Daneman R, Ransohoff RM. Development, maintenance and disruption of the blood-brain barrier. Nat Med. 2013;19:1584–96.
29. Bauer HC, Bauer H, Lametschwandtner A, Amberger A, Ruiz P, Steiner M. Neo-vascularization and the appearance of morphological characteristics of the blood-brain barrier in the embryonic mouse central nervous system. Brain Res Dev Brain Res. 1993;75:269–78.
30. Hagan N, Ben-Zvi A. The molecular, cellular, and morphological components of blood–brain barrier development during embryogenesis. Semin Cell Dev Biol. 2015;38:7–15.
31. Blanchette Marie, Daneman Richard. Formation and maintenance of the BBB. Mech Dev. 2015;138(Pt 1):8–16.
32. Engelhardt B, Liebner S. Novel insights into the development and maintenance of the blood–brain barrier. Cell Tissue Res. 2014;355:687–99.
33. Zhao Z, Nelson AR, Betsholtz C, Zlokovic BV. Establishment and dysfunction of the blood-brain barrier. Cell. 2015;163:1064–78.
34. Daneman R. The blood–brain barrier in health and disease. Ann Neurol. 2012;72:648–72.
35. Nelson AR, Sweeney MD, Sagare AP, Zlokovic BV. Neurovascular dysfunction and neurodegeneration in dementia and Alzheimer's disease. Biochim Biophys Acta. 2016;1862:887–900.
36. Marchi N, Granata T, Ghosh C, Janigro D. Blood-brain barrier dysfunction and epilepsy: pathophysiologic role and therapeutic approaches. Epilepsia. 2012;53:1877–86.
37. Grontoft O. Intracranial haemorrhage and blood-brain barrier problems in the new-born a pathologico-anatomical and experimental investigation. Acta Pathol Microbiol Scand Suppl. 1954;100:8–109.
38. Virgintino D, Errede M, Robertson D, Capobianco C, Girolamo F, Vimercati A, Bertossi M, Roncali L. Immunolocalization of tight junction proteins in the adult and developing human brain. Histochem Cell Biol. 2004;122:51–9.
39. Virgintino D, Robertson D, Benagiano V, Errede M, Bertossi M, Ambrosi G, Roncali L. Immunogold cytochemistry of the blood-brain barrier glucose transporter GLUT1 and endogenous albumin in the developing human brain. Dev Brain Res. 2000;123:95e101.
40. Liebner S, Plate KH. Differentiation of the brain vasculature: the answer came blowing by the Wnt. J Angiogenes Res. 2010;2:1.
41. Daneman R, Angalliu D, Agalliu D, Zhou L, Kuhnert F, Kuo CJ, Barres BA. Wnt/beta-catenin signaling is required for CNS, but not non-CNS, angiogenesis. Proc Natl Acad Sci USA. 2009;106:641–6.
42. Stenman JM, Rajagopal J, Carroll TJ, Ishibashi M, McMahon J, McMahon AP. Canonical Wnt signaling regulates organ-specific assembly and differentiation of CNS vasculature. Science. 2008;322:1247–50.
43. Krizbai IA, Deli MA. Signalling pathways regulating the tight junction permeability in the blood-brain barrier. Cell Mol Biol. 2003;49:23–31.
44. Ben-Zvi A, Lacoste B, Kur E, Andreone BJ, Mayshar Y, Yan H, Gu C. Mfsd2a is critical for the formation and function of the blood-brain barrier. Nature. 2014;22:507–11.
45. Cullen M, Elzarrad MK, Seaman S, Zudaire E, Stevens J, Yang MY, Li X, Chaudhary A, Xu L, Hilton MB, Logsdon D, Hsiao E, Stein EV, Cuttitta F, Haines DC, Nagashima K, Tessarollo L, St Croix B. GPR124, an orphan G protein-coupled receptor, is required for CNS-specific vascularization and establishment of the blood–brain barrier. Proc Natl Acad Sci USA. 2011;108:5759–64.
46. Stewart PA, Hayakawa EM. Early ultrastructural changes in blood-brain barrier vessels of the rat embryo. Brain Res Dev Brain Res. 1994;78:25–34.
47. Nico B, Quondamatteo F, Herken R, Marzullo A, Corsi P, Bertossi M, Russo G, Ribatti D, Roncali L. Developmental expression of ZO-1 antigen in the mouse blood-brain barrier. Dev Brain Res. 1999;114:161–9.
48. Bauer H, Sonnleitner U, Lamet-schwandtner A, Steiner M, Adam H, Bauer HC. Ontogenic expression of the erythroid type glucose transporter (Glut1) in the telencephalon of the mouse: correlation to the tightening of the blood-brain barrier. Dev Brain Res. 1995;86:317–25.
49. Braun LD, Cornford EM, Oldendorf WH. Newborn rabbit blood–brain barrier is selectively permeable and differs substantially from the adult. J Neurochem. 1980;34:147–52.
50. Wakai S, Hirokawa N. Development of the blood brain barrier to horseradish peroxidase in the chick embryo. Cell Tissue Res. 1978;195:195–203.
51. Dziegielewska KM, Evans CAN, Malinowska DH, Møllgård K, Reynolds JM, Reynolds ML, Saunders NR. Studies of the development of brain barrier systems to lipid insoluble molecules in fetal sheep. J Physiol (Lond). 1979;292:207–31.
52. Goasdoué K, Miller SM, Colditz PB, Björkman ST. Review: The blood-brain barrier; protecting the developing fetal brain. Placenta. 2016.
53. Saunders NR, Dreifuss JJ, Dziegielewska KM, Johansson PA, Habgood MD, Møllgård K, Bauer HC. The rights and wrongs of blood-brain barrier permeability studies: a walk through 100 years of history. Front Neurosci. 2014;8:404.
54. Ribatti D, Nico B, Crivellato E, Artico M. Development of the blood-brain barrier: a historical point of view. Anat Rec. 2006;289:3–8.
55. Moretti R, Pansiot J, Bettati D, Strazielle N, Ghersi-Egea JF, Damante G, Fleiss B, Titomanlio L, Gressens P. Blood-brain barrier dysfunction in disorders of the developing brain. Front Neurosci. 2015;9:40.
56. Ochocinska MJ, Zlokovic BV, Searson PC, Crowder AT, Kraig RP, Ljubimova JY, Mainprize TG, Banks WA, Warren RQ, Kindzelski A, Timmer W, Liu CH. NIH workshop report on the trans-agency blood-brain interface workshop 2016: exploring key challenges and opportunities associated with the blood, brain and their interface. Fluids Barriers CNS. 2017;14:12.
57. Bystron I, Blakemore C, Rakic P. Development of the human cerebral cortex: boulder committee revisited. Nat Rev Neurosci. 2008;9:110–22.
58. Dehay C, Kennedy H, Kosik KS. The outer subventricular zone and primate-specific cortical complexification. Neuron. 2015;85:683–94.
59. Lewitus E, Kelava I, Huttner WB. Conical expansion of the outer subventricular zone and the role of neocortical folding in evolution and development. Front Hum Neurosci. 2013;7:424.
60. Hansen DV, Lui JH, Parker PR, Kriegstein AR. Neurogenic radial glia in the outer subventricular zone of human neocortex. Nature. 2010;464:554–61.
61. Smart IH, Dehay C, Giroud P, Berland M, Kennedy H. Unique morphological features of the proliferative zones and postmitotic compartments of the neural epithelium giving rise to striate and extrastriate cortex in the monkey. Cereb Cortex. 2002;12:37–53.
62. Ortloff A. Mecanismo celular del denudamiento ependimario en mutantes que desarrollan hidrocefalia congénita. Ph.D. Thesis, Universidad Austral de Chile; 2008.
63. Jiménez AJ, Rodríguez-Pérez LM, Domínguez-Pinos MD, Gómez-Roldán MC, García-Bonilla M, Ho-Plagaro A, Roales-Buján R, Jiménez S, Roquero-Mañueco MC, Martínez-León MI, García-Martín ML, Cifuentes M, Ros B, Arráez MÁ, Vitorica J, Gutiérrez A, Pérez-Fígares JM. Increased levels of tumour necrosis factor alpha (TNFα) but not transforming growth factor-beta 1 (TGFβ1) are associated with the severity of congenital hydrocephalus in the hyh mouse. Neuropathol Appl Neurobiol. 2014;40:911–32.
64. Sival DA, Felderhoff-Müser U, Schmitz T, Hoving EW, Schaller C, Heep A. Neonatal high pressure hydrocephalus is associated with elevation of pro-inflammatory cytokines IL-18 and IFNgamma in cerebrospinal fluid. Cerebrospinal Fluid Res. 2008;5:21.
65. Thyboll J, et al. Deletion of the laminin alpha4 chain leads to impaired microvessel maturation. Mol Cell Biol. 2002;22:1194–202.
66. Yao Y, Chen ZL, Norris EH, Strickland S. Astrocytic laminin regulates pericyte differentiation and maintains blood brain barrier integrity. Nat Commun. 2014;5:3413. doi:10.1038/ncomms4413.

67. Gautam J, Zhang X, Yao Y. The role of pericytic laminin in blood brain barrier integrity maintenance. Sci Rep. 2016;6:36450.
68. Sada Y, Moriki T, Kuwahara S, Yamane T, Hara H. Immunohistochemical study on blood-brain barrier in congenitally hydrocephalic HTX rat brain. Zentralbl Pathol. 1994;140:289–98.
69. Verkman AS, Tradtrantip L, Smith AJ, Yao X. Aquaporin water channels and hydrocephalus. Pediatr Neurosurg. 2016 [Epub ahead of print].
70. Owler BK, Pitham T, Wang D. Aquaporins: relevance to cerebrospinal fluid physiology and therapeutic potential in hydrocephalus. Cerebrospinal Fluid Res. 2010;7:15.
71. Zador Z, Bloch O, Yao X, Manley GT. Aquaporins: role in cerebral edema and brain water balance. Prog Brain Res. 2007;161:185–94.
72. Shen XQ, Miyajima M, Ogino I, Arai H. Expression of the water-channel protein aquaporin 4 in the H-Tx rat: possible compensatory role in spontaneously arrested hydrocephalus. J Neurosurg. 2006;105(6 Suppl):459–64.
73. Paul L, Madan M, Rammling M, Chigurupati S, Chan SL, Pattisapu JV. Expression of aquaporin 1 and 4 in a congenital hydrocephalus rat model. Neurosurgery. 2011;68:462–73.
74. Skjolding AD, Holst AV, Broholm H, Laursen H, Juhler M. Differences in distribution and regulation of astrocytic aquaporin-4 in human and rat hydrocephalic brain. Neuropathol Appl Neurobiol. 2013;39:179–91.
75. Schmidt MJ, Rummel C, Hauer J, Kolecka M, Ondreka N, McClure V, Roth J. Increased CSF aquaporin-4, and interleukin-6 levels in dogs with idiopathic communicating internal hydrocephalus and a decrease after ventriculo-peritoneal shunting. Fluids Barriers CNS. 2016;13:12.
76. Castañeyra-Ruiz L, González-Marrero I, Carmona-Calero EM, Abreu-Gonzalez P, Lecuona M, Brage L, Rodríguez EM, Castañeyra-Perdomo A. Cerebrospinal fluid levels of tumor necrosis factor alpha and aquaporin 1 in patients with mild cognitive impairment and idiopathic normal pressure hydrocephalus. Clin Neurol Neurosurg. 2016;146:76–81.
77. Filippidis AS, Kalani MY, Rekate HL. Hydrocephalus and aquaporins: lessons learned from the bench. Childs Nerv Syst. 2011;27:27–33.
78. Zhang S, Chen D, Huang C, Bao J, Wang Z. Expression of HGF, MMP-9 and TGF-β1 in the CSF and cerebral tissue of adult rats with hydrocephalus. Int J Neurosci. 2013;123:392–9.
79. Sosvorova L, Kanceva R, Vcelak J, Kancheva L, Mohapl M, Starka L, Havrdova E. The comparison of selected cerebrospinal fluid and serum cytokine levels in patients with multiple sclerosis and normal pressure hydrocephalus. Neuro Endocrinol Lett. 2015;36:564–71.
80. Dudvarski Stankovic N, Teodorczyk M, Ploen R, Zipp F, Schmidt MH. Microglia-blood vessel interactions: a double-edged sword in brain pathologies. Acta Neuropathol. 2016;131:347–63.
81. Ueno M, Chiba Y, Murakami R, Matsumoto K, Kawauchi M, Fujihara R. Blood-brain barrier and blood-cerebrospinal fluid barrier in normal and pathological conditions. Brain Tumor Pathol. 2016;33:89–96.
82. Williams JL, Holman DW, Klein RS. Chemokines in the balance: maintenance of homeostasis and protection at CNS barriers. Front Cell Neurosci. 2014;8:154.
83. Petty MA, Lo EH. Junctional complexes of the blood–brain barrier: permeability changes in neuroinflammation. Prog Neurobiol. 2002;68:311–23.
84. van der Flier M, Hoppenreijs S, van Rensburg AJ, Ruyken M, Kolk AH, Springer P, Hoepelman AI, Geelen SP, Kimpen JL, Schoeman JF. Vascular endothelial growth factor and blood-brain barrier disruption in tuberculous meningitis. Pediatr Infect Dis J. 2004;23:608–13.
85. Rodewald M, Herr D, Fraser HM, Hack G, Kreienberg R, Wulff C. Regulation of tight junction proteins occludin and claudin 5 in the primate ovary during the ovulatory cycle and after inhibition of vascular endothelial growth factor. Mol Hum Reprod. 2007;13:781–9.
86. Shim JW, Sandlund J, Han CH, Hameed MQ, Connors S, Klagsbrun M, Madsen JR, Irwin N. VEGF, which is elevated in the CSF of patients with hydrocephalus, causes ventriculomegaly and ependymal changes in rats. Exp Neurol. 2013;247:703–9.
87. Tietz S, Engelhardt B. Brain barriers: Crosstalk between complex tight junctions and adherens junctions. J Cell Biol. 2015;209:493–506.
88. Brouwer AJ, Groenendaal F, Benders MJ, de Vries LS. Early and late complications of germinal matrix-intraventricular haemorrhage in the preterm infant: what is new? Neonatology. 2014;106:296–303.
89. Pikus HJ, Levy ML, Gans W, Mendel E, McComb JG. Outcome, cost analysis, and long-term follow-up in preterm infants with massive grade IV germinal matrix hemorrhage and progressive hydrocephalus. Neurosurgery. 1997;40:983–8.
90. Reinprecht A, Dietrich W, Berger A, Bavinzski G, Weninger M, Czech T. Posthemorrhagic hydrocephalus in preterm infants: long term follow-up and shunt-related complications. Childs Nerv Syst. 2001;17:663–9.
91. Ballabh P. Pathogenesis and prevention of intraventricular hemorrhage. Clin Perinatol. 2014;41:47–67.
92. Cherian S, Whitelaw A, Thoresen M, Love S. The pathogenesis of neonatal post-hemorrhagic hydrocephalus. Brain Pathol. 2004;14:305–11.
93. Ballabh P. Intraventricular hemorrhage in premature infants: mechanism of disease. Pediatr Res. 2010;67:1–8.
94. El-Khoury N, Braun A, Hu F, Pandey M, Nedergaard M, Lagamma EF, Ballabh P. Astrocyte end-feet in germinal matrix, cerebral cortex, and white matter in developing infants. Pediatr Res. 2006;59:673–9.
95. Baburamani AA, Ek CJ, Walker DW, Castillo-Melendez M. Vulnerability of the developing brain to hypoxic-ischemic damage: contribution of the cerebral vasculature to injury and repair? Front Physiol. 2012;3:424.
96. Ballabh P, Braun A, Nedergaard M. Anatomic analysis of blood vessels in germinal matrix, cerebral cortex, and white matter in developing infants. Pediatr Res. 2004;56:117–24.
97. Braun A, Xu H, Hu F, Kocherlakota P, Siegel D, Chander P, Ungvari Z, Csiszar A, Nedergaard M, Ballabh P. Paucity of pericytes in germinal matrix vasculature of premature infants. J Neurosci. 2007;27:12012–24.
98. Del Bigio MR, Di Curzio DL. Nonsurgical therapy for hydrocephalus: a comprehensive and critical review. Fluids Barriers CNS. 2016;13:3.
99. Patel MM, Goyal BR, Bhadada SV, Bhatt JS, Amin AF. Getting into the brain: approaches to enhance brain drug delivery. CNS Drugs. 2009;23:5–58.
100. Soni V, Jain A, Khare P, Gulbake A, Jain SK. Potential approaches for drug delivery to the brain: past, present, and future. Crit Rev Ther Drug Carrier Syst. 2010;27:187–236.
101. Lu CT, Zhao YZ, Wong HL, Cai J, Peng L, Tian XQ. Current approaches to enhance CNS delivery of drugs across the brain barriers. Int J Nanomed. 2014;9:2241–57.
102. Guerra M. Neural stem cells: are they the hope of a better life for patients with fetal-onset hydrocephalus? Fluids Barriers CNS. 2014;11:7.
103. Yuan Q, Bu X, Yan Z, Liu X, Wei Z, Ma C, Qu M. Combination of endogenous neural stem cell mobilization and lithium chloride treatment for hydrocephalus following intraventricular haemorrhage. Exp Ther Med. 2016;12:3275–81.
104. Cacci E, Villa A, Parmar M, Cavallaro M, Mandahl N, Lindvall O, Martinez-Serrano A, Kokaia Z. Generation of human cortical neurons from a new immortal fetal neural stem cell line. Exp Cell Res. 2007;313:588–601.
105. Monni E, Cusulin C, Cavallaro M, Lindvall O, Kokaia Z. Human fetal striatum-derived neural stem (NS) cells differentiate to mature neurons in vitro and in vivo. Curr Stem Cell Res Ther. 2014;9:338–46.
106. Rohban R, Pieber TR. Mesenchymal Stem and Progenitor Cells in Regeneration: tissue Specificity and Regenerative Potential. Stem Cells Int. 2017;2017:5173732.
107. Das M, Sundell IB, Koka PS. Adult mesenchymal stem cells and their potency in the cell-based therapy. J Stem Cells. 2013;8:1–16.
108. Fu L, Zhu L, Huang Y, Lee TD, Forman SJ, Shih CC. Derivation of neural stem cells from mesenchymal stem cells: evidence for a bipotential stem cell population. Stem Cells Dev. 2008;17:1109–21.
109. Murphy SV, Atala A. Amniotic fluid and placental membranes: unexpected sources of highly multipotent cells. Semin Reprod Med. 2013;31:62–8.
110. Hass R, Kasper C, Böhm S, Jacobs R. Different populations and sources of human mesenchymal stem cells (MSC): a comparison of adult and neonatal tissue-derived MSC. Cell Commun Signal. 2011;9:12.
111. Castro-Manrreza ME, Montesinos JJ. Immunoregulation by mesenchymal stem cells: biological aspects and clinical applications. J Immunol Res. 2015;2015:394917.
112. Drago D, Cossetti C, Iraci N, Gaude E, Musco G, Bachi A, Pluchino S. The stem cell secretome and its role in brain repair. Biochimie. 2013;95:2271–85.

113. Hofer HR, Tuan RS. Secreted trophic factors of mesenchymal stem cells support neurovascular and musculoskeletal therapies. Stem Cell Res Ther. 2016;7:131.
114. Ahn SY, Chang YS, Park WS. Mesenchymal stem cells transplantation for neuroprotection in preterm infants with severe intraventricular haemorrhage. Korean J Pediatr. 2014;57:251–6.
115. Björklund A, Lindvall O. Replacing dopamine neurons in Parkinson's disease: how did it happen? J Parkinsons Dis. 2017;7(s1):S23–33.
116. Li W, Englund E, Widner H, Mattsson B, van Westen D, Lätt J, Rehncrona S, Brundin P, Björklund A, Lindvall O, Li JY. Extensive graft-derived dopaminergic innervation is maintained 24 years after transplantation in the degenerating parkinsonian brain. Proc Natl Acad Sci USA. 2016;113:6544–9.
117. Kefalopoulou Z, Politis M, Piccini P, Mencacci N, Bhatia K, Jahanshahi M, Widner H, Rehncrona S, Brundin P, Björklund A, Lindvall O, Limousin P, Quinn N, Foltynie T. Long-term clinical outcome of fetal cell transplantation for Parkinson disease: two case reports. JAMA Neurol. 2014;71:83–7.
118. Malik S, Vinukonda G, Vose LR, Diamond D, Bhimavarapu BBR, Hu F, Zia MT, Hevner R, Zecevic N, Ballabh P. Neurogenesis continues in the third trimester of pregnancy and is suppressed by premature birth. J Neurosci. 2013;33:411–23.
119. Adzick NS, Thom EA, Spong CY, Brock JW, Burrows PK, Johnson MP, Howell LJ, Farrell JA, Dabrowiak ME, Sutton LN, Gupta N, Tulipan NB, D'Alton ME, Farmer DL, MOMS Investigators. A randomized trial of prenatal versus postnatal repair of myelomeningocele. N Engl J Med. 2011;364:993–1000.
120. Benjaminy S, Lo C, Illes J. Social responsibility in stem cell research-is the news all bad? Stem Cell Rev. 2016;12:269–75.
121. Dimmeler S, Ding S, Rando TA, Trounson A. Translational strategies and challenges in regenerative medicine. Nat Med. 2014;20:814–21.
122. Imitola J, Khoury SJ. Neural stem cells and the future treatment of neurological diseases: raising the standard. Methods Mol Biol. 2008;438:9–16.
123. Singh AK, Arya RK, Maheshwari S, Singh A, Meena S, Pandey P, Dormond O, Datta D. Tumor heterogeneity and cancer stem cell paradigm: updates in concept, controversies and clinical relevance. Int J Cancer. 2015;136:1991–2000.
124. Haarer J, Johnson CL, Soeder Y, Dahlke MH. Caveats of mesenchymal stem cell therapy in solid organ transplantation. Transpl Int. 2015;28:1–9.
125. Fiore EJ, Mazzolini G, Aquino JB. Mesenchymal stem/stromal cells in liver fibrosis: recent findings, old/new caveats and future perspectives. Stem Cell Rev. 2015;11:586–97.
126. Roybal JL, Santore MT, Flake AW. Stem cell and genetic therapies for the fetus. Semin Foetal Neonatal Med. 2010;15:6.
127. Merianos D, Heaton T, Flake AW. In utero hematopoietic stem cell transplantation: progress toward clinical application. Biol Blood Marrow Transpl. 2008;14:729–40.
128. Li H, Gao F, Ma L, Jiang J, Miao J, Jiang M, Fan Y, Wang L, Wu D, Liu B, Wang W, Lui VC, Yuan Z. Therapeutic potential of in utero mesenchymal stem cell (MSCs) transplantation in rat foetuses with spina bifida aperta. J Cell Mol Med. 2012;16:1606–17.
129. Fauza DO, Jennings RW, Teng YD, Snyder EY. Neural stem cell delivery to the spinal cord in an ovine model of foetal surgery for spina bifida. Surgery. 2008;144:367–73.
130. Ahn SY, Chang YS, Sung DK, Sung SI, Yoo HS, Im GH, Choi SJ, Park WS. Optimal route for mesenchymal stem cells transplantation after severe intraventricular hemorrhage in newborn rats. PLoS ONE. 2015;10(7):e0132919.
131. Porada CD, Almeida-Porada G. Mesenchymal stem cells as therapeutics and vehicles for gene and drug delivery. Adv Drug Deliv Rev. 2010;62:1156–66.
132. Glage S, Klinge PM, Miller MC, Wallrapp C, Geigle P, Hedrich HJ, Brinker T. Therapeutic concentrations of glucagon-like peptide-1 in cerebrospinal fluid following cell-based delivery into the cerebral ventricles of cats. Fluids Barriers CNS. 2011;8:18.
133. Rodríguez EM. The cerebrospinal fluid as a pathway in neuroendocrine integration. J Endocrinol. 1976;71:407–43.
134. Zappaterra MW, Lehtinen MK. The cerebrospinal fluid: regulator of neurogenesis, behavior, and beyond. Cell Mol Life Sci. 2012;69:2863–78.
135. Kaur C, Rathnasamy G, Ling EA. The Choroid plexus in healthy and diseased brain. J Neuropathol Exp Neurol. 2016;75:198–213.
136. Spector R, Keep RF, Robert Snodgrass S, Smith QR, Johanson CE. A balanced view of choroid plexus structure and function: focus on adult humans. Exp Neurol. 2015;267:78–86.
137. Galarza M. Evidence of the subcommissural organ in humans and its association with hydrocephalus. Neurosurg Rev. 2002;25:205–15.
138. Huh MS, Todd MA, Picketts DJ. SCO-ping out the mechanisms underlying the etiology of hydrocephalus. Physiology (Bethesda). 2009;24:117–26.
139. Lehtinen MK, Bjornsson CS, Dymecki SM, Gilbertson RJ, Holtzman DM, Monuki ES. The choroid plexus and cerebrospinal fluid: emerging roles in development, disease, and therapy. J Neurosci. 2013;33:17553–9.
140. Richardson SJ, Wijayagunaratne RC, D'Souza DG, Darras VM, Van Herck SL. Transport of thyroid hormones via the choroid plexus into the brain: the roles of transthyretin and thyroid hormone transmembrane transporters. Front Neurosci. 2015;9:66.
141. Gomes JR, Nogueira RS, Vieira M, Santos SD, Ferraz-Nogueira JP, Relvas JB, Saraiva MJ. Transthyretin provides trophic support via megalin by promoting neurite outgrowth and neuroprotection in cerebral ischemia. Cell Death Differ. 2016;23:1749–64.
142. Alshehri B, D'Souza DG, Lee JY, Petratos S, Richardson SJ. The diversity of mechanisms influenced by transthyretin in neurobiology: development, disease and endocrine disruption. J Neuroendocrinol. 2015;27:303–23.
143. Skinner SJ, Geaney MS, Rush R, Rogers ML, Emerich DF, Thanos CG, Vasconcellos AV, Tan PL, Elliott RB. Choroid plexus transplants in the treatment of brain diseases. Xenotransplantation. 2006;13:284–8.
144. Sandrof MA, Emerich DF, Thanos CG. Primary choroid plexus tissue for use in cellular therapy. Methods Mol Biol. 2017;1479:237–49.
145. Thanos CG, Bintz B, Emerich DF. Microencapsulated choroid plexus epithelial cell transplants for repair of the brain. Adv Exp Med Biol. 2010;670:80–91.
146. Skinner SJ, Geaney MS, Lin H, Muzina M, Anal AK, Elliott RB, Tan PL. Encapsulated living choroid plexus cells: potential long-term treatments for central nervous system disease and trauma. J Neural Eng. 2009;6:065001.
147. Ide C, Nakano N, Kanekiyo K. Cell transplantation for the treatment of spinal cord injury - bone marrow stromal cells and choroid plexus epithelial cells. Neural Regen Res. 2016;11:1385–8.
148. Rodríguez EM, Oksche A, Hein S, Yulis CR. Cell biology of the subcommissural organ. Int Rev Cytol. 1992;135:39–121.
149. Guerra MM, González C, Caprile T, Jara M, Vío K, Muñoz RI, Rodríguez S, Rodríguez EM. Understanding how the subcommissural organ and other periventricular secretory structures contribute via the cerebrospinal fluid to neurogenesis. Front Cell Neurosci. 2015;9:480.
150. Rodríguez S, Rodríguez EM, Jara P, Peruzzo B, Oksche A. Single injection into the cerebrospinal fluid of antibodies against the secretory material of the subcommissural organ reversibly blocks formation of Reissner's fiber: immunocytochemical investigations in the rat. Exp Brain Res. 1990;81:113–24.
151. Vio K, Rodríguez S, Navarrete EH, Pérez-Fígares JM, Jiménez AJ, Rodríguez EM. Hydrocephalus induced by immunological blockage of the subcommissural organ-Reissner's fiber (RF) complex by maternal transfer of anti-RF antibodies. Exp Brain Res. 2000;135:41–52.
152. Ortloff AR, Vío K, Guerra M, Jaramillo K, Kaehne T, Jones H, McAllister JP 2nd, Rodríguez EM. Role of the subcommissural organ in the pathogenesis of congenital hydrocephalus in the HTx rat. Cell Tissue Res. 2013;352:707–25.
153. Montecinos HA, Richter H, Caprile T, Rodriguez EM. Synthesis of transthyretin by the ependymal cells of the subcommissural organ. Cell Tissue Res. 2005;320:487–99.
154. Cuevas P, Reimers D, Giménez-Gallego G. Loss of basic fibroblast growth factor in the subcommissural organ of old spontaneously hypertensive rats. Neurosci Lett. 1996;221:25–8.
155. Schöbitz K, Gonzalez C, Peruzzo B, Yulis CR, Rodríguez EM. Organ culture of the bovine subcommissural organ: evidence for synthesis and release of the secretory material. Microsc Res Tech. 2001;52:496–509.
156. Rodríguez S, Navarrete EH, Vio K, González C, Schöbitz K, Rodríguez EM. Isograft and xenograft of the subcommissural organ into the lateral ventricle of the rat and the formation of Reissner's fiber. Cell Tissue Res. 1999;296:457–69.

157. Morris PJ. Immunoprotection of therapeutic cell transplants by encapsulation. Trends Biotechnol. 1996;14:163–7.
158. Begley DJ. Delivery of therapeutic agents to the central nervous system: the problems and the possibilities. Pharmacol Ther. 2004;104:29–45.
159. Orive G, Santos E, Poncelet D, Hernández RM, Pedraz JL, Wahlberg LU, De Vos P, Emerich D. Cell encapsulation: technical and clinical advances. Trends Pharmacol Sci. 2015;36:537–46.
160. Brinker T, Spader H. A translational view of peptide treatment of neurological disorders. Curr Med Chem. 2014;21:2583–90.
161. Acarregui A, Orive G, Pedraz JL, Hernández RM. Therapeutic applications of encapsulated cells. Methods Mol Biol. 2013;1051:349–64.
162. Koch S, Schwinger C, Kressler J, Heinzen Ch, Rainov NG. Alginate encapsulation of genetically engineered mammalian cells: comparison of production devices, methods and microcapsule characteristics. J Microencapsul. 2003;20:303–16.
163. Zimmermann H, Shirley SG, Zimmermann U. Alginate-based encapsulation of cells: past, present and future. Curr Diabet Rep. 2007;7:314–20.
164. Wahlberg LU, Lind G, Almqvist PM, Kusk P, Tornøe J, Juliusson B, Söderman M, Selldén E, Seiger Å, Eriksdotter-Jönhagen M, Linderoth B. Targeted delivery of nerve growth factor via encapsulated cell biodelivery in Alzheimer disease: a technology platform for restorative neurosurgery. J Neurosurg. 2012;117:340–7.
165. Fernandez-Espejo E. Pathogenesis of Parkinson's disease: prospects of neuroprotective and restorative therapies. Mol Neurobiol. 2004;29:15–30.
166. Kanter-Schlifke I, Fjord-Larsen L, Kusk P, Angehagen M, Wahlberg L, Kokaia M. GDNF released from encapsulated cells suppresses seizure activity in the epileptic hippocampus. Exp Neurol. 2009;216:413–9.
167. Kuramoto S, Yasuhara T, Agari T, Kondo A, Jing M, Kikuchi Y, Shinko A, Wakamori T, Kameda M, Wang F, Kin K, Edahiro S, Miyoshi Y, Date I. BDNF-secreting capsule exerts neuroprotective effects on epilepsy model of rats. Brain Res. 2011;1368:281–9.
168. Borlongan CV, Skinner SJ, Geaney M, Vasconcellos AV, Elliott RB, Emerich DF. CNS grafts of rat choroid plexus protect against cerebral ischemia in adult rats. NeuroReport. 2004;15:1543–7.
169. Winn SR, Emerich DF. Managing chronic pain with encapsulated cell implants releasing catecholamines and endogenous opiods. Front Biosci. 2005;10:367–78.

9

A 3D subject-specific model of the spinal subarachnoid space with anatomically realistic ventral and dorsal spinal cord nerve rootlets

Lucas R. Sass[1], Mohammadreza Khani[1], Gabryel Connely Natividad[1], R. Shane Tubbs[3], Olivier Baledent[2] and Bryn A. Martin[1,4*]

Abstract

Background: The spinal subarachnoid space (SSS) has a complex 3D fluid-filled geometry with multiple levels of anatomic complexity, the most salient features being the spinal cord and dorsal and ventral nerve rootlets. An accurate anthropomorphic representation of these features is needed for development of in vitro and numerical models of cerebrospinal fluid (CSF) dynamics that can be used to inform and optimize CSF-based therapeutics.

Methods: A subject-specific 3D model of the SSS was constructed based on high-resolution anatomic MRI. An expert operator completed manual segmentation of the CSF space with detailed consideration of the anatomy. 31 pairs of semi-idealized dorsal and ventral nerve rootlets (NR) were added to the model based on anatomic reference to the magnetic resonance (MR) imaging and cadaveric measurements in the literature. Key design criteria for each NR pair included the radicular line, descending angle, number of NR, attachment location along the spinal cord and exit through the dura mater. Model simplification and smoothing was performed to produce a final model with minimum vertices while maintaining minimum error between the original segmentation and final design. Final model geometry and hydrodynamics were characterized in terms of axial distribution of Reynolds number, Womersley number, hydraulic diameter, cross-sectional area and perimeter.

Results: The final model had a total of 139,901 vertices with a total CSF volume within the SSS of 97.3 cm^3. Volume of the dura mater, spinal cord and NR was 123.1, 19.9 and 5.8 cm^3. Surface area of these features was 318.52, 112.2 and 232.1 cm^2 respectively. Maximum Reynolds number was 174.9 and average Womersley number was 9.6, likely indicating presence of a laminar inertia-dominated oscillatory CSF flow field.

Conclusions: This study details an anatomically realistic anthropomorphic 3D model of the SSS based on high-resolution MR imaging of a healthy human adult female.

Keywords: Spinal subarachnoid space, Intrathecal drug delivery, 3D reconstruction, Cerebrospinal fluid, Spinal cord, Dura mater, Nerve roots, Spinal cord injury, Neurapheresis, Cerebrospinal fluid hypothermia

Background

Detailed analysis of cerebrospinal fluid (CSF) dynamics is thought to be of importance to help understand diseases of the central nervous system such as Chiari malformation [1], hydrocephalus [2, 3] and intracranial hypertension [4]. CSF therapeutic interventions have also been investigated such as intrathecal drug delivery [5], CSF filtration or "neurapheresis" (also previously termed liquorpheresis) [6, 7] and CSF hypothermia (cooling) treatment [8]. The exact relation, if any, of CSF dynamics to these disorders and treatments is under investigation. There

*Correspondence: brynm@uidaho.edu
[4] Department of Biological Engineering, University of Idaho, 875 Perimeter Dr. MC0904, Moscow, ID 83844-0904, USA
Full list of author information is available at the end of the article

are many opportunities for researchers to make a contribution to the field.

A significant contribution to our understanding of CSF dynamics has been made by the use of computational fluid dynamics (CFD) modeling; an engineering technique that allows detailed analysis of the CSF flow field that is not possible by MRI measurements or invasive means. In addition, CFD allows for variational analysis, where specific parameters in the model can be altered to understand their distinct contribution. Major CFD-based contributions to our knowledge of CSF physiology have been made in the areas of CSF ventricular dynamics [9], drug transport [10, 11], filtration [12], alterations in brain pathologies [13–15], spinal cord pathology [16] and wave mechanics [17, 18].

Computational fluid dynamics modeling relies on accurate representation of boundary conditions that are difficult to define because of the intricate spinal subarachnoid space (SSS) geometry, complex CSF flow field and lack of material property information about the central nervous system tissues. Each CFD modeling approach has necessitated varying degrees of boundary condition simplification with respect to anatomy and physiology. When considering anatomy, CFD models that attempt to accurately imitate the spinal geometry are generally built from subject-specific MRI scans. However, even for experts in spinal neuroanatomy, magnetic resonance (MR) imaging resolution and artifacts make subject-specific anatomical reconstruction of the SSS difficult, particularly for engineers who often have limited anatomical knowledge. Herein, we provide to the research community an open-source subject-specific 3D model of the complete SSS with idealized spinal cord nerve rootlets (NR) licensed under the Creative Commons Attribution-ShareAlike 4.0 International license (CC BY-SA 4.0). This also includes the in vivo measured CSF flow waveforms along the spine. The open-source model can allow multiple researchers a tool to investigate and compare results for CSF dynamics related phenomena and technologies such as pharmacokinetics of intrathecal drug distribution, neurapheresis and hypothermia.

Methods

Subject selection

A single, representative healthy, 23-year-old, female Caucasian subject was enrolled in this study. The subject had no previous history of neurological or cardiovascular disorders.

MRI CSF flow measurement protocol

All MRI measurements were obtained with a General Electric 3T scanner (Signa HDxt, software 15.0_M4_0910.a). CSF flow data were collected at three vertebral levels, C2–C3, C7–T1 and T10–T11, using phase-contrast MRI with retrospective electrocardiogram (ECG) gating and 32 cardiac phases [14]. Each slice had a thickness of 5.0 mm and an in-plane resolution of 0.54 × 0.54 mm. Orientation of the slice was made perpendicular to the CSF flow direction and positioned vertically by intersection with a vertebral disk (i.e. C2–C3). A flip angle, TR, TE and VENC was used with a value of 25°, 13.4, 8.26 and 8 cm/s respectively. Detailed information on imaging parameters is provided by Baledent et al. [19].

CSF flow quantification

Oscillatory cardiac-related CSF flow was quantified for the axial locations located at the vertebral disk at the C2–C3, C7–T1 and T10–T11 vertebral levels. As detailed in our previous studies [14, 20], Matlab was used to compute the CSF flow waveform, $Q_{(t)}$, based on integration of the pixel velocities with $Q(t) = \sum A_{pixel}\,[V_{pixel}(t)]$, where A_{pixel} is the area of one MRI pixel, V_{pixel} is the velocity for the corresponding pixel, and $Q_{(t)}$ is the summation of the flow for each pixel of interest. A smooth distribution of CSF flow along the spine was achieved by interpolating CSF flow between each axial measurement location [21]. Similar to previous studies, the diastolic CSF flow cycle phase was extended in cases when necessary [22]. For correcting eddy current offsets, the cyclic net CSF flow was offset to produce zero net flow over a complete flow cycle [14].

MRI CSF space geometry protocol

To collect geometric measurements with improved CSF signal, 3D fast imaging employing steady state acquisition (3D FIESTA) was used, and acquisitions were realized with free breathing. The coils used were the HD Neck-Spine Array with 16 Channels for the spine and the 29 element phased array for the upper-neck. Images were collected in three volumes, from the top of the brain to C7, from C5 to T9, and from T9 to S5, with each section containing 140, 104 and 104 sagittal T2-weighted images respectively. The field of view (FOV) size was 30 cm × 30 cm × 7 cm for the craniocervical volume, and 30 cm × 30 cm × 5.25 cm for both the thoracic and lumbosacral volumes. In-plane voxel spacing was 0.547 × 0.547 mm and slice thickness was 1 mm with slice spacing set at 0.499 mm. Echo times (TE) were 1.944, 2.112, 2.100 and repetition times (TR) were 5.348, 5.762, 5.708 for the craniocervical, thoracic, and lumbosacral volumes respectively. Total imaging time for the three levels was ~ 45 min.

CSF space segmentation

The open-source program, ITK-SNAP (Version 3.4.0, University of Pennsylvania, USA) [23], was used to segment the MRI data. Similar to our previous work [24], the cervical, thoracic and lumbar MR image sets were manually segmented in the axial orientation using the semi-automatic contrast-based segmentation tool. The segmented region extended from the foramen magnum to the end of the dural sac. One expert operator completed the segmentation, as our previous study showed strong inter-operator reliability of SSS geometric parameters [24]. A second expert operator reviewed the images to confirm region selection, and in areas of disagreement, discussed in detail with respect to the anatomy. Hyperintensities in the T2-weighted image sets near the epidural space were excluded from the model segmentation (Fig. 1). MRI data were not collected in high-resolution for the entire brain, and thus the cortical and ventricular CSF spaces were not included in the model. After completion, each segmentation was exported as an .STL file with Gaussian smoothing option applied (standard deviation = 0.80 and maximum approximation error = 0.03).

Model alignment

The open source program, Blender (Version 2.77a, Amsterdam, Netherlands), was used for the majority of mesh modifications and all modeling operations in this study. After segmentation, the .STL files generated were imported into Blender. Because of the global reference coordinate set by the MRI, segmentations generated from different image series were automatically registered. However, 3D rigid

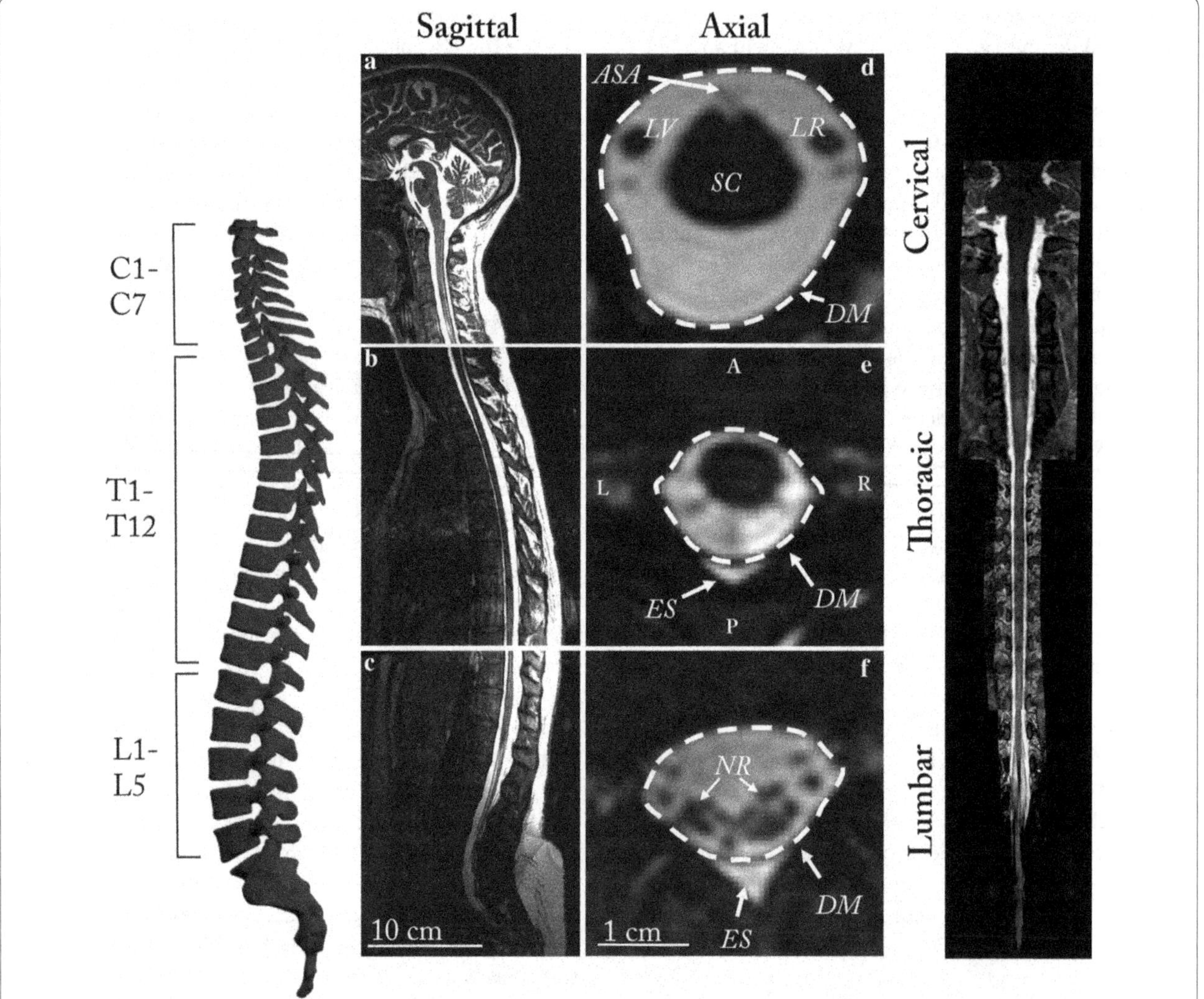

Fig. 1 T2-weighted MRI data were collected as three volumes, **a** craniocervical, **b** thoracic, **c** Lumbosacral. A variety of artifacts exist in and around the SSS, **d–f** including the anterior spinal artery (ASA), left and right vertebral arteries (LV and LR), epidural space (ES), dura mater (DM), spinal cord (SC), and dorsal and ventral nerve rootlets (NR) in particular near the cauda equina. Note: the 3D geometry provided in this manuscript only includes the CSF within the spine below the foramen magnum (*L* left, *R* right, *A* anterior, *P* posterior)

body translation (~ 5 mm maximum) was required to align each model section due to a small degree of subject movement between the MR image acquisitions. These translations were performed based on a visual best fit.

Geometry remeshing and smoothing

The following operations were completed to create a lowest-resolution semi-regular surface mesh of the spinal cord and dura while maintaining an accurate representation of the original geometry. After alignment, the triangulated .STL segmentations were converted to quadrilateral meshes using the automatic conversion tool "tris to quads" in Blender. The spinal cord and dural surfaces were separated, and an array of planes was placed along the entire spinal segmentation at a roughly orthogonal orientation to the spinal trajectory. Vertical spacing of these planes was determined by choosing an inter-plane interval (~ 5 mm) that preserved surface contours; this required a minimum of three planes to preserve a change in surface concavity. The circumferential contour of the spinal cord and dura was obtained at each plane using the "intersect (knife)" operation in Blender. The original geometry was then removed. Each surface contour was then vertically extruded ~ 1 mm. Simple circle meshes were place at each contour using the "add circle" command, the "shrink wrap" modifier was then used to form these circles around each profile. The number of vertices in the circles wrapped to the dural and spinal cord profiles was specified to be 55 and 32 respectively. These parameters were determined based on visual inspection of the shrink-wrap fit at the largest profile diameter located at the foramen magnum. Manual adjustment of individual vertices was made to preserve a uniform vertex distribution and surface contour at each slice. To create a continuous quadrilateral mesh of both the spinal cord and dura, the "bridge edge loops" command was used between adjacent contours (Fig. 2).

Manual adjustments were then made by sculpting the remeshed surfaces within the "sculpt mode" workspace in Blender to produce ~ 50% visual interference with the original segmentation surface (Fig. 3). To further improve surface accuracy, a combination of a shrink-wrap and "smooth" modifiers were used simultaneously. Importantly, the "keep above surface" option and "offset" options on the shrink-wrap modifier were used. The values for shrink-wrap offset and smoothing factor in their respective modifier menus must be determined by a trial and error method for each unique mesh until the desired smoothness is justified with overall volume. In this study, values of 0.04 and 0.900 were used for offset and smoothing factor respectively.

Nerve root modeling

The 31 NR pairs, starting from the craniocervical junction, were modeled using the following methodology. For each rootlet, a "circle" mesh was extruded from the SC junction to the dural exit location in Blender. The curvature, radicular line (RL) and descending angle (DA) for each rootlet were determined based on the subject specific segmentation, average cadaveric measurements from the literature and anatomic reference imagery [25–28] (Fig. 4). The exact method varied by location due to variations in the completeness of the data types; these differences are described below. Note: the 31st nerve root, or coccygeal nerve did not bifurcate into a nerve root pair until after leaving the intrathecal CSF space.

In the left side of the cervical spine, segmentations of the NR were possible to obtain directly from the anatomic MR imaging. These were imported and aligned with the existing model in Blender. A "circle" mesh was

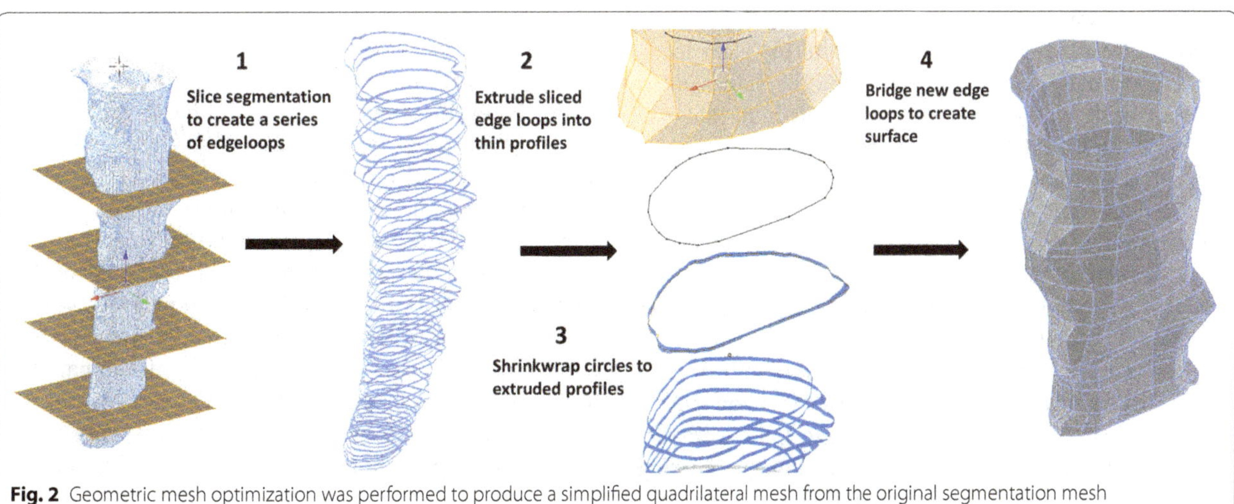

Fig. 2 Geometric mesh optimization was performed to produce a simplified quadrilateral mesh from the original segmentation mesh

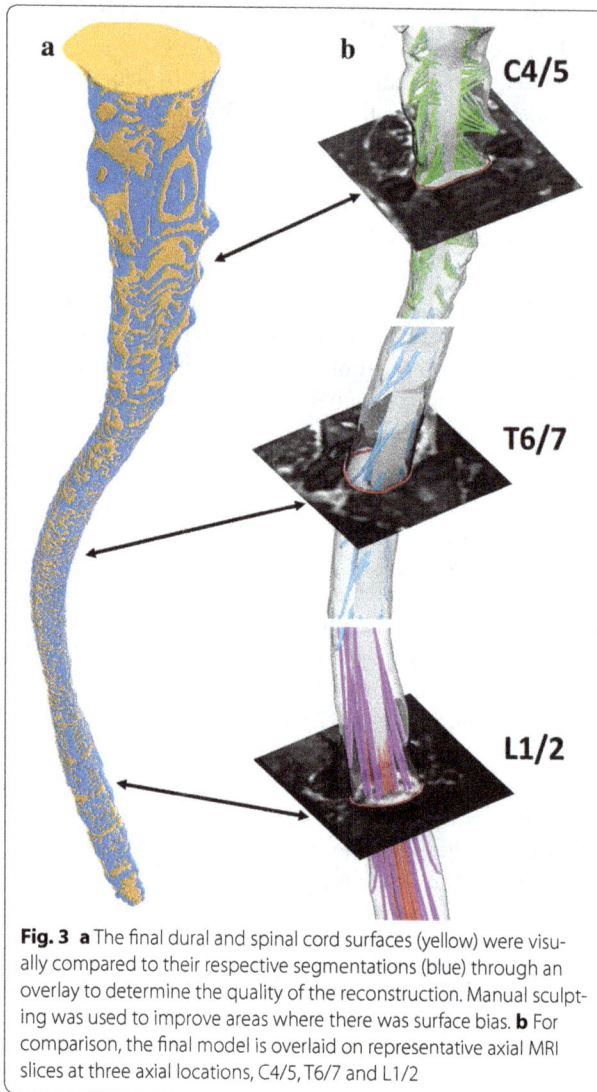

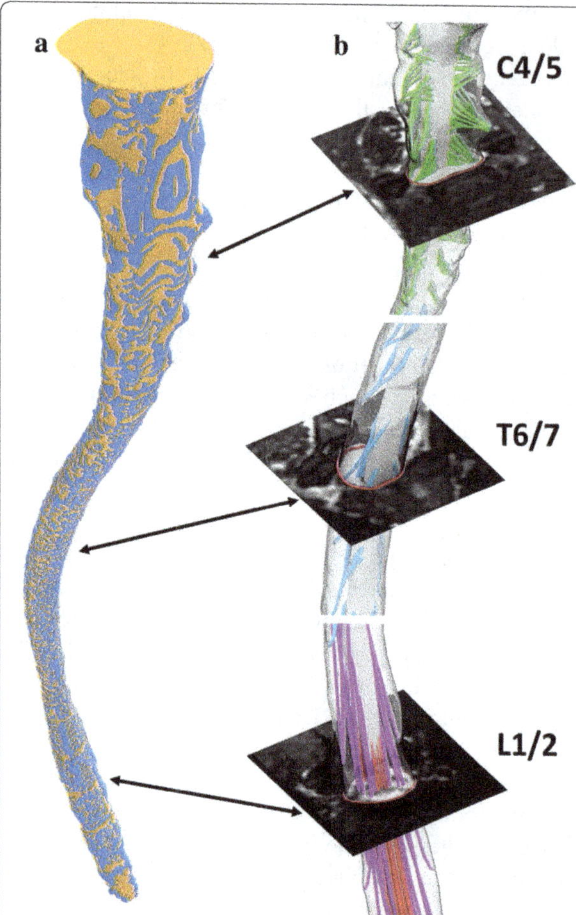

Fig. 3 **a** The final dural and spinal cord surfaces (yellow) were visually compared to their respective segmentations (blue) through an overlay to determine the quality of the reconstruction. Manual sculpting was used to improve areas where there was surface bias. **b** For comparison, the final model is overlaid on representative axial MRI slices at three axial locations, C4/5, T6/7 and L1/2

extruded along each segmented path and the diameter of this circle was defined as the average NR diameter or thickness from cadaveric measurements for each location. Additionally, in the cervical spine the spinal entry point of each rootlet cylinder was scaled in the cranial direction (~ 150%) along the spinal cord to create a blended transition. Finally, cervical rootlets were mirrored left to right and small adjustments were made to fit them to the correct exit points on the right side of the dura. Mirroring was applied as the NR intersection location at the spinal cord and dura was nearly identical for the left and right side NR.

In the thoracic spine, segmentations were only able to inform NR entry and exit points, and by extension, DA. It is possible that NR points in the thoracic spine were difficult to visualize within this region due to image blurring stemming from respiratory-related tissue motion. NR morphology in the thoracic spine is a steeply descending and tightly packed bundle. Therefore, to reduce unnecessary mesh complexity, a standard NR set was developed as a simplified cylinder with a diameter based on the average NR bundle size in the thoracic region. In addition to this main cylinder, a secondary cylinder was incorporated at the SC entry point to more closely imitate NR branching near the spinal cord. This cylinder extends from just below the primary rootlet entry point to a location approximately one-third of way along the primary rootlet; overall a steeply descending deltoid morphology is created. As in the cervical spine, a blended transition was created at the SC entry point for each NR. This standard NR set was mirrored left to right of the SC and duplicated along the SC for the entire thoracic region.

In the lumbosacral spine, the NR form the cauda equina. High MR image contrast made complete segmentations of this region possible and NR modeling was completed as in the cervical spine. NR were again simplified as a single cylinder of average diameter. Because of this, RLs for this region were not possible to define.

Geometric analysis

Geometric parameters were calculated along the complete spinal mesh at 1 mm intervals [21]. SSS cross-sectional area, $A_{cs} = A_d - A_c - A_{nr}$, was determined based on cross-sectional area of the NR (A_{nr}), SC (A_c) and dura (A_d). Hydraulic diameter for internal flow within a tube, $D_H = 4A_{cs}/P_{cs}$, was determined based on the cross-sectional area and wetted perimeter, $P_{cs} = P_d + P_c + P_{nr}$. Wetted perimeter was computed as the sum of the NR (P_{nr}), SC (P_c) and dura (P_d) perimeters. Each of these parameters was calculated within a user defined function compiled in ANSYS FLUENT (Ver. 18.1, ANSYS inc, Canonsburg, PA). Note, for geometric analysis, the coccygeal nerve (spinal nerve) was considered to be a part of the spinal cord.

Hydrodynamic analysis

The hydrodynamic environment at 1 mm slice intervals along the entire spine was assessed by Reynolds number based on peak flow rate, $\mathrm{Re} = \frac{Q_{sys} D_H}{\nu A_{cs}}$, and Womersley number based on hydraulic diameter. For Reynolds number, Q_{sys} is the temporal maximum of the local flow at each axial interval along the spine obtained by interpolation from the experimental data and ν is the kinematic viscosity of the fluid. Similar to previous studies, CSF viscosity was assumed to be that of water at body temperature. To evaluate the presence of laminar flow, ($Re < 2300$), similar to previous studies in CSF and biofluids mechanics, Reynolds number was evaluated at peak systolic flow along the spine. Womersley number, $\alpha = \frac{D_h}{2}\sqrt{\omega/\nu}$, where ω is the angular velocity of the

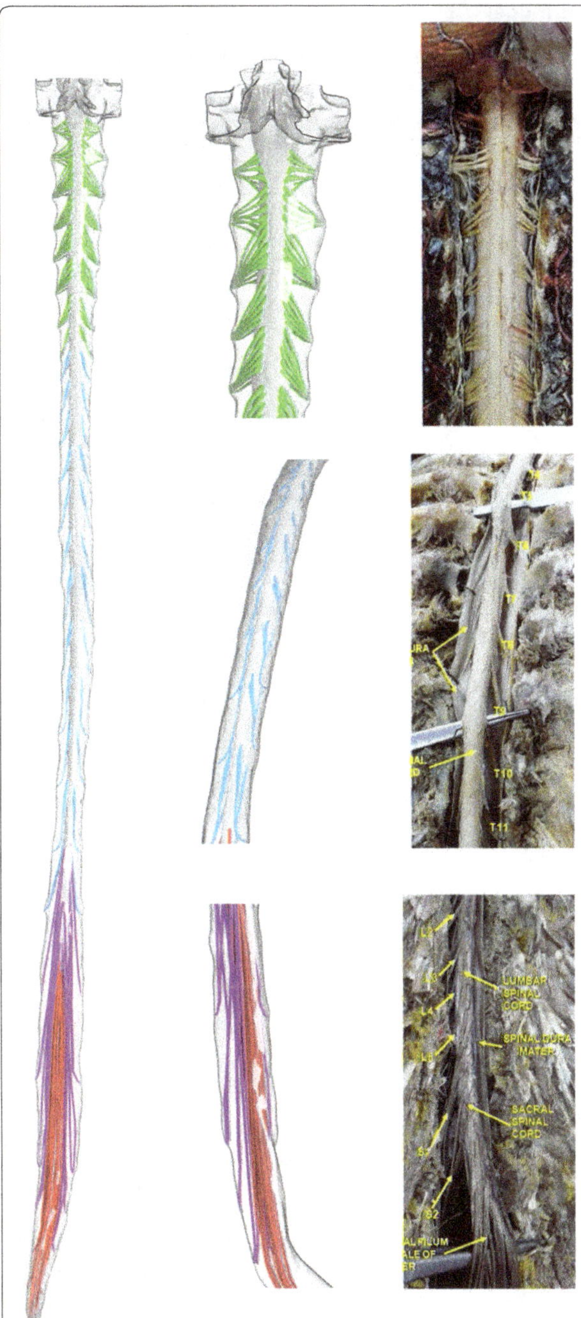

Fig. 4 Complete spinal geometry showing detail in the cervical (green), thoracic (blue), lumbar (violet), and sacral (red) regions compared to anatomic imagery of respective locations [84–86]. Note: all model calculations are made for SSS region located below the foramen magnum only (picture shows part of foramen magnum for illustration of connection to brain)

volume flow waveform $\omega = 2\pi/T$, was used to quantify the ratio of unsteady inertial forces to viscous forces. This ratio was previously found to be large relative to viscous forces by Loth et al. [29]. A value greater than 5 for Womersley number indicates transition from parabolic to "m-shaped" velocity profiles for oscillatory flows [30]. CSF pulse wave velocity (PWV) was quantified as an indicator of CSF space compliance. Timing of peak systolic CSF flow rate along the spine was determined based on our previously published method [31]. In brief, a linear fit was computed based on the peak systolic flow rate arrival time with the slope being equivalent to the PWV.

Results

The final model includes the 31 pairs of dorsal and ventral NR, spinal cord with coccygeal nerve and dural wall (Fig. 4). Final values for the vertical location where the NR join into the dura (Z position), radicular line, descending angle, root thickness, and number of rootlets for both dorsal and ventral NR are provided (Table 1). The percent difference of the final remeshed dura volume compared to the original dura segmentation was 2.7% (original segmentation volume = 100.5 cm^3 and a final remeshed volume = 103.2 cm^3). Addition of NR reduced the final remeshed volume to 97.3 cm^3. A 3D visualization of the internal geometry is shown in Fig. 5.

Geometric parameters

Total intrathecal CSF volume below the foramen magnum was 97.3 cm^3 (Table 3). Volumes of the dura mater, spinal cord and 31 NR pairs were 123.0, 19.9 and 5.8 cm^3 respectively. The surface areas for the dura mater, spinal cord and NR were 318.5, 112.2 and 232.1 cm^2 respectively. The average cross-sectional areas of the dura mater, spinal cord and NR were 2.03, 0.33 and 0.10 cm^2 respectively. The length of the spinal cord down to the conus and spinal dura mater were ~44.8 cm and 60.4 cm respectively. Note, geometric parameters for the spinal cord were computed based on the spinal cord with the coccygeal nerve included as one continuous structure.

3D model files

Both quadrilateral and triangulated meshes for NR, spinal cord, and dura are provided (six files in total) with Creative Commons Attribution-ShareAlike 4.0 International (CC BY-SA 4.0) license (Additional file 1, note: file units are in millimeters). The number of polygons in the quadrilateral meshes of the NR, spinal cord and dura wall was 61,749, 35,905 and 27,281 respectively for a total of 124,935 quadrangles. The number of polygons in the triangulated meshes of the NR, spinal cord, and dura were 199,372, 71,870 and 54,613 respectively for a total of 325,855 triangles. In addition, to allow reduced order modeling of intrathecal CSF flow [32], a 1D graph of model x, y, z-coordinates for the dura and spinal cord centroids are provided in a Additional file 1. This file also contains the corresponding numeric values for all

Table 1 Anatomic measurements obtained from the final 3D spine model

		Dorsal rootlet measurements (average of left and right)				Ventral rootlet measurements (average of left and right)			
Nerve root #	Z position (mm from FM)	Descending angle (°)	Radicular line (mm)	Diameter (mm)	Number of rootlets	Descending angle (°)	Radicular line (mm)	Diameter (mm)	Number of rootlets
C1	6.1	6.8	10.1	0.7	4	− 7.8	8.3	0.7	3
C2	19.8	19.4	10.6	0.7	4	− 8.5	11.1	0.7	4
C3	38.9	45.2	15.5	0.7	6	28.3	13.7	0.7	5
C4	55.3	42.9	17.1	0.8	5	37.0	13.3	0.8	5
C5	71.1	47.5	13.9	0.8	5	37.3	10.7	0.8	5
C6	87.3	51.9	12.6	0.9	4	39.5	12.8	0.9	4
C7	105.4	54.8	11.5	1.0	4	59.6	4.9	1.0	4
C8	118.3	68.9	7.4	0.9	2	58.6	5.2	0.9	2
T1	132.3	70.2	6.1	1.1	3	64.3	7.5	1.1	3
T2	148.7	72.3	7.2	1.1	2	69.9	6.0	1.1	2
T3	169.2	70.4	7.1	1.1	2	68.6	7.2	1.1	2
T4	187.8	69.2	8.0	1.1	2	65.8	6.1	1.1	2
T5	209.9	73.5	10.5	1.1	2	73.1	9.7	1.1	2
T6	230.5	76.8	8.1	1.1	2	76.2	6.4	1.1	2
T7	258.0	78.7	8.2	1.1	2	78.7	8.5	1.1	2
T8	277.2	79.8	8.0	1.1	2	79.8	10.5	1.1	2
T9	307.5	79.7	8.3	1.1	2	79.7	6.1	1.1	2
T10	333.3	77.7	8.5	1.1	2	77.7	8.3	1.1	2
T11	366.2	77.4	8.5	1.1	2	77.4	6.5	1.1	2
T12	401.6	74.8	10.6	1.1	1	74.8	6.9	1.1	1
L1	436.3	82.7	1.1	1.1	1	82.6	1.1	1.1	1
L2	474.9	84.7	1.1	1.1	1	85.1	1.1	1.1	1
L3	510.7	87.1	1.5	1.5	1	88.0	1.5	1.5	1
L4	543.9	87.0	1.3	1.3	1	87.6	1.3	1.3	1
L5	570.6	87.3	1.2	1.2	1	86.9	1.2	1.2	1
S1	585.5	86.9	1.0	1.0	1	87.0	1.0	1.0	1
S2	595.3	86.6	0.5	0.5	1	87.5	0.5	0.5	1
S3	599.4	86.6	0.5	0.5	1	87.0	0.5	0.5	1
S4	602.0	86.8	0.5	0.5	1	87.3	0.5	0.5	1
S5	602.6	87.3	0.5	0.5	1	87.5	0.5	0.5	1

geometric and hydrodynamic parameters at 1 mm intervals along the spine.

CSF flow

Peak-to-peak CSF flow amplitude measured at the C2–C3, C7–C8 and T10–T11 was 4.75, 3.05 and 1.26 cm^3/s respectively (Fig. 6a). These were measured at an axial position relative to the model end (foramen magnum) of 4.0, 12.5, and 35.4 cm respectively. Based on the interpolated CSF flow waveform between MRI measurement locations, the maximum peak and mean CSF velocities were present at 38 mm (~ C4–C5, Fig. 7f). Minimum value of peak and mean CSF velocities occurred in the lower lumbar spine and within the thoracic spine from 390 to 410 mm (~ T7–T10, Fig. 7f).

Cerebrospinal fluid flow oscillation had a decreasing magnitude and considerable variation in waveform shape along the spine (Fig. 6a). Spatial temporal distribution of CSF flow rate along the SSS showed that maximum CSF flow rate occurred caudal to C3–C4 at ~ 40 mm (Fig. 6b). CSF pulse wave velocity (PWV) was estimated to be 19.4 cm/s (Fig. 6b).

Hydrodynamic parameters

Average Reynolds and Womersley number was 68.5 and 9.6 respectively. Womersley number ranged from 1.6 to 22.96 (Table 2, Fig. 7d). Maximum Womersley number was present near the foramen magnum ($\alpha = 22.96$). Womersley number had local minima within the cervical spine and just rostral to the intrathecal sac.

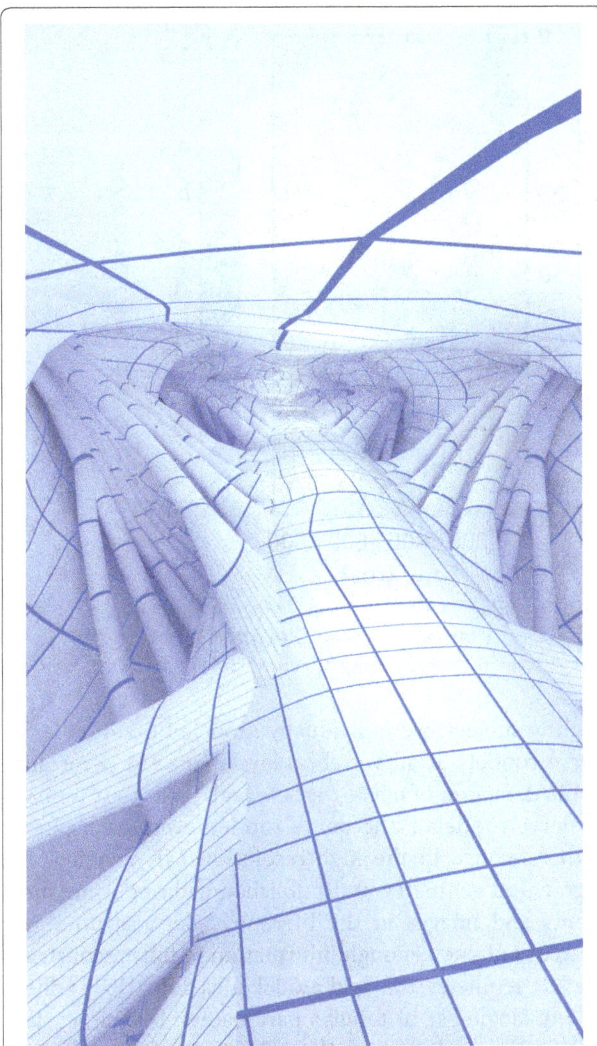

Fig. 5 Visualization of the final quadrilateral surface mesh showing internal view of the spinal cord NR in the cervical spine with view in the caudal direction

Maximum Reynolds number was 174.9 and located at C3–C4.

Discussion

The intrathecal CSF space is a complex 3D fluid-filled geometry with multiple levels of anatomic complexity, the most salient features being the spinal cord, dura mater and dorsal and ventral spinal cord NR. An accurate anthropomorphic representation of these features is needed as a tool for development of in vitro and numerical models of CSF dynamics that can be used to inform and optimize CSF-based therapeutics. In this paper, we provide a detailed and downloadable anthropomorphic 3D model (Additional file 1) of the intrathecal CSF space that is licensed for re-use under the Creative Commons Attribution-ShareAlike 4.0 International license (CC BY-SA 4.0). CSF flow data, measured by PCMRI, is provided as a validation data set for numerical modeling. The model is characterized in terms of axial distribution of intrathecal CSF dynamics with detailed information on various hydrodynamic parameters including Reynolds number, Womersley number, hydraulic diameter and CSF velocities. Herein, we discuss the model in terms of its segmentation, remeshing, key modeling considerations and comparison to previous anatomic and modeling studies and in vivo CSF dynamics measurements.

Segmentation of the intrathecal CSF space

A variety of software exists to help reconstruct MRI DICOM image files in 3D. Many segmentation software platforms provide automatic segmentation algorithms that can deliver relatively quick visualizations but these segmentations are often not suitable to create 3D models that can be used for CFD modeling or easily exported for 3D printing [33]. In this study, we used the open-source program ITK-SNAP ("The Insight Segmentation and Registration Toolkit", http://www.itk.org) that supports automatic, semi-automatic and manual approaches. The final model was constructed based on manual segmentation of each slice along the spine by an expert operator previously trained in intrathecal CSF segmentation procedures.

Despite the popularity of CFD studies conducted in the SSS, there is a lack of detailed information on intrathecal segmentation methods based on anatomic MR imaging. The craniocervical junction is highly vascularized with relatively large blood vessels that transverse the region, including the vertebral arteries (3.7 mm diameter for the left vertebral artery and 3.4 mm diameter for the right vertebral artery [34]) and the anterior spinal artery (0.3–1.3 mm diameter [35]). Spinal cord NR can sometimes be seen as dark regions crossing the SSS (Fig. 1d–f). Their length and obliqueness increases progressively moving towards the feet [36]. Denticulate ligaments are located between adjacent sets of NR in the cervical and thoracic spinal cord segments. These structures are too small to be quantified by MRI (thickness of ~ 0.1 mm) but may also appear as slightly darkened regions of SSS on each side of the spinal cord. The CSF on the anterior or posterior side of the spinal cord near the foramen magnum may appear dark in coloration due to flow void artifacts resulting from elevated CSF velocities at this region (and others along the SSS, Fig. 1). Although these regions can appear relatively dark on MR imaging, they should be considered as fluid.

Along the entire spine, the epidural space can appear hyper intense due to the presence of epidural fat (Fig. 1e–f). Care should be taken to not confuse these areas with

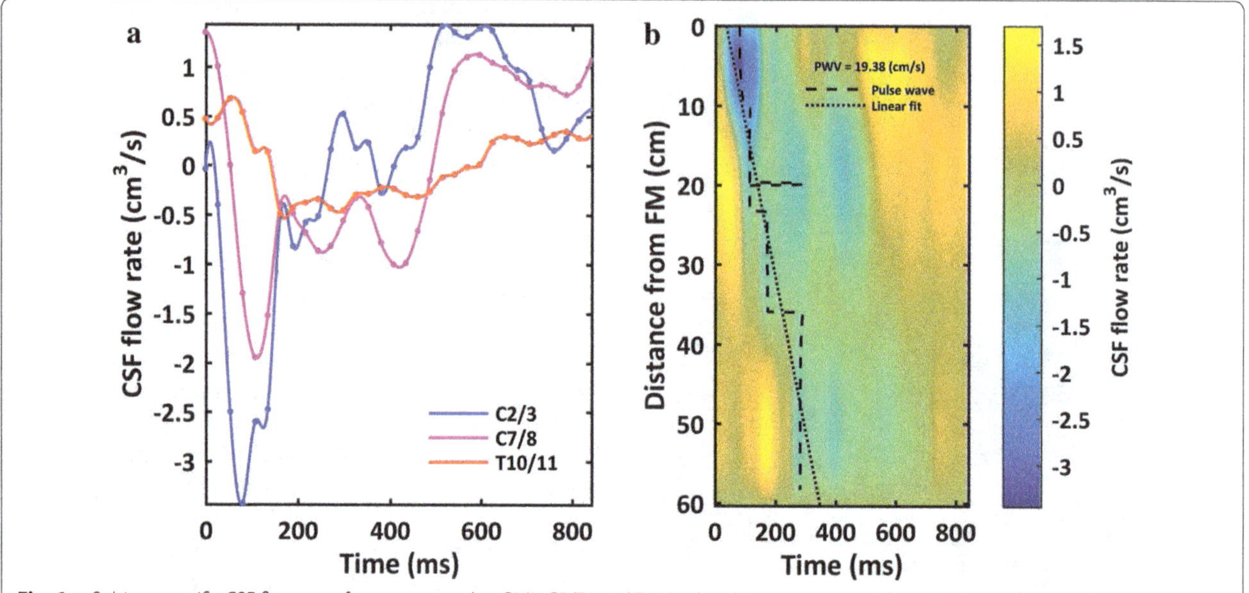

Fig. 6 **a** Subject-specific CSF flow waveforms measured at C2/3, C7/T1 and T10/11 by phase contrast MRI. **b** Subject-specific quantification of CSF pulse wave velocity (PWV) along the spine estimated to be ~ 19.4 cm/s based on a linear fit (dotted line) of peak flow rate arrival times (dashed line)

CSF as it can be difficult to visualize the relatively thin dura mater that separates the two spaces. This ambiguity often confounds automatic segmentation tools and thresholding should be reviewed in detail to ensure accuracy. From our experience, no presently available automated algorithm can avoid over-segmentation of epidural fat, as there can be virtually no border visible between these two regions at many locations along the spine due to MR image resolution limits that do not allow visualization of the relatively thin dura.

The cauda equina begins around the conus medullaris that is located near the lower border of the first lumbar vertebra. This structure is formed by the long rootlets of the lumbar, sacral and coccygeal nerves that run vertically downward to their exit. Similar to the spinal cord NR, ligaments and blood vessels, these small bundles of nerves are not possible to accurately quantify with the current MR image resolution through segmentation alone. In the presented model, they are modeled as curving cylinders as described in our methods with reference to cadaveric studies in the literature and visual interpretation and measurement of NR insertion at the spinal cord and dura.

Modeling considerations with small anatomy

Although the spinal cord and dura mater were easily visible, smaller structures such as NR were not clearly discernible in the MRI scans used in this study. In our previous study [36], we grossly modeled spinal cord NR as single airfoil shaped structures within the cervical spine only. For the present complete spine model for a healthy subject, we individually modeled the number of nerve rootlets at all vertebral levels (see Fig. 4 for anatomic depiction of nerve rootlets and Table 1 for number of nerve rootlets). The nerve rootlets were each placed with reference to the high-resolution MR imaging, 3D segmented geometry and published cadaveric measurements and images in the literature. Because no single source contained enough information to fully reconstruct the NR geometry, the final model does not strictly adhere to any single set of tabular parameters, but rather, is a best judgment based on the collective information (see Table 1 for parameters). Furthermore, due to limitations in the data as well as the time intensive nature of the modeling process, NR were mirrored left to right along the spinal cord. The duplicate side was subjected to < 3.0 mm translation as necessary to best fit rootlets to the spinal and dural geometry. NR vertical positioning is only referenced by the corresponding vertebral level in the literature. Therefore, vertical positioning was based solely on segmentation data marking SSS entry and exits locations. The resulting model is subject-specific in terms of NR location and orientation, but idealized in terms of the exact structure (Fig. 4).

Volumetric differences in geometry

A large portion of this work is centered on the quadrilateral remeshing of the spinal and dural surfaces. In this case, introducing volumetric error was a primary concern during this process. This was largely compensated by selectively increasing mesh resolution in areas with higher degree of curvature while reducing resolution in

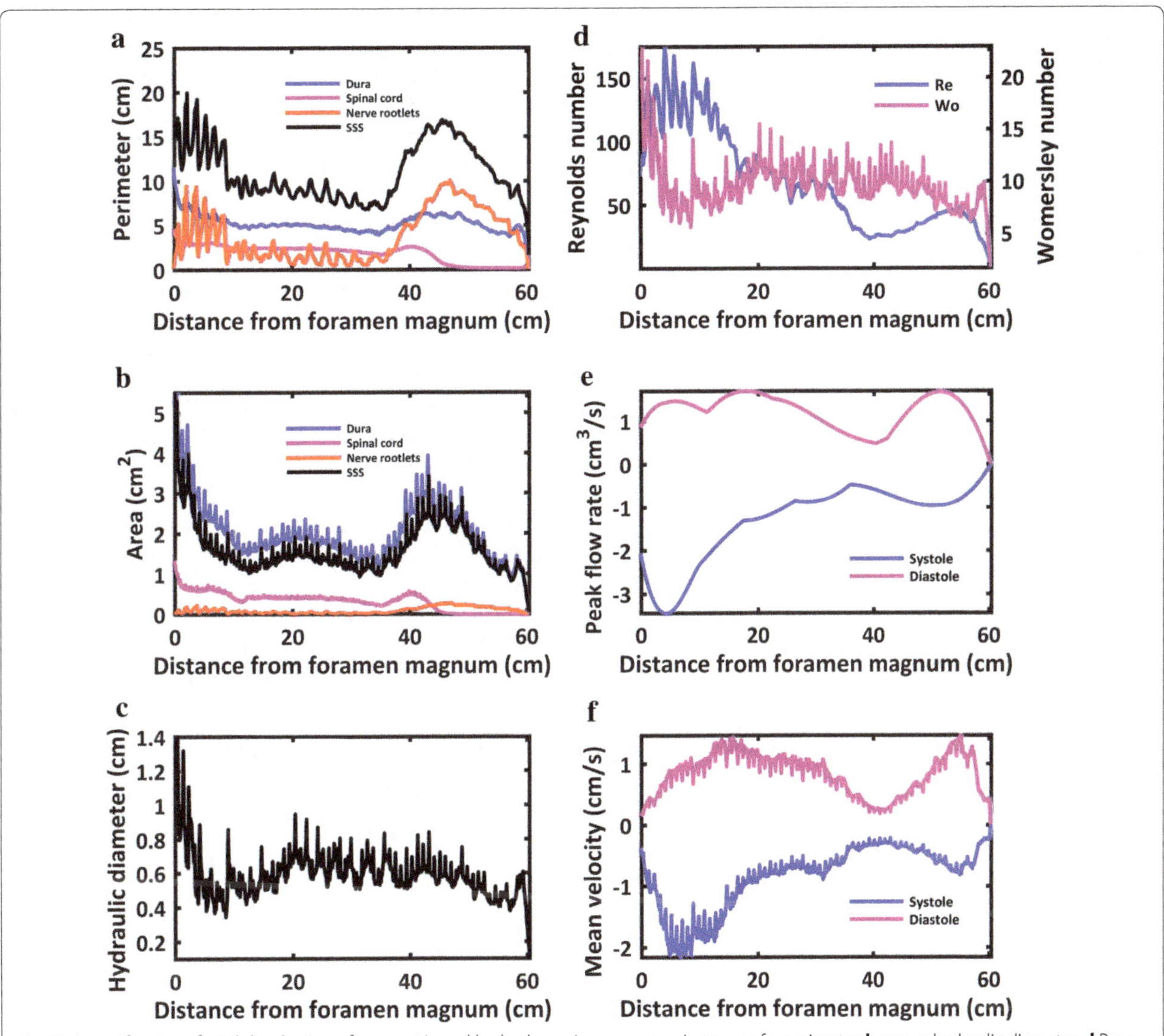

Fig. 7 Quantification of axial distribution of geometric and hydrodynamic parameters in terms of **a** perimeter, **b** area, **c** hydraulic diameter, **d** Reynolds and Womersley number, **e** peak flow rate in the caudal direction (systole) and rostral direction (diastole), **f** mean velocity of CSF flow at peak systole and diastole

locations with little curvature. However, discrepancies still occurred and it was necessary to further modify the entire surface fit as described in the "Methods". Excluding the NR, which were not originally segmented, the final difference between segmented and remeshed SSS volumes is 2.7% (Fig. 3). Our previous study showed inter-operator volumetric error for SSS CSF segmentation to be < 2.7% [24], a value comparable to the percent difference in the remeshed volume for the present study. In an in vitro cervical SSS model, segmentation inaccuracy was quantified to be 15% larger than the original geometry STL file used to create the model [37]. In combination, these findings indicate a high-degree of segmentation and remeshing reliability, but do not rule out the possibility for significant degree of segmentation inaccuracy. Unfortunately, the true SSS geometry is not known and therefore not possible to validate for accuracy.

Comparison of model CSF volume to measurements in the literature

While the provided model is subject-specific, it can be compared to other MRI-based studies to help understand its similarity to the general population. Overall, the provided model had a SSS volume of 97.34 cm^3 and showed a strong similarity with the previous studies cited that, on average, reported SSS volume to be 90.3 cm^3 [38–45]. Table 3 gives a review of studies that used MRI to quantify the volume of anatomical features within the

Table 2 Summary of geometric and hydrodynamic parameters obtained from the final 3D spine model

Parameter	Average ± std.	Maximum	Minimum
Perimeter SC[a] (cm)	1.85 ± 1.00	4.62	0.14
Perimeter DM (cm)	5.26 ± 1.01	11.59	1.25
Perimeter NR (cm)	3.84 ± 2.81	10.08	0.00
Perimeter SSS (cm)	10.96 ± 3.12	19.91	1.6
Area SC[a] (cm^2)	0.33 ± 0.23	1.34	0.00
Area DM (cm^2)	2.03 ± 0.79	6.95	0.04
Area NR (cm^2)	0.10 ± 0.08	0.28	0.00
Area SSS (cm^2)	1.61 ± 0.65	5.62	0.04
Hydraulic diameter HD (cm)	0.59 ± 0.14	1.40	0.10
Re	68.46 ± 39.00	174.9	0.00
α	9.59 ± 2.27	22.96	1.64
U_{sys} (cm/s)	− 0.83 ± 0.51	N/A	− 2.16
U_{dia} (cm/s)	0.83 ± 0.34	1.47	N/A
Q_{sys} (cm^3/s)	− 1.29 ± 0.87	N/A	− 3.44
Q_{dia} (cm^3/s)	1.22 ± 0.39	1.69	N/A
PWV (cm/s)	19.4	N/A	N/A

[a] Average, maximum and minimum values are based 1 mm slice intervals along the entire spine including the coccygeal nerve

full spine and lumbosacral spine for healthy subjects. In collection, these published studies indicate a decreasing trend in CSF volume with age given by: $SSS_{volume(ml)} = (- 0.27 \times age) + 102$ (Fig. 8). The provided model had a volume that was on the higher end of the average reported values, however it was also for a relatively young 23-year-old subject (Table 3). It should be noted that the model was based on high-resolution 0.5 mm isotropic MR images, whereas all cited studies were based on MR images with considerably lower resolution. In addition, many of these studies used axial images with ~ 8 mm slice spacing and a relatively large slice thickness.

The provided subject-specific 3D model was based on a combination of subject-specific MR imaging (Fig. 1) and cadaveric measurements by Bozkurt et al. [25], Zhou et al. [26], Hauck et al. [27] and Lang et al. [28]. The cadaveric studies used to define the NR specifications were selected based on their completeness of information that included spinal cord NR descending angle, radicular line and diameter. As expected, a local enlargement of the spinal cord cross-sectional area was present near the lumbosacral (L2–S2) and cervical (C5–T1) enlargements located near 13 and 40 cm respectively below the

Table 3 Review of studies that include volumetric quantification of anatomic regions within the spine using MR imaging

Source	Region	SC (cm^3)	NR (cm^3)	SSS (cm^3)	N	Mean age	Segmentation method	Subject type
Current study (Sass et al. (2017))	Full spine	19.9	5.8	97.3	1	23	Manual	Healthy
Hogan et al. [38]	Full spine	–	–	107[a]	2	35	Manual	Healthy
Edsbagge et al. [39]	Full spine	20	–	81 ± 13	22	70	Semi-automated	Healthy elderly
Bagci et al. [43]	Full spine	–	–	86	1	–	Automated	Idiopathic intracranial hypertension
Hsu et al. [40]	Full spine	–	–	122	1	29	Manual	Healthy
Lebret et al. [44]	Full spine	–	–	99 ± 27	6	70.2	Automated	Non-communicating hydrocephalus
Lebret et al. [44]	Full spine			80 ± 28	12	54.5[b]	Automated	Healthy
Lebret et al. [44]	Full spine	–	–	65 ± 18	20	43.8[b]	Automated	Communicating hydrocephalus
Alperin et al. [41]	Full spine	21.0	–	78 ± 8	8	29	Automated	Obese women only
Levi Chazen et al. [42]	Full spine	–	–	84 ± 15	15	39	Automated	Healthy
Current study (Sass et al. (2017))	Lumbosacral	3.8	4.0	51.0	1	23	Manual	
Hogan et al. [38]	Lumbosacral	–	7.31	49.9	25	35	Manual	
Carpenter et al. [47]	Lumbosacral	–	–	53.7[a]	41	33	Manual	
Higuchi et al. [48]	Lumbosacral	–	–	41.7[a]	41	30	Manual	
Sullivan et al. [45]	Lumbosacral	–	–	35.8	71	48	Automated	
Edsbagge et al. [39]	Lumbosacral	–	13	25	22	70	Semi-automated	
Martyr et al. [46]	Lumbosacral	–	9.2	31.8	16	72	Automated	
Puigdellivol et al. [49], [87]	Lumbosacral	–	–	34.4	7	37	Semi-automated	
Prats Galino et al. [50]	Lumbosacral	–	10.4	34.3	7	38	Semi-automated	
Hsu et al. [40]	Lumbosacral	–	–	53.0	1	29	Manual	

[a] Indicates studies where NR volume was included in the calculation

[b] Value obtained from personal correspondence with author

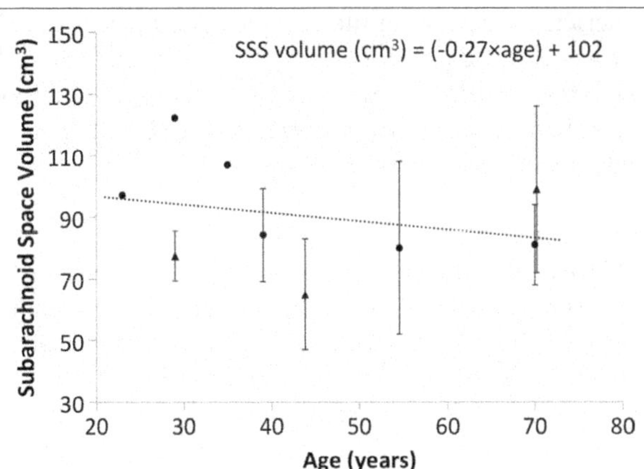

Fig. 8 Summary of spinal subarachnoid space (SSS) volumes computed in published studies in the literature using MR imaging applied for adult-aged subjects (studies in Table 3). A decreasing trend in SSS CSF volume occurs with age (error bars represent standard deviations, triangles indicate studies with patients and circles indicate studies with healthy controls)

foramen magnum (Fig. 7). These locations corresponded to the expected enlargement due to gray matter increase within those regions.

The exact 3D structure of the 31 NR pairs and coccygeal nerve were idealized based on the literature as it was not possible to extract their exact detailed geometry directly from MR imaging. However, it was possible to place each NR pair on a subject-specific basis at the insertion point in the spinal cord and exit point at the dura (details in "Methods"). The resulting model had a total NR volume of 5.8 cm^3. This value is similar to that quantified by Hogan et al. (1996) and Martyr et al. (2011) with 7.31 and 9.2 cm^3 respectively [38, 46]. The relatively smaller volume in our model is likely due to the smaller size of NR between the L2–S2 levels in comparison to Hogan's cadaveric measurements [40]. In addition to the noted wide individual variability, Hogan et al. [38] estimated NR volume assuming estimate root lengths from relatively low resolution MRI data. Other studies quantifying cauda equina volume also based their results solely on estimations from MRI segmentations [39, 45–50].

Total CSF volume in healthy adults

Total CSF volume in healthy adults has been reported to be ~ 150 mL in many standard medical textbooks [42, 51, 52] and recently published review articles [53, 54]. This value has become ubiquitous within the literature to the point of often not being cited with reference to any empirical study. Methods for CSF volume estimation by relatively crude casting techniques were originally applied [55]. These estimates were later criticized as being prone to significant degree of error [56, 57]. Review of more recent literature using non-invasive MRI-based methods indicates that total CSF volume in healthy adults to range from ~ 250 to 400 cm^3 [42, 58–61]. The difference in CSF volume determined from MRI versus invasive techniques is likely an underlying reason for the discrepancy. The referenced CSF volumetric studies using non-invasive techniques with high-resolution MR imaging may provide a more accurate estimate of total CSF volume. However, invasive measurements provide a lower bound for total CSF volume. More research is needed to fully establish detailed information about CSF volumetric distribution throughout the intracranial cisterns and subarachnoid space of the brain and spine.

Comparison of 3D model with previous geometries used for CFD modeling

At present, all models of the spinal SSS rely on varying degrees of simplification or idealization, often neglecting realistic spinal canal geometry and/or microanatomy. The simplest geometries are coaxial circular annuli employed by Lockey et al. [62], Berkouk et al. [63], Hettiarachchi et al. [64] and Elliott [65] that in some cases also included pathological variations, as well as in Bertram et al. [17] which used an idealized axial distribution for SSS area. Stockman [66] used an elliptical annuli and included microanatomical features, whereas Kuttler [67] modeled an elliptical annulus based on work by Loth et al. [29] who created a SSS from realistic SSS cross sections. The axial distribution of our model spinal cord and dura shows strong similarity to Loth et al. [29], Fig. 3, with a peak SSS area located at the FM and dural sac lumbar enlargement (Fig. 7b). Hsu et al. [40], Pahlavian et al. [36] and Tangen et al. [10, 12] developed CFD models with a subject specific geometry of the SSS reconstructed from MR data. The Pahlavian and Tangen CFD models also included varying degrees of NR detail. Pahlavian idealized NR as smooth airfoil-shaped flat objects and limited the model to the cervical spine. Yiallourou et al. [68] conducted a CFD study to investigate alterations in craniocervical CSF hydrodynamics in healthy controls versus patients with Chiari malformation. In that study, NR were not included in the CFD geometry. The CFD-based velocity profile results were found to lack similarity with in vivo 4D Flow MRI measurements. It was concluded that NR or other relatively small anatomic features are likely needed to accurately reflect CSF velocities within the cervical spine.

The geometric model presented in this study contributes NR microanatomy as discreet rootlets and cauda equina within a complete subject-specific SSS geometry. The model geometry is provided in a downloadable format with the dura, spinal cord and NR as separate files in the .STL (triangular) and .OBJ (quadrilateral) formats (six files in total). This allows modification of each surface separately for modeling purposes. For example, the model could be altered locally to increase the thecal sac volume during upright posture.

CSF dynamics quantification

The computed parameters for CSF dynamics in terms peak flow rate, mean velocity and Reynolds number (Fig. 7) compare favorably to previous studies. The measured CSF flow rate waveforms (Fig. 6a) had similar magnitude as previous studies in the literature by Loth et al. [29], Linninger et al. [69] and Greitz [70, 71]. For those studies, average value of the peak CSF velocity at C2 vertebral level was ~ 2.5 cm/s. In the present model, peak CSF velocity at C2 vertebral level was 2.16 cm/s (Fig. 7f, towards feet). CSF pulse wave velocity (PWV), was estimated to be 19.4 cm/s in the healthy subject based on feature points of the CSF flow waveform measured along the entire spine (Fig. 6b). This value is lower than those previously reported in the literature that include 4.6 ± 1.7 m/s by Kalata et al. in the cervical spine [31] and ~ 40 m/s by Greitz in a patient [72]. It is difficult to directly compare these results with the present study, as they varied in technique, measurement location and type of subject.

Peak Reynolds number was predicted to be 175 and located within the cervical spine. This value suggests the presence of laminar CSF flow throughout the intrathecal space. However, it should be noted that that the SSS is a highly complex geometry that also contains microscopic structures called arachnoid trabeculae that were not included in the flow calculations. Previous biofluids studies have shown that geometric complexity can allow flow to become partially turbulent at Re > 600 in a stenosis [73], at Re 200–350 in aneurysms [74, 75], in the heart [76] and within CSF in the SSS [77, 78]. More research is needed to define the nature of CSF flow dynamics with respect to turbulence.

Cerebrospinal fluid flow data was collected at three distinct axial locations along the spine for a single subject. Data from these three locations was spatial-temporally interpolated (Fig. 6b) and used in combination with the geometry to quantify axial distribution of CSF dynamics along the spine (Fig. 7). While only representative of the single subject analyzed, the provided parameters give insight into CSF dynamics for a single healthy subject within a complete SC model containing detailed nerve root geometry. For example, the detailed geometry showed that Reynolds number varies significantly along the spine due to the presence of NR (see Fig. 7d Reynolds number variation in cervical spine). Note: validation of numerical models using the provided downloadable CSF flow waveform data should only take into account CSF flow rates measured at the three distinct axial locations (Fig. 6a). Interpolated values are not empirical data to be used for validation purposes.

Limitations

The provided anthropomorphic model of intrathecal CSF has several important limitations. Our model included the dorsal and ventral spinal cord NR with semi-idealized geometry that was mirrored across the spinal cord for a healthy subject. For a diseased case, such as in patients with syringomyelia or Chiari malformation, it is expected that the exact NR position may be altered. In the case of syringomyelia, the SSS has been found to narrow near the syrinx [79] and would likely result in local displacement of NR towards the dura. The present model may not be relevant for representing such a diseased case.

We sought to render the NR structures as near as possible to reality based on a combination of referencing the in vivo MR imaging and cadaveric measurements in the literature. However, the resulting model cannot be considered truly subject-specific, as the exact locations and geometry of each NR was not possible to directly visualize. Higher resolution MRI would be required to construct such a model. In addition, several additional anatomic features are missing in the model including: denticulate ligaments and tiny blood vessels that transverse the intrathecal CSF spaces. Additional work could be made to add these features to the model in an idealized way.

The provided model only includes CSF within the intrathecal space. This was due to MRI scanning time limitations. The protocol used in the present study required 45 min of scanning time to obtain the necessary high-resolution complete spine imaging. Future studies should quantify the entire CSF space geometry in detail to allow modeling of Chiari malformation and other intracranial central nervous system diseases.

Cerebrospinal fluid flow data used for calculation of CSF dynamics along the spine was measured at three axial positions along the spine. An improved method would include measurement of CSF flow at more axial levels and with higher temporal resolution. The exact reproducibility of these CSF flow waveforms could be tested by conducting a reliability study on the same subject. In this study, cardiac-related CSF flow was quantified using retrospective gated PCMRI measurements. Therefore, Fig. 7 results indicate CSF hydrodynamics under cardiac-related CSF oscillations. Impact of the respiratory cycle on CSF flow dynamics could be quantified using real-time PCMRI [80–83].

Conclusions

This study provides an anatomically realistic anthropomorphic 3D model of the complete intrathecal space based on high-resolution MR imaging of a healthy human adult female. The axial distribution of CSF dynamics within the model are quantified in terms of key hydrodynamic and geometric variables and likely indicate laminar CSF flow throughout the SSS. The model (Additional file 1) is provided for re-use under the Creative Commons Attribution-ShareAlike 4.0 International license (CC BY-SA 4.0) and can be used as a tool for development of in vitro and numerical models of CSF dynamics for design and optimization of intrathecal drug delivery, CSF filtration, CSF hypothermia and central nervous system diseases of the SC such as syringomyelia and spinal arachnoiditis.

Abbreviations

3D: three-dimensional; ASA: anterior spinal artery; CFD: computational fluid dynamics; CSF: cerebrospinal fluid; DM: dura mater; DA: descending angle; ES: epidural space; FIESTA: fast imaging employing steady-state acquisition; FM: foramen magnum; FOV: field of view; LV: left vertebral artery; MR: magnetic resonance; MRI: magnetic resonance imaging; NR: nerve rootlets; PWV: pulse wave velocity; RL: radicular line; RV: right vertebral artery; SC: spinal cord; SSS: spinal subarachnoid space; TE: echo time; TR: repetition time.

Authors' contributions

Study conception and design: BAM. Acquisition of data: OB, RST, GCN, LRS, MK. Analysis and interpretation of data: BAM, LRS, RST, OB, MK, GCN. Drafting of manuscript: BAM, LRS. Critical revision: BAM, LRS, RST, OB, MK, GCN. All authors read and approved the final manuscript.

Author details

[1] Neurophysiological Imaging and Modeling Laboratory, University of Idaho, 875 Perimeter Dr. MC1122, Moscow, ID 83844-1122, USA. [2] Bioflow Image, Service de Biophysique et de Traitement de l'Image médicale, Bâtiment des écoles, CHU Nord Amiens-Picardie, Place Victor Pauchet, 80054 Amiens Cedex 1, France. [3] Seattle Science Foundation, 200 2nd Ave N, Seattle, WA 98109, USA. [4] Department of Biological Engineering, University of Idaho, 875 Perimeter Dr. MC0904, Moscow, ID 83844-0904, USA.

Competing interests

BAM has received research funding from Alcyone Lifesciences Inc., Minnetronix Inc. and Voyager Therapeutics.

Funding

This work was supported by an Intuitional Development Award (IDeA) from the National Institute of General Medical Sciences (NIGMS) of the National Institutes of health (NIH) under Grant #P20GM1033408 and #4U54GM104944-04TBD, The National Institutes of Mental Health Grant #1R44MH112210-01A1, and University of Idaho Vandal Ideas Project.

References

1. Bunck AC, Kroeger JR, Juettner A, Brentrup A, Fiedler B, Crelier GR, Martin BA, Heindel W, Maintz D, Schwindt W, Niederstadt T. Magnetic resonance 4D flow analysis of cerebrospinal fluid dynamics in Chiari I malformation with and without syringomyelia. Eur Radiol. 2012;22:1860–70.
2. Bradley WG Jr, Scalzo D, Queralt J, Nitz WN, Atkinson DJ, Wong P. Normal-pressure hydrocephalus: evaluation with cerebrospinal fluid flow measurements at MR imaging. Radiology. 1996;198:523–9.
3. Woodworth GF, McGirt MJ, Williams MA, Rigamonti D. Cerebrospinal fluid drainage and dynamics in the diagnosis of normal pressure hydrocephalus. Neurosurgery. 2009;64:919–25 **(discussion 925–916)**.
4. Sklar FH, Beyer CW Jr, Ramanathan M, Cooper PR, Clark WK. Cerebrospinal fluid dynamics in patients with pseudotumor cerebri. Neurosurgery. 1979;5:208–16.
5. Papisov MI, Belov VV, Gannon KS. Physiology of the intrathecal bolus: the leptomeningeal route for macromolecule and particle delivery to CNS. Mol Pharm. 2013;10:1522–32.
6. Abhi V, Minnetronix I. Devices and systems for access and navigation of cerebrospinal fluid space. 2016. Patent US20160051801 A1. https://www.google.com/patents/US20160051801
7. Finsterer J, Mamoli B. Cerebrospinal fluid filtration in amyotrophic lateral sclerosis. Eur J Neurol. 1999;6:597–600.
8. Meylaerts SA, Kalkman CJ, de Haan P, Porsius M, Jacobs MJ. Epidural versus subdural spinal cord cooling: cerebrospinal fluid temperature and pressure changes. Ann Thorac Surg. 2000;70:222–7 **(discussion 228)**.
9. Siyahhan B, Knobloch V, de Zelicourt D, Asgari M, Schmid Daners M, Poulikakos D, Kurtcuoglu V. Flow induced by ependymal cilia dominates near-wall cerebrospinal fluid dynamics in the lateral ventricles. J R Soc Interface. 2014;11:20131189.
10. Tangen KM, Hsu Y, Zhu DC, Linninger AA. CNS wide simulation of flow resistance and drug transport due to spinal microanatomy. J Biomech. 2015;48:2144–54.
11. Stockman HW. Effect of anatomical fine structure on the flow of cerebrospinal fluid in the spinal subarachnoid space. J Biomech Eng. 2006;128:106–14.
12. Tangen K, Narasimhan NS, Sierzega K, Preden T, Alaraj A, Linninger AA. Clearance of subarachnoid hemorrhage from the cerebrospinal fluid in computational and in vitro models. Ann Biomed Eng. 2016;44:3478–94.
13. Clarke EC, Fletcher DF, Stoodley MA, Bilston LE. Computational fluid dynamics modelling of cerebrospinal fluid pressure in Chiari malformation and syringomyelia. J Biomech. 2013;46:1801–9.
14. Martin BA, Kalata W, Shaffer N, Fischer P, Luciano M, Loth F. Hydrodynamic and longitudinal impedance analysis of cerebrospinal fluid dynamics at the craniovertebral junction in type I Chiari malformation. PLoS ONE. 2013;8:e75335.
15. Helgeland A, Mardal KA, Haughton V, Reif BA. Numerical simulations of the pulsating flow of cerebrospinal fluid flow in the cervical spinal canal of a Chiari patient. J Biomech. 2014;47:1082–90.
16. Cheng S, Stoodley MA, Wong J, Hemley S, Fletcher DF, Bilston LE. The presence of arachnoiditis affects the characteristics of CSF flow in the spinal subarachnoid space: a modelling study. J Biomech. 2012;45:1186–91.
17. Bertram CD, Bilston LE, Stoodley MA. Tensile radial stress in the spinal cord related to arachnoiditis or tethering: a numerical model. Med Biol Eng Comput. 2008;46:701–7.
18. Elliott NSJ, Bertram CD, Martin BA, Brodbelt AR. Syringomyelia: a review of the biomechanics. J Fluids Struct. 2013;40:1–24.
19. Baledent O, Henry-Feugeas MC, Idy-Peretti I. Cerebrospinal fluid dynamics and relation with blood flow: a magnetic resonance study with semiautomated cerebrospinal fluid segmentation. Investig Radiol. 2001;36:368–77.
20. Martin BA, Kalata W, Loth F, Royston TJ, Oshinski JN. Syringomyelia hydrodynamics: an in vitro study based on in vivo measurements. J Biomech Eng Trans Asme. 2005;127:1110–20.
21. Khani M, Xing T, Gibbs C, Oshinski JN, Stewart GR, Zeller JR, Martin BA. Nonuniform moving boundary method for computational fluid dynamics simulation of intrathecal cerebrospinal flow distribution in a Cynomolgus Monkey. J Biomech Eng. 2017;139:081005.
22. Yiallourou T, Schmid Daners M, Kurtcuoglu V, Haba-Rubio J, Heinzer R, Fornari E, Santini F, Sheffer DB, Stergiopulos N, Martin BA. Continuous

positive airway pressure alters cranial blood flow and cerebrospinal fluid dynamics at the craniovertebral junction. Interdiscip Neurosurg Adv Tech Case Manag. 2015;2:152–9.
23. Yushkevich PA, Piven J, Hazlett HC, Smith RG, Ho S, Gee JC, Gerig G. User-guided 3D active contour segmentation of anatomical structures: significantly improved efficiency and reliability. Neuroimage. 2006;31:1116–28.
24. Martin BA, Yiallourou TI, Pahlavian SH, Thyagaraj S, Bunck AC, Loth F, Sheffer DB, Kroger JR, Stergiopulos N. Inter-operator reliability of magnetic resonance image-based computational fluid dynamics prediction of cerebrospinal fluid motion in the cervical spine. Ann Biomed Eng. 2016;44:1524–37.
25. Bozkurt M, Canbay S, Neves GF, Akture E, Fidan E, Salamat MS, Baskaya MK. Microsurgical anatomy of the dorsal thoracic rootlets and dorsal root entry zones. Acta Neurochir. 2012;154:1235–9.
26. Zhou MW, Wang WT, Huang HS, Zhu GY, Chen YP, Zhou CM. Microsurgical anatomy of lumbosacral nerve rootlets for highly selective rhizotomy in chronic spinal cord injury. Anat Rec. 2010;293:2123–8.
27. Hauck EF, Wittkowski W, Bothe HW. Intradural microanatomy of the nerve roots S1–S5 at their origin from the conus medullaris. J Neurosurg Spine. 2008;9:207–12.
28. Lang J, Bartram CT. Fila radicularia of the ventral and dorsal radices of the human spinal cord. Gegenbaurs Morphol Jahrb. 1982;128:417–62.
29. Loth F, Yardimci MA, Alperin N. Hydrodynamic modeling of cerebrospinal fluid motion within the spinal cavity. J Biomech Eng. 2001;123:71–9.
30. San O, Staples AE. An improved model for reduced-order physiological fluid flows. J Mech Med Biol. 2012;12:1250052.
31. Kalata W, Martin BA, Oshinski JN, Jerosch-Herold M, Royston TJ, Loth F. MR measurement of cerebrospinal fluid velocity wave speed in the spinal canal. IEEE Trans Biomed Eng. 2009;56:1765–8.
32. Martin BA, Reymond P, Novy J, Baledent O, Stergiopulos N. A coupled hydrodynamic model of the cardiovascular and cerebrospinal fluid system. Am J Physiol Heart Circ Physiol. 2012;302:H1492–509.
33. De Leener B, Taso M, Cohen-Adad J, Callot V. Segmentation of the human spinal cord. MAGMA. 2016;29:125–53.
34. Seidel E, Eicke BM, Tettenborn B, Krummenauer F. Reference values for vertebral artery flow volume by duplex sonography in young and elderly adults. Stroke. 1999;30:2692–6.
35. Biglioli P, Roberto M, Cannata A, Parolari A, Fumero A, Grillo F, Maggioni M, Coggi G, Spirito R. Upper and lower spinal cord blood supply: the continuity of the anterior spinal artery and the relevance of the lumbar arteries. J Thorac Cardiovasc Surg. 2004;127:1188–92.
36. Pahlavian SH, Yiallourou T, Tubbs RS, Bunck AC, Loth F, Goodin M, Raisee M, Martin BA. The impact of spinal cord nerve roots and denticulate ligaments on cerebrospinal fluid dynamics in the cervical spine. PLoS ONE. 2014;9:e91888.
37. Thyagaraj S, Pahlavian SH, Sass LR, Loth F, Vatani M, Choi JW, Tubbs RS, Giese D, Kroger JR, Bunck AC, Martin BA. An MRI-compatible hydrodynamic simulator of cerebrospinal fluid motion in the cervical spine. IEEE Trans Biomed Eng. 2017. 10.1109/TBME.2017.2756995
38. Hogan QH, Prost R, Kulier A, Taylor ML, Liu S, Mark L. Magnetic resonance imaging of cerebrospinal fluid volume and the influence of body habitus and abdominal pressure. Anesthesiology. 1996;84:1341–9.
39. Edsbagge M, Starck G, Zetterberg H, Ziegelitz D, Wikkelso C. Spinal cerebrospinal fluid volume in healthy elderly individuals. Clin Anat. 2011;24:733–40.
40. Hsu Y, Hettiarachchi HD, Zhu DC, Linninger AA. The frequency and magnitude of cerebrospinal fluid pulsations influence intrathecal drug distribution: key factors for interpatient variability. Anesth Analg. 2012;115:386–94.
41. Alperin N, Bagci AM, Lee SH, Lam BL. Automated quantitation of spinal CSF volume and measurement of craniospinal CSF redistribution following lumbar withdrawal in idiopathic intracranial hypertension. AJNR Am J Neuroradiol. 2016;37:1957–63.
42. Levi Chazen J, Dyke JP, Holt RW, Horky L, Pauplis RA, Hesterman JY, David Mozley P, Verma A. Automated segmentation of MR imaging to determine normative central nervous system cerebrospinal fluid volumes in healthy volunteers. Clin Imaging. 2017;43:132–5.
43. Bagci AM, Ranganathan S, Gomez JR, Lam BL, Alperin N. Automated quantitation of CSF volumes in central nervous system by MRI. In: Proceedings of the International Society for Magnetic Resonance in Medicine. 2012.
44. Lebret A, Hodel J, Rahmouni A, Decq P, Petit E. Cerebrospinal fluid volume analysis for hydrocephalus diagnosis and clinical research. Comput Med Imaging Graph. 2013;37:224–33.
45. Sullivan JT, Grouper S, Walker MT, Parrish TB, McCarthy RJ, Wong CA. Lumbosacral cerebrospinal fluid volume in humans using three-dimensional magnetic resonance imaging. Anesth Analg. 2006;103:1306–10.
46. Martyr JW, Song SJ, Hua J, Burrows S. The correlation between cauda equina nerve root volume and sensory block height after spinal anaesthesia with glucose-free bupivacaine. Anaesthesia. 2011;66:590–4.
47. Carpenter RL, Hogan QH, Liu SS, Crane B, Moore J. Lumbosacral cerebrospinal fluid volume is the primary determinant of sensory block extent and duration during spinal anesthesia. Anesthesiology. 1998;89:24–9.
48. Higuchi H, Hirata J, Adachi Y, Kazama T. Influence of lumbosacral cerebrospinal fluid density, velocity, and volume on extent and duration of plain bupivacaine spinal anesthesia. Anesthesiology. 2004;100:106–14.
49. Puigdellivol-Sanchez A, Prats-Galino A, Reina MA, Maches F, Hernandez JM, De Andres J, van Zundert A. Three-dimensional magnetic resonance image of structures enclosed in the spinal canal relevant to anesthetists and estimation of the lumbosacral CSF volume. Acta Anaesthesiol Belg. 2011;62:37–45.
50. Prats-Galino A, Reina MA, Puigdellivol-Sanchez A, Juanes Mendez JA, De Andres JA, Collier CB. Cerebrospinal fluid volume and nerve root vulnerability during lumbar puncture or spinal anaesthesia at different vertebral levels. Anaesth Intensiv Care. 2012;40:643–7.
51. Guyton AC, Hall JE. Textbook of medical physiology. 9th ed. Philadelphia: W.B. Saunders; 1996.
52. Davson H, Segal MB. Physiology of the CSF and blood-brain barriers. Boca Raton: CRC Press; 1996.
53. Johanson CE, Duncan JA 3rd, Klinge PM, Brinker T, Stopa EG, Silverberg GD. Multiplicity of cerebrospinal fluid functions: new challenges in health and disease. Cerebrospinal Fluid Res. 2008;5:10.
54. Sakka L, Coll G, Chazal J. Anatomy and physiology of cerebrospinal fluid. Eur Ann Otorhinolaryngol Head Neck Dis. 2011;128:309–16.
55. Last RJ, Tompsett DH. Casts of the cerebral ventricles. Br J Surg. 1953;40:525–43.
56. Wyper DJ, Pickard JD, Matheson M. Accuracy of ventricular volume estimation. J Neurol Neurosurg Psychiatry. 1979;42:345–50.
57. Grant R, Condon B, Lawrence A, Hadley DM, Patterson J, Bone I, Teasdale GM. Human cranial CSF volumes measured by MRI: sex and age influences. Magn Reson Imaging. 1987;5:465–8.
58. Hodel J, Lebret A, Petit E, Leclerc X, Zins M, Vignaud A, Decq P, Rahmouni A. Imaging of the entire cerebrospinal fluid volume with a multistation 3D SPACE MR sequence: feasibility study in patients with hydrocephalus. Eur Radiol. 2013;23:1450–8.
59. Courchesne E, Chisum HJ, Townsend J, Cowles A, Covington J, Egaas B, Harwood M, Hinds S, Press GA. Normal brain development and aging: quantitative analysis at in vivo MR imaging in healthy volunteers. Radiology. 2000;216:672–82.
60. Coffey CE, Lucke JF, Saxton JA, Ratcliff G, Unitas LJ, Billig B, Bryan RN. Sex differences in brain aging: a quantitative magnetic resonance imaging study (vol 55, pg 169, 1998). Arch Neurol. 1998;55:627.
61. Pfefferbaum A, Mathalon DH, Sullivan EV, Rawles JM, Zipursky RB, Lim KO. A quantitative magnetic resonance imaging study of changes in brain morphology from infancy to late adulthood. Arch Neurol. 1994;51:874–87.
62. Lockey P, Poots G, Williams B. Theoretical aspects of the attenuation of pressure pulses within cerebrospinal-fluid pathways. Med Biol Eng. 1975;13:861–9.
63. Berkouk K, Carpenter PW, Lucey AD. Pressure wave propagation in fluid-filled co-axial elastic tubes. Part 1: basic theory. J Biomech Eng. 2003;125:852–6.
64. Hettiarachchi HD, Hsu Y, Harris TJ Jr, Penn R, Linninger AA. The effect of pulsatile flow on intrathecal drug delivery in the spinal canal. Ann Biomed Eng. 2011;39:2592–602.
65. Elliott NS. Syrinx fluid transport: modeling pressure-wave-induced flux across the spinal pial membrane. J Biomech Eng. 2012;134:031006.
66. Stockman HW. Effect of anatomical fine structure on the dispersion of solutes in the spinal subarachnoid space. J Biomech Eng. 2007;129:666–75.

67. Kuttler A, Dimke T, Kern S, Helmlinger G, Stanski D, Finelli LA. Understanding pharmacokinetics using realistic computational models of fluid dynamics: biosimulation of drug distribution within the CSF space for intrathecal drugs. J Pharmacokinet Pharmacodyn. 2010;37:629–44.
68. Yiallourou TI, Kroger JR, Stergiopulos N, Maintz D, Martin BA, Bunck AC. Comparison of 4D phase-contrast MRI flow measurements to computational fluid dynamics simulations of cerebrospinal fluid motion in the cervical spine. PLoS ONE. 2012;7:e52284.
69. Linninger AA, Tsakiris C, Zhu DC, Xenos M, Roycewicz P, Danziger Z, Penn R. Pulsatile cerebrospinal fluid dynamics in the human brain. IEEE Trans Biomed Eng. 2005;52:557–65.
70. Greitz D. Cerebrospinal fluid circulation and associated intracranial dynamics. A radiologic investigation using MR imaging and radionuclide cisternography. Acta Radiol Suppl. 1993;386:1–23.
71. Greitz D, Franck A, Nordell B. On the pulsatile nature of intracranial and spinal CSF-circulation demonstrated by MR imaging. Acta Radiol. 1993;34:321–8.
72. Greitz D, Ericson K, Flodmark O. Pathogenesis and mechanics of spinal cord cysts—a new hypothesis based on magnetic resonance studies of cerebrospinal fluid dynamics. Int J Neuroradiol. 1999;5:61–78.
73. Ahmed SA, Giddens DP. Pulsatile poststenotic flow studies with laser Doppler anemometry. J Biomech. 1984;17:695–705.
74. Valen-Sendstad K, Steinman DA. Mind the gap: impact of computational fluid dynamics solution strategy on prediction of intracranial aneurysm hemodynamics and rupture status indicators. AJNR Am J Neuroradiol. 2014;35:536–43.
75. Valen-Sendstad K, Mardal KA, Mortensen M, Reif BAP, Langtangen HP. Direct numerical simulation of transitional flow in a patient-specific intracranial aneurysm. J Biomech. 2011;44:2826–32.
76. Tagliabue A, Dede L, Quarteroni A. Complex blood flow patterns in an idealized left ventricle: a numerical study. Chaos. 2017;27:093939.
77. Jain K, Universität Siegen. universi-Universitätsverlag Siegen. Transition to turbulence in physiological flows: direct numerical simulation of hemodynamics in intracranial aneurysms and cerebrospinal fluid hydrodynamics in the spinal canal. 1st ed. Siegen: universi-Universitätsverlag Siegen; 2016.
78. Jain K, Ringstad G, Eide PK, Mardal KA. Direct numerical simulation of transitional hydrodynamics of the cerebrospinal fluid in Chiari I malformation: the role of cranio-vertebral junction. Int J Numer Method Biomed Eng. 2017;33.
79. Thompson A, Madan N, Hesselink JR, Weinstein G, del Rio AM, Haughton V. The cervical spinal canal tapers differently in patients with Chiari I with and without syringomyelia. AJNR Am J Neuroradiol. 2016;37:755–8.
80. Chen L, Beckett A, Verma A, Feinberg DA. Dynamics of respiratory and cardiac CSF motion revealed with real-time simultaneous multi-slice EPI velocity phase contrast imaging. Neuroimage. 2015;122:281–7.
81. Takizawa K, Matsumae M, Sunohara S, Yatsushiro S, Kuroda K. Characterization of cardiac- and respiratory-driven cerebrospinal fluid motion based on asynchronous phase-contrast magnetic resonance imaging in volunteers. Fluids Barriers CNS. 2017;14:25.
82. Yatsushiro S, Sunohara S, Takizawa K, Matsumae M, Kajihara N, Kuroda K. Characterization of cardiac- and respiratory-driven cerebrospinal fluid motions using correlation mapping with asynchronous 2-dimensional phase contrast technique. In: Engineering in Medicine and Biology Society (EMBC), 2016 IEEE 38th Annual International Conference. 2016. p. 3867–70.
83. Yildiz S, Thyagaraj S, Jin N, Zhong X, Heidari Pahlavian S, Martin BA, Loth F, Oshinski J, Sabra KG. Quantifying the influence of respiration and cardiac pulsations on cerebrospinal fluid dynamics using real-time phase-contrast MRI. J Magn Reson Imaging. 2017;46:431–9.
84. Penrod KE. A stereoscopic atlas of human anatomy-Bassett DL. J Med Educ. 1959;34:75.
85. File:Slide5rer.JPG-Wikimedia Commons. https://commons.wikimedia.org/wiki/File:Slide5rer.JPG.
86. Filum terminale-Wikipedia. 2017. https://en.m.wikipedia.org/wiki/Filum_terminale. Accessed 1 June 2017.
87. Puigdellivol-Sanchez A, Reina MA, San-Molina J, Escobar JM, Castedo J, Prats-Galino A. Threshold selection criteria for quantification of lumbosacral cerebrospinal fluid and root volumes from MRI. J Neuroimaging. 2015;25:488–93.

10

A change in brain white matter after shunt surgery in idiopathic normal pressure hydrocephalus: a tract-based spatial statistics study

Shigenori Kanno[1,2*], Makoto Saito[2], Tomohito Kashinoura[2], Yoshiyuki Nishio[2], Osamu Iizuka[2], Hirokazu Kikuchi[2], Masahito Takagi[2], Masaki Iwasaki[3], Shoki Takahashi[4] and Etsuro Mori[2]

Abstract

Background: The aim of this study was to elucidate changes in cerebral white matter after shunt surgery in idiopathic normal pressure hydrocephalus (INPH) using diffusion tensor imaging (DTI).

Methods: Twenty-eight consecutive INPH patients whose symptoms were followed for 1 year after shunt placement and 10 healthy control (HC) subjects were enrolled. Twenty of the initial 28 INPH patients were shunt-responsive (SR) and the other 8 patients were non-responsive (SNR). The cerebral white matter integrity was detected by assessing fractional anisotropy (FA) and mean diffusivity (MD). The mean hemispheric DTI indices and the ventricular sizes were calculated, and a map of these DTI indices was created for each subject. The DTI maps were analysed to compare preshunt INPH with HC and preshunt INPH with 1 year after shunt placement in each INPH group, using tract-based spatial statistics. We restricted analyses to the left hemisphere because of shunt valve artefacts.

Results: The ventricles became significantly smaller after shunt placement both in the SR and SNR groups. In addition, there was a significant interaction between clinical improvement after shunt and decrease in ventricular size. Although the hemispheric DTI indices were not significantly changed after shunt placement, there was a significant interaction between clinical improvement and increase in hemispheric MD. Compared with the HC group, FA in the corpus callosum and in the subcortical white matter of the convexity and the occipital cortex was significantly lower in SR at baseline, whereas MD in the periventricular and peri-Sylvian white matter was significantly higher in the SR group. Compared with the pre-operative images, the post-operative FA was only decreased in the corona radiata and only in the SR group. There were no significant regions in which DTI indices were altered after shunt placement in the SNR group.

Conclusions: Brain white matter regions in which FA was decreased after shunt placement were in the corona radiata between the lateral ventricles and the Sylvian fissures. This finding was observed only in shunt-responsive INPH patients and might reflect the plasticity of the brain for mechanical pressure changes from the cerebrospinal fluid system.

Keywords: Idiopathic normal pressure hydrocephalus, Diffusion tensor imaging, White matter, Ventriculoperitoneal shunt, Lumboperitoneal shunt

*Correspondence: s-kanno@med.tohoku.ac.jp
[1] Department of Neurology, Southmiyagi Medical Center, 38-1, Aza-nishi, Shibata, Miyagi 989-1253, Japan
Full list of author information is available at the end of the article

Background

Neuropathological findings in idiopathic normal pressure hydrocephalus (INPH) are generally consistent with white matter damage, regardless of the underlying, yet unknown, pathophysiological mechanisms involved in INPH [1–5]. Diffusion tensor imaging (DTI) has recently been applied to evaluate white matter damage in INPH because DTI is a useful MRI technique that can reflect the structural integrity and interstitial space of the white matter by detecting the directionality of extracellular water diffusion [fractional anisotropy (FA)] and of free water diffusion [mean diffusivity (MD)] [6–9]. However, it has been found that these DTI indices could not only reflect the microstructural damage of fibres, such as axonal degeneration or ischaemic demyelination, which is generally represented by a low FA value, because several recent DTI studies reported that FA values of the periventricular corticospinal tract (CST) in INPH patients were higher compared to those in healthy controls [10–12]. Hattigen et al. postulated that mechanical compaction of the CST due to ventricular dilatation might increase fibre density and directionality of diffusion [10]. Hattori et al. noted that the decreased integrity of the superior longitudinal fasciculus, which crosses the CST at a level of the corona radiata, might increase the FA value of the CST [11]. Therefore, interpretations of FA value abnormalities in INPH patients should be affected by the different effects of mechanical pressure depending on the orientation and organization of the fibre bundles. Investigation of regional changes of DTI indices after shunt placement is needed.

Another issue among DTI studies in INPH is that most of the studies were limited by inhomogeneity in aetiology and differences in DTI analysis methods [9–13]. In the DTI studies for INPH, anatomical region of interest (ROI) approaches have been used because of the severe morphological changes that occur in the brain. However, the brain regions selected for analyses in these studies were often arbitrary and inconsistent with each other. On the other hand, although at present there is no established method for achieving accurate registration of images in INPH patients, tract-based spatial statistics (TBSS) [14], which was developed for analysing FA images from multiple subjects with INPH, have been used for voxel-based DTI analysis. The TBSS has a function that can reverse each voxel in normalized space back to its original location in native space (back-projection). This function is useful for confirming accurate registration of images in which severe deformations occur, such as in INPH patients [15]. In the present study, we attempted to elucidate a change in brain white matter involvement in INPH patients by shunt placement using DTI. We also investigated the difference between shunt responders and non-responders by applying TBSS including back-projection for tract-based DTI and mean hemispheric DTI analyses [9].

Methods

Subjects

Fifty (20 female/30 male) consecutive patients with INPH who underwent shunt surgery at Tohoku University Hospital between August 2006 and October 2010 and 10 healthy control (HC) subjects (mean age: 65.1 $\pm$ 3.6 years, 5 females and 5 males) were enrolled in this study. The patients were diagnosed with probable INPH by board-certified neurologists based on the diagnostic criteria established according to the Japanese Clinical Guidelines for INPH [16]. The criteria for probable INPH are as follows: (1) >60 years of age; (2) gait disturbance, dementia, and/or urinary incontinence; (3) ventricular dilatation (Evans index >0.3) with a narrow cerebrospinal fluid (CSF) space in the superior convexity; (4) CSF pressure <200 mm H_2O with normal CSF cell counts and protein levels; (5) the absence of other diseases that may account for such symptoms; (6) the lack of a previous history of illness that may cause ventricular dilatation; and (7) a positive CSF tap test.

Shunt implantation was conducted using a Codman-Hakim programmable valve with a Siphon-Guard (Codman and Shurtleff, Johnson and Johnson Inc.). A shunt tube was inserted in the right anterior horn of the lateral ventricle in all the patients who underwent a ventriculoperitoneal (VP) shunt procedure and in the lumbar subarachnoid space in all the patients who underwent a lumboperitoneal (LP) shunt procedure. Post-operatively, the patients were followed at the outpatient clinic, and the pressure setting of their programmable value was adjusted in a stepwise manner. Pressure adjustments were made repeatedly until the optimal pressure for each patient was attained. Thirty-five (18 female/17 male) of the initial 50 INPH patients were re-evaluated approximately 1 year after shunt surgery. The other 15 patients withdrew because of refusal, heart attack, cancer, or residential relocation. Twenty-seven (10 female/17 male) of the re-evaluated INPH patients showed significant shunt responsiveness, which is defined as an improvement by one or more points on the total score of the idiopathic Normal pressure hydrocephalus grading scale (iNPHGS) [17] at 1 year after shunt placement. However, we excluded 7 patients with cerebral vascular lesions, either focal or multiple lesions, both with abnormal intensity as observed by fluid attenuated inversion recovery (FLAIR) images and with hypointensity as observed by T1-weighted images, to avoid the possibility that the DTI parameters and clinical symptoms would be affected by a vascular brain disease. However, we did not exclude the patients only with periventricular hyperintensity as observed by FLAIR images. Consequently, the improving 20 patients (shunt responders: SR) and not improving 8 patients (shunt non-responders: SNR) with INPH after shunt placement were included in this study. The demographic characteristics of the patients with INPH at baseline are shown in Table 1.

Clinical assessments

In the present study, clinical measures were assessed prior to performing both CSF removal and shunt placement and re-assessed approximately 1 year after shunt placement. In addition to the iNPHGS, we administered a gait test and a series of standard neuropsychological tests, including the Timed Up and Go (TUG) test [18], the Mini-Mental State Examination (MMSE) [19], and the frontal assessment battery (FAB) [20]. We used the FAB because it has been reported that executive dysfunction is a characteristic feature of the cognitive impairment in patients with INPH [21, 22].

MRI procedure

Similar to the clinical assessment, cranial MRI scans were performed at baseline and approximately 1 year after shunt placement in the patients with INPH. Three-dimensional spoiled gradient echo (3D-SPGR) imaging and diffusion-weighted imaging (DWI) data were acquired via a single-shot spin echo-type echo planar imaging sequence with a GE Signa 1.5 Tesla MRI unit (General Electric Company, Milwaukee, WI, USA). The imaging parameters used for 3D-SPGR imaging were TR 20 ms, TE 4.1 ms, 1.5 mm thickness/0.0 sp by 108 slices and no intersection gap, FOV 21 × 21 cm, and matrix 256 × 256. The imaging parameters used for the acquisition of the DWI data were TR 15,000 ms, TE 52.8 ms, 2.5 mm thickness/0.0 sp by 50 slices and no insertion gap, FOV 23 × 23 cm, and matrix 256 × 256. The DWI data were acquired along 13 gradient directions with $b = 1000\ s/mm^2$. One volume was acquired with no diffusion weighting ($b = 0\ s/mm^2$). Two sets of the DWI (each set using same gradient directions) and no diffusion weighting data were acquired for subsequent averaging to improve the signal-to-noise ratio.

MRI data processing

We restricted analyses to the left brain because the postoperative images of the right brain could be distorted by shunt valve artefacts except when comparing between

Table 1 Demographics of patients at baseline

Variables	INPH (n = 20) Responder (SR)	INPH (n = 8) Non-responder (SNR)	df	p value[a]
Age in years, mean (SD)	75.5 (5.2)	76.6 (3.9)	26	NS
Sex, female/male	8/12	1/7	1	0.023
Education years, mean (SD)	10.4 (2.9)	8.8 (3.2)	26	NS
CSF shunt placement (VP/LP)	13/7	6/2	1	NS
TUG, mean (SD)				
Time to complete (s)	14.7 (4.1)	15.6 (3.1)	26	NS
Number of steps	21.9 (7.0)	22.6 (4.0)	26	NS
iNPHGS, median (range)				
Gait disturbance	2.0 (2–3)	2.0 (1–4)		NS
Cognitive disturbance	3.0 (0–3)	2.5 (1–3)		NS
Urinary disturbance	1.5 (0–3)	2.0 (0–4)		NS
Total	6.5 (2–9)	7.0 (4–9)		NS
MMSE, mean (SD)	21.5 (4.6)	22.3 (5.1)	26	NS
FAB, mean (SD)	10.7 (2.3)	12.9 (3.1)	26	NS
Left VV/ICV ratio (%), mean (SD)	8.29 (1.99)	7.19 (1.64)	26	NS
Left hemispheric FA, mean (SD)	0.386 (0.022)	0.380 (0.024)	26	NS
Left hemispheric MD ($\times 10^{-3}$ mm^2/s), mean (SD)	0.813 (0.036)	0.829 (0.068)	26	NS

INPH idiopathic normal pressure hydrocephalus, iNPHGS idiopathic normal pressure hydrocephalus grading scale, *VP* ventriculoperitoneal, *LP* lumboperitoneal, *TUG* Timed "Up and GO" test, *MMSE* Mini-Mental State Examination, *FAB* frontal assessment battery, *Left VV/ICV ratio* the ratio of the volume of the left lateral ventricle + the cerebral aqueduct + the left side region of the third and fourth ventricles and the volume of the left half intracranial space, *FA* fractional anisotropy, *MD* mean diffusivity, *SD* standard deviation, *df* degrees of freedom, *NS* not significant

[a] Paired Student's t test was used except for iNPHGS (Mann–Whitney U test)

[b] Pearson's Chi squared test was used for sex and CSF shunt placement ratios

the pre-operative DTI measures of the patients with INPH and those of the HC subjects. The left half volumes of the intracranial space and of the ventricles (the left lateral ventricle, the cerebral aqueduct, and the left side region of the third and fourth ventricles) that were obtained via 3D-SPGR imaging were measured manually using MRIcron [23] and Wacom™ tablets (Cintiq 12WX). The left volume of ventricles/intracranial volume (VV/ICV) ratio, which is calculated by dividing the left half volume of the ventricles (VV) by the left half volume of the intracranial space (ICV) and expressed as a percentage of ICV, was used as an index of the ventricular dilatation for each subject.

All diffusion images in each subject were aligned with the initial b0 image, and we used motion correction and registration software (eddy current correction) from the FSL software package [24]. The corrected images for each direction, which were acquired in two scans, were averaged to improve the signal-to-noise ratio. MD and FA maps were calculated from the mean diffusion weighted images for each direction using DTI calculation software from the FSL software package (DTIFIT Reconstruct diffusion tensors software). The mean MD and FA values of all of the left supratentorial white matter (the left hemispheric FA and MD), which was defined as the regions of the voxels with white matter probability values greater than 0.95 based on the SPM8 segmentation results of 3D-SPGR images (new segmentation software), were calculated from the co-registered MD and FA maps for each subject according to the method of Kanno et al. [9].

TBSS analyses

Regional comparisons of the FA and MD maps between baseline and 1 year after shunt placement were performed using TBSS. The initial step of TBSS consisted of determining the most representative FA map (the most typical map of the subject in the analysed groups) as the one needing the least warping for all the other maps to align to it. This map was used as the target image, and the FA maps of all the patients and the HC subjects were nonlinearly transformed into the space of the target image. The transformed FA maps were averaged to create a mean FA skeleton of white matter tracts using an algorithm that found local FA maxima along the perpendicular direction of a white matter tract. An FA threshold of 0.2 was then used to differentiate between grey and white matter. Each patient's warped FA map was projected onto the mean FA skeleton, and the final image was normalized to the Montreal Neurological Institute (MNI) space using FLIRT [25]. We used the TBSS results for the FA maps to analyse the MD maps of all the patients and the HC subjects.

Statistical analyses and back-projection

Comparisons of the baseline MMSE scores, FAB scores, TUG completion times, TUG numbers of steps, left VV/ICV ratios, and left hemispheric FAs and MDs between the SR and SNR groups were performed using a two-tailed Student's t test except for iNPHGS total and sub-scores (using the Mann–Whitney U test). For the baseline left VV/ICV ratio and left hemispheric DTI measures, comparisons were made between the SR or SNR groups, and the HC group. A two-tailed Student's t test was used for comparison of the baseline and post-operative data between the patients following VP shunt surgery and those following LP shunt surgery in the SR group except for sex (using the Chi squared test) and iNPHGS total and sub-scores (using the Mann–Whitney U test).

A paired two-tailed Student's *t* test was used for comparison between the baseline and post-operative data except for iNPHGS total and sub-scores (using the Wilcoxon signed rank test) in the SR and SNR groups. In addition, a repeated measure of analysis of variance (ANOVA) was used to analyse influences of shunt effectiveness on the change in ventricle size and hemispheric DTI measures. Statistical analyses were performed using JMP pro statistics software (version 11.00; SAS Institute Inc., Cary, NC, USA), and the statistical significance was defined for p values <0.05.

In the TBSS analyses, the baseline FA and MD maps of the SR and SNR groups were compared to those of the HC group using two sample t tests. In addition, comparisons of the baseline FA and MD maps between the SR and SNR groups were performed using two sample t tests. In these analyses, age and sex were included as nuisance variables [26, 27]. Furthermore, the FA and MD maps in the patients with INPH were compared between baseline and 1 year after shunt placement in each group using a paired t test. All the analyses were performed using the threshold-free cluster enhancement (TFCE) option of the randomize program in TBSS, which performs a permutation test developed for a general linear model. The number of permutations was set at 5000, and the significance threshold of the comparisons was set at $p < 0.05$ (family-wise error correction).

The locations of the clusters were determined first by using the Harvard-Oxford Subcortical Structural Atlas and JHU ICBM-DTI-81 White-Matter Labels (implemented in FSLView, http://www.cma.mgh.harvard.edu/fsl_atlas.html). However, there was insufficient accuracy for warping from the MNI space (Fig. 1a), such that two neurologists (S.K. and E.M.) eventually identified the locations of the clusters by consulting with each other and using the mean colour-coded FA skeleton

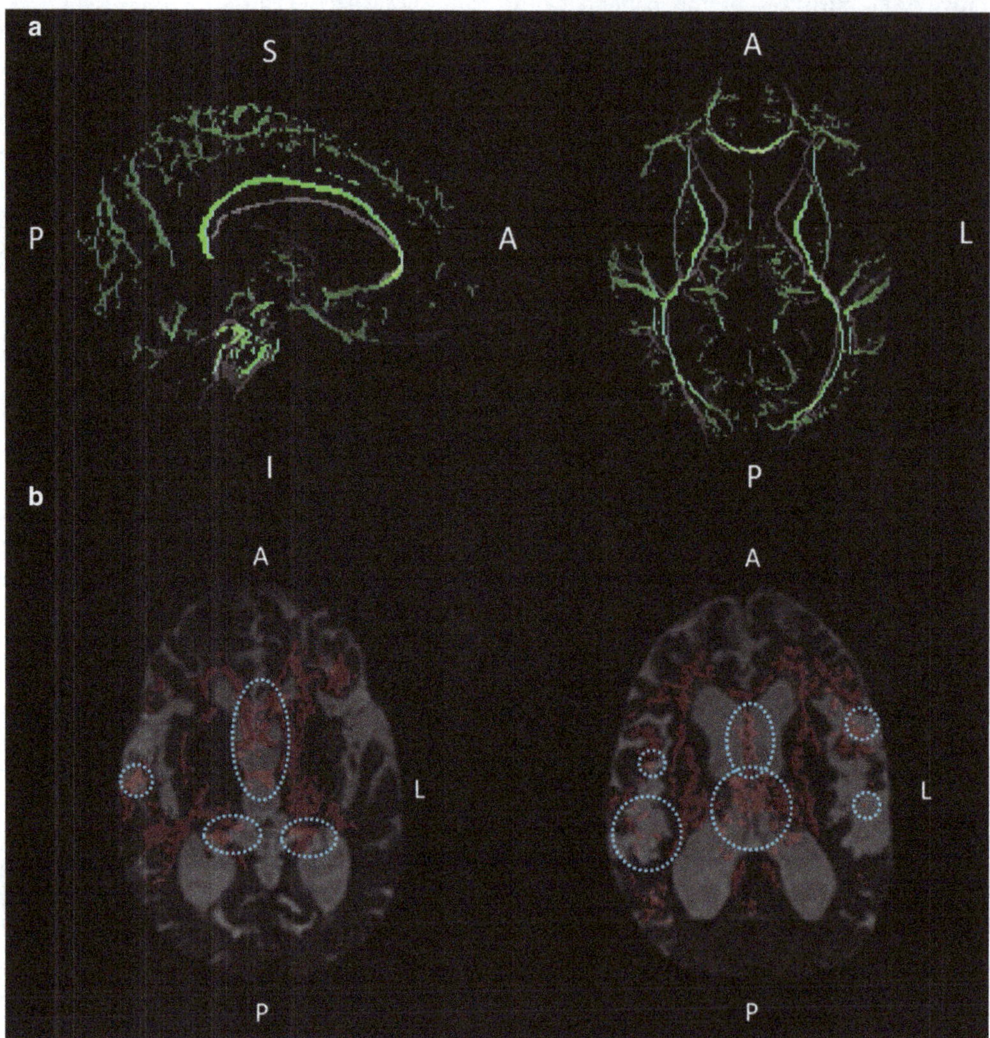

Fig. 1 Comparison of skeletons and mis-registrations observed in TBSS analysis. **a** Demonstrates the mean FA skeleton (*green*) derived from the study (the comparison between the patients with INPH and the healthy control subjects) and the FMRIB58 FA standard space skeleton (*grey*). The periventricular tracks in the mean FA skeleton (the internal capsules and the corpus callosum in particular) are out of position. **b** Shows a sample of mis-registration that occurred in the comparison of MD maps between the patients with INPH and the healthy control subjects. The back-projected voxels (*red*) in the columns, bodies, and crura of the bilateral fornixes were positioned on each side of the lateral ventricle, and those in a peri-Sylvian portion of the SWM of bilateral frontal operculums were on each side of the Sylvian fissure. *A* anterior, *I* inferior, *L* left, *P* posterior, *S* superior

map (directionally encoded) and the mean normalized b0 image in reference to the MRI atlas of Human White Matter made by Mori et al. [28].

To confirm whether the results of TBSS analyses were based on accurate registrations, the back-projection in TBSS was performed. The back-projection can investigate where one or more voxels of the mean FA skeleton originally came from in each subject's FA map. Two neurologists (S.K. and E.M.) examined the clusters independently to determine whether the back-projected TBSS results were positioned on tract-centre points and were anatomically the same among the patients with INPH and the HC subjects. If both neurologists judged that some clusters in the back-projected TBSS results were positioned on the outside of tract-centre points or were different among the patients with INPH, these clusters were excluded from the data set for significant regions. In addition, anatomical ROI analyses of the regions in which FA or MD were significantly altered after shunt placement were performed using a paired two-tailed Student's t test to validate the results of the TBSS analyses. Statistical significance was defined for p values <0.05 (using Bonferroni correction).

Results

Clinical assessments, ventricular size, and hemispheric DTI measures

The results of the baseline demographics and the iNPHGS, TUG, MMSE, FAB, left VV/ICV ratio, and left hemispheric FA and MD for the patients with INPH are summarized in Table 1. There were no significant differences between the SR and SNR groups, except that the number of females in the SNR group was significantly smaller than that in the SR group. The left VV/ICV ratio in the HC group (mean ratio: 1.511 ± 0.520) was significantly smaller than those in the SR ($p < 0.001$) and SNR ($p < 0.001$) groups. The left hemispheric FA in the HC group (mean FA: 0.4105 ± 0.014) was significantly larger than those in the SR ($p = 0.036$) and SNR ($p = 0.005$) groups. The left hemispheric MD (mean MD: 0.7460 ± 0.031) in the HC group was significantly smaller than those in the SR ($p < 0.001$) and SNR ($p = 0.004$) groups (data not shown). There were no significant differences in the baseline data or in the post-operative changes between the VP shunt and the LP shunt groups in the SR group (Additional file 1: Table S1).

The changes after shunt surgery in clinical and DTI measures in the patients with INPH are shown in Table 2A (SR group) and 2B (SNR group). The total and sub-scores of the iNPHGS, the total scores of the MMSE and the FAB, and the TUG complete time and number of steps in the SR group were significantly improved 1 year after shunt placement compared with those at baseline, whereas those in the SNR group were largely unchanged. The left VV/ICV ratios measured at 1 year after shunt placement were significantly smaller than those measured at baseline in both the SR and SNR groups. On the other hand, the left hemispheric FAs and MDs were not significantly changed between baseline and 1 year after shunt placement in either group. Repeated measure of ANOVA of the left VV/ICV ratio revealed a significant main effect of shunt surgery for the decrease in ventricular size [$F(1, 26) = 45.11$, $p < 0.001$] and a significant interaction between shunt effectiveness for clinical improvement and decrease in ventricular size [$F(1, 26) = 5.92$, $p = 0.022$] (Fig. 2). Although there was no significant interaction between shunt effectiveness for clinical improvement and change in the left hemispheric FA, there was a significant interaction between shunt effectiveness for clinical improvement and change in left hemispheric MD [$F(1, 26) = 6.01$, $p = 0.021$] (Fig. 2).

TBSS analyses

The comparison between FA maps for the SR group at baseline and the HC group and the regional peaks for significant clusters (t value >2.0) are demonstrated in Fig. 3 and Table 3A. The FA values of the SR group were significantly lower in the middle and posterior parts of the cingulum, genu, body, and splenium of the corpus callosum, the crus of the right fornix, and the subcortical white matter (SWM) of the right frontal operculum, right precuneus, bilateral superior parietal lobules, right occipital cortex, right primary motor cortex, and left primary motor cortex. However, as the result of the back-projection, the back-projected voxels in a peri-Sylvian portion of the SWM of the right frontal operculum were positioned on the right Sylvian fissure (incidence: HC 4/10; SR 19/20; SNR 4/10), and those in the crus of the right fornix were on the right lateral ventricle or right thalamus (incidence: HC 9/10; SR 20/20; SNR 8/8). Therefore, these regions were excluded from the FA data set. There were no regions in which the SR group presents significantly higher FA values than the HC group. In addition, there were no regions in which the FA values were significantly different between the SNR group and the HC group and between the SR group and SNR group (data not shown).

Figure 4 and Table 3B show the results of the group comparison for MD between the baseline SR and HC groups and the regional peaks for significant clusters (t value >2.0). The MD values of the SR group were significantly higher in the columns, bodies, and crura of the bilateral fornixes, the hippocampal part of the right cingulum, the genu, body, and splenium of the corpus callosum, and the subcortical white matter (SWM) of the bilateral frontal operculum, bilateral orbitofrontal cortex, bilateral primary motor and sensory cortex, posterior part of temporal cortex, bilateral superior and inferior parietal lobules, right precuneus, and right occipital cortex, as well as the right external capsule, the bilateral cerebral peduncles, and the bilateral internal capsules. However, as a result of the back-projection, the back-projected voxels in the columns, bodies, and crura of the bilateral fornixes were positioned on each side of the lateral ventricle (incidence: HC 10/10; SR 20/20; SNR 8/8), those in a peri-Sylvian portion of the SWM of bilateral frontal operculums were on each side of the Sylvian fissure [incidence (right): HC 5/10; SR 20/20; SNR 8/8, incidence (left): HC 0/10; SR 20/20; SNR 8/8], and those in the SWM of posterior part of the right temporal cortex were on the right Sylvian fissure (incidence: HC 0/10; SR 20/20; SNR 8/8). Therefore, these regions were excluded from the MD data set (Fig. 1b). There were no regions in which the SR group presented a significantly lower MD than the HC group. Furthermore, there were no regions in which the MD values were significantly different between the SNR group and the HC group and between the SR group and SNR group (data not shown).

The comparison of FA maps between baseline and 1 year after shunt placement in the SR group are shown

Table 2 Changes in clinical and MRI variables after shunt placement

Variables	Baseline	Post-operative	df	p value[a]
A. Shunt responders (SR, n = 20)				
TUG, mean (SD)				
Time to complete (s)	14.7 (4.1)	11.2 (4.3)	19	<0.001
Number of steps	21.9 (7.0)	18.1 (7.2)	19	0.001
iNPHGS, median (range)				
Gait disturbance	2.0 (2–3)	1.0 (0–3)		<0.001
Cognitive disturbance	3.0 (0–3)	2.0 (0–3)		0.001
Urinary disturbance	1.5 (0–3)	0.0 (0–2)		0.004
Total	6.5 (2–9)	3.0 (1–7)		<0.001
MMSE, mean (SD)	21.5 (4.6)	24.0 (4.3)	19	0.008
FAB, mean (SD)	10.7 (2.3)	12.9 (3.1)	19	0.002
Left VV/ICV ratio (%), mean (SD)	8.29 (1.99)	6.59 (2.03)	19	<0.001
Left hemispheric FA, mean (SD)	0.386 (0.022)	0.382 (0.026)	19	NS
Left hemispheric MD ($\times 10^{-3}$ mm^2/s), mean (SD)	0.813 (0.036)	0.816 (0.035)	19	NS
Mean FA of the left corona radiata, mean (SD)	0.624 (0.041)	0.592 (0.048)	19	<0.001
B. Shunt non-responders (SNR, n = 8)				
TUG, mean (SD)				
Time to complete (s)	15.6 (3.1)	14.2 (3.5)	7	NS
Number of steps	22.6 (4.0)	20.5 (5.0)	7	NS
iNPHGS, median (range)				
Gait disturbance	2.0 (1–4)	2.0 (1–4)		NS
Cognitive disturbance	2.5 (1–3)	2.0 (1–3)		NS
Urinary disturbance	2.0 (0–4)	2.0 (0–4)		NS
Total	7.0 (4–9)	7.0 (4–9)		NS
MMSE, mean (SD)	22.3 (5.0)	22.3 (5.0)	7	NS
FAB, mean (SD)	11.0 (3.8)	11.0 (3.7)	7	NS
Left VV/ICV ratio (%), mean (SD)	7.19 (1.99)	6.40 (1.79)	7	0.005
Left Hemispheric FA, mean (SD)	0.380 (0.024)	0.375 (0.030)	7	NS
Left Hemispheric MD ($\times 10^{-3}$ mm^2/s), mean (SD)	0.829 (0.068)	0.876 (0.099)	7	NS
Mean FA of the left corona radiata, mean (SD)	0.612 (0.043)	0.607 (0.044)	7	NS

DTI diffusion tensor imaging, *INPH* idiopathic normal pressure hydrocephalus, *iNPHGS* idiopathic normal pressure hydrocephalus grading scale, *TUG* Timed "Up and GO" test, *MMSE* Mini-Mental State Examination, *FAB* frontal assessment battery, *Left VV/ICV ratio* the volume of the left lateral ventricle + the cerebral aqueduct + the left side region of the third and fourth ventricles/the left half volume of the intracranial space, *FA* fractional anisotropy, *MD* mean diffusivity, *SD* standard deviation, *df* degrees of freedom, *NS* not significant

[a] Paired Student's t test was used except for iNPHGS (Wilcoxon signed rank test)

in Fig. 5a and Table 3C. The FA values were significantly decreased in the left corona radiata. In addition, the result of the back-projection revealed the precise registration of each FA map. The anatomical ROI of the left corona radiata of each SR or SNR patient was placed using colour-coded FA map and referring to the result of the TBSS analysis (Fig. 5b). The anatomical ROI analysis showed that the mean FA value of the regions in the left corona radiata was significantly decreased after shunt placement only in the SR group (Table 2A). There were no other regions in which the FA values were significantly increased after shunt placement in the SR group. In the comparison of the FA map between baseline and 1 year after shunt placement in the SNR group, there were no regions in which the FA values were significantly altered. In the comparison of MD maps between baseline and 1 year after shunt placement, there were no regions in which the MD values were significantly altered in either the SR or the SNR groups.

Discussion

In the present study, we investigated the differences between shunt responders and non-responders after shunt placement by applying the TBSS including back-projection and hemispheric DTI analyses to elucidate brain white matter changes in INPH patients with shunt

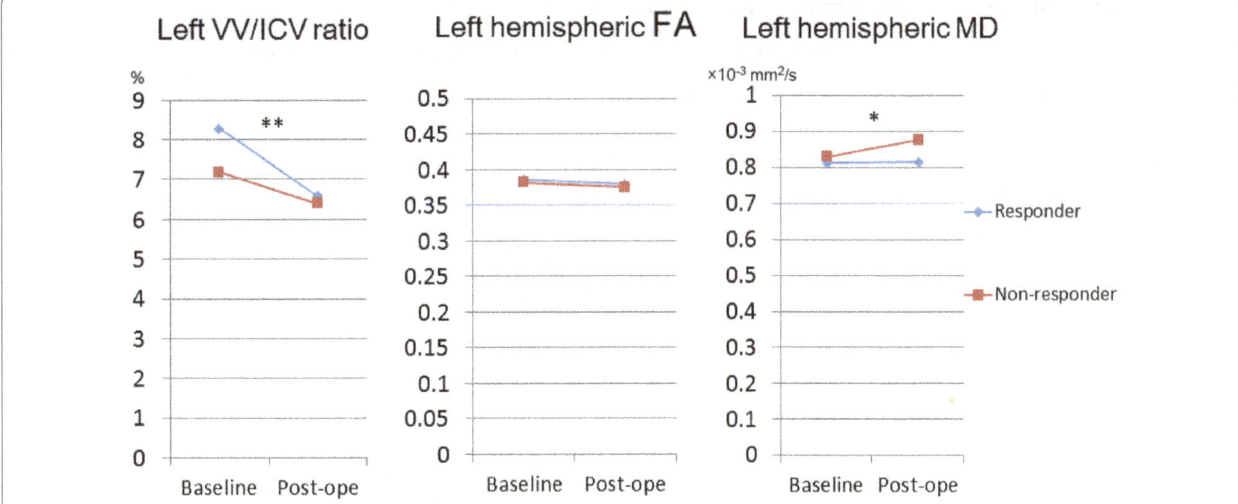

Fig. 2 Changes in left VV/ICV ratio, hemispheric FA, and hemispheric MD after shunt placement. Significance of interaction between shunt effectiveness for clinical improvement and for each index is denoted as follows: *$p < 0.05$; **$p < 0.001$

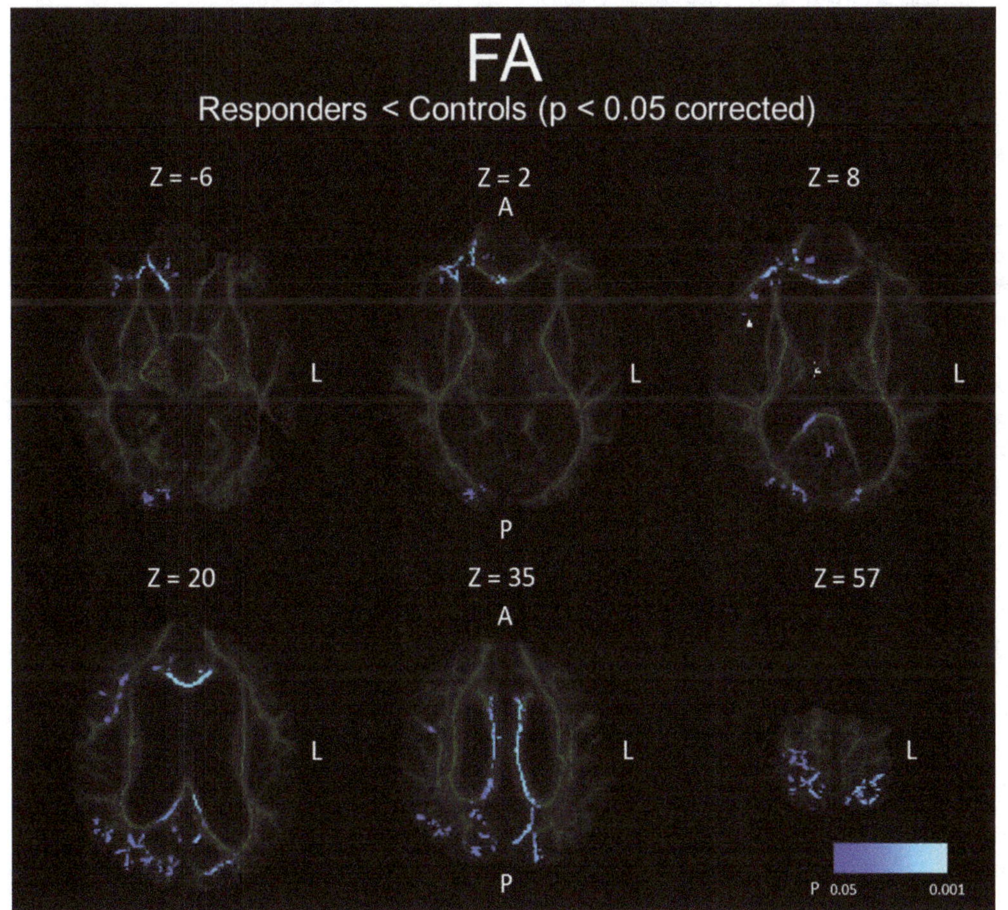

Fig. 3 White matter regions in which FA values were significantly lower in shunt-responsive INPH. The areas with significantly lower FA values are demonstrated by colours ranging from *blue* to *light-blue* in the shunt-responsive INPH patients compared to control subjects ($p < 0.05$, corrected for multiple comparisons by using TFCE). The mis-registered regions are shown in *white*. *A* anterior, *L* left, *P* posterior

Table 3 Regions of the peaks for significant clusters in TBSS analyses

	Hemisphere	MNI coordinate (x, y, z)	T value[a]	Cluster size
A. FA for shunt responders (SR) at baseline compared to healthy controls (HC)				
Region				
Middle part of cingulum	Right	5, −12, 35	6.88	7210
Middle part of corpus callosum	Left	−10, −25, 38	5.56	
SWM of superior parietal lobule	Left	−22, −51, 56	5.33	
Posterior part of corpus callosum	Left	−10, −43, 33	5.31	
Posterior part of corpus callosum	Right	12, −48, 20	6.29	713
Posterior part of cingulum	Right	10, −39, 37	4.63	
Splenium of corpus callosum	Right	10, −46, 13	4.58	
SWM of precuneus	Right	9, −56, 27	5.63	113
SWM of superior parietal lobule	Right	15, −47, 52	5.55	4177
SWM of primary motor cortex	Right	23, −27, 57	4.99	
SWM of cuneus	Right	16, −74, 33	4.57	
SWM of frontal operculum	Right	43, 4, 18	4.66	387
SWM of frontal operculum	Right	42, 20, 16	4.47	358
Excluded regions				
SWM of frontal operculum	Right	41, 22, 6	7.01	39
Perithalamic white matter	Right	6, −14, 7	5.68	8
B. MD for shunt responders (SR) at baseline compared to healthy controls (HC)				
Region				
SWM of primary motor cortex	Left	−30, −14, 53	3.72	118
SWM of superior parietal lobule	Left	−13, −59, 49	3.48	119
SWM of primary motor cortex	Right	13, −20, 56	3.47	117
SWM of precuneus	Right	10, −53, 24	3.40	115
SWM of orbitofrontal cortex	Left	−26, 21, −18	3.37	114
SWM of lateral occipital cortex	Right	38, −63, 27	3.35	111
Cingulum (cingulate gyrus)	Right	7, −26, 37	3.01	106
Cerebral peduncle	Left	−10, −17, −7	2.74	108
SWM of middle temporal gyrus	Right	51, −42, 4	2.74	101
External capsule	Right	23, 20, −4	2.73	112
SWM of superior frontal gyrus	Left	−18, −1, 47	2.63	103
SWM of superior parietal lobule	Right	42, −53, 39	2.58	94
Posterior corona radiata	Right	35, −40, 36	2.43	87
Superior longitudinal fasciculus	Left	−30, 15, 30	2.38	100
Perithalamic white matter	Left	−18, −22, 9	2.32	83
SWM of inferior parietal lobule	Right	58, −28, 31	2.28	105
SWM of superior temporal gyrus	Right	51, −16, −2	2.17	98
SWM of primary sensory cortex	Left	−9, −45, 59	2.14	39
SWM of precuneus	Left	−8, −58, 42	2.10	96
Excluded regions				
Cingulum (hippocampus)	Right	26, −41, −6	14.4	120
Fornix	Right	3, −20, 20	10.6	120
Fornix	Left	0, −20, 21	10.6	
SWM of frontal operculum	Right	54, −10, 14	5.57	116
C. FA in shunt responders (SR) post-operation compared to baseline				
Corona radiata	Left	−27, −10, 15	6.93[b]	66

DTI diffusion tensor imaging, *INPH* idiopathic normal pressure hydrocephalus, *HC* healthy controls, *MNI* Montreal Neurological Institute, *FA* fractional anisotropy, *MD* mean diffusivity, *SR* shunt responder, *SWM* subcortical white matter

[a] The number of degrees of freedom is 28

[b] The number of degrees of freedom is 19

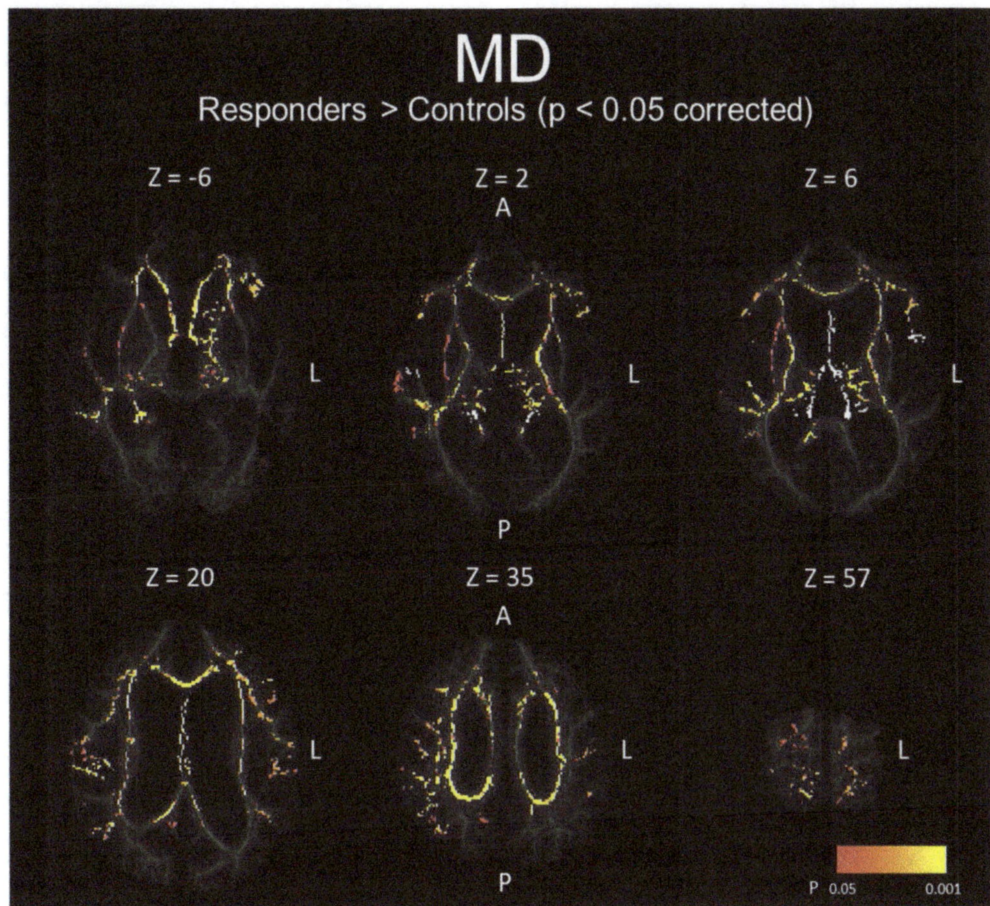

Fig. 4 White matter regions in which MD values were significantly higher in shunt-responsive INPH. The areas with significantly higher MD values are demonstrated by colours ranging from *red* to *yellow* in the shunt-responsive INPH patients compared to control subjects ($p < 0.05$, corrected for multiple comparisons by using TFCE). The mis-registered regions are shown in *white*. *A* anterior, *L* left, *P* posterior

placement. We showed that FA values in the corona radiata were decreased by shunt placement in patients that had a good response to shunt treatment. In the back-projection analysis of the TBSS, mis-registration was observed in the periventricular or intraventricular structures such as the fornix, hippocampal part of the cingulum, perithalamic area, and peri-Sylvian SWM. These regions appear to be strongly associated with the typical deformation of the brain in patients with INPH [30]. The back-projected voxels in the fornix, cingulum, and perithalamic area were positioned on each side of lateral ventricle. These findings of mis-registration were also reported in the previous INPH study applying the TBSS analysis [15]. Hattori et al. speculated that the fornix might be displaced by the elevated and stretched corpus callosum because the fornix is attached to the posterior part of the body and splenium of the corpus callosum [15]. Not only the ventricles but also the Sylvian fissures are commonly dilated in INPH, which might cause inhibition of lateral expansion of the lateral ventricles represented by the narrowing of the callosal angle [31, 32]. The dilation of the Sylvian fissures might be one cause of the elevation of the corpus callosum.

On the other hand, the results of back-projection revealed the precise registration of the corpus callosum, the cerebral peduncles, the internal capsule, the corona radiata, and the SWM except for the frontal and temporal operculum. The DTI measures of the corpus callosum and the CST using the TBSS were validated by anatomical ROI analysis in several previous studies [10, 15]. The results of the current study suggested that the TBSS is a useful tool for detecting white matter abnormalities in these regions.

FA values in the corpus callosum and in the SWM of the convexity and occipital cortex were significantly lower in SR than in HC, whereas MD values in the periventricular and peri-Sylvian white matter were significantly higher. These findings were frequently reported in the

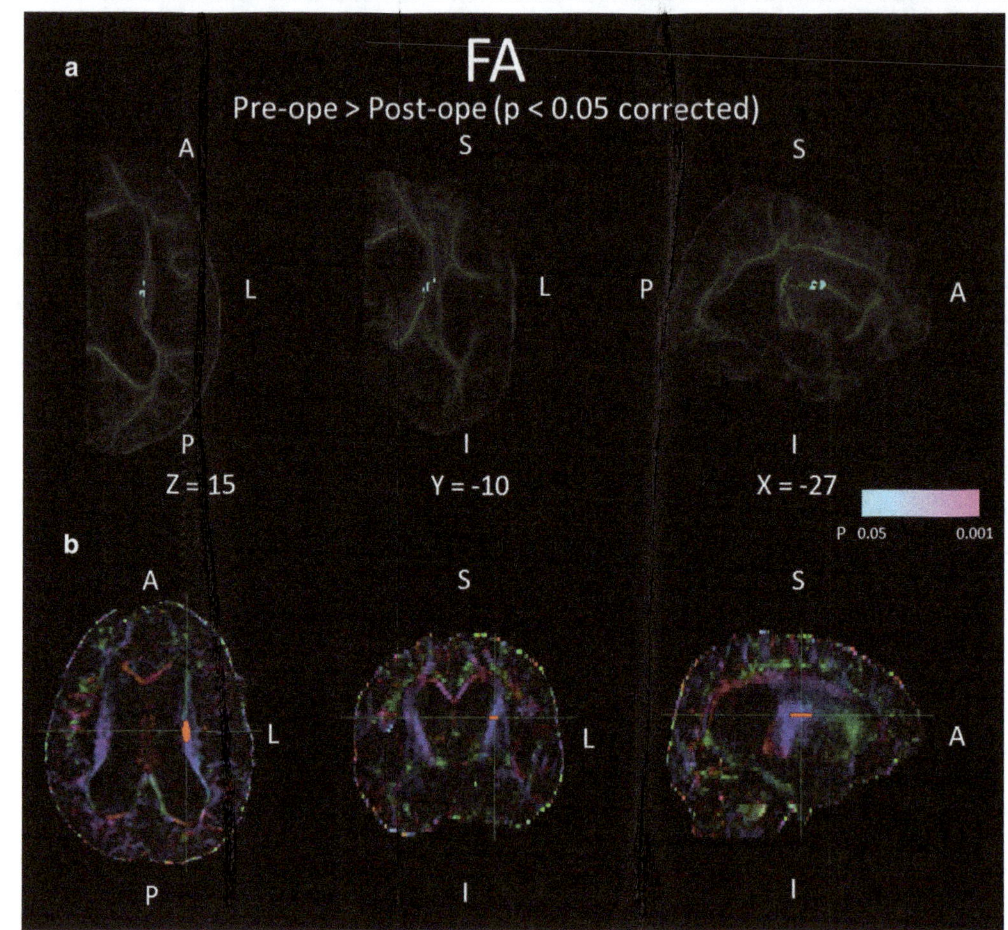

Fig. 5 White matter regions in which FA values significantly changed after shunt placement. **a** Demonstrates the areas with significantly decreased FA values after shunt placement in the shunt-responsive INPH patients using colours ranging from *light-blue* to *pink* ($p < 0.05$, corrected for multiple comparisons by using TFCE). **b** Shows the position of the anatomical ROI. On colour-coded FA map, *red*, *green*, and *blue* represent the direction of fibres (*red*, *right-left*; *green*, anterior-posterior; *blue*, superior-inferior). The ROI was placed on the *blue* regions in the left radiata on the axial slice that included the genu of the corpus callosum. *A* anterior, *L* left, *P* posterior

previous DTI studies [10, 15]. The white matter regions in which FA values were decreased after shunt placement were distributed in the left corona radiata. These regions were located between the lateral ventricle and the Sylvian fissure, and therefore may have been severely compressed. Recent studies reported that the FA values of the CST near the lateral ventricles in INPH were higher compared with those in healthy controls, although this result was not confirmed in the present study [10, 11]. Hattori et al. detected the increase of axial eigenvalues and unaltered radial eigenvalues in the CST and suggested that mechanical pressure from ventricular dilatation could enhance directional water diffusivity parallel to the axon in the CST in INPH [11]. In addition, we speculated that dilatation of the Sylvian fissures could play a role of counterfort against mechanical pressure from the ventricular dilatation in INPH. It is considered that the release of compression to the corona radiata including the CST and projection fibre to the medial frontal cortex, which is thought to play a role in planning or programming voluntary movements including gait, is associated with clinical improvement after shunt placement [9, 33, 34].

Although the left hemispheric FA and MD of the INPH patients were not significantly changed after shunt placement, it was identified that left hemispheric MDs of the SNR patients increased after shunt placement when compared to those of the SR patients. In addition, it was revealed that the ventricles of the SNR patients decreased to a lesser extent after shunt placement compared to those of the SR patients which started from a higher pre-shunt ratio. One of the possible reasons is insufficiency of pressure adjustments in clinical practice. In the study, all the patients in the SNR group fulfilled the clinical criteria of the Japanese Clinical Guidelines for INPH. In previous cohort studies in Japan using the same criteria, the efficiency of the shunt operation (both VP and LP shunts) was 80%. Because the efficiency in the current study was 71% (20/28), there was no apparent evidence that the pressure adjustments were insufficient [29, 30]. Another possible reason is that these findings reflected progression of brain atrophy in SNR. Poor contraction of ventricles and an expansion of the interstitial oedema represented by an increase in the MD value might be related to a decline in compliance of the brain, which is associated with co-morbidity with other central nervous system diseases. Hamilton et al. reported that Alzheimer disease pathology observed in cortical biopsies obtained during shunt insertion was associated with worse baseline cognitive performance and diminished postoperative improvement in patients with hydrocephalus [35]. We excluded the patients with vascular brain disease from the study by neuroradiological criteria. However, the severity of ischaemic brain injuries might be relevant to shunt responsiveness because micropathological findings of ischaemic demyelination and infarction have been observed in the brains of patients with normal pressure hydrocephalus [5]. In the future, we need to investigate whether the pre-operative hemispheric FA and MD can predict the effectiveness of shunt surgery in a large-scale cohort study, which will lead us to better outcomes and further discussions about neuropathological changes of the cerebral white matter in INPH.

In our previous study, we reported that the hemispheric FA in INPH was lower than that in disease controls (Alzheimer's disease and idiopathic Parkinson's disease), was correlated with severity of gait and cognitive disturbances, and was not correlated with degree of ventricular dilation [9]. According these findings, it was suggested that the hemispheric FA might be altered depending on improvement of gait and cognitive disturbances. However, the results in the present study were inconsistent with our expectation. Although the hemispheric FA in INPH might strongly reflect the severity of irreversible white matter involvement, further studies are needed to clarify this issue.

There were several limitations in the current study: one is that we could not detect a change in white matter in the right brain after shunt placement because of shunt valve artefacts. It is possible that the change in white matter after shunt placement is different between the right and left brains, although the brain ventricular system consists of a semi-enclosed cavity. One solution to this problem may be to analyse DTI of only subjects who underwent lumboperitoneal (LP) shunt surgery. In this study, there were no significant differences in the changes of the clinical and hemispheric DTI data after shunt placement between the LP and VP shunt groups. A recent study revealed the benefit of LP shunt surgery for patients with INPH [29]. However, there were insufficient patient numbers to conclude whether the effectiveness of an LP shunt is equivalent to that of a VP shunt. In addition, regional statistical comparisons of the change in the DTI parameters after shunt placement between the LP and VP shunt groups could not be performed because of insufficient sample sizes. Further larger-scale studies are needed to confirm whether there are significant differences in clinical effectiveness and of regional changes in DTI parameters between the LP and VP shunts.

Another limitation is that the mean age of the HC subjects was significantly lower than that of the INPH patients. Previous studies suggested that the FA values tend to decline and the MD value tend to elevate with ageing [26]. Although we applied age as nuisance variable in the comparison analysis, the results of the DTI analyses might overestimate the cerebral white matter change in INPH. The other limitation is the small sample size of the SNR group. There is some possibility that we could not detect the difference in white matter alterations between the SR and SNR groups and between the SNR and HC groups. Moreover, another limitation is that we applied the non-isotropic voxels and only 13 gradient directions in the DTI scan. The FA values measured using non-isotropic voxels tend to result in underestimation in regions with crossing fibres such as the centrum semiovale (crossing interhemispheric, projection, and association fibres) [36]. In addition, the analysis of high resolution DTI using non-isotropic voxels may not be sufficiently precise because the signal-to noise ratio is prone to decline with a decrease in the voxel size [37]. Melhem et al. suggested that more than 20 gradient directions were needed to obtain highly reproducible FA values [37]. These problems might be solved by using isotropic voxels or a many gradient directions scan. However, this seems to be difficult in clinical settings.

Conclusions

Our study demonstrated that fractional anisotropy in the corona radiata was decreased by shunt placement. The regions were distributed between the enlarged lateral ventricles and Sylvian fissures. This finding was observed only in shunt-responsive INPH patients and might reflect the plasticity of the brain for mechanical pressure from the cerebrospinal fluid system.

Abbreviations

CSF: cerebrospinal fluid; CST: corticospinal tract; DTI: diffusion tensor imaging; DWI: diffusion-weighted image; FA: fractional anisotropy; FAB: frontal assessment battery; FLAIR: fluid attenuated inversion recovery; HC: healthy control; INPH: idiopathic normal pressure hydrocephalus; iNPHGS: idiopathic Normal Pressure Hydrocephalus Grading Scale; LP: lumboperitoneal; MD: mean diffusivity; MMSE: Mini-Mental State Examination; MNI: Montreal Neurological Institute; ROI: region of interest; SNR: shunt non-responder; SR: shunt responder; SWM: subcortical white matter; TBSS: tract-based spatial statistics; TFCE: threshold-free cluster enhancement; 3D-SPGR: three-dimensional spoiled gradient echo; TUG: Timed Up and Go Test; VP: ventriculoperitoneal; VV/ICV: volume of ventricles/intracranial volume.

Authors' contributions

SK: Study design, data acquisition, data analysis, and manuscript writing. MS, TK: Data acquisition and data analysis. OI, YN, HK, MT: Data acquisition. MI: Data acquisition and shunt operation. ST: Manuscript editing. EM: Study design, data analysis, and manuscript editing. All authors have read and approved the final manuscript.

Author details

[1] Department of Neurology, Southmiyagi Medical Center, 38-1, Aza-nishi, Shibata, Miyagi 989-1253, Japan. [2] Department of Behavioural Neurology and Cognitive Neuroscience, Tohoku University Graduate School of Medicine, Sendai, Japan. [3] Department of Neurosurgery, Tohoku University Graduate School of Medicine, Sendai, Japan. [4] Department of Diagnostic Radiology, Tohoku University Graduate School of Medicine, Sendai, Japan.

Acknowledgements

We thank the patients and their families for their participation in this study. We also thank Takeo Kondo and Kazunori Nishijima for their constant support. This study was supported by a Grant-in-Aid for Scientific Research on Priority Areas—System study on higher-order brain functions from the MECSSR Japan (20020004) and by the Ministry of Health, Labor, and Welfare of Japan.

Competing interests

The authors declare that they have no competing interests.

References

1. Adams RD, Fisher CM, Hakim S, Ojemann RG, Sweet WH. Symptomatic occult hydrocephalus with "normal" cerebrospinal-fluid pressure. A treatable syndrome. N Engl J Med. 1965;273:117–26.
2. Akai K, Uchigasaki S, Tanaka U, Komatsu A. Normal pressure hydrocephalus. Neuropathological study. Acta Pathol Jpn. 1987;37:97–110.
3. Del Bigio MR. Neuropathological changes caused by hydrocephalus. Acta Neuropathol. 1993;85:573–85.
4. Di Rocco C, Di Trapani G, Maira G, Bentivoglio M, Macchi G, Rossi GF. Anatomo-clinical correlations in normotensive hydrocephalus. Reports on three cases. J Neurol Sci. 1977;33:437–52.
5. Del Bigio MR, Wilson MJ, Enno T. Chronic hydrocephalus in rats and humans: white matter loss and behavior changes. Ann Neurol. 2003;53:337–46.
6. Chabriat H, Pappata S, Poupon C, et al. Clinical severity in CADASIL related to ultrastructural damage in white matter: in vivo study with diffusion tensor MRI. Stroke. 1999;30:2637–43.
7. Le Bihan D, Mangin JF, Poupon C, Clark CA, Vahedi K, Poupon F, et al. Diffusion tensor imaging: concepts and applications. J Magn Reson Imaging. 2001;13:534–46.
8. van Gelderen P, de Vleeschouwer MH, DesPres D, Pekar J, van Zijl PC, Moonen CT. Water diffusion and acute stroke. Magn Reson Med. 1994;31:154–63.
9. Kanno S, Abe N, Saito M, Takagi M, Nishio Y, Hayashi A, et al. White matter involvement in idiopathic normal pressure hydrocephalus: a voxel-base diffusion tensor imaging study. J Neurol. 2011;258:1949–57.
10. Hattingen E, Jurcoane A, Melber J, Blasel S, Zanella FE, Neumann-Haefelin T, et al. Diffusion tensor imaging in patients with adult chronic hydrocephalus. Neurosurgery. 2010;66:917–24.
11. Hattori T, Yuasa T, Aoki S, Sato R, Sawaura H, Mori T, et al. Altered microstructure in corticospinal tract in idiopathic normal pressure hydrocephalus: comparison with Alzheimer disease and Parkinson disease with dementia. AJNR Am J Neuroradiol. 2011;32:1681–7.
12. Kim MJ, Seo SW, Lee KM, Kim ST, Lee JI, Nam DH, et al. Differential diagnosis of idiopathic normal pressure hydrocephalus from other dementias using diffusion tensor imaging. AJNR Am J Neuroradiol. 2011;32:1496–503.
13. Scheel M, Diekhoff T, Sprung C, Hoffmann KT. Diffusion tensor imaging in hydrocephalus-findings before and after shunt surgery. Acta Neurochir (Wien). 2012;154:1699–706.
14. Smith SM, Jenkinson M, Johansen-Berg H, Rueckert D, Nichols TE, Mackay CE, et al. Tract-based spatial statistics: voxelwise analysis of multi-subject diffusion data. Neuroimage. 2006;31:1487–505.
15. Hattori T, Ito K, Aoki S, Yuasa T, Sato R, Ishikawa M, et al. White matter alteration in idiopathic normal pressure hydrocephalus: tract-based spatial statistics study. AJNR Am J Neuroradiol. 2012;33:97–103.
16. Ishikawa M, Hashimoto M, Kuwana N, Mori E, Miyake H, Wachi A, et al. Guidelines for management of idiopathic normal pressure hydrocephalus. Neurol Med Chir. 2012;48(Suppl):S1–23.
17. Kubo Y, Kazui H, Yoshida T, Kito Y, Kimura N, Tokunaga H, et al. Validation of grading scale for evaluating symptoms of idiopathic normal pressure hydrocephalus. Dement Geriatr Cogn Disord. 2008;25:37–45.
18. Podsiadlo D, Richardson S. The timed "Up & Go": a test of basic functional mobility for frail elderly persons. J Am Geriatr Soc. 1991;39:142–8.
19. Folstein MF, Folstein SE, McHugh PR. "Mini-mental state". A practical method for grading the cognitive state of patients for the clinician. J Psychiatr Res. 1975;12:189–98.
20. Dubois B, Slachevsky A, Litvan I, Pillon B. The FAB: a frontal assessment battery at bedside. Neurology. 2000;55:1621–6.
21. Miyoshi N, Kazui H, Ogino A, Ishikawa M, Miyake H, Tokunaga H, et al. Association between cognitive impairment and gait disturbance in patients with idiopathic normal pressure hydrocephalus. Dement Geriatr Cogn Disord. 2005;20:71–6.
22. Kanno S, Saito M, Hayashi A, Uchiyama M, Hiraoka K, Nishio Y, et al. Counting-backward test for executive function in idiopathic normal pressure hydrocephalus. Acta Neurol Scand. 2012;126:279–86.
23. Rorden C, Karnath HO, Bonilha L. Improving lesion-symptom mapping. J Cogn Neurosci. 2007;19:1081–8.
24. Smith SM, Jenkinson M, Woolrich MW, Beckmann CF, Behrens TE, Johansen-Berg H, et al. Advances in functional and structural MR image analysis and implementation as FSL. Neuroimage. 2004;23(Suppl 1):S208–19.
25. Jenkinson M, Smith SM. A global optimisation method for robust affine registration of brain images. Med Image Anal. 2001;5:143–56.
26. Keneddy KM, Raz N. Aging white matter and cognition: differential effects of regional variations in diffusion properties on memory, executive functions, and speed. Neuropsychologia. 2009;47:916–27.
27. Szeszko PR, Vogel J, Ashtari M, Malhotra AK, Bates J, Kane JM, et al. Sex differences in frontal lobe white matter microstructure: a DTI study. Neuroreport. 2003;14:2469–73.
28. Oishi K, Faria AV, VanZijl PCM, Mori S. MRI atlas of human white matter. 2nd ed. Amsterdam: Elsevier; 2011.

29. Kazui H, Miyajima M, Mori E, Ishikawa M, SINPHONI-2 Investigators. Lumboperitoneal shunt surgery for idiopathic normal pressure hydrocephalus (SINPHONI-2): an open-label randomised trial. Lancet Neurol. 2015;14:585–94.
30. Hashimoto M, Ishikawa M, Mori E, Kuwana N. Study of INPH on neurological improvement (SINPHONI). Diagnosis of idiopathic normal pressure hydrocephalus is supported by MRI-based scheme: a prospective cohort study. Cerebrospinal Fluid Res. 2010;7:18.
31. Kitagaki H, Mori E, Ishii K, Yamaji J, Hirono N, Imamura T. CSF spaces in idiopathic normal pressure hydrocephalus: morphology and volumetry. AJNR Am J Neuroradiol. 1998;19:1277–84.
32. Ishii K, Kanda T, Harada A, Miyamoto N, Kawaguchi T, Shimada K, et al. Clinical impact of the callosal angle in the diagnosis of idiopathic normal pressure hydrocephalus. Eur Radiol. 2008;18:2678–83.
33. Lenfeldt N, Larsson A, Nyberg L, Birgander R, Eklund A, Malm J. Diffusion tensor imaging reveals supplementary lesions to frontal white matter in idiopathic normal pressure hydrocephalus. Neurosurgery. 2011;68:1586–93.
34. Fukuyama H, Ouchi Y, Matsuzaki S, Nagahama Y, Yamauchi H, Ogawa M, et al. Brain functional activity during gait in normal subjects: a SPECT study. Neurosci Lett. 1997;228:183–6.
35. Hamilton R, Patel S, Lee EB, Jackson EM, Lopinto J, Arnold SE, et al. Lack of shunt response in suspected idiopathic normal pressure hydrocephalus with Alzheimer disease pathology. Ann Neurol. 2010;68:535–40.
36. Dyrby TB, Søgaard LV, Parker GJ, Alexander DC, Lind NM, Baaré WF, et al. Validation of in vitro probabilistic tractography. Neuroimage. 2007;37:1266–77.
37. Melhem ER, Itoh R, Jones L, Barker PB. Diffusion tensor MR imaging of the brain: effect of diffusion weighting on trace and anisotropy measurements. AJNR Am J Neuroradiol. 2000;21:1813–20.

11

In vitro characterization of pralidoxime transport and acetylcholinesterase reactivation across MDCK cells and stem cell-derived human brain microvascular endothelial cells (BC1-hBMECs)

Erin Gallagher[1,2], Il Minn[3], Janice E. Chambers[4] and Peter C. Searson[1,2*]

Abstract

Background: Current therapies for organophosphate poisoning involve administration of oximes, such as pralidoxime (2-PAM), that reactivate the enzyme acetylcholinesterase. Studies in animal models have shown a low concentration in the brain following systemic injection.

Methods: To assess 2-PAM transport, we studied transwell permeability in three Madin-Darby canine kidney (MDCKII) cell lines and stem cell-derived human brain microvascular endothelial cells (BC1-hBMECs). To determine whether 2-PAM is a substrate for common brain efflux pumps, experiments were performed in the MDCKII-MDR1 cell line, transfected to overexpress the P-gp efflux pump, and the MDCKII-FLuc-ABCG2 cell line, transfected to overexpress the BCRP efflux pump. To determine how transcellular transport influences enzyme reactivation, we developed a modified transwell assay where the inhibited acetylcholinesterase enzyme, substrate, and reporter are introduced into the basolateral chamber. Enzymatic activity was inhibited using paraoxon and parathion.

Results: The permeability of 2-PAM is about 2×10^{-6} cm s^{-1} in MDCK cells and about 1×10^{-6} cm s^{-1} in BC1-hBMECs. Permeability is not influenced by pre-treatment with atropine. In addition, 2-PAM is not a substrate for the P-gp or BCRP efflux pumps.

Conclusions: The low permeability explains poor brain penetration of 2-PAM and therefore the slow enzyme reactivation. This elucidates one of the reasons for the necessity of sustained intravascular (IV) infusion in response to organophosphate poisoning.

Background

The blood–brain barrier (BBB) is a dynamic system responsible for maintaining homeostasis by regulating the chemical environment, immune cell transport, and the entry of toxins into the CNS [1–3]. Neurotoxins are microorganisms, viruses, bacterial toxins, and chemicals that disrupt neurological function [2, 4]. Organophosphates (OPs) are a class of chemical neurotoxicants comprised of a central phosphate surrounded by electronegative atoms, such as oxygen and sulfur. While widely used as insecticides, nerve agents such as sarin and VX, are also organophosphates [5]. In the brain and body, organophosphates persistently bind to the active site of acetylcholinesterase, blocking breakdown of the neurotransmitter acetylcholine [6, 7].

Organophosphate poisoning is usually treated with oximes, such as pralidoxime (2-PAM), that reactivate acetylcholinesterase [7]. The FDA protocol for organophosphate poisoning involves immediate intramuscular

*Correspondence: searson@jhu.edu
[1] Institute for Nanobiotechnology Johns Hopkins University, 3400 North Charles Street, Baltimore, MD 21218, USA
Full list of author information is available at the end of the article

(IM) injection followed by intravascular (IV) administration [6, 8]. IM injection of 2-PAM is usually co-administered with atropine and/or diazepam. Typical IV dosing of 2-PAM, depending on symptoms and exposure pathway, involves administration of 1 g in 100 mL^{-1} saline over 15–30 min followed by continuous infusion of 500 mg h^{-1} (about 700 μM in blood) [6, 7].

2-PAM is an ionic molecule and hence the permeability across the blood–brain barrier has been assumed to be very low [9, 10]. Clinical trials have shown that 2-PAM is rapidly cleared from the body [11, 12], highlighting the need for continuous infusion to maintain a therapeutic dose [11, 13–15]. Based on animal studies, the minimum effective concentration in blood is reported to be around 4 mg L^{-1} (about 30 μM) [9, 15].

Therefore, to assess transport into the brain we studied permeability of 2-PAM in four cell lines: MDCKII, MDCKII-MDR1, MDCKII-FLuc-ABCG2, and BC1-hBMECs. Madin-Darby canine kidney epithelial cells (MDCKs) are widely used for in vitro assessment of brain penetration and the permeability values for a wide range of solutes have been reported [16]. The MDCKII-MDR1 cell line is transfected to express the human P-gp efflux pump, and the MDCKII-FLuc-ABCG2 line is transfected to overexpress BCRP efflux pump. Human brain microvascular endothelial cells (BC1-hBMECs) are derived from human-induced pluripotent stem cells (hiPSCs) [17–19].

Materials

Cell lines

MDCKII and MDCKII-MDR1 cells were obtained from the Netherlands Cancer Institute (NKI) [20]. Following NKI's protocol, cells were cultured in DMEM (High Glucose, GlutaMAX) with 10 % Fetal Bovine Serum (FBS, ATCC, Manassas, VA, USA), and 1 % penicillin–streptomycin (ATCC). MDCKII/ABCG2 cells expressing ABCG2/BCRP were provided by the Pomper Group (JHU). MDCKII cells were transfected with pGL4.16 [luc2cp/Hygro] (Promega, Madison, WI, USA) [21, 22]. Cells were maintained in MEM-L-glutamine (Life Tech, Carlsbad, CA, USA), 10 % FBS HI, 1 mg mL^{-1} G418 (Geneticin, Life Tech), and 100 μg mL^{-1} Hygromycin B (Life Tech) [22].

Human brain microvascular endothelial cells (BC1-hBMECs) were derived from iPSCs, based on a protocol reported by Lippmann et al. [17, 18]. Briefly, BC1 iPSCs [23] were cultured for 4 days in TeSR-E8 Basal Medium (05940, Stem Cell Technologies, Vancouver, BC, Canada) on growth factor-reduced Matrigel, 40 μg mL^{-1} (354230, Fisher Scientific, Pittsburgh, PA, USA) [19]. Once cells formed substantial colonies, they were placed in UM/F- unconditioned media (DMEM/F12, 20 % KOSR, 0.5 % L-glutamine, 1 % NEAA, 0.836 μM Beta-Mercaptoethanol) for 6 days. For the final 2 days of differentiation, the cells were placed in endothelial cell serum-free media (EC, 1 % human platelet poor-derived serum, 20 ng mL^{-1} bFGF) with 10 μM all trans retinoic acid (Sigma, St. Louis, MO, USA) to promote preferential growth of the BC1-hBMECs. The cells were then sub-cultured onto the transwell supports coated with collagen IV (100 μg mL^{-1}; Sigma) and fibronectin (50 μg mL^{-1}; Sigma) and cultured for two more days prior to performing permeability experiments [19]. Characterization of the BC1-hBMEC cells has been reported elsewhere [19].

Permeability measurements

2-PAM

MDCK cells were seeded on transwells (24 well; PE; 0.33 cm^2 area; 0.4 μm pore diameter, Corning, Corning, NY, USA) coated with collagen I (rat tail, 10 μg cm^{-2}, Corning) at a density of 6×10^5 cells cm^{-2}. Permeability experiments were performed 4 days after seeding. The medium was changed 2 h before the experiment and transepithelial electrical resistance (TEER) was measured before all experiments (Endohm/EVOM2). For MDCK cells, permeability measurements were performed if the TEER was ≥90 Ω cm^2 (see Additional file 1: Table S1: TEER values for transwell experiments) [24, 25]. To confirm the integrity of the MDCK monolayers, the permeability of Lucifer yellow, 100 μM, was measured for up to 2 h. In all cases the permeability was $\leq 1 \times 10^{-6}$ cm s^{-1}: $0.71 \pm 0.34 \times 10^{-6}$ cm s^{-1} (MDCKII), $0.38 \pm 0.20 \times 10^{-6}$ cm s^{-1} (MDCKII-MDR1), and $0.46 \pm 0.21 \times 10^{-6}$ cm s^{-1} (MDCKII-FLuc-ABCG2). The measured permeability for Lucifer yellow under the same conditions in transwells without cells, was 4.35×10^{-5} cm s^{-1}.

All experiments with MDCK cells were performed in Hank's balanced salt solution (HBSS) with 10 mM HEPES (Sigma) and 15 mM glucose (Sigma), pH 7.4. After incubation in media for 2 h, cell monolayers were immersed in fresh HBSS for 30 min to remove any traces of media. Then 100 μM or 10 μM 2-PAM (pralidoxime chloride, Sigma) in HBSS was pipetted into either the apical or basolateral chamber, with HBSS on the receiving side. Cell monolayers with test solutes were incubated at 37 °C with 5 % CO_2 on a rocker to ensure good mixing.

For experiments with BC1-hBMECs, cells were seeded on transwells (24 well; PE; 0.33 cm^2 area; 0.4 μm pore diameter, Corning) coated overnight with a 50/50 mixture collagen IV (100 μg mL^{-1}; Sigma) and fibronectin (50 μg mL^{-1}; Sigma) at a density of 1×10^6 cells mL^{-1}. For BC1-hBMECs, permeability measurements were performed with cells that had a TEER of ≥1500 Ω cm^2. Experiments were performed in transport buffer (distilled Millipore water with 0.12 M NaCl, 25 mM $NaHCO_3$, 3 mM KCl, 2 mM $MgSO_4$, 2 mM $CaCl_2$, 0.4 mM K_2HPO_4,

1 mM HEPES, and 0.1 % human platelet poor-derived serum) without the pre-incubation of media or rocking of the cells. After 2 days in EC media, 100 μM of 2-PAM in transport buffer was pipetted into the apical or basolateral well with transport buffer on the receiving side.

The concentration of 2-PAM was determined by HPLC (1260 Infinity HPLC, Agilent, Santa Clara, CA, USA) with UV Vis detection at 296 nm. Solvents were degassed by sonication for 45 min before use and all samples were run at room temperature. An isocratic flow of 44 vol.% acetonitrile (HPLC grade, Chromasolv, Sigma) and 56 vol.% ammonium acetate (0.03 M; HPLC grade, Sigma), pH 4.5, was used with a PolyCAT A column (100 × 2.1 mm, 5 μM, 300 Å, 102CT05-03, Poly LC Inc, Columbia, MD, USA) [26]. Calibration curves were constructed from standard solutions with concentrations of 0.1, 1, 10 and 100 μM. Due to the simplicity of the procedure, no internal standard was used.

2-PAM/atropine

To assess whether atropine, which is often co-administered with 2-PAM, modulates the transport of 2-PAM we performed experiments where MDCK cells were pretreated with atropine. After 2 h incubation in media, and 30 min rinse in HBSS, MDCKII monolayers were pretreated with 1 μM atropine for 30 min, rinsed in HBSS for 5 min, and then incubated in 100 μM 2-PAM for permeability measurements using the same procedure as described above. 2-PAM concentrations were measured by HPLC with an isocratic flow of 55 vol.% acetonitrile and 45 vol.% ammonium acetate (0.03 M).

Rhodamine 123

To confirm the up-regulation and polarization of P-gp efflux pumps to the apical face, we measured the permeability of Rhodamine 123, a known P-gp substrate, across MDCKII and MDCKII. MDR1 monolayers [27]. Permeability experiments were performed for 60 min at a concentration of 50 μM. The concentration of Rhodamine 123 (excitation 486 and emission 523) was measured by fluorescence (Fluorolog, Horiba Scientific, Edison, NJ, USA). Calibration curves were generated over the concentration range from 0.001 to 1 μM.

Coupled permeability and acetylcholinesterase reactivation

To assess coupled 2-PAM transport and enzyme reactivation, experiments were performed in a transwell device with acetylcholinesterase in the basolateral chamber. Confluent monolayers of MDCKII cells were formed as described above. Electric eel acetylcholinesterase (AChE, 1U or about 1 μL, >1000 U/mg, Sigma) was placed into the basolateral chamber (24 well plate). A mixture of Ellman's reagent (DTNB), final concentration 300 μM, and acetylthiocholine (ASCh), final concentration 450 μM, dissolved in HBSS, was introduced into the basolateral chamber, to give a final volume of 600 μL. The time-dependent activity of the enzyme was determined from the absorbance of the DTNB reporter at 412 nm using a plate reader (Spectramax M3). Results were normalized to the activity of the uninhibited enzyme, unnormalized data are provided in the Additional file 1 (Figure S1: Non-normalized reactivation data).

Inhibition was achieved by incubating the enzyme with 0.72 mM parathion (PESTANAL-grade, Sigma) or 4.6 μM paraoxon (PESTANAL-grade, Sigma) for 20 min prior to experiments. In inhibition experiments, the enzyme was inhibited with parathion. Paraoxon, a metabolite of parathion, is about three orders of magnitude more potent as an anticholinesterase inhibitor [28]. The parathion concentration was 157-fold higher than the paraoxon concentration, reflecting their different activities. For reactivation experiments, 2-PAM was introduced into either the apical or basolateral chamber in HBSS. Introducing 2-PAM into the basolateral chamber simulates reactivation alone, whereas introduction of 2-PAM into the apical chamber simulates coupled trans-endothelial transport and reactivation.

Positive control (uninhibited enzyme + substrate)

To assess the kinetics of enzyme interaction with the substrate, uninhibited enzyme (AChE), along with substrate (ASCh), and reporter (DTNB) in HBSS were introduced into the basolateral chamber. An apical transwell chamber with a monolayer of MDCK cells was located on the top of the basolateral chamber to ensure that the control was performed in the same way as the other experiments.

Negative control (inhibited enzyme + substrate)

To assess the efficiency of enzyme inhibition, AChE was mixed for 20 min with concentrated parathion (0.72 mM final concentration) or paraoxon (4.6 μM final concentration) organophosphates (OP). The inhibited enzyme (AChE-OP) was then placed in the basolateral chamber with substrate (ASCh) and reporter (DTNB) in HBSS. An apical transwell chamber was located on the top of the basolateral chamber as described above.

Direct interaction of 2-PAM (inhibited enzyme + substrate + reactivator)

To assess the kinetics of direct reactivation of inhibited enzyme, 100 μM 2-PAM was introduced in the basolateral chamber with the inhibited enzyme (AChE-OP), substrate (ASCh) and reporter (DTNB) in HBSS. An apical transwell chamber was located on the top of the basolateral chamber as described above.

Coupled transport of 2-PAM and reactivation

To evaluate the coupled transport of 2-PAM across a cell monolayer and reactivation of inhibited enzyme, 100 μM of 2-PAM was introduced into the apical chamber, with inhibited enzyme (AChE-OP), reporter (DTNB), and substrate (ASCH) in the basolateral chamber.

Statistics

Permeability, activity, and reactivation half-time represent the mean ± standard deviation. Statistical significance was determined using a student's t test (two-tailed with unequal variance) with $p < 0.01$ ** and $p < 0.001$ ***. The average permeability values for the MDCK cell lines were calculated from analysis of all of the replicates. Due to variations between differentiations, the average permeability across the BC1-hBMECs was calculated from the average values from each differentiation. Similarly, the efflux ratio was calculated from the average value obtained from each differentiation.

Results

Permeability of 2-PAM

To assess the transport of 2-PAM and to determine whether 2-PAM is an efflux pump substrate, transwell experiments were performed in three cell lines: MDCKII, MDCKII-MDR1, MDCKII-FLuc-ABCG2 at concentrations of 10 and 100 μM (Table 1; Fig. 1). In 10 μM 2-PAM, the average apical-to-basolateral permeability in MDCKII and MDCKII-MDR1 monolayers was about 2×10^{-6} cm s^{-1}. The average permeability of MDCKII-ABCG2 monolayers was slightly lower, 0.83×10^{-6} cm s^{-1}, although the difference compared to the MDCKII and MDCKII-MDR1 monolayers was not significant. For 100 μM 2-PAM, the average permeability in MDCKII and MDCKII-MDR1 monolayers increased to about 3×10^{-6} cm s^{-1}; this increase was significant in MDCKII cells ($p = 0.05$), but not significant in MDCKII-MDR1 cells. The average permeability in MDCKII-ABCG2 cells was 0.76×10^{-6} cm s^{-1}, very close to the value in 10 μM 2-PAM. The average basolateral-to-apical permeability was very close to the apical-to-basolateral value in all three cell lines with no statistical difference. The apical-to-basolateral permeability of 2-PAM across the stem-cell derived BC1-hBMECs was $1.12 \pm 0.80 \times 10^{-6}$ cm s^{-1}, comparable to the permeability across the MDCKII cells. The basolateral-to-apical permeability ($0.49 \pm 0.16 \times 10^{-6}$ cm s^{-1}) was lower ($p = 0.05$).

Influence of atropine on 2-PAM permeability

To determine whether atropine, co-administered with 2-PAM, modulates the permeability of 2-PAM, we measured the permeability of 2-PAM following pre-treatment of the MDCKII monolayer with atropine. The permeability of 2-PAM was $2.54 \pm 0.33 \times 10^{-6}$ cm s^{-1}, which was not significantly different to the value of $2.99 \pm 1.12 \times 10^{-6}$ cm s^{-1} obtained without pre-treatment with atropine (Table 1).

Table 1 Permeability of pralidoxime (2-PAM), rhodamine 123 R123) and Lucifer yellow (Ly) across MDCKII, MDCKII-MDR1, MDCKII-FLuc-ABCG2, and BC1-hBMEC monolayers

	P_{app} A→B (cm s^{-1})	N	P_{app} B→A (cm s^{-1})	N	Efflux ratio
100 μM 2-PAM					
MDCKII	$2.99 \pm 1.12 \times 10^{-6}$	11	$2.48 \pm 1.30 \times 10^{-6}$	8	0.82
MDCKII-MDR1	$3.01 \pm 1.27 \times 10^{-6}$	8	$2.51 \pm 1.08 \times 10^{-6}$	7	0.83
MDCKII-FLuc-ABCG2	$0.76 \pm 0.05 \times 10^{-6}$	7	$0.98 \pm 0.40 \times 10^{-6}$	7	1.30
BC1-hBMECs	$1.12 \pm 0.80 \times 10^{-6}$ (n = 5)	18	$0.49 \pm 0.16 \times 10^{-6}$ (n = 3)	12	0.84
10 μM 2-PAM					
MDCKII	$1.62 \pm 0.21 \times 10^{-6}$	6	$1.29 \pm 1.76 \times 10^{-6}$	7	0.80
MDCKII-MDR1	$2.03 \pm 0.14 \times 10^{-6}$	8	$1.18 \pm 0.45 \times 10^{-6}$	8	0.58
MDCKII-FLuc-ABCG2	$0.83 \pm 0.35 \times 10^{-6}$	7	$0.99 \pm 0.62 \times 10^{-6}$	7	1.18
50 μM R123					
MDCKII	$0.30 \pm 0.20 \times 10^{-6}$	6	$3.18 \pm 0.60 \times 10^{-6}$	5	10.7
MDCKII-MDR1	$0.21 \pm 0.21 \times 10^{-6}$	12	$4.36 \pm 0.41 \times 10^{-6}$	11	20.3
100 μM LY					
MDCKII	$0.71 \pm 0.34 \times 10^{-6}$	7			
MDCKII-MDR1	$0.38 \pm 0.20 \times 10^{-6}$	7			
MDCKII-FLuc-ABCG2	$0.46 \pm 0.21 \times 10^{-6}$	8			
2-PAM atropine					
MDCKII	$2.54 \pm 0.33 \times 10^{-6}$	7			

A→B represents apical-to-basolateral permeability, and B→A represents basolateral-to-apical permeability. Permeability values are reported as mean ± standard deviation. The efflux ratio is the ratio of basolateral-to-apical permeability divided by the apical-to-basolateral permeability. For MDCK cells, permeabilities and efflux ratios were calculated from the total number of replicates (N). Data were obtained from at least three independent experiments each with two or more replicates. For the BC1-hBMECs, the permeabilities and efflux ratios were calculated from the average of each differentiation, where N represents the number of independent differentiations

Permeability of rhodamine 123

To confirm the polarization of the P-gp efflux pumps to the apical surface of the MDCK cells, we measured the permeability of 50 μM rhodamine 123, a known substrate for the P-gp efflux pump [27, 29], in MDCKII and MDCKII-MDR1 cells (Table 1). The basolateral-to-apical permeability of rhodamine 123 in MDCKII was 3.18×10^{-6} cm s^{-1}, with an apical-to-basolateral permeability of 0.30×10^{-6} cm s^{-1} ($p = 0.001$), corresponding to an efflux ratio of 10.7. For the MDCKII-MDR1 cells, the basolateral-to-apical permeability was 4.36×10^{-6} cm s^{-1}, with an apical-to-basolateral permeability of 0.22×10^{-6} cm s^{-1} ($p = 0.001$) corresponding to an efflux ratio of 20.3. The basolateral-to-apical permeabilities to

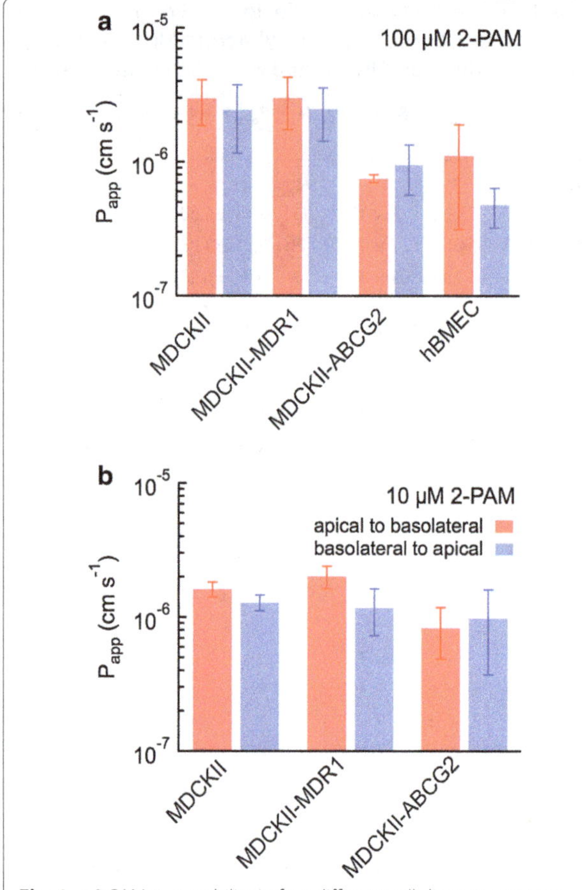

Fig. 1 **a** 2-PAM permeability in four different cells lines at a concentration of 100 μM. **b** 2-PAM permeability of in three different cells lines at a concentration of 10 μM. Basolateral-to-apical (*red*), basolateral-to-apical (*blue*). Permeability is reported as mean ± standard deviation. Experiments were performed in HBSS (MDCKII, MDCKII-MDR1, MDCKII-ABCG2) or transport buffer (BC1-hBMEC)

rhodamine in MDCKII and MDCKII. MDR1 cells were significantly different ($p = 0.02$) supporting upregulation and polarization of P-gp efflux pumps to the apical side of the MDCKII.MDR1 cells. Apical-to-basolateral permeabilities of 0.83×10^{-6} and 0.89×10^{-6} cm s^{-1}, with corresponding efflux ratios of 9 and 115, have been reported for transport of 5 μM rhodamine 123 across MDCKII. MDR1 cells [27, 29]. The reported efflux ratio for rhodamine in BC1-hBMEC cells is approximately 4 [19].

Coupled transport and acetylcholinesterase (AChE) reactivation

To assess the coupled transcellular transport and AChE reactivation, we performed transwell experiments with a monolayer of MDCKII cells and inhibited enzyme in the basolateral chamber (Fig. 2a). Acetylcholinesterase was inhibited with an organophosphate (parathion or paraoxon) for 20 min and then introduced into the basolateral chamber of a transwell device, along with acetylthiocholine (ASCh) and the colorimetric reporter (DTNB). Control experiments were performed to confirm the activity of the enzyme and effectiveness of the inhibitor.

In the absence of 2-PAM, the activity of the inhibited enzyme (AChE-OP) increased very slowly during the 2 h experiment (Fig. 2b). When 2-PAM was introduced into the basolateral chamber with inhibited enzyme, reactivation occurred much more quickly (Parathion: inhibited enzyme and direct reactivation $p < 0.001$, Paraoxon: inhibited enzyme and direct reactivation $p < 0.01$). However, when 2-PAM was introduced into the apical chamber, reactivation of the inhibited enzyme was slowed considerably due to the coupled transport and reactivation (Parathion: direct reactivation and transport reactivation $p < 0.001$, paraoxon: direct reactivation and transport reactivation $p < 0.01$).

The activity of the enzyme following transcellular transport of 2-PAM across MDCKII monolayers (3.49×10^{-4} abs s^{-1}) was about four fold lower than when the inhibited enzyme was directly exposed to 2-PAM (1.35×10^{-3} abs s^{-1}) (Fig. 2c). Similarly, the half-time for reactivation of the substrate increased sixfold from 680 s for direct reactivation to 4100 s following transcellular transport (Fig. 2d).

Discussion

Transendothelial transport

The permeability of 2-PAM was between 1×10^{-6} and 2×10^{-6} cm s^{-1} in all three MDCK cell lines, lower than for most central nervous system drugs, which typically have permeabilities greater than 1×10^{-5} cm s^{-1} [30]. However several CNS drugs have permeabilities similar to 2-PAM, including the antipsychotics perphenazine ($p = 1.8 \times 10^{-6}$ cm s^{-1}) and fluphenazine ($p = 3.5 \times 10^{-6}$ cm s^{-1}), the anti-anxiety drug sertralin (Zoloft) ($p = 2.1 \times 10^{-6}$ cm s^{-1}), and the analgesic, morphine ($p = 2 \times 10^{-6}$ cm s^{-1}) [16]. While morphine has a low permeability in MDCK cells, the therapeutic dose is particularly low [16]. The low permeability of 2-PAM explains the reported low concentration in the brain in animal studies [10] and the recommended sustained clinical infusion in a clinical setting [6].

MDCK cells are widely used to assess brain penetration of small molecules. Although MDCK cell lines are epithelial in origin and not human, they express tight junction proteins, which limit paracellular transport. Variants such as MDCKII-MDR1 can be used to determine whether a solute is an efflux pump substrate. The stem cell derived BC1-hBMECs exhibit high transendothelial electrical resistance (TEER > 1000 Ω cm^2), low permeability to solutes such as Lucifer yellow, and

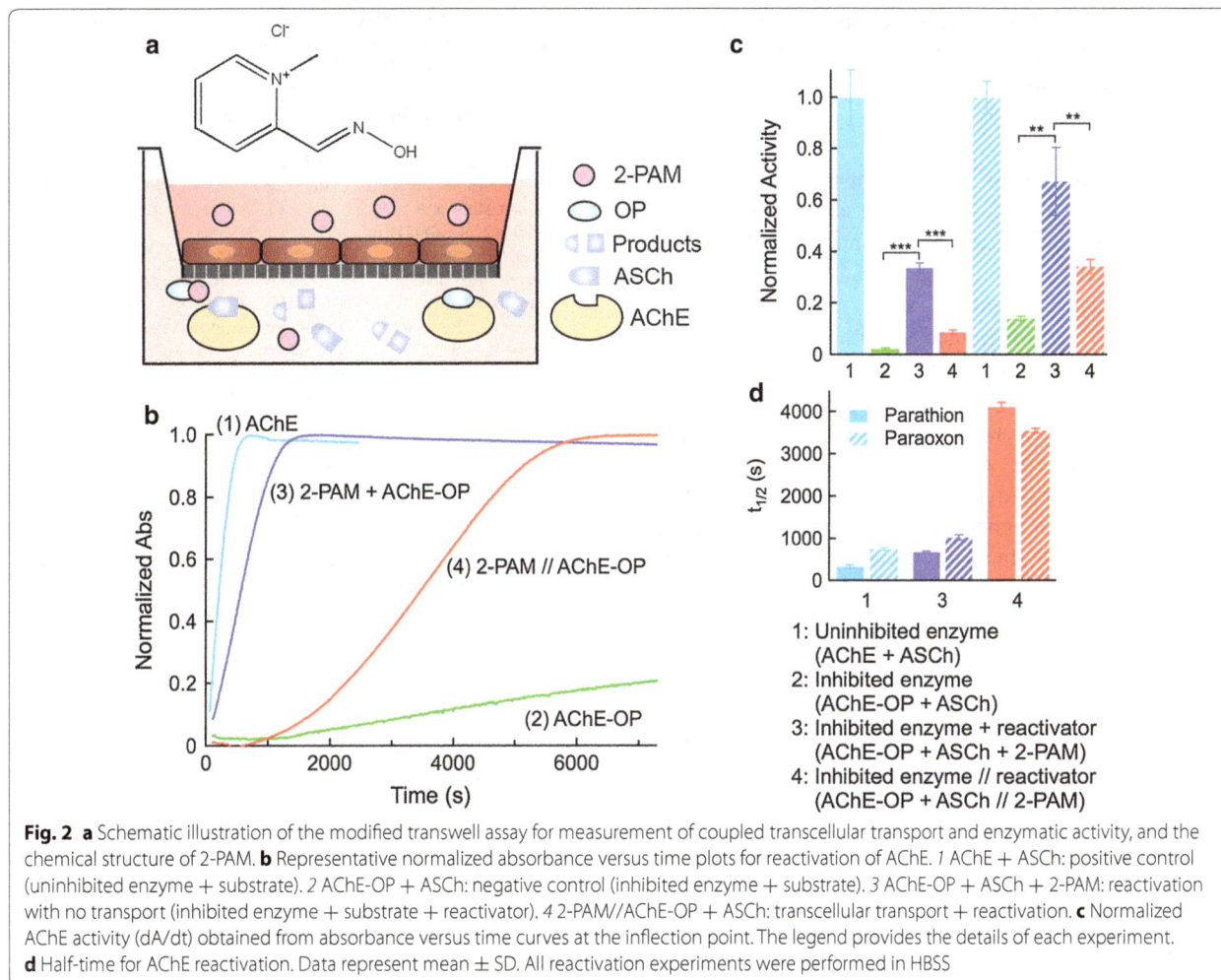

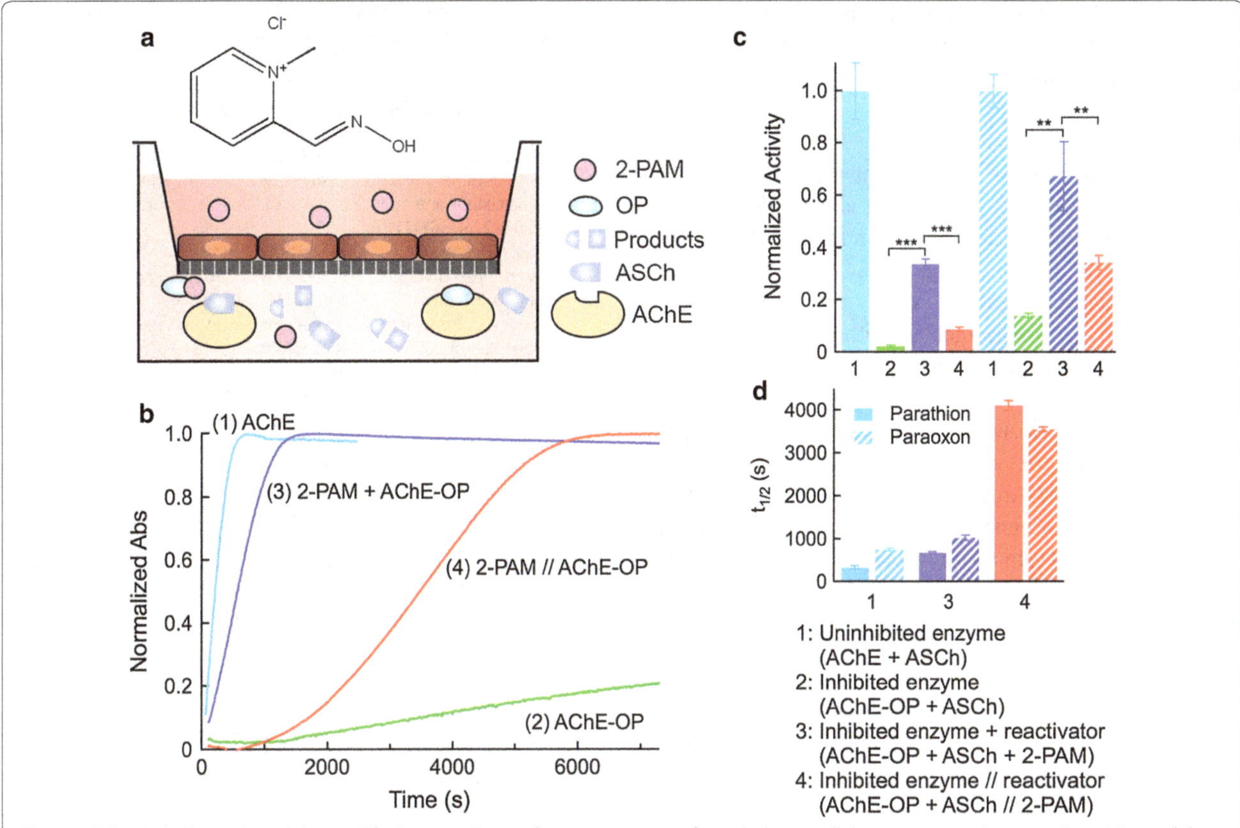

Fig. 2 **a** Schematic illustration of the modified transwell assay for measurement of coupled transcellular transport and enzymatic activity, and the chemical structure of 2-PAM. **b** Representative normalized absorbance versus time plots for reactivation of AChE. *1* AChE + ASCh: positive control (uninhibited enzyme + substrate). *2* AChE-OP + ASCh: negative control (inhibited enzyme + substrate). *3* AChE-OP + ASCh + 2-PAM: reactivation with no transport (inhibited enzyme + substrate + reactivator). *4* 2-PAM//AChE-OP + ASCh: transcellular transport + reactivation. **c** Normalized AChE activity (dA/dt) obtained from absorbance versus time curves at the inflection point. The legend provides the details of each experiment. **d** Half-time for AChE reactivation. Data represent mean ± SD. All reactivation experiments were performed in HBSS

express tight junction proteins (e.g. claudin-5), transporters (e.g. LAT-1), and efflux pumps (e.g. P-gp) [17, 19]. The permeability of the stem cell derived BC1-hBMECs ($p = 1.12 \pm 0.80 \times 10^{-6}$ cm s^{-1}) was slightly lower than values obtained in MDCK cells, but in the range that is consistent with slow accumulation in the brain.

High permeability values are usually associated with small molecular weight and moderate lipophilicity [31, 32]. While 2-PAM has a molecular weight under 500 Da (172 Da), fewer than 5 hydrogen bond donors (1), and fewer than 10 hydrogen bond acceptors (2), the charge results in a low lipophilicity and hence 2-PAM is not expected to have a high permeability.

There was no significant difference between apical-and-basolateral and basolateral-to-apical permeabilities in MDCK cells, indicating that 2-PAM is not a substrate of the P-gp or ABCG2 pumps. To confirm the polarized expression and activity of the P-gp efflux pumps, we determined efflux ratios of 10.7 and 20.3 for the MDCKII and MDCKII. MDR1 cell lines for the known P-gp substrate rhodamine 123.

Treatment for organophosphate poisoning involves co-administration of 2-PAM and atropine. The permeability of 2-PAM was the same in MDCKII cells and cells pretreated with atropine, showing that atropine does not modulate the permeability of 2-PAM.

Coupled transcellular transport and enzyme reactivation

To study coupled transcellular transport of the neurotoxin antidote 2-PAM with enzyme reactivation, we developed a modified transwell assay with inhibited enzyme (AChE-OP), substrate (ASCh), and reporter (DTNB) in the basolateral chamber. When 2-PAM was introduced into the apical chamber of the transwell device, the activity of the enzyme decreased four fold compared to the case where 2-PAM was introduced directly into the basolateral chamber. Similarly, the half-time for reactivation of the enzyme increased six fold when coupled to transcellular transport. These results highlight the difficulty in maintaining a therapeutic dose when the permeability is low.

Conclusions

The permeability of the nerve agent reactivator 2-PAM is $1 \times 10^{-6} - 2 \times 10^{-6}$ cm s^{-1} and is not influenced by pre-treatment with atropine. In addition, 2-PAM is not a substrate for the P-gp or BCRP/ABCG2 efflux pumps. Similar permeability values were obtained for human brain microvascular endothelial cells derived from induced pluripotent stem cells. In a modified transwell assay to couple transcellular transport and enzyme reactivation, we showed that transcellular transport decreased enzymatic activity four fold and increased the reactivation half-time six fold. The low permeability explains poor brain penetration of 2-PAM and the necessity for sustained IV infusion in response to organophosphate poisoning.

Abbreviations

MDCK: Madin-Darby canine kidney epithelial cells; 2-PAM: pralidoxime chloride; BC1-hBMEC: stem cell derived human brain microvascular endothelial cells; TEER: transendothelial electrical resistance; MDR1: multi-drug resistance gene; P-gp: P-glycoprotein; ABCG2: ATP-binding cassette sub-family G member 2; BCRP: breast cancer resistance protein; ASCh: acetylthiocholine; AChE: acetylcholinesterase; AChE-OP: inhibited enzyme; DTNB: 5,5′-dithiobis-(2-nitrobenzoic acid) (Ellman's reagent).

Authors' contributions

EG performed the experiments. EG and PS analyzed the data. EG, IM, JC, and PS wrote the manuscript. All authors read and approved the final manuscript.

Author details

[1] Institute for Nanobiotechnology Johns Hopkins University, 3400 North Charles Street, Baltimore, MD 21218, USA. [2] Department of Materials Science and Engineering, Johns Hopkins University, 3400 North Charles Street, Baltimore, MD 21218, USA. [3] Department of Radiology and Radiological Science, Johns Hopkins University, 3400 North Charles Street, Baltimore, MD 21231, USA. [4] College of Veterinary Medicine, Mississippi State University, Mississippi State, MS 39762-6100, USA.

Acknowledgements

The authors gratefully acknowledge support from DTRA (HDTRA1-15-1-0046).

Competing interests

The authors declare that they have no competing interests.

References

1. Pardridge WM. Drug transport across the blood–brain barrier. J Cereb Blood Flow Metab. 2012;32(11):1959–72. doi:10.1038/jcbfm.2012.126.
2. Salinas S, Schiavo G, Kremer EJ. A Hitchhiker's guide to the nervous system: the complex journey of viruses and toxins. Nat Rev Microbiol. 2010;8(9):645–55. doi:10.1038/nrmicro2395.
3. Abbott NJ, Ronnback L, Hansson E. Astrocyte-endothelial interactions at the blood–brain barrier. Nat Rev Neurosci. 2006;7(1):41–53. doi:10.1038/nrn1824.
4. Dando SJ, Mackay-Sim A, Norton R, Currie BJ, St John JA, Ekberg JA, et al. Pathogens penetrating the central nervous system: infection pathways and the cellular and molecular mechanisms of invasion. Clin Microbiol Rev. 2014;27(4):691–726. doi:10.1128/CMR.00118-13.
5. Colovic MB, Krstic DZ, Lazarevic-Pasti TD, Bondzic AM, Vasic VM. Acetylcholinesterase inhibitors: pharmacology and toxicology. Curr Neuropharmacol. 2013;11(3):315–35. doi:10.2174/1570159X11311030006.
6. Holstege CP, Dobmeier SG. Nerve agent toxicity and treatment. Curr Treat Options Neurol. 2005;7(2):91–8. doi:10.1007/s11940-005-0018-y.
7. Wiener SW, Hoffman RS. Nerve agents: a comprehensive review. J Intensive Care Med. 2004;19(1):22–37. doi:10.1177/0885066603258659.
8. FDA. PROTOPAM Chloride (pralidoxime chloride) for injection. New Drug Application (NDA): U.S. Food and Drug Administration 2010 September 8, 2010 Contract No.: 014134/S-022.
9. Kassa J. Review of oximes in the antidotal treatment of poisoning by organophosphorus nerve agents. J Toxicol Clin Toxic. 2002;40(6):803–16.
10. Lorke DE, Nurulain SM, Hasan MY, Kuca K, Musilek K, Petroianu GA. Eight new bispyridinium oximes in comparison with the conventional oximes pralidoxime and obidoxime: in vivo efficacy to protect from diisopropylfluorophosphate toxicity. J Appl Toxicol. 2008;28(7):920–8. doi:10.1002/jat.1359.
11. Medicis JJ, Stork CM, Howland MA, Hoffman RS, Goldfrank LR. Pharmacokinetics following a loading plus a continuous infusion of pralidoxime compared with the traditional short infusion regimen in human volunteers. J Toxicol Clin Toxic. 1996;34(3):289–95.
12. Abbara C, Rousseau JM, Lelievre B, Turcant A, Lallement G, Ferec S, et al. Pharmacokinetic analysis of pralidoxime after its intramuscular injection alone or in combination with atropine–avizafone in healthy volunteers. Br J Pharmacol. 2010;161(8):1857–67. doi:10.1111/j.1476-5381.2010.01007.x.
13. Jovanovic D. Pharmacokinetics of pralidoxime chloride: a comparative study in healthy volunteers and in organophosphorus poisoning. Arch Toxicol. 1989;63(5):416–8.
14. Willems JL, Debisschop HC, Verstraete AG, Declerck C, Christiaens Y, Vanscheeuwyck P, et al. Cholinesterase reactivation in organophosphorus poisoned patients depends on the plasma-concentrations of the oxime pralidoxime methylsulfate and of the organophosphate. Arch Toxicol. 1993;67(2):79–84. doi:10.1007/Bf01973675.
15. Schexnayder S, James LP, Kearns GL, Farrar HC. The pharmacokinetics of continuous infusion pralidoxime in children with organophosphate poisoning. J Toxicol Clin Toxic. 1998;36(6):549–55.
16. Summerfield SG, Read K, Begley DJ, Obradovic T, Hidalgo IJ, Coggon S, et al. Central nervous system drug disposition: the relationship between in situ brain permeability and brain free fraction. J Pharmacol Exp Ther. 2007;322(1):205–13. doi:10.1124/jpet.107.121525.
17. Lippmann ES, Azarin SM, Kay JE, Nessler RA, Wilson HK, Al-Ahmad A, et al. Derivation of blood-brain barrier endothelial cells from human pluripotent stem cells. Nat Biotechnol. 2012;30(8):783–91. doi:10.1038/nbt.2247.
18. Lippmann ES, Al-Ahmad A, Azarin SM, Palecek SP, Shusta EV. A retinoic acid-enhanced, multicellular human blood-brain barrier model derived from stem cell sources. Sci Rep. 2014;4:4160. doi:10.1038/srep04160.
19. Katt ME, Xu ZS, Gerecht S, Searson PC. Human brain microvascular endothelial cells derived from the BC1 iPS cell line exhibit a blood-brain barrier phenotype. PLoS ONE. 2016;11(4):e0152105. doi:10.1371/journal.pone.0152105.
20. Evers R, Kool M, Smith AJ, Van Deemter L, De Haas M, Borst P. Inhibitory effect of the reversal agents V-104, GF120918 and Pluronic L61 on MDR1 Pgp-, MRP1- and MRP2-mediated transport. Br J Cancer. 2000;83(3):366–74. doi:10.1054/bjoc.2000.1260.
21. Zhang YM, Bressler JP, Neal J, Lal B, Bhang HEC, Laterra J, et al. ABCG2/BCRP expression modulates D-luciferin-based bioluminescence imaging. Cancer Res. 2007;67(19):9389–97. doi:10.1158/0008-5472.CAN-07-0944.

22. Zhang Y, Byun Y, Ren YR, Liu JO, Laterra J, Pomper MG. Identification of inhibitors of ABCG2 by a bioluminescence imaging-based high-throughput assay. Cancer Res. 2009;69(14):5867–75. doi:10.1158/0008-5472.CAN-08-4866.
23. Chou BK, Mali P, Huang X, Ye Z, Dowey SN, Resar LM, et al. Efficient human iPS cell derivation by a non-integrating plasmid from blood cells with unique epigenetic and gene expression signatures. Cell Res. 2011;21(3):518–29. doi:10.1038/cr.2011.12.
24. Dukes JD, Whitley P, Chalmers AD. The MDCK variety pack: choosing the right strain. Bmc Cell Biol. 2011;12:1. doi:10.1186/1471-2121-12-43.
25. Avdeef A, Deli MA, Neuhaus W. In vitro assays for assessing BBB permeability: artificial membrane and cell culture models. In: Di L, Kerns EH, editors. Blood–brain barrier in drug discovery: optimizing brain exposure of CNS drugs and minimizing brain side effects for peripheral drugs. New York: Wiley; 2015. p. 188–237.
26. Singh H, Moorad-Doctor D, Ratcliffe RH, Wachtel K, Castillo A, Garcia GE. A rapid cation-exchange HPLC method for detection and quantification of pyridinium oximes in plasma and tissue. J Anal Toxicol. 2007;31(2):69–74.
27. Tang F, Ouyang H, Yang JZ, Borchardt RT. Bidirectional transport of rhodamine 123 and Hoechst 33342, fluorescence probes of the binding sites on P-glycoprotein, across MDCK-MDR1 cell monolayers. J Pharm Sci. 2004;93(5):1185–94. doi:10.1002/jps.20046.
28. Monnet-Tschudi F, Zurich M-G, Schilter B, Costa LG, Honegger P. Maturation-dependent effects of chlorpyrifos and parathion and their oxygen analogs on acetylcholinesterase and neuronal and glial markers in aggregating brain cell cultures. Toxicol Appl Pharm. 2000;165(3):175–83. doi:10.1006/taap.2000.8934.
29. Wang Q, Rager JD, Weinstein K, Kardos PS, Dobson GL, Li J, et al. Evaluation of the MDR-MDCK cell line as a permeability screen for the blood–brain barrier. Int J Pharm. 2005;288(2):349–59. doi:10.1016/j.ijpharm.2004.10.007.
30. Wong AD, Ye M, Levy AF, Rothstein JD, Bergles DE, Searson PC. The blood–brain barrier: an engineering perspective. Front Neuroeng. 2013;6:7. doi:10.3389/fneng.2013.00007.
31. Lipinski CA, Lombardo F, Dominy BW, Feeney PJ. Experimental and computational approaches to estimate solubility and permeability in drug discovery and development settings. Adv Drug Deliv Rev. 2001;46(1–3):3–26.
32. Leeson P. Drug discovery: chemical beauty contest. Nature. 2012;481(7382):455–6. doi:10.1038/481455a.

12

The effect of an adenosine A_{2A} agonist on intra-tumoral concentrations of temozolomide in patients with recurrent glioblastoma

Sadhana Jackson[1,9*], Jon Weingart[2], Edjah K. Nduom[3], Thura T. Harfi[4], Richard T. George[5], Dorothea McAreavey[6], Xiaobu Ye[2], Nicole M. Anders[7], Cody Peer[8], William D. Figg[8], Mark Gilbert[9], Michelle A. Rudek[7] and Stuart A. Grossman[1]

Abstract

Background: The blood–brain barrier (BBB) severely limits the entry of systemically administered drugs including chemotherapy to the brain. In rodents, regadenoson activation of adenosine A_{2A} receptors causes transient BBB disruption and increased drug concentrations in normal brain. This study was conducted to evaluate if activation of A_{2A} receptors would increase intra-tumoral temozolomide concentrations in patients with glioblastoma.

Methods: Patients scheduled for a clinically indicated surgery for recurrent glioblastoma were eligible. Microdialysis catheters (MDC) were placed intraoperatively, and the positions were documented radiographically. On post-operative day #1, patients received oral temozolomide (150 mg/m^2). On day #2, 60 min after oral temozolomide, patients received one intravenous dose of regadenoson (0.4 mg). Blood and MDC samples were collected to determine temozolomide concentrations.

Results: Six patients were enrolled. Five patients had no complications from the MDC placement or regadenoson and had successful collection of blood and dialysate samples. The mean plasma AUC was 16.4 ± 1.4 h μg/ml for temozolomide alone and 16.6 ± 2.87 h μg/ml with addition of regadenoson. The mean dialysate AUC was 2.9 ± 1.2 h μg/ml with temozolomide alone and 3.0 ± 1.7 h μg/ml with regadenoson. The mean brain:plasma AUC ratio was 18.0 ± 7.8 and 19.1 ± 10.7% for temozolomide alone and with regadenoson respectively. Peak concentration and T_{max} in brain were not significantly different.

Conclusions: Although previously shown to be efficacious in rodents to increase varied size agents to cross the BBB, our data suggest that regadenoson does not increase temozolomide concentrations in brain. Further studies exploring alternative doses and schedules are needed; as transiently disrupting the BBB to facilitate drug entry is of critical importance in neuro-oncology.

Keywords: Temozolomide, Adenosine A_{2A} agonist, Regadenoson, Microdialysis, Glioblastoma, High grade glioma, Blood–brain barrier

*Correspondence: Sadhana.jackson@nih.gov
[1] Brain Cancer Program, Johns Hopkins University, David H. Koch Cancer Research Building II, 1550 Orleans Street, Room 1M16, Baltimore, MD 21287, USA
Full list of author information is available at the end of the article

Background

The integrity of the blood brain barrier (BBB) is one of the major obstacles to effective chemotherapy for malignant brain tumors. Previous research has focused on how to circumvent the BBB with direct delivery of chemotherapy to the tumor or by mechanically opening the BBB using focused ultrasound or intra-arterial mannitol [1–6]. These direct methods are often associated with comorbidities, hospitalization or added expenses. Very few systemic pharmacologic agents have been evaluated for effectiveness of transient BBB disruption [7–9]. Yet, there is a significant need to identify agents that can transiently disrupt the BBB to improve chemotherapy delivery for patients with such CNS malignancies.

Previous studies have demonstrated the limited permeability of an intact blood–brain barrier [10–12]. However with the presence of tumor cells the BBB becomes heterogeneously disrupted and has been noted as the blood-tumor barrier (BTB) [10]. The BTB and BBB provide a physical barrier with collaborative cells that inhibit entry of toxins, including chemotherapy. Specifically, the BTB amongst malignant gliomas is unique with a high proliferative index of microvasculature and evident alterations in astrocytic endfeet and transcytotic mechanisms; making the BTB more leaky in certain areas of the tumor but peritumoral brain less permeable with a normal BBB [10, 13–15]. These factors collectively play a role in restricting drug entry and have guided extensive research on how best to enhance transport to the CNS.

Adenosine appears to play an important role in the integrity of the BBB [16–21]. The function of adenosine is controlled by four G-protein coupled receptors: A_1, A_{2A}, A_{2B} and A_3. A_1 and A_3 receptors inhibit and A_{2A} and A_{2B} stimulate downstream activation of adenylate cyclase resulting in calcium influx and vasodilation [17, 22]. Inhibitory receptor A_1 and stimulating receptor A_{2A} exhibit high expression and functionality within the heart and brain; specifically impacting local vasodilation [18, 21, 23]. Regadenoson is an FDA-approved A_{2A} receptor agonist which is routinely used for pharmacologic stress testing in patients with suspected cardiac disease and an inability to perform an exercise stress test. Single-photon emission computed tomography (SPECT) is often performed with a radiotracer to measure myocardial perfusion both at rest and then at the time of stress induced by regadenoson administration. Pre-clinical models have demonstrated the effectiveness of A_1 and/or A_{2A} receptor agonism to increase BBB permeability to a 70 kD dextran molecule in both mice and rat brains [24]. The large dextran was detected in the brain for up to 180 min following a single injection in both mice and rats. In additional studies that evaluated CNS barrier permeability with regadenoson, there was a 60% increase in temozolomide brain concentrations in non-tumor bearing rats, without changing the systemic pharmacology of temozolomide [19]. These findings prompted clinical studies of regadenoson followed by brain SPECT and CT imaging to evaluate CNS permeability differences, but there was no detectable change in permeability of the BBB in patients [25]. However, no previous study has directly investigated whether regadenoson is capable of increasing temozolomide concentrations in the human brain.

Temozolomide is an FDA approved oral alkylating agent used in newly diagnosed and recurrent high grade gliomas. While temozolomide with radiotherapy has modestly improved overall survival rates in high grade gliomas, previous studies have proven that levels of temozolomide in the brain are only 20% of systemic drug levels [26, 27]. The peak concentration of temozolomide in the brain occurs approximately 1–2 h after ingestion. Once ingested, temozolomide undergoes degradation from its prodrug form to the highly reactive alkylating agent, methyl-triazenyl imidazole carboxamide (MTIC). Previous studies have utilized CSF sampling and intracerebral microdialysis catheters (MDC) to measure temozolomide brain extracellular concentrations in primary or metastatic brain tumors. Use of an indwelling MDC for long term tissue monitoring in the cerebrum is not new, and this technique has been utilized mainly in the traumatic brain injury setting. Prolonged catheter placement allows for continued fluid collections in alert and mobile patients [28–30]. These catheters are often placed in the operating room with verification of placement determined by brain CT. The presence of a gold filament at the catheter tip allows for easy visibility on non-contrast CT brain imaging. The semi-permeable catheter performs similarly to a capillary when perfusion fluid is pumped continuously through it. The presence of the microvial at the end of the catheter allows for regular interval sampling of the dialysate fluid. Then, drug recovery is assessed in each dialysate sample as an indirect measurement of free drug concentration.

Limited clinical studies have been performed in brain tumor patients evaluating drug delivery to the tumor bed using intracerebral microdialysis measurements [26, 31–34]. To date, the only chemotherapeutic agents evaluated have been methotrexate, temozolomide, bafetinib and 5-flucytosine [26, 32, 33, 35]. Portnow and colleagues studied serum and brain extracellular concentrations of temozolomide via MDC collected at 30 min time intervals post oral drug administration over 24 h. This study evaluated temozolomide drug delivery to the peritumoral non-contrast enhancing area in both primary and metastatic patients (n = 10). Collectively, they found that oral administration of temozolomide yielded an average brain:plasma AUC ratio of 17.8 ± 13.3%, with a peak drug concentration of approximately 2–3 h after administration and undetectable concentrations by 18 h [26]. We designed this study to determine if FDA-approved doses of regadenoson would increase the temozolomide concentration in human brains with malignant glioma as measured by serial brain interstitial fluid assessments.

In this pilot feasibility study, we utilized MDC to determine the neuropharmacokinetics of temozolomide co-administered with regadenoson to assess temozolomide drug entry. We hypothesized that regadenoson would transiently impact the permeability of temozolomide as it did in rodents resulting in increased brain interstitium (BI) and brain:plasma AUC ratio. The primary aim of this trial was to measure brain interstitial temozolomide concentrations pre and post regadenoson using MDC in patients with recurrent high grade glioma. The secondary endpoint was to evaluate tolerability of temozolomide with a single dose of regadenoson in the post-operative setting.

Methods

Study subjects

This study was approved by Institutional Review Boards at Johns Hopkins and the National Institutes of Health, and all patients provided informed consent. Eligible patients were ≥ 18 years old with a diagnosis of recurrent high grade glioma suspected by MRI findings. All patients had a clinically indicated need for surgical intervention. Patients were required to have: Karnofsky performance status (KPS) of ≥ 60%; normal liver and kidney function; absolute neutrophil count ≥ 1500 cells/mm^3; and a platelet count ≥ 100,000 cells/mm^3. Patients were excluded if they were currently receiving chemotherapy or radiation therapy, allergic to temozolomide, pregnant or breast-feeding, had a serious medical or psychiatric illness or social situation that could interfere with catheter placement/monitoring. Patients with a prior use of VEGF or VEGFR-targeted therapy, use of investigational agents within the past 4 weeks, NCI CTC grade 3 or greater baseline neurologic symptoms, history of cardiac, bronchospastic lung disease, or a contraindication to adenosine were all excluded from study participation. Additionally, patients were asked to refrain for caffeine use at least 24 h prior to regadenoson administration, secondary to its ability to blunt the effect of regadenoson.

Study design

Once intra-operative pathology was confirmed, one to two MDialysis 70 Microdialysis Brain Catheters (membrane length 10 mm; shaft length 60 mm; ref. no. P00049) were placed into contrast-enhancing and/or non-contrast peritumoral tissue (within 5 mm from the resection cavity). Post-operative non-contrast CT imaging confirmed catheter placement with identification of an enhancing gold tip. After transfer to the intensive critical care unit, the inlet tubing of the catheter was connected to a portable syringe pump (MDialysis 107 Microdialysis Pump, ref no. P000127), containing artificial CSF (Perfusion Fluid CNS, ref no. P000151) at a rate of 1 μl/min. A microvial was connected at the end of the outlet tubing to continuously collect dialysate samples. To account for the correction factor, fractional recovery of temozolomide by ICMD was calculated based on previous in vitro sampling using CMA 70 Microdialysis catheter [26]. All microdialysis supplies were purchased from MDialysis, (Stockholm, Sweden).

Once the patient was clinically stable, at least 24 h after the completion of surgery on post-operative day 1, and tolerating oral intake, they were administered temozolomide 150 mg/m^2 orally once. On post-operative day 2, each patient was again given temozolomide 150 mg/m^2 orally, and approximately 60 min later, each patient was administered intravenous regadenoson 0.4 mg once over 10 s. Previous studies have demonstrated temozolomide peak brain concentrations occur 90–120 min after administration [26, 27]. Additionally, preclinical studies with regadenoson have demonstrated the peak effect on barrier permeability occurs 30–60 min after administration [19, 24, 36]. Thus, we opted to administer regadenoson 60 min after temozolomide to ensure peak concentration of temozolomide in the brain and optimal mechanism of regadenoson action on brain vasculature simultaneously. Regadenoson was given with continuous ECG monitoring for a total of 10 min post injection, in the presence of a staff cardiologist (standard cardiac dosing regimen). Pre-temozolomide blood samples were collected 15 min prior to drug administration and then 1, 2, 3, 4, 8, and 18 h after the dose of temozolomide (5 ml per collection). The samples of blood were collected in heparinized syringes, promptly mixed by inversion, and then placed on wet ice until centrifugation at 1300×*g* for 10 min at 4 °C (within 1 h). The samples were processed to plasma within 30 min from centrifugation, and the pH of each sample was adjusted to < 4 with the use of 8.5% phosphoric acid. Plasma was then stored frozen at − 70 °C or below until subsequent batch analysis via liquid chromatography-tandem mass spectrometry (LC–MS/MS).

Dialysate samples were continuously collected with microvial changes every 3 h after portable syringe pump connection on post-operative day 0. At least 24 h after surgery, the microvial was changed pre-temozolomide ingestion and then 1, 2, 3, 4, 6, 8, 10, 12, 14, 16, and 18 h after temozolomide intake on post-operative day 1 and 2. For temozolomide stabilization each microvial was pre-filled with 6–12 µl of acetic acid. Microvials containing dialysate samples were stored on dry ice until all microdialysis samples were collected from the patient. Thereafter, the dialysate samples were stored at or below − 70 °C until LC–MS/MS analysis.

Analytical method to evaluate temozolomide concentrations

Temozolomide concentrations were quantified in acidified sodium heparin plasma and acidified brain interstitial dialysate. For plasma, 15 µl of 8.5% phosphoric acid was added per 0.5 ml of plasma. For microdialysis fluid, 1 µl of glacial acetic acid was added for every 10 µl of the dialysate. Perfusion fluid CNS (artificial CSF) was used as a surrogate matrix for dialysate standards and QCs. Temozolomide was extracted from samples (50 µl of acidified plasma or 20 µl of acidified microdialysis fluid) by adding 600 µl of ethyl acetate containing IS (20 ng/ml of caffeine-$^{13}C_3$) (Sigma–Aldrich, St. Louis, MO). Samples were vortex-mixed and centrifuged at 2000 rpm for 10 min. The top layer was transferred to a clean glass tube and dried under a nitrogen air stream. Samples were reconstituted with 200 µl of 0.5% formic acid in water and stored in the autosampler at 5 °C for LC–MS/MS analysis.

Liquid chromatography-tandem mass spectrometry analysis was performed on an AB Sciex 5500 QTrap mass spectrometer (Sciex, Foster City, CA) coupled with an Acquity UPLC system (Waters, Milford MA). The LC separation was achieved using a Zorbax XDB C_{18} column (4.6 × 50 mm, 5 µm) (Agilent, Santa Clara, CA) at room temperature. The mobile phase solvent A was water containing 0.1% formic acid and mobile phase solvent B was methanol containing 0.1% formic acid. The mobile phase was delivered at a flow rate of 0.3 ml/min. The initial mobile phase composition was 60% solvent A and 40% solvent B. From 0.5 to 4.0 min, solvent B was increased to 100% and conditions held until 5.0 min. At 5.1 min, the mobile phase composition was then returned to 40% solvent B until 6.0 min. The total runtime was 6 min.

The column eluent was monitored using a Sciex 5500 QTrap mass spectrometer using electrospray ionization operating in positive mode. The mass spectrometer was programmed to monitor the following multiple reaction monitoring (MRM) *m/z* transitions: 195.15 → 138.10 and 198.00 → 140.00 for temozolomide and IS, respectively. Calibration curves for temozolomide were computed using the area ratio peak of the analysis to the internal standard by using a quadratic regression with 1/x^2 weighting for plasma and 1/x weighting for artificial CSF, both with a calibration range of 0.005–1.0 µg/ml, and dilutions up to 1:10 (v/v) were accurately quantitated.

Pharmacokinetic analysis

Using non-compartmental methods, the pharmacokinetic parameters within plasma and dialysate temozolomide were determined by concentrations vs. time. While the maximum concentration (C_{max}) and time maximum concentration (T_{max}) were determined directly from the measured data points, half-lives ($t_{1/2}$) were calculated from the elimination rate constant derived from the terminal slope. The $AUC_{0-18\,h}$ for each day was estimated by standard non-compartmental analysis performed by Phoenix® WinNonlin version 6.3 (Pharsight Corporation, Mountain View, CA, USA). The pharmacokinetics variables were tabulated, using descriptive statistics calculated pre and post regadenoson. The differences of the AUCs were summarized by mean and standard deviation. Means and standard deviations were presented for peak drug concentration (C_{max}), time of peak drug concentration (T_{max}), drug half-life ($t_{1/2}$) and area under the curve from time 0–18 h after temozolomide administration ($AUC_{0-18\,h}$).

Results

Feasibility/safety and tolerability

Six patients were enrolled on the study from May 2015 to April 2017. Five of the patients were deemed as evaluable. One patient was deemed unevaluable due to microdialysis catheter displacement, which occurred approximately 24 h after insertion. This displacement was attributed to manipulation of the patient's surgical head dressing post-operatively. This patient was removed from study before any study medications were administered. Table 1 summarizes patient demographics. All patients underwent surgical debulking for their recurrent high grade glioma. Each catheter was placed in peritumoral tissue that was

Table 1 Clinical demographics

Patient	Age	Gender	Diagnosis	Catheter(s) tip placement area
1	49	M	Glioblastoma	Non-contrast and contrast enhancing
2	68	M	Glioblastoma	Non-contrast enhancing
3	32	M	Glioblastoma	Non-contrast and contrast enhancing
4	60	M	Glioblastoma	Non-contrast enhancing
5	51	M	Glioblastoma	Non-contrast enhancing
6	70	F	Glioblastoma	Non-contrast enhancing

All patients diagnosed with recurrent glioblastoma and catheter tips were placed in non-contrast enhancing tumor. In patients 1 and 3, tips were also placed in contrast enhancing tissue

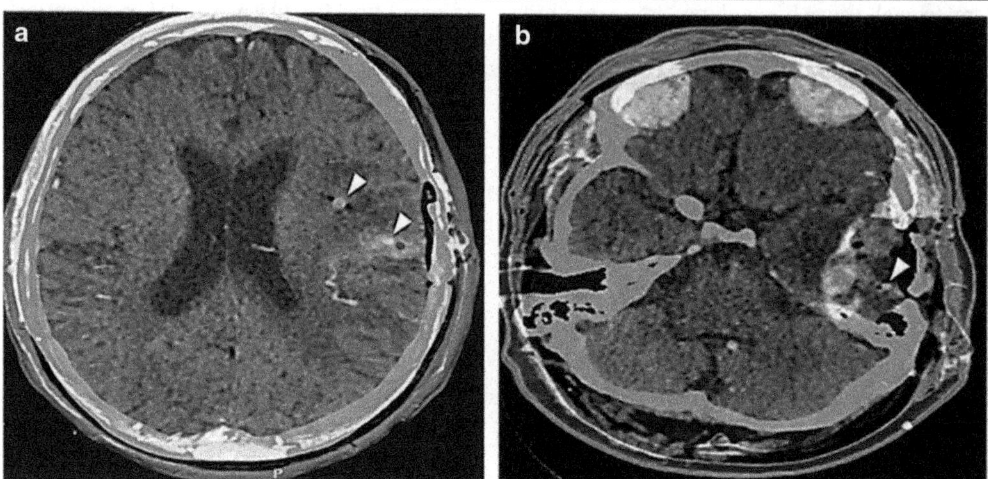

Fig. 1 Catheter placement imaging. Brain CT and MRI superimposed delineating catheter placement and tumor margins. Patient 1 had one catheter tip placed in non-contrast enhancing area and the second in contrast enhancing tissue (**a**). Patient 2 had one catheter placed in non-contrast enhancing tissue (**b**). Superimposed images denote contrast enhancement in green. The white triangle indicates placement of catheter tips

deemed to be non-contrast enhancing tissue by pre-operative MRI. In two patients, catheters were also placed in contrast enhancing areas approximately 5 mm from the surgical bed due to a subtotal resection. Catheter tip locations were accurately determined by superimposed CT and MRI imaging (Fig. 1). All evaluable patients tolerated microdialysis catheter insertion without associated bleeding, infection, pain or other incidents attributable to foreign material placement.

Post-operatively, each patient was transferred and cared for in the intensive care unit during the entire duration of the microdialysis sampling period. Dialysate samples were obtained from 5 patients, with sampling obtained for approximately 72 h from catheter insertion. Drug administration and monitoring while in the ICU included regadenoson administration by the trial-associated cardiologist. Each patient received temozolomide 150 mg/m^2 daily for 2 days and on day 2 was administered regadenoson by the cardiologist; who noted expected regadenoson side effects of transient tachycardia, elevated blood pressure and flushing. Only two patients experienced grade 1 headaches, (patient 2 and 4) which resolved within 30 min from regadenoson administration. No subjects required aminophylline as a reversal agent to regadenoson. No unanticipated adverse events were noted from temozolomide, regadenoson drug administrations, or microdialysis catheter sample collections.

Dexamethasone was administered to each patient as part of their standard post-operative care; in an effort to minimize post-operative vasogenic brain edema. For each patient on study, dexamethasone was given via intravenous administration every 8 h. Specifically, on the days of study, all patients except patient 4 received dexamethasone approximately 2 h after temozolomide administration (1 h after regadenoson administration). For patient 4, dexamethasone was given at the same time as temozolomide (1 h prior to regadenoson administration).

Temozolomide neuropharmacokinetic analysis

Additional file 1: Table S1 summarizes the plasma and brain interstitial pharmacokinetic data for each patient, accounting for in vitro fractional recovery [26]. We opted to only assess plasma and brain dialysate samples for temozolomide because the active temozolomide metabolite, MTIC, was associated with poor acid stabilization and recovery [26]. Comparing plasma concentrations of temozolomide alone vs. temozolomide with regadenoson, neither the C_{max} nor AUCs were impacted by regadenoson (Fig. 2, Additional file 2: Fig S1). Peak temozolomide plasma concentrations with temozolomide alone or combined with regadenoson were: 3.5 ± 1.6 µg/ml vs. 4.8 ± 1.2 µg/ml, respectively. Non-contrast enhancing brain concentrations for temozolomide alone or combined with regadenoson were: 0.55 ± 0.26 µg/ml vs. 0.57 ± 0.32 µg/ml, respectively. The non-contrast enhancing brain:plasma AUC ratio was 19.1 ± 10.7% when temozolomide was administered alone and 18.0 ± 7.8% when combined with regadenonson Three patients (patients 2, 3 and 5) demonstrated a rise in non-contrast enhancing mean brain AUC with regadenoson by approximately 53%. But this increase can be mostly attributed to patient 2 who demonstrated a significant rise in temozolomide brain AUC concentration with regadenoson; doubling AUC from 0.6 to 1.2 µg/ml h.

Overall, evaluation of non-enhancing brain interstitium mean concentrations for all 5 patients demonstrated no significant difference in C_{max} or AUCs between treatment groups, but individual variations existed.

Two patients (patients 1 and 3) had catheters placed in contrast enhancing brain. The dialysate AUCs increased slightly by 10.0 and 19.1% when temozolomide was administered with regadenoson. For patient 1, brain AUC increased from 4.4 to 5.4 μg/ml h with temozolomide alone to combination with regadenoson, respectively. And for patient 3, brain AUC increased from 3.2 to 4.2 μg/ml h with temozolomide alone to combination with regadenoson, respectively. Generally, treatment with regadenoson exhibited a quicker rise to peak concentration but failed to demonstrate a prolonged increase of brain interstitial temozolomide concentrations (Fig. 2). The variations in peak time, T_{max} and AUC can be seen in individual patient neuropharmacokinetics with temozolomide alone vs. temozolomide + regadenoson (Fig. 3, Additional file 1: Table S1).

Discussion

Despite numerous clinical studies using chemotherapeutic agents, novel biologics and immunotherapeutic agents, the overall survival of patients with high grade gliomas has not changed drastically over the last decade [37]. The clinical impact of many cytotoxic agents has likely been limited in patients with malignant gliomas by their inability to cross the BBB. This poses an issue not only for primary brain tumors but also for metastatic brain disease. Unfortunately, while systemic therapy options have improved over the years for solid tumors, metastatic tumor cells are able to invade the CNS and proliferate with shelter from an impermeable BBB. Thus, with a lack of effective drug entry of varied chemotherapy agents, there has been no improvements in the

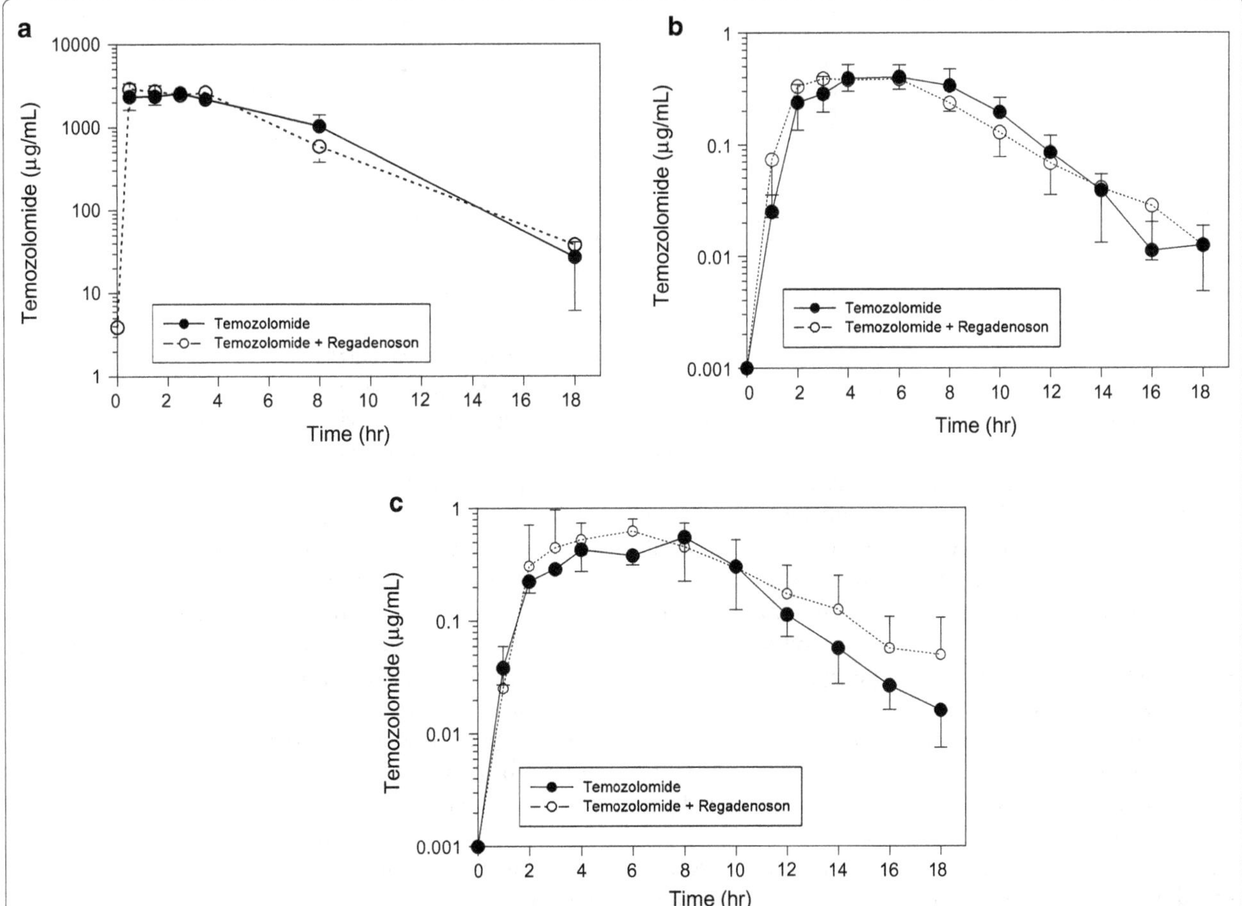

Fig. 2 Mean temozolomide concentrations. Plasma temozolomide systemic concentrations unchanged with regadenoson treatment (**a**). Non-contrast enhancing brain interstitium (BI) temozolomide concentration over time failed to increase with regadenoson (**b**). Contrast enhancing BI temozolomide concentration demonstrated a slight increase in temozolomide concentration over time (**c**). Error bars represent standard error of mean values

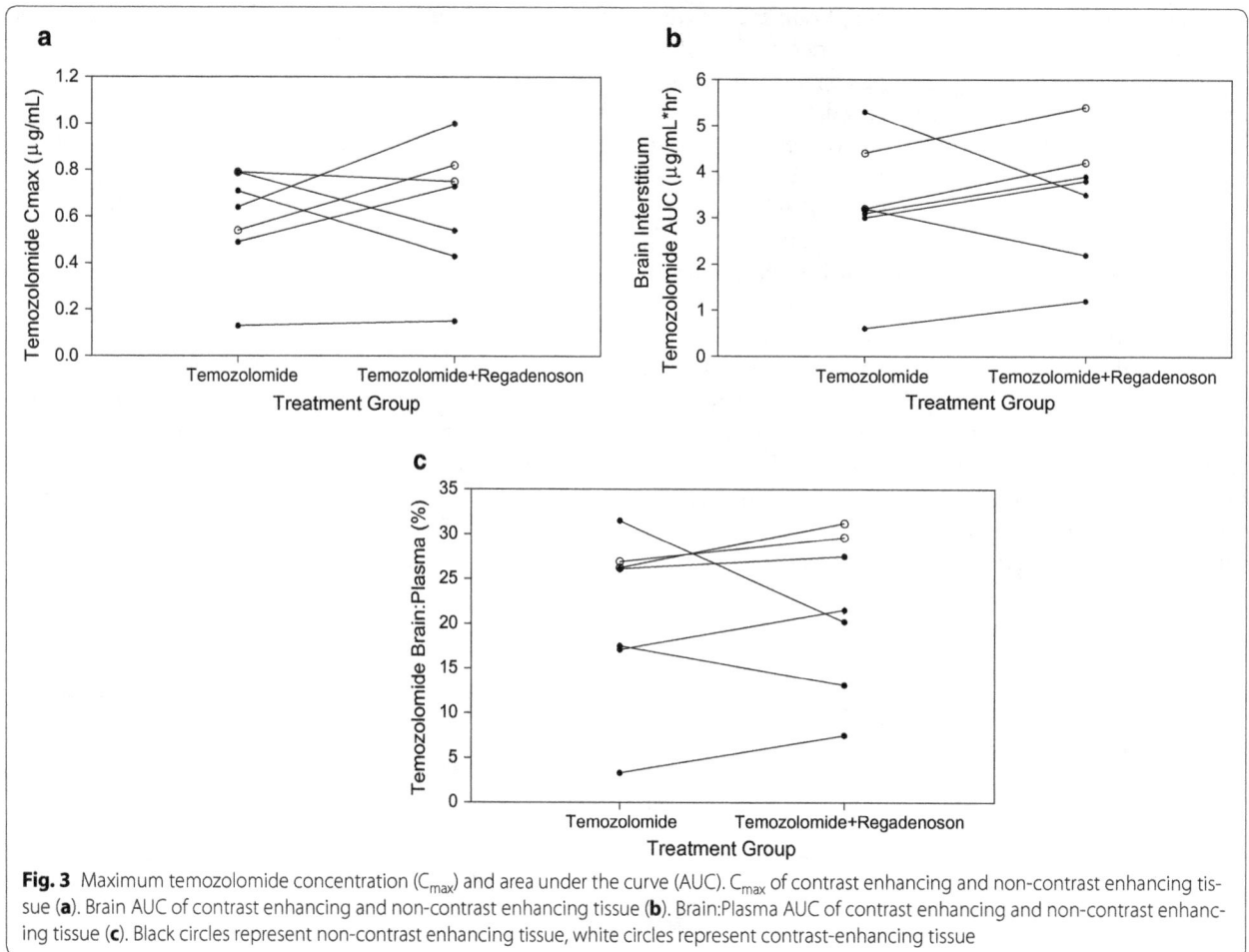

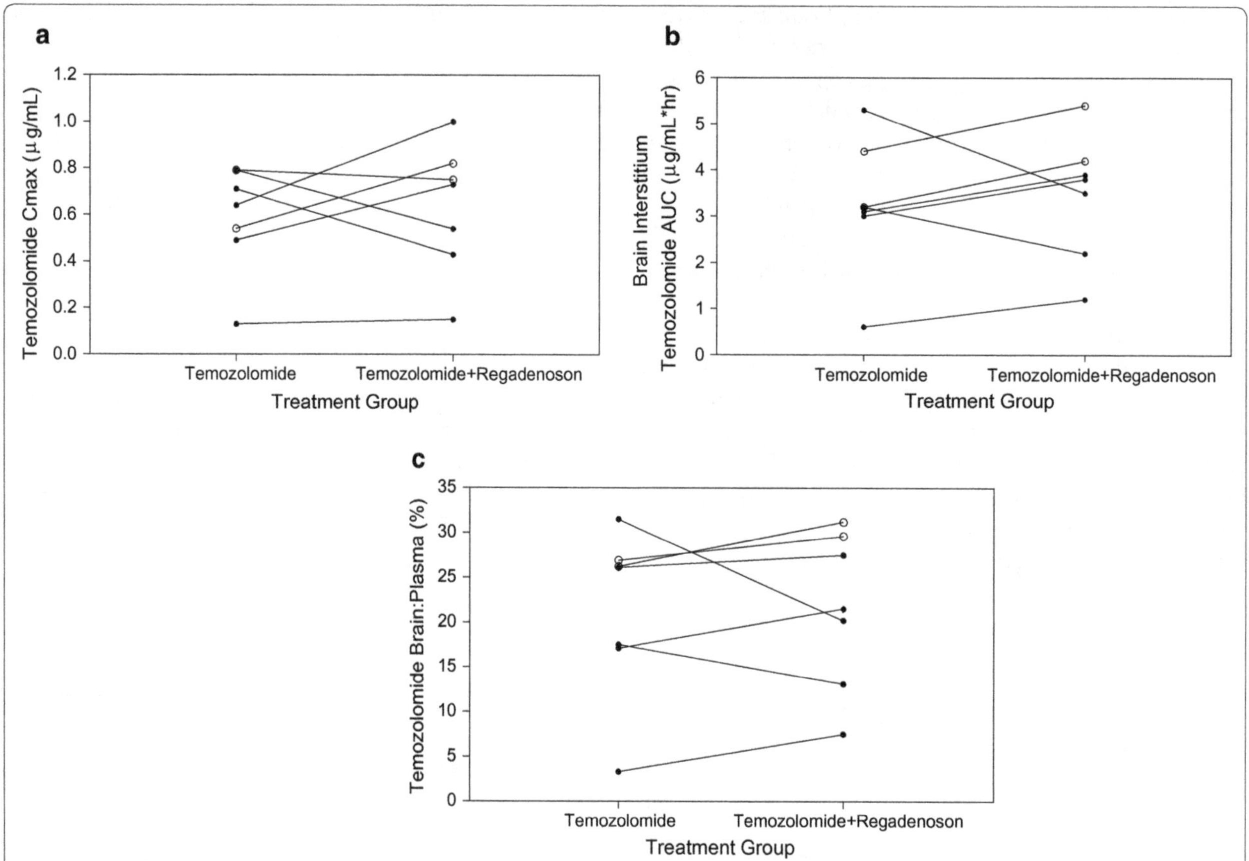

Fig. 3 Maximum temozolomide concentration (C_{max}) and area under the curve (AUC). C_{max} of contrast enhancing and non-contrast enhancing tissue (**a**). Brain AUC of contrast enhancing and non-contrast enhancing tissue (**b**). Brain:Plasma AUC of contrast enhancing and non-contrast enhancing tissue (**c**). Black circles represent non-contrast enhancing tissue, white circles represent contrast-enhancing tissue

overall survival of both malignant glioma and metastatic brain tumors. With this small clinical study, we evaluated regadenoson as a tool to facilitate CNS entry of a mildly permeable agent, temozolomide, from the proposed mechanism of enabling transient BBB disruption.

Overall, our study failed to demonstrate that brain interstitial temozolomide concentrations were increased by use of standard dose regadenoson; which we prespecified as an increase in temozolomide brain concentration by $\geq$ 50%. Importantly, regadenoson did not alter temozolomide plasma concentrations which could result in changes in temozolomide related efficacy or toxicity. Although these results are consistent with our previous negative imaging study [25], they are at odds with the preclinical data that demonstrated increased drug delivery with one small dose of regadenoson [16, 19, 24, 36]. This difference in effect has raised further questions regarding BBB differences between mice and humans relating to expression and function of CNS adenosine A_{2A} receptors. Alternatively, activation of A_{2A} receptors and subsequent BBB disruption in the brains of glioblastoma patients may differ from the activation of A_{2A} receptors in the normal brain vasculature. Previous preclinical studies demonstrated regadenoson's ability to decrease cell–cell adhesion integrity while potentially modifying efflux transporter expression within 0.5–2 h after administration [19, 36, 38]. While we anticipated that regadenoson might increase drug entry across the BBB, drug exit from the CNS could also be facilitated resulting in decreased temozolomide concentrations in brain interstitium. The effect on transport is further compounded by the studies by that demonstrated temozolomide's ability to bind to the multi-drug resistance protein, P-glycoprotein; which likely plays a significant role in glioblastoma temozolomide resistance [39]. Interestingly, regadenoson has been shown to downregulate P-glycoprotein expression in brain endothelial cells thus increasing CNS drug delivery in in vitro *BBB* models and non-tumor bearing rodents [36]. Thus, these combined findings add to the plausibility of temozolomide efflux by P-glycoprotein along with inadequate P-glycoprotein inhibition within brain/brain tumor parenchyma by regadenoson, thereby not causing a significant increase in brain interstitial temozolomide concentrations.

The early rapid rise of temozolomide seen with regadenoson administration can be attributed to the fast acting modulation that results from adenosine receptor activation [16, 24, 36]. Preclinical studies demonstrated the effect of regadenoson on brain vasculature with 0.05 mg/kg dosage per mouse (human equivalent dosing of 0.004 mg/kg); which is less than the standard cardiac stress dosing of 0.006 mg/kg per patient. Yet, despite these preclinical studies utilizing lower than standard regadenoson dosing, increased CNS penetration of 70 kD dextran and temozolomide was observed [16, 19, 24]. Interestingly, these studies in rodents demonstrated a bell shaped dose/effect curve, suggesting that regadenoson doses too high or too low result in minimal changes in BBB disruption. With this clinical study, we opted to use the standard clinical dosing of regadenoson (0.4 mg). This FDA approved agent is used daily in the clinical setting of patients with suspected heart disease to induce vasodilation. Clinically, patients receive one dose with associated cardiac imaging. We hypothesized that because approximately 26% of patients with suspected cardiac disease experience brief headaches after regadenoson administration, it is possible that headaches may be a direct correlate/biomarker for the presence or degree of BBB disruption. We opted to start with the clinical dosing of regadenoson as a means to increase temozolomide CNS entry. While optimal dosing has been determined for cardiac stress testing, optimal dosing and schedule of administration has yet to be determined with a focus on BBB permeability. Thus, it is plausible that increased or decreased standard regadenoson dosing could optimally augment CNS temozolomide entry. These studies of varied regadenoson dosing impacting the BBB permeability have not been performed to date in humans.

Conclusions

Given the importance of transiently opening the BBB to facilitate drug entry, further research in this area is desperately needed to improve the outcome of patients with CNS malignancies. For both primary and metastatic tumors, treatment options are very limited and/or exhibit poor sustainability for growth inhibition, and invasion. Several agents have been investigated in the past as a means to transiently "open" the BBB, but very few studies or laboratory investigations are being conducted to identify optimal genes, signaling pathways, or receptors so as to design drugs to influence CNS permeability. Regadenoson may be a potential agent, but more studies are needed to define the optimal dose and dosing schedule with the desired effect on CNS vasculature. These questions, along with the proper dosing and schedule of regadenoson, remain to be further studied, in order to explain our negative findings and improve chances of future success in enhancing transient BBB permeability.

Abbreviations

CNS: central nervous system; BBB: blood brain barrier; MDC: microdialysis catheter; SPECT: single-photon emission computed tomography; AUC: area under the curve; MTIC: methyl-triazenyl imidazole carboxamide; CSF: cerebral spinal fluid; MRM: multiple reaction monitoring.

Authors' contributions

JW and EN performed neurosurgical tumor resection and catheter placement in all patients. TH, RTG and DM provided Cardiology support for all patients, assisted with protocol design and manuscript writing. XY performed statistical design of the trial. NMA, CP, WDF, MAR, performed pharmacologic analysis of patient samples. SJ, SAG, MG, MAR, XY, DM, RTG and EN were all involved in the design of the protocol and intellectual content. SJ, MAR, NMA and SAG were involved in the data analysis and interpretation for graphical display. SJ, MG, and SAG consented patients, provided neuro-oncology support, coordinated supportive staff engagement and were major contributors in writing the manuscript. All authors read and approved the final manuscript.

Author details

[1] Brain Cancer Program, Johns Hopkins University, David H. Koch Cancer Research Building II, 1550 Orleans Street, Room 1M16, Baltimore, MD 21287, USA. [2] School of Medicine, Department of Neurosurgery, Johns Hopkins University, Baltimore, MD 21287, USA. [3] Surgical Neurology Branch, NINDS/NIH, 10 Center Drive, 3D20, Bethesda, MD 20814, USA. [4] David Heart & Lung Research Institute, The Ohio State University, 374 12th Avenue, Suite 200, Columbus, OH 43210, USA. [5] Heart and Vascular Institute, Johns Hopkins University, 600 N. Wolfe Street, Sheikh Zayed Tower, Baltimore, MD 21287, USA. [6] Critical Care Medicine Department, Nuclear Cardiology Section, NIH Clinical Center, 10 Center Drive, Bethesda, MD 20892, USA. [7] Cancer Chemical and Structural Biology and Analytical Pharmacology Core Laboratory, Johns Hopkins University, Bunting-Blaustein Cancer Research Building I, 1650 Orleans Street, CRB1 Room 1M52, Baltimore, MD 21231, USA. [8] Clinical Pharmacology, NCI/NIH, 10 Center Drive, 5A01, Bethesda, MD 20814, USA. [9] Neuro-Oncology Branch, NCI/NIH, 9030 Old Georgetown Rd, Building 82, Bethesda, MD 20892, USA.

Acknowledgements

We are appreciative of the patients and families who agreed to participate on the study requiring ICU admission, catheter placement and frequent neurologic monitoring. We are also thankful for the supportive ICU, nursing surgical and research staff who assisted with clinical care, trial execution and enrollment assessment of study patients.

Competing interests

The authors declare that they have no competing interests.

Funding

This work was supported by fellowship support T32GM066691 in Johns Hopkins Clinical pharmacology training program (Sadhana Jackson) and by the National Institutes of Health Clinical Center. The project described was supported in part by the Analytical Pharmacology Core of the Sidney Kimmel Comprehensive Cancer Center at Johns Hopkins (NIH grants P30CA006973 and UL1 TR 001079). Grant Number UL1 TR 001079 is from the National Center for Advancing Translational Sciences (NCATS) a component of the NIH, and NIH Roadmap for Medical Research. Its contents are solely the responsibility of the authors and do not necessarily represent the official view of the Johns Hopkins ICTR, NCATS or NIH.

References

1. Saunders NR, et al. The biological significance of brain barrier mechanisms: help or hindrance in drug delivery to the central nervous system? F1000Res. 2016;5. https://doi.org/10.12688/f1000research.7378.
2. Yang FY, et al. Pharmacokinetic analysis of 111 in-labeled liposomal doxorubicin in murine glioblastoma after blood-brain barrier disruption by focused ultrasound. PLoS ONE. 2012;7(9):e45468.
3. Doolittle ND, et al. Delivery of chemotherapeutics across the blood-brain barrier: challenges and advances. Adv Pharmacol. 2014;71:203–43.
4. Abraham T, Feng J. Evolution of brain imaging instrumentation. Semin Nucl Med. 2011;41(3):202–19.
5. Fortin D, et al. Enhanced chemotherapy delivery by intraarterial infusion and blood-brain barrier disruption in malignant brain tumors: the Sherbrooke experience. Cancer. 2005;103(12):2606–15.
6. Oberoi RK, et al. Strategies to improve delivery of anticancer drugs across the blood-brain barrier to treat glioblastoma. Neuro Oncol. 2016;18(1):27–36.
7. Borlongan CV, Emerich DF. Facilitation of drug entry into the CNS via transient permeation of blood brain barrier: laboratory and preliminary clinical evidence from bradykinin receptor agonist. Cereport Brain Res Bull. 2003;60(3):297–306.
8. Warren K, et al. Pharmacokinetics of carboplatin administered with lobradimil to pediatric patients with brain tumors. Cancer Chemother Pharmacol. 2004;54(3):206–12.
9. Emerich DF, et al. The development of the bradykinin agonist labradimil as a means to increase the permeability of the blood-brain barrier: from concept to clinical evaluation. Clin Pharmacokinet. 2001;40(2):105–23.
10. van Tellingen O, et al. Overcoming the blood-brain tumor barrier for effective glioblastoma treatment. Drug Resist Updat. 2015;19:1–12.
11. Abbott NJ, et al. Structure and function of the blood-brain barrier. Neurobiol Dis. 2010;37(1):13–25.
12. Dubois LG, et al. Gliomas and the vascular fragility of the blood brain barrier. Front Cell Neurosci. 2014;8:418.
13. Zhou W, et al. Targeting glioma stem cell-derived pericytes disrupts the blood-tumor barrier and improves chemotherapeutic efficacy. Cell Stem Cell. 2017;21(5):591–603.
14. Watkins S, et al. Disruption of astrocyte-vascular coupling and the blood-brain barrier by invading glioma cells. Nat Commun. 2014;5:4196.
15. Verbeek MM, et al. Induction of alpha-smooth muscle actin expression in cultured human brain pericytes by transforming growth factor-beta 1. Am J Pathol. 1994;144(2):372–82.
16. Bynoe MS, et al. Adenosine receptor signaling: a key to opening the blood-brain door. Fluids Barriers CNS. 2015;12:20.
17. Dixon AK, et al. Tissue distribution of adenosine receptor mRNAs in the rat. Br J Pharmacol. 1996;118(6):1461–8.
18. Fried NT, Elliott MB, Oshinsky ML. The role of adenosine signaling in headache: a review. Brain sci. 2017;7(3):30.
19. Jackson S, et al. The effect of regadenoson-induced transient disruption of the blood-brain barrier on temozolomide delivery to normal rat brain. J Neurooncol. 2016;126(3):433–9.
20. Kochanek PM, et al. Characterization of the effects of adenosine receptor agonists on cerebral blood flow in uninjured and traumatically injured rat brain using continuous arterial spin-labeled magnetic resonance imaging. J Cereb Blood Flow Metab. 2005;25(12):1596–612.
21. Latini S, Pedata F. Adenosine in the central nervous system: release mechanisms and extracellular concentrations. J Neurochem. 2001;79(3):463–84.
22. Fredholm BB, et al. International Union of Basic and Clinical Pharmacology. LXXXI. Nomenclature and classification of adenosine receptors-an update. Pharmacol Rev. 2011;63(1):1–34.
23. Gariboldi V, et al. Expressions of adenosine A_{2A} receptors in coronary arteries and peripheral blood mononuclear cells are correlated in coronary artery disease patients. Int J Cardiol. 2017;230:427–31.
24. Carman AJ, et al. Adenosine receptor signaling modulates permeability of the blood-brain barrier. J Neurosci. 2011;31(37):13272–80.
25. Jackson S, et al. The effect of regadenoson on the integrity of the human blood-brain barrier, a pilot study. J Neurooncol. 2017;132(3):513–9.
26. Portnow J, et al. The neuropharmacokinetics of temozolomide in patients with resectable brain tumors: potential implications for the current approach to chemoradiation. Clin Cancer Res. 2009;15(22):7092–8.
27. Ostermann S, et al. Plasma and cerebrospinal fluid population pharmacokinetics of temozolomide in malignant glioma patients. Clin Cancer Res. 2004;10(11):3728–36.
28. Guyot LL, et al. Cerebral monitoring devices: analysis of complications. Acta Neurochir Suppl. 1998;71:47–9.
29. Thelin EP, et al. Microdialysis monitoring in clinical traumatic brain injury and its role in neuroprotective drug development. AAPS J. 2017;19(2):367–76.
30. Patet C, et al. Cerebral lactate metabolism after traumatic brain injury. Curr Neurol Neurosci Rep. 2016;16(4):31.
31. Blakeley J, Portnow J. Microdialysis for assessing intratumoral drug disposition in brain cancers: a tool for rational drug development. Expert Opin Drug Metab Toxicol. 2010;6(12):1477–91.
32. Blakeley JO, et al. Effect of blood brain barrier permeability in recurrent high grade gliomas on the intratumoral pharmacokinetics of methotrexate: a microdialysis study. J Neurooncol. 2009;91(1):51–8.
33. Portnow J, et al. Neural stem cell-based anticancer gene therapy: A first-in-human study in recurrent high-grade glioma patients. Clin Cancer Res. 2016;23(12):2951–60.
34. Bergenheim AT, et al. Distribution of BPA and metabolic assessment in glioblastoma patients during BNCT treatment: a microdialysis study. J Neurooncol. 2005;71(3):287–93.
35. Portnow J, et al. A neuropharmacokinetic assessment of bafetinib, a second generation dual BCR-Abl/Lyn tyrosine kinase inhibitor, in patients with recurrent high-grade gliomas. Eur J Cancer. 2013;49(7):1634–40.
36. Kim DG, Bynoe MS. A_{2A} adenosine receptor modulates drug efflux transporter P-glycoprotein at the blood-brain barrier. J Clin Invest. 2016;126(5):1717–33.
37. Stupp R, et al. Radiotherapy plus concomitant and adjuvant temozolomide for glioblastoma. N Engl J Med. 2005;352(10):987–96.
38. Kim DG, Bynoe MS. A_{2A} adenosine receptor regulates the human blood-brain barrier permeability. Mol Neurobiol. 2015;52(1):664–78.
39. Munoz JL, et al. Temozolomide competes for P-glycoprotein and contributes to chemoresistance in glioblastoma cells. Cancer Lett. 2015;367(1):69–75.

13

Permeability across a novel microfluidic blood-tumor barrier model

Tori B. Terrell-Hall[1], Amanda G. Ammer[2], Jessica I. G. Griffith[1] and Paul R. Lockman[1*]

Abstract

Background: The lack of translatable in vitro blood-tumor barrier (BTB) models creates challenges in the development of drugs to treat tumors of the CNS and our understanding of how the vascular changes at the BBB in the presence of a tumor.

Methods: In this study, we characterize a novel microfluidic model of the BTB (and BBB model as a reference) that incorporates flow and induces shear stress on endothelial cells. Cell lines utilized include human umbilical vein endothelial cells co-cultured with CTX-TNA2 rat astrocytes (BBB) or Met-1 metastatic murine breast cancer cells (BTB). Cells were capable of communicating across microfluidic compartments via a porous interface. We characterized the device by comparing permeability of three passive permeability markers and one marker subject to efflux.

Results: The permeability of Sulforhodamine 101 was significantly ($p < 0.05$) higher in the BTB model ($13.1 \pm 1.3 \times 10^{-3}$, $n = 4$) than the BBB model ($2.5 \pm 0.3 \times 10^{-3}$, $n = 6$). Similar permeability increases were observed in the BTB model for molecules ranging from 600 Da to 60 kDa. The function of P-gp was intact in both models and consistent with recent published in vivo data. Specifically, the rate of permeability of Rhodamine 123 across the BBB model ($0.6 \pm 0.1 \times 10^{-3}$, $n = 4$), increased 14-fold in the presence of the P-gp inhibitor verapamil ($14.7 \pm 7.5 \times 10^{-3}$, $n = 3$) and eightfold with the addition of Cyclosporine A ($8.8 \pm 1.8 \times 10^{-3}$, $n = 3$). Similar values were noted in the BTB model.

Conclusions: The dynamic microfluidic in vitro BTB model is a novel commercially available model that incorporates shear stress, and has permeability and efflux properties that are similar to in vivo data.

Keywords: Efflux, p-glycoprotein, Permeability, Metastasis

Background

The occurrence of brain metastases in breast cancer patients is approximately 10–16% [1]. Due to improvements in chemotherapy, the overall survival of breast cancer patients has increased. Unfortunately with prolonged survival the incidence of patients developing symptomatic brain metastases has also increased. One of the leading complications of brain metastases is the inability of drugs to reach the tumor at concentrations adequate to induce cytotoxicity. This is due, in part, to the presence of a partially intact blood–brain barrier (BBB).

*Correspondence: prlockman@hsc.wvu.edu
[1] Department of Basic Pharmaceutical Sciences, School of Pharmacy, West Virginia University HSC, 1 Medical Center Dr., Morgantown, WV 26506, USA
Full list of author information is available at the end of the article

The BBB is a complex anatomical network, functioning to strictly regulate the movement of molecules and ions from the blood to the brain and back. In addition, the BBB serves as the conduit to supply the brain with the essential nutrients it needs, while facilitating the excretion of waste products through efflux [2]. The hallmark of the BBB is the presence of endothelial cells that are tightly connected by tight junction protein complexes, which are composed of claudins, occludins, and junction adhesion molecules [3]. In addition to endothelia, the BBB has a thick basal membrane with pericytes and astrocytic foot processes in close proximity [4, 5]. The net effect of this anatomical structure results in the transendothelial electrical resistance (TEER) of brain capillaries being ~2000 O*cm^2, in comparison to 2–20 O*cm^2 in peripheral capillaries [6, 7]. In addition to the structural components, the BBB is highly enriched in efflux transporters that actively restrict the entry a large and diverse set of lipophilic solutes from accumulating in the brain [8, 9].

When metastatic cancer cells invade the CNS, they may eventually colonize and proliferate into a larger tumor mass. Once the lesion has grown to a point that it has areas of hypoxia, the tumor will secrete high amounts of vascular endothelial growth factor in an attempt to develop a new blood supply [10, 11]. This vasculature (blood-tumor barrier; BTB) is different than the BBB predominantly because astrocytes, pericytes, and neurons are no longer in close proximity to the capillary. It is hypothesized that these anatomical changes result in vasculature that has greater permeability than the BBB [12]. The BTB may also have a somewhat different and varied expression of efflux transporters depending on the CNS malignancy [13–15]. Despite the apparent breakdown of the BBB in the presence of a tumor [16], the BTB still limits drug movement into the CNS lesion significantly more than in peripheral tumors.

Currently, there are no widely validated in vitro models of the BTB. The most widely used in vitro BBB model, which also has been used to model the BTB, is a transwell insert system. Briefly, the model consists of an upper chamber with endothelial cells grown on the surface separated from a lower chamber that may or may not contain astrocytes and or cancer cells. The two chambers are separated by a porous membrane [17, 18]. Drug movement is modeled by measuring accumulation in the lower chamber versus time.

However, the transwell model has limitations. First, there is a lack of flow exerted on the endothelia resulting in poor cell morphology and a "leakier" barrier compared to in vivo data [17–21]. Second, endothelial cells do not uniformly attach to the outer walls of the insert, leaving gaps between endothelial cells and the edge of the insert, also resulting in increased permeability [22]. Third, an unstirred water later forms on the surface of the endothelia, which results in increased permeability for hydrophilic drugs and decreased permeability for lipid soluble drugs [23, 24].

Herein we characterize novel in vitro microfluidic model of the BTB and BBB (as a reference point) using a co-culture of human umbilical endothelial cells (one of a number of endothelial cell lines used in a number of BBB studies [25, 26]) and brain metastases cells. This model incorporates flow during culture of the endothelia and has a micro-tubular lumen, which in other work has substantially reduced limitations seen in transwells [27–31]. This model is unique from other flow based models in that it allows for a co-culture or triple culture of relevant cells, it is easily duplicated, it is commercially available and provides a cost-effective solution for running multiple and parallel assays.

Methods

Microfluidic device

Co-culture idealized microvascular networks used in this study were obtained from SynVivo Inc. Huntsville, AL. The device consists of a central compartment (basolateral) that is comprised of the brain tissue cells (astrocytes, pericytes, neurons) and the outer compartment (apical) that is comprised of the endothelial cells and provides perfusion similar to physiological fluid flow conditions. The outer compartments and central compartment are separated by an interface with a series of 3 μm pores along the length, replacing the use of membranes in conventional models.

Chemicals

Sulforhodamine 101 acid chloride (Free TRD), Rhodamine 123 (Rho123), Texas Red 3000 MW Dextran (TRD 3 kDa), and Texas Red 70,000 MW Dextran (TRD 70 kDa) were purchased from ThermoFisher Scientific (Grand Island, NY). Verapamil was purchased from Sigma (St. Louis, MO). Cyclosporine A was purchased from Toronto Research Chemicals Inc. (Toronto, Canada). All other chemicals used were of analytical grade and were used as supplied.

Cell culture

Human umbilical vein endothelial cells (HUVECs) were purchased from Lonza (Allendale, NJ). CTX-TNA2 rat brain astrocytes were kindly donated by Dr. Jim Simpkins (West Virginia University, Morgantown, WV). Met-1 murine metastatic breast cancer cells were a kind gift from Dr. Alexander Borowsky (UC Davis, Sacramento, CA). All cells were maintained in endothelial basal medium-2 (EBM-2) supplemented with the EGM-2 BulletKit from Lonza (Allendale, NJ). Cells were grown in a 37 °C humidified incubator with 5% CO_2 until ~85% confluent.

Cell culture in microfluidic chip

Matrigel (40 μg cm^{-2}, EMD Milipore, Billerica MA) was injected into the central compartment and allowed to sit covered in ice for approximately 1 h, after which serum-free media was promptly injected to wash the central compartment. Fibronectin (200 μg mL^{-1}, EMD Milipore, Billerica MA) was then injected into one of the outer sides of the device and allowed to incubate at 37 °C overnight. Prior to the seeding of all cells, the device was flushed with EBM-2 media. Astrocytes/Met-1 cells were harvested using TrypLE Select (ThermoFisher, Waltham MA) and re-suspended into a final concentration of ~1×10^7 mL^{-1} cells for injection, and were seeded at a flow rate of 10 μL min^{-1} in the central compartment using a Pump 11 Elite Nanomite programmable syringe pump (Harvard Apparatus, Holliston MA). The inlet port tubing was clamped when cells reached a central compartment density of ~50%, and chip was transferred to a CO_2 incubator at 37 °C to allow cells to attach for 2 h. HUVECs were harvested using TrypLE Select (ThermoFisher, Waltham MA) in the same process described above, re-suspended to a concentration of ~1×10^7 mL^{-1}, and seeded into the outer compartment previously coated with Fibronectin at a flow rate of 6 μL min^{-1} using a Pump 11 Elite Nanomite programmable syringe pump (Harvard Apparatus, Holliston MA). Inlet port tubing was clamped when HUVECs reached an intra-outer compartment density of ~90%, then chip was transferred to a CO_2 incubator at 37 °C and cells were allowed to attach for 24 h, with the exception of media refreshment. After 6 h of incubation, medium in central and both outer compartments was replaced with fresh EBM-2 medium. Media replacement was repeated again at 24 h. Astrocyte/Met-1 cells were maintained in the central compartment under static conditions in EBM-2 medium while EBM-2 medium was prepared in syringes mounted on a programmable PHD 2000 syringe pump (Harvard Apparatus, Holliston MA) and then connected to the chips through ~12 in. of sterile Tygon tubing (Harvard Apparatus, Holliston MA). This medium was flowed at a flow rate of 0.02 μL min^{-1} over the seeded HUVECs in the outer compartment for 4 h, then increased to 0.05 μL min^{-1} after 4 h, and finally to 0.1 μL min^{-1} after 4 more hours, equivalent to 1.9×10^{-3} dynes cm^{-2} [32] This flow rate of 0.1 μL min^{-1} was then maintained for 24 h.

In vitro transport studies

EBM-2 Medium was incubated in a BD Luer-Lok Syringe with either Free TRD (600 mg mL^{-1}), TRD 3 kDa (600 mg mL^{-1}), TRD 70 kDa (600 mg mL^{-1}), or with R123 (600 mg mL^{-1}) in the presence or absence of known P-gp inhibitors (verapamil: 50 mM, Cyclosporine A: 10 mM) and mounted on a programmable PHD 2000 syringe pump (Harvard Apparatus, Holliston MA), with syringes connected to chips through sterile Tygon tubing (Harvard Apparatus, Holliston MA). Permeability was measured through the injection of desired tracer into the outer compartment at 0.1 μL min^{-1} for a total of 90 min while brightfield images (acquired at a 25 ms exposure) and fluorescent images (acquired at a 200 ms exposure) were acquired every 2 min. Permeability of each tracer was determined using NIS Elements Imaging Software. Using linear regression (Prism 6.0), the slope of the best-fit line was used to represent the relative k_{in}, or rate of accumulation, of fluorescence in the central compartment (comparable to the concentration of drug found in normal brain) divided by the accumulation of fluorescence in the outer compartment (comparable to the concentration of drug found in the plasma of the BBB vasculature). Unless otherwise stated, data are presented as mean ± SEM.

Quantification of fluorescent tracers using fluorescent microscopy

Chips were mounted on an automated stage enclosure, maintained at 37 °C with 5% CO_2, on a Nikon Eclipse TE2000-E Live Cell Sweptfield Confocal microscope (Melville, NY). Acquisition of images and fluorescence was achieved through the utilization of a Photometrics CoolSnap HQ2 Monochrome CCD Camera (Tucson, AZ) with a 20×/0.75 Plan Fluor Phase Contrast objective with a total field of 6 × 8, stitching images using brightfield with a 10% overlay. Brightfield and fluorescent images were taken every 2 min for 90 min. Excitation and emission of Free Texas Red, Texas Red 3 and 70 kDa, was obtained using the TRITC epiflourescence filter (peak fluorophore excitation is 596 nm and emission is 615 nm); excitation filter wheel of 555/25×, emission filter wheel of 605/52 m and dichromatic mirror at 89,000 sedat quad. The excitation and emission of Rhodamine 123 (±Cyclosporine A or Verapamil) was obtained using the FITC epiflourescence filter (peak fluorophore excitation is 511 nm and emission is 534 nm); excitation filter wheel of 490/20×, emission filter wheel of 525/36 m and dichromatic mirror at 89,000 sedat quad.

Kinetic analysis

Unidirectional uptake transfer constants (k_{in}) were calculated from the following relationship to the linear portion of the uptake curve:

$$(C_{CC} + C_{PF}) / C_{PF} = k_{in}(t) + O_C \quad (1)$$

where C_{CC} is the sum intensity of fluorophore in the region of interest in the central compartment (au) at the end of perfusion, C_{PF} is the sum intensity of fluorophore (au) in the region of interest within the outer compartment, t is the perfusion time in minutes, and O_C is the extrapolated intercept [T = 0 min; "outer compartment volume" (au)]. After the determination of a perfusion time where an adequate amount of fluorescent marker was allowed to pass into brain, while still remaining in the linear uptake zone, k_{in} was determined [33].

Statistical analysis

The slope of the line (k_{in}) was determined with linear regression using best-fit values. One-way ANOVA analysis and unpaired t test with Welch's correction, followed by an F test to compare variances were used for the comparison of the k_{in} values between unrestricted diffusion, BBB, and BTB among each tracer and with Rho123 in absence and presence of inhibitors. For all data, errors are reported as standard error of the mean unless otherwise indicated. Differences were considered statistically significant at the $p < 0.05$ levels (GraphPad Prism version 6.00 for Mac, GraphPad Software, San Diego, CA, USA).

Results

In this study, we evaluate transfer rates of Free TRD, Texas Red 3 kDa, Texas Red 70 kDa, and Rho123 (with and without inhibitors) (Fig. 1) in a novel microfluidic BBB and BTB model as validation to previously published literature [34]. Briefly in this model, endothelial cells are seeded in the outer compartments, while astrocytes (BBB) or brain seeding breast cancer cells (BTB) are seeded in the central compartment. The porous architecture between the two compartments allows for cellular crosstalk and biochemical exchanges, while shear stress from perfusate flow facilitates development of endothelial morphology [19]. Confocal brightfield images show the differences in morphology between endothelial cells with and without flow (Fig. 1b, c). In order to verify a confluent 360° coating of endothelial cells within the outer compartment, we used a Nikon A1R Confocal on Eclipse TiE Microscope to acquire a 3D z-stack of the outer compartment. Utilizing this system, DAPI stained endothelial cells were imaged from the bottom (Fig. 2a), through to the top (Fig. 2b) showing HUVECs wrapping around the sides of the outer compartment (Fig. 2c) connecting the HUVECs on the top to the HUVECs on the bottom, verifying confluent formation of a tubular in vitro microvasculature.

In initial kinetic experiments, we determined unrestricted diffusion rates of difference sized molecules by perfusing solutes through microfluidic chips without endothelial cells or astrocytes/cancer cells. To quantify tracer accumulation, regions of interest were selected to determine sum fluorescence intensity in the outer compartment (ROI 136), central compartment (ROI 139), and background (ROI 165) over time (1D). ROI 165 was taken to ensure data received in the outer and central compartments were significant when compared to the background sum fluorescence. We observed (Fig. 3) that small tracers (<1000 Da) had a diffusion rate of $22.8 \pm 2.5 \times 10^{-3}$, $n = 6$, which was not significantly different compared to tracers of molecular weights between 3 and 5 kDa ($22.1 \pm 8.5 \times 10^{-3}$, $n = 3$) and >60 kDa ($17.5 \pm 4.2 \times 10^{-3}$, $n = 3$).

In our next experiments, we qualitatively imaged Texas Red accumulation from 0 to 90 min in the BBB model (Fig. 4a–d). Linear accumulation of the dye in the central chamber of the BBB model is quantitatively shown in Fig. 4e. We then determined k_{in} values for each tracer in both the BBB and BTB model, given in units of (μL min^{-1}) according to the equation found in our methods. Free Texas Red k_{in} values (Fig. 5a) for the BBB ($2.5 \pm 0.3 \times 10^{-3}$, $n = 6$) and BTB ($13.1 \pm 1.3 \times 10^{-3}$, $n = 4$) were significantly different ($p < 0.05$) between each other. Texas Red 3 kDa values (Fig. 5b) for the BBB ($0.1 \pm 0.1 \times 10^{-3}$, $n = 3$) and BTB ($1.8 \pm 1.0 \times 10^{-3}$, $n = 3$) and Texas Red 70 kDa values (Fig. 5c) for the BBB ($1.1 \pm 0.9 \times 10^{-3}$, $n = 3$) and BTB ($4.5 \pm 2.4 \times 10^{-3}$, $n = 3$) were also significant ($p < 0.05$) when compared to the unrestricted diffusion k_{in}, but significance was not observed between the BBB and BTB models of these dyes.

To determine if P-gp inhibitors alter the accumulation of P-gp sensitive fluorescent dye accumulation into the central compartment we perfused Rho123 in the absence and presence of P-gp inhibitors Cyclosporine A (10 mM), and Verapamil (50 mM)—concentrations that ensured maximal inhibition [34]. We qualitatively observed an increase in dye accumulation in the central compartment over the course of 90 min in both the BBB (Fig. 6a) and BTB (Fig. 6b) models (Fig. 6c). Quantitatively, we observed a 14-fold increase of Rho123 in the central compartment, in the presence of P-gp inhibitor Verapamil ($14.7 \pm 7.5 \times 10^{-3}$, $n = 3$), and a significant ($p < 0.05$) eight fold increase of Rho123 with Cyclosporine A ($8.8 \pm 1.8 \times 10^{-3}$, $n = 3$) when compared to control Rho123 ($0.6 \pm 0.1 \times 10^{-3}$, $n = 4$) in the BBB model (Fig. 6d). Similarly in the BTB model, a threefold increase was observed in Rhodamine 123 permeability in the presence of P-gp inhibitor Verapamil ($10.3 \pm 3.1 \times 10^{-3}$, $n = 3$), and a twofold increase with Cyclosporine A ($7.1 \pm 5.2 \times 10^{-3}$, $n = 3$) when compared to Rho123 control ($3.2 \pm 2.8 \times 10^{-3}$, $n = 3$) (Fig. 6e).

Discussion

The results of the studies presented herein suggest that a novel microfluidic chip in part mimics the in vivo BTB with regard to passive permeability and efflux [16]. Importantly, this study demonstrates that perfusion flow through the luminal compartment improves endothelial function. This model also has potential to be used in screening assays for drug discovery and development for central nervous system disease.

Predominant in vitro BBB models have some key similarities. First, there is a presence of some type of "barrier" cell in a luminal or outer compartment (representing the vascular lumen). These cells range from primary or immortalized brain endothelial cells (most commonly rat, mouse, or human), peripheral endothelial (HUVECs), or stem-cell derived cells. In this study HUVECs were chosen as they are commonly used by a number of labs, and using a co-culture of astrocytes or even astrocyte-conditioned media alone has been shown to induce BBB-like

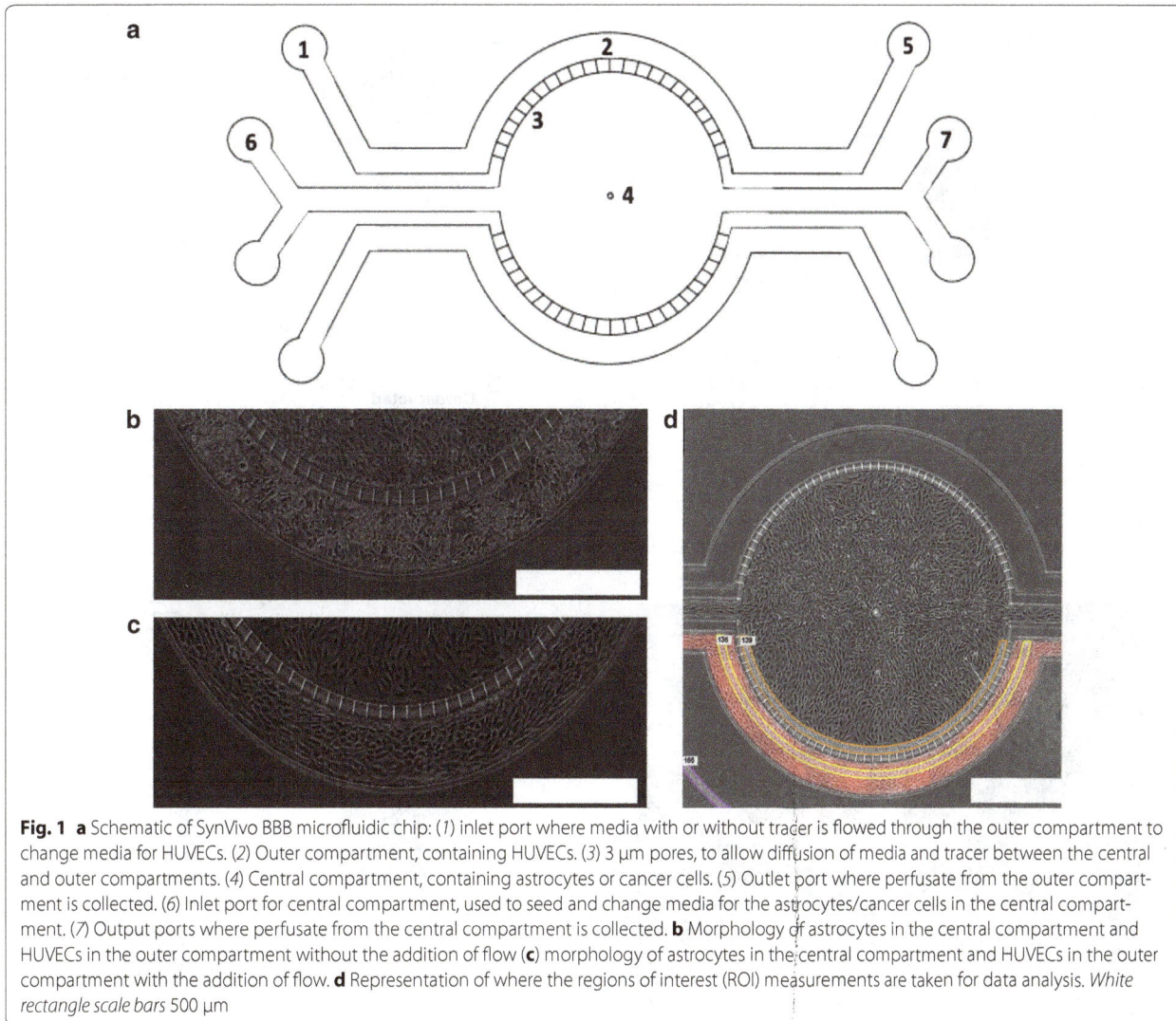

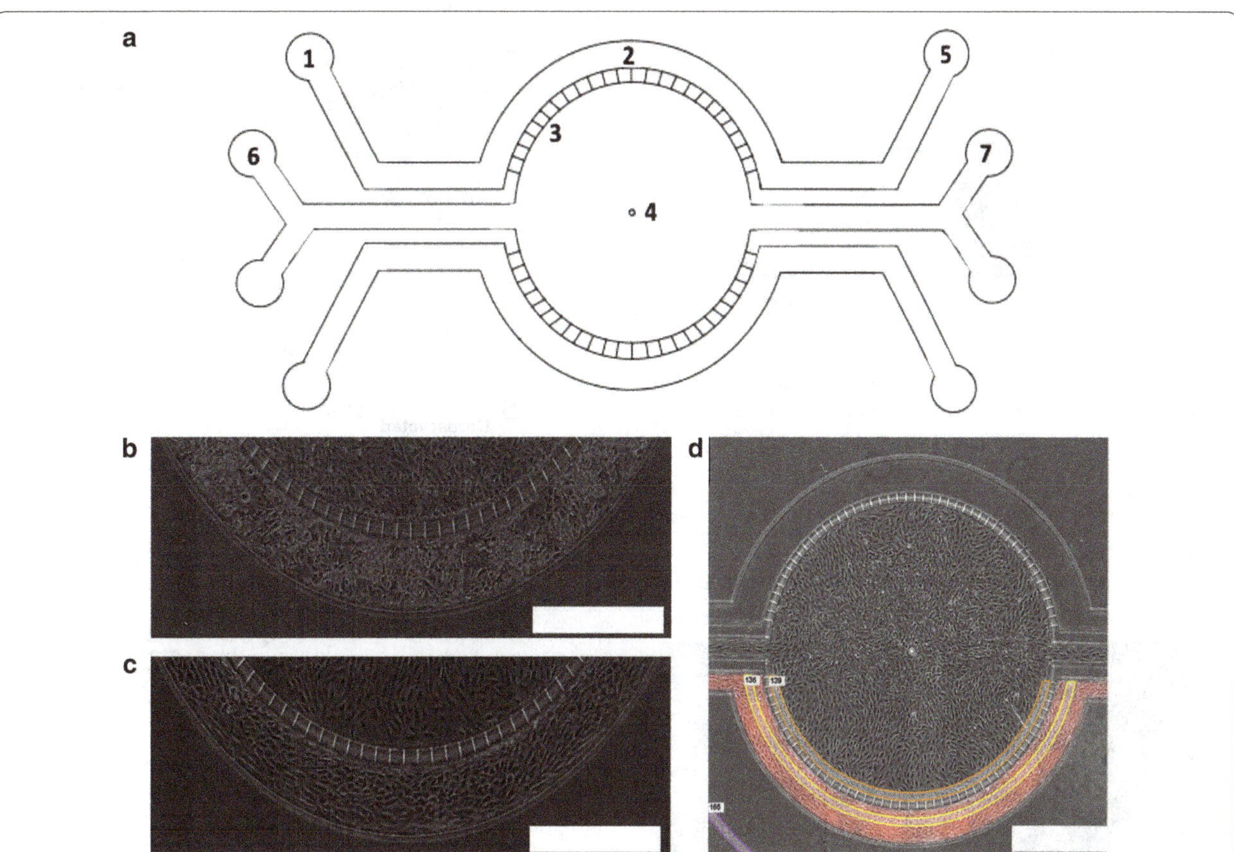

Fig. 1 **a** Schematic of SynVivo BBB microfluidic chip: (*1*) inlet port where media with or without tracer is flowed through the outer compartment to change media for HUVECs. (*2*) Outer compartment, containing HUVECs. (*3*) 3 μm pores, to allow diffusion of media and tracer between the central and outer compartments. (*4*) Central compartment, containing astrocytes or cancer cells. (*5*) Outlet port where perfusate from the outer compartment is collected. (*6*) Inlet port for central compartment, used to seed and change media for the astrocytes/cancer cells in the central compartment. (*7*) Output ports where perfusate from the central compartment is collected. **b** Morphology of astrocytes in the central compartment and HUVECs in the outer compartment without the addition of flow (**c**) morphology of astrocytes in the central compartment and HUVECs in the outer compartment with the addition of flow. **d** Representation of where the regions of interest (ROI) measurements are taken for data analysis. *White rectangle scale bars* 500 μm

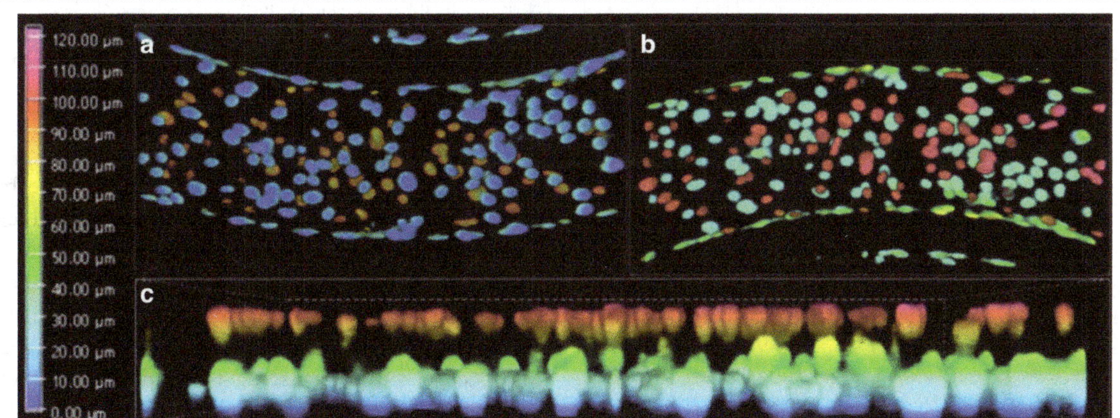

Fig. 2 3-dimensional confocal images of DAPI labeled HUVECs in the outer compartment demonstrating a 360° coating of cells. The nuclei of the HUVECs are seen on the *bottom* (**a**) and *top* (**b**) and in a *side view* (**c**)

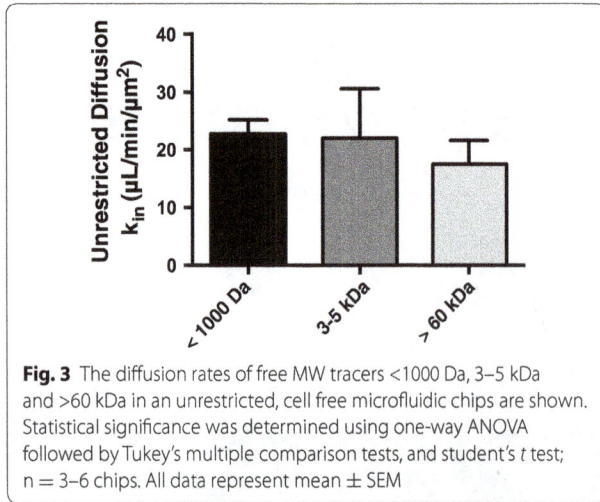

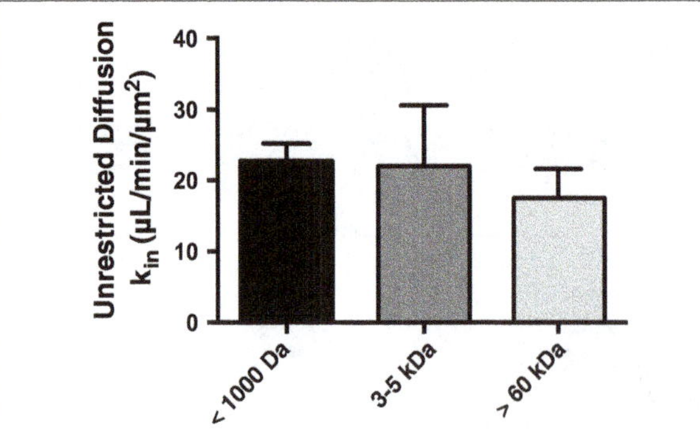

Fig. 3 The diffusion rates of free MW tracers <1000 Da, 3–5 kDa and >60 kDa in an unrestricted, cell free microfluidic chips are shown. Statistical significance was determined using one-way ANOVA followed by Tukey's multiple comparison tests, and student's *t* test; n = 3–6 chips. All data represent mean ± SEM

expression of tight junctions and barrier tightness in

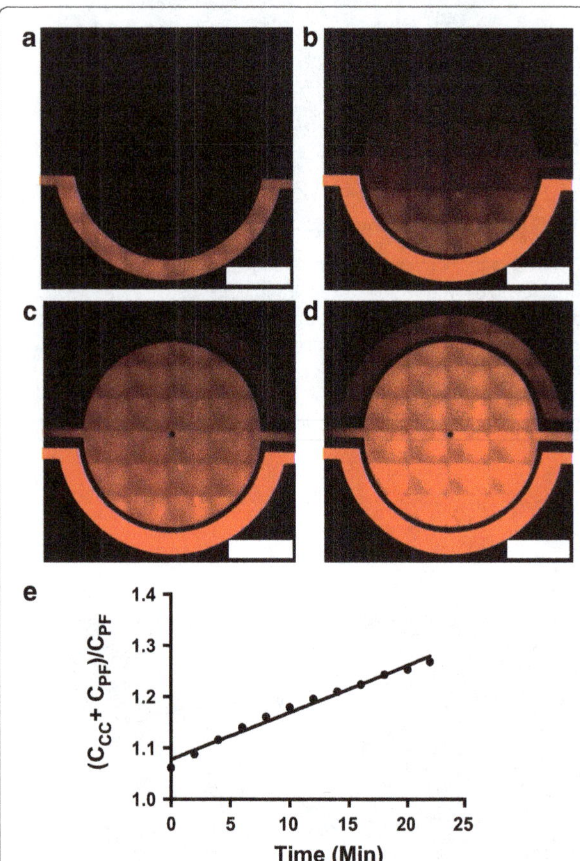

Fig. 4 Representative timelapse images showing passive diffusion of Free TRD from the outer to the central compartment. Intensity of fluorescence increases linearly over time 0 min (**a**), 30 min (**b**), 60 min (**c**), and 90 min (**d**). **e** Linear concentration of tracer movement versus time to determine diffusion constants (K_{in}). *White rectangle scale bars* 500 μm

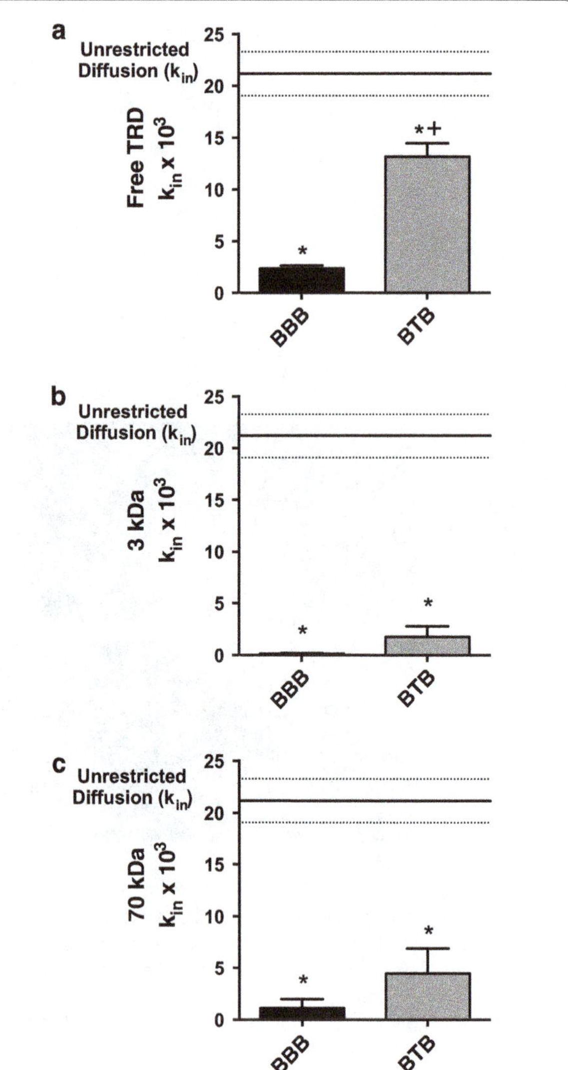

Fig. 5 Linear central compartment accumulation of Free Texas Red (**a**), Texas Red 3 kDa (**b**), and Texas Red 70 kDa (**c**) in BBB and BTB SynVivo chip models. Images show rate of each tracer within each model. Statistical significance was determined using one-way ANOVA followed by Tukey's multiple comparison tests, and student's *t* test; *$p < 0.05$ significance between tracer and unrestricted diffusion k_{in}, n = 3–6; $^{+}p < 0.05$ significance between BBB and BTB models, n = 3–6. All data represent mean ± SEM

a variety of endothelial cells [20, 29, 35]. These barrier cells typically express tight junction proteins, which seal the endothelial cells together and produce higher TEER values [36]. Second, the models usually include the presence of a semipermeable basement membrane separating the outer (lumen) and central (brain side) compartments. Lastly, cells, typically astrocytes and or pericytes, are seeded in the central compartment in an effort to mimic the brain microenvironment. The addition of these cells

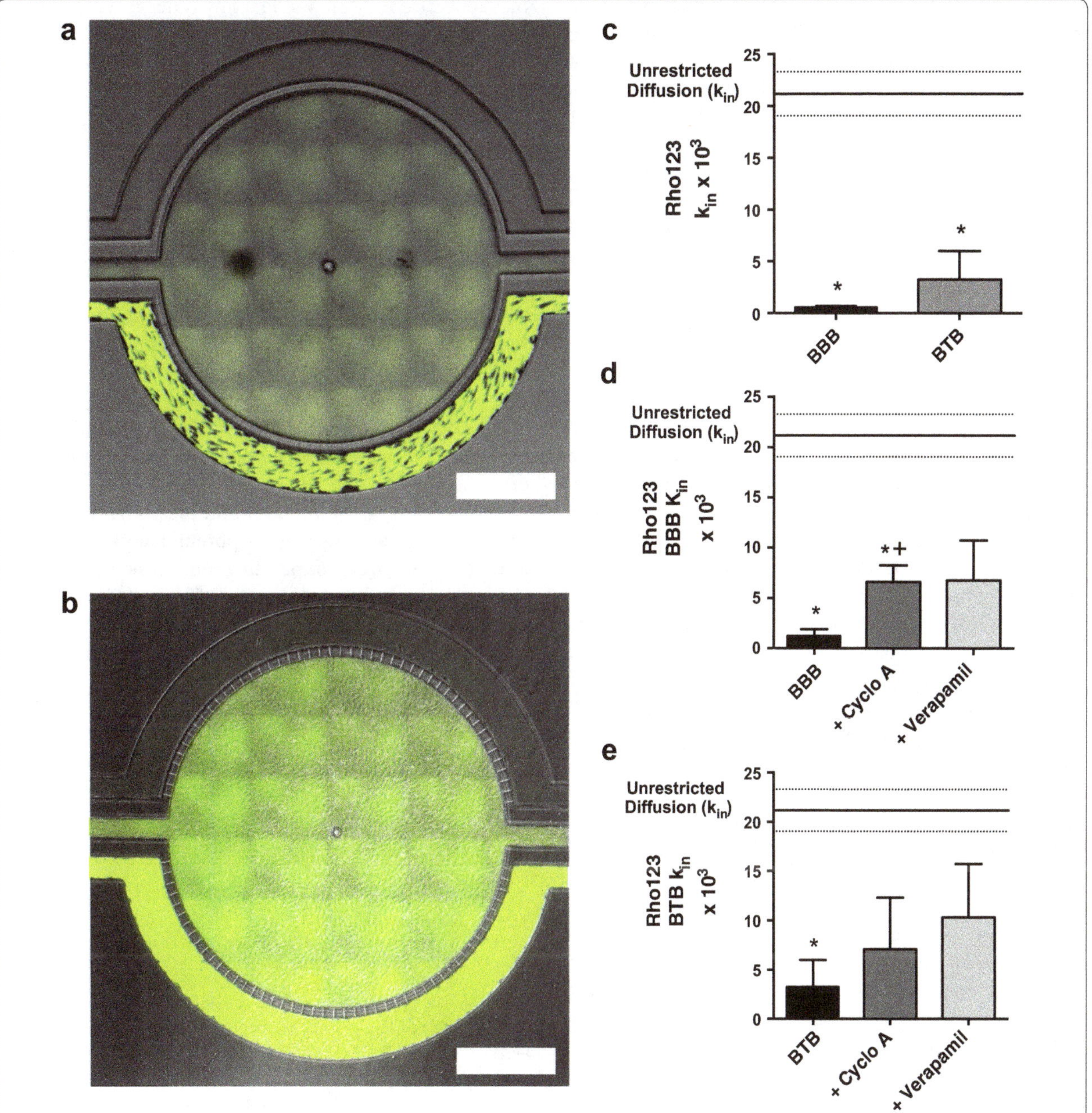

Fig. 6 Representative brightfield image of Rhodamine 123 dye accumulation in the central compartment after 90 min of perfusion in the BBB model without an inhibitor (**a**) and with an inhibitor (**b**). Rate of fluorescent dye accumulation of Rho123 into central compartment after 90 min of dye perfusion in BBB, and BTB chips (**c**). Rate of fluorescent dye accumulation in BBB (**d**) and BTB (**e**) chips perfused with Rho123 ± P-gp inhibitors (Cyclosporine A or Verapamil). Statistical significance was determined using one-way ANOVA followed by Tukey's multiple comparison tests, and student's *t* test; *$p < 0.05$ significance between tracer and unrestricted diffusion k_{in}, n = 3–4; $^{+}p < 0.05$ significance between BBB/BTB models and the addition of inhibitor, n = 3–6. All data represent mean ± SEM. *White rectangle scale bars* 500 μm

provide cell to cell communication to the endothelial cells in the outer compartment, resulting in the formation of tighter barrier and an increase in TEER [4, 17, 37]. Germane to this work, to re-create the BTB, astrocytes and or pericytes are replaced with tumor cells in the central compartment. In vivo, angiogenesis occurs with the establishment of tumor tissue, resulting in the presence of fenestrations, gaps between the endothelial cells, varied expression of efflux transporters, and an increase in permeability [10, 38].

The use of dyes has been a long-standing method to evaluate the integrity of the BBB and the breakdown of the BTB [39]. Some of the earliest work using dyes dates back to the nineteenth century, where Paul Ehrlich and Edwin Goldmann intravenously injected water-soluble dyes and observed that dyes did not have the ability to freely exchange between the vascular and brain parenchyma compartment (reviewed in [34]). Dyes have also been used as a tool to visualize and qualitatively measure disruption at the BBB [40–44] as well as the BTB [16, 34]. Passive permeability dyes are a simple way to compare rates of diffusion between different models in vivo and in vitro.

In measuring the unrestricted diffusion (the absence of cells) of molecules from the outer chamber to the center chamber, we observed that the diffusion rates (k_{in}), from the outer compartment to the central compartment, of all three sized molecules were not significantly different from each other. This data is consistent with previous work showing that if the diameter of each molecule being tested is at least 12× less than the barrier defects, then diffusion will remain constant for all molecules [45].

An interesting aspect of our observations was the similarity of efflux function that existed in the microfluidic model compared to the in vivo BBB [9]. Rhodamine 123 is subject to P-gp mediated efflux at both the BBB and the BTB. When rhodamine 123 and an inhibitor of P-gp are administered concurrently, dye accumulates in brain ~10- to 12-fold higher than in the absence of efflux inhibition [34]. Similarly, in this work, when Verapamil or Cyclosporine A was added to the outer chamber of the microfluidic device, Rhodamine 123 accumulation increased similar to in vivo reports [9]. Further, P-gp function retains function despite barrier breakdown in a number of pathologies [9, 46]. The data herein agree that the degree of efflux function for the BTB, though disrupted, is intact and it retains the ability to restrict drug and dye movement from the vasculature to the brain compartment.

Transwells are a widely used in vitro method to study the BBB. Transwells are cheap, available in high throughput assays, and easy to use. However, there are substantial limitations. First, transport kinetics in transwell systems are strongly influenced by an unstirred water layer that exists on the outer side of the endothelial cells. The unstirred water layer may decrease the apparent permeability rate of lipid soluble and increase to some extent water-soluble molecules. Second, because the cells are grown in a static media, there is no shear stress (or flow) forced on the endothelial cells, which may contribute to the low passive permeability measurements which can be as low as ~74 Ω cm^2 [47], compared to in vivo values of ~2000 Ω cm^2 [48]. While a few other in vitro models and microfluidic devices have a flow component [27–31], this microfluidic device is the first commercially available blood-tumor barrier using a microfluidic model seeded with brain-seeking cells and with shear stress similar to that observed in vivo [19] in addition to real-time visualization and quantitation.

Conclusions

This novel and dynamic microfluidic in vitro BTB model mimics the in vivo barrier with regard to shear stress, permeability, and efflux. Permeability of large molecule dextrans, as well as small molecule dextrans and Rhodamine 123 (with and without inhibitors) were characteristic and relatable to what is seen in vivo. The shear stress from adding flow over HUVECs eliminates the unstirred water layer and allows for different tracers to be added and followed in real time from outer to central compartment. Based on these characteristics, this microfluidic chip shows potential for use in BBB and BTB research. Expanding on these data, future work should entail the use of different drugs, and the comparison of different endothelial cell models to in vivo data with regards to passive permeability and influx/efflux.

Abbreviations

BBB: blood–brain barrier; P-gp: P-glycoprotein; BTB: blood-tumor barrier; TEER: transendothelial electrical resistance; Free TRD: sulforhodamine 101 Acid Chloride; Rho123: rhodamine 123; TRD 3kDa: Texas Red 3000 MW Dextran; TRD 70 kDa: Texas Red 70,000 MW Dextran; HUVEC: human umbilical vein endothelial cells; EBM-2: endothelial basal medium-2; k_{in}: unidirectional uptake transfer constants.

Authors' contributions

TTH participated in the design of the study, performed all of the experiments, as well as data processing and analysis, interpretation of data, statistical analysis, and manuscript drafting, revision, and finalizing. AA contributed to data processing and analysis, and interpretation of data. JG contributed data processing and analysis. PRL conceived and designed the study, and contributed to data processing and analysis, interpretation of data, statistical analysis, and manuscript drafting, revision, and finalizing. All authors read and approved the final manuscript.

Author details

[1] Department of Basic Pharmaceutical Sciences, School of Pharmacy, West Virginia University HSC, 1 Medical Center Dr., Morgantown, WV 26506, USA. [2] WVU Cancer Institute Research Laboratories, West Virginia University HSC, Morgantown, WV 26506, USA.

Acknowledgements

The authors would like to thank Ashley Smith (Kiyatec Inc., Greenville, S) and Dr. Prabhakar Pandian (CFDRC, Huntsville, AL) for their generosity in troubleshooting the microfluidic devices, Dr. Alexander Borowsky (UC Davis, Sacramento, CA) for his generosity in supplying the Met-1 murine metastatic breast cancer cells, and Dr. Jim Simpkins (West Virginia University, Morgantown, WV) for his generosity in supplying the CTX-TDR2 rat brain astrocyte cell line.

Competing interests

The authors declare that they have no competing interests.

Funding

This research was supported by grants from the National Cancer Institute (R01CA166067-01A1) awarded to P. Lockman. Additional support for this research was provided by WVCTSI through the National Institute of General Medical Sciences of the National Institutes of Health (U54GM104942).

References

1. Lin NU, et al. CNS metastases in breast cancer: old challenge, new frontiers. Clin Cancer Res. 2013;19(23):6404–18.
2. Daneman R, Prat A. The blood–brain barrier. Cold Spring Harb Perspect Biol. 2015;7(1):a020412.
3. Serlin Y, et al. Anatomy and physiology of the blood–brain barrier. Semin Cell Dev Biol. 2015;38:2–6.
4. Pardridge WM. Molecular biology of the blood–brain barrier. Mol Biotechnol. 2005;30(1):57–70.
5. Golden PL, Pardridge WM. P-Glycoprotein on astrocyte foot processes of unfixed isolated human brain capillaries. Brain Res. 1999;819(1–2):143–6.
6. Crone C, Christensen O. Electrical resistance of a capillary endothelium. J Gen Physiol. 1981;77(4):349–71.
7. Olesen SP, Crone C. Electrical resistance of muscle capillary endothelium. Biophys J. 1983;42(1):31–41.
8. Loscher W, Potschka H. Role of drug efflux transporters in the brain for drug disposition and treatment of brain diseases. Prog Neurobiol. 2005;76(1):22–76.
9. Adkins CE, et al. P-glycoprotein mediated efflux limits substrate and drug uptake in a preclinical brain metastases of breast cancer model. Front Pharmacol. 2013;4:136.
10. Plate KH, Scholz A, Dumont DJ. Tumor angiogenesis and anti-angiogenic therapy in malignant gliomas revisited. Acta Neuropathol. 2012;124(6):763–75.
11. Folkman J. Tumor angiogenesis: therapeutic implications. N Engl J Med. 1971;285(21):1182–6.
12. Liebner S, et al. Claudin-1 and claudin-5 expression and tight junction morphology are altered in blood vessels of human glioblastoma multiforme. Acta Neuropathol. 2000;100(3):323–31.
13. Sawada T, et al. Expression of the multidrug-resistance P-glycoprotein (Pgp, MDR-1) by endothelial cells of the neovasculature in central nervous system tumors. Brain Tumor Pathol. 1999;16(1):23–7.
14. Demeule M, et al. Expression of multidrug-resistance P-glycoprotein (MDR1) in human brain tumors. Int J Cancer. 2001;93(1):62–6.
15. Lockman PR, et al. Heterogeneous blood-tumor barrier permeability determines drug efficacy in experimental brain metastases of breast cancer. Clin Cancer Res. 2010;16(23):5664–78.
16. Adkins CE, et al. Characterization of passive permeability at the blood-tumor barrier in five preclinical models of brain metastases of breast cancer. Clin Exp Metastasis. 2016;33(4):373–83.
17. Helms HC, et al. In vitro models of the blood–brain barrier: an overview of commonly used brain endothelial cell culture models and guidelines for their use. J Cereb Blood Flow Metab. 2016;36(5):862–90.
18. Czupalla CJ, Liebner S, Devraj K. In vitro models of the blood–brain barrier. Methods Mol Biol. 2014;1135:415–37.
19. Deosarkar SP, et al. A novel dynamic neonatal blood–brain barrier on a chip. PLoS ONE. 2015;10(11):e0142725.
20. Prabhakarpandian B, et al. SyM-BBB: a microfluidic blood brain barrier model. Lab Chip. 2013;13(6):1093–101.
21. Cucullo L, et al. The role of shear stress in blood–brain barrier endothelial physiology. BMC Neurosci. 2011;12:40.
22. Santaguida S, et al. Side by side comparison between dynamic versus static models of blood–brain barrier in vitro: a permeability study. Brain Res. 2006;1109(1):1–13.
23. Loftsson T. Drug permeation through biomembranes: cyclodextrins and the unstirred water layer. Pharmazie. 2012;67(5):363–70.
24. Korjamo T, Heikkinen AT, Monkkonen J. Analysis of unstirred water layer in in vitro permeability experiments. J Pharm Sci. 2009;98(12):4469–79.
25. Lutgendorf MA, et al. Effect of dexamethasone administered with magnesium sulfate on inflammation-mediated degradation of the blood–brain barrier using an in vitro model. Reprod Sci. 2014;21(4):483–91.
26. Adriani G, et al. Modeling the blood–brain barrier in a 3D triple co-culture microfluidic system. Conf Proc IEEE Eng Med Biol Soc. 2015;2015:338–41.
27. Booth R, Kim H. Characterization of a microfluidic in vitro model of the blood–brain barrier (muBBB). Lab Chip. 2012;12(10):1784–92.
28. Cucullo L, et al. A dynamic in vitro BBB model for the study of immune cell trafficking into the central nervous system. J Cereb Blood Flow Metab. 2011;31(2):767–77.
29. Herland A, et al. Distinct contributions of astrocytes and pericytes to neuroinflammation identified in a 3D human blood–brain barrier on a chip. PLoS ONE. 2016;11(3):e0150360.
30. Neuhaus W, et al. A novel flow based hollow-fiber blood–brain barrier in vitro model with immortalised cell line PBMEC/C1-2. J Biotechnol. 2006;125(1):127–41.
31. Griep LM, et al. BBB on chip: microfluidic platform to mechanically and biochemically modulate blood–brain barrier function. Biomed Microdevices. 2013;15(1):145–50.
32. Cucullo L, et al. A new dynamic in vitro modular capillaries-venules modular system: cerebrovascular physiology in a box. BMC Neurosci. 2013;14:18.
33. Koziara JM, et al. In situ blood–brain barrier transport of nanoparticles. Pharm Res. 2003;20(11):1772–8.
34. Mittapalli RK, et al. Quantitative fluorescence microscopy provides high resolution imaging of passive diffusion and P-gp mediated efflux at the in vivo blood–brain barrier. J Neurosci Methods. 2013;219(1):188–95.
35. Patabendige A, Skinner RA, Abbott NJ. Establishment of a simplified in vitro porcine blood–brain barrier model with high transendothelial electrical resistance. Brain Res. 2013;1521:1–15.
36. Zlokovic BV. The blood–brain barrier in health and chronic neurodegenerative disorders. Neuron. 2008;57(2):178–201.
37. Stanimirovic DB, et al. Blood–brain barrier models: in vitro to in vivo translation in preclinical development of CNS-targeting biotherapeutics. Expert Opin Drug Discov. 2015;10(2):141–55.
38. Schlageter KE, et al. Microvessel organization and structure in experimental brain tumors: microvessel populations with distinctive structural and functional properties. Microvasc Res. 1999;58(3):312–28.
39. Hawkins BT, Egleton RD. Fluorescence imaging of blood–brain barrier disruption. J Neurosci Methods. 2006;151(2):262–7.
40. Bakay L, et al. Ultrasonically produced changes in the blood–brain barrier. AMA Arch Neurol Psychiatry. 1956;76(5):457–67.
41. Lin SR, Kormano M. Cerebral circulation after cardiac arrest. Microangiographic and protein tracer studies. Stroke. 1977;8(2):182–8.
42. da Costa JC. Influence of electroconvulsions on the permeability of the blood–brain barrier to trypan blue. Arq Neuropsiquiatr. 1972;30(1):1–7.
43. Nemeroff CB, Crisley FD. Monosodium L-glutamate-induced convulsions: temporary alteration in blood–brain barrier permeability to plasma proteins. Environ Physiol Biochem. 1975;5(6):389–95.
44. Schettler T, Shealy CN. Experimental selective alteration of blood–brain barrier by x-irradiation. J Neurosurg. 1970;32(1):89–94.
45. Mittapalli RK, Adkins CE, Bohn KA, Mohammad AS, Lockman JA, Lockman PR. Quantitative fluorescence microscopy measures vascular pore size in primary and metastatic brain tumors. Cancer Res. 2017;77(2):238–46. doi:10.1158/0008-5472.CAN-16-1711.
46. Cordon-Cardo C, et al. Expression of the multidrug resistance gene product (P-glycoprotein) in human normal and tumor tissues. J Histochem Cytochem. 1990;38(9):1277–87.
47. Man S, et al. Human brain microvascular endothelial cells and umbilical vein endothelial cells differentially facilitate leukocyte recruitment and utilize chemokines for T cell migration. Clin Dev Immunol. 2008;2008:384982.
48. Crone C, Olesen SP. Electrical resistance of brain microvascular endothelium. Brain Res. 1982;241(1):49–55.

14

Early and delayed assessments of quantitative gait measures to improve the tap test as a predictor of shunt effectiveness in idiopathic normal pressure hydrocephalus

Masatsune Ishikawa[1,2*], Shigeki Yamada[2,3] and Kazuo Yamamoto[3]

Abstract

Background: To improve the diagnostic performance of the cerebrospinal fluid (CSF) tap test (TT), early and delayed assessments of gait were performed after the removal of 30 ml of CSF in patients with probable idiopathic normal pressure hydrocephalus. Assessments of gait included the 3-m timed up and go test (TUG), and the 10-m walk in time (10Ti) and in step (10St) tests.

Methods: Quantitative data for the TUG, the 10Ti, and the 10St were obtained before CSF removal and on days 1 and 4 after removal of 30 ml CSF. CSF shunt surgery was performed in 61 patients within one month after the TT. The gait outcome was assessed 3 months after surgery. The area under the curve (AUC), sensitivity, specificity, and cutoff values were computed for the TUG, the 10Ti, and the 10St on day 1 and day 4 using receiver operating characteristic (ROC) curve analysis.

Results: The positive response rate in three measures on day 4 was equal to or higher than the values on day 1. Times were reduced significantly in the TUG and the 10mTi tests between baseline and both days 1 and 4 after TT. No significant differences were noted in the number of steps for the 10St test. The percent change in TUG on day 1 had the highest AUC value among all other variables (0.808). Although this was not statistically different from other variables in the TUG and the 10Ti, it had a good balance of high sensitivity (78.3%) and high specificity (80.0%), with a cutoff value of 11.3%. The change in the measured value in the day 1 TUG had the second highest AUC value at 0.770. The variables on day 4 tended to have high specificities of around 90%, although their sensitivities were low.

Conclusions: The percent change of TUG on day 1 showed the highest diagnostic accuracy. Delayed assessments on day 4 were not superior to those on day 1. Thus, the TUG on day 1 is useful as a simple quantitative measure for predicting shunt effectiveness.

Keywords: Hydrocephalus, Aged population, Tap test, Gait disturbance

Background

Idiopathic normal pressure hydrocephalus (iNPH) is a disorder resulting in abnormal gait, cognition, and urination in the aged population [1, 2]. CSF shunt surgery is effective in improving the symptoms of iNPH, especially those concerning gait [2]. The cerebrospinal fluid (CSF) tap test (TT), which involves the removal of 30–50 ml of CSF, is useful for the diagnosis of iNPH [3]. However, its diagnostic accuracy has been reported to vary between low and high [4–8]. This may be due to inconsistencies in various factors, such as the volume of CSF removed, the timing of the assessment, qualitative vs. quantitative assessments, and the use of single vs. multiple examiners. Virhammar et al. [9] recommend early assessment within 24 h of CSF removal. However, delayed improvement of

*Correspondence: rakuwadr1001@rakuwadr.com
[1] Rakuwa Villa Ilios, 186 Jyrakumawari-nishimachi, Nakagyouku, Kyoto 604-8402, Japan
Full list of author information is available at the end of the article

symptoms is often observed. Recently, Schniepp et al. [10] reported a maximal increase in gait velocity 24–48 h after the TT using quantitative measures of gait. Assessment of gait is performed using clinical grading scales in most studies. However, categorical scales lack reliability. Since quantitative measures for gait are more reliable and have good objectivity, we investigated the clinical usefulness of quantitative measures of gait. We used the timed up and go test (TUG), the 10-m walk in time (10Ti), and the 10-m walk in step (10St) tests. In order to improve the diagnostic performance of the CSF TT, we focused on the following clinical questions: (1) When is a better time for the assessment: day 1 or day 4? (2) Which is the best measure of gait among the above three popular measures? (3) Which is the best variable to use for the measured values: the change in the measured value, or its percent change? Diagnostic performances of the three measures were investigated using multiple receiver operating characteristic (ROC) curve analyses.

Methods

Study population

This study was approved by the institutional board in Rakuwakai Otowa Hospital, Kyoto, Japan (Rakuoto1023). To study the usefulness of the TT, it was performed in 101 patients with possible iNPH as defined by the Japanese guidelines for iNPH [11] from January 2012 to December 2015 in Rakuwakai Otowa hospital. Brain and spine magnetic resonance imaging (MRI) was performed in all patients. There was a positive response to TT in 75 of the patients. A positive response was defined as an improvement of one point or more on the Japanese iNPH grading scale (GS) [12] or an improvement of 10% or more above baseline in quantitative measures of the TT made according to a proposal of the Japanese guidelines for iNPH [11]. Among the 75 patients with a positive response, 61 patients with subsequent shunt surgery were included in this analysis. Patients who did not receive surgery due to patient's unwillingness and 5 patients who had severe gait disturbance requiring support at assessment, were excluded. Among the 61 patients, 51 had both early and delayed assessments of the TT. The remaining ten patients did not undergo the delayed assessment of the TT, due to the patient's unwillingness or difficulty with the examiners' time schedules. However, to exclude the possibility of selection bias, statistical analyses were performed on all 61 patients who had undergone surgery and in whom quantitative measures of gait could be obtained without any support.

MRI

The brain MRI studies included T2-weighted images, T2-star weighted images, fluid attenuation inversion recovery images, constructive interference in steady state (CISS) images, and magnetic resonance angiography. MRIs with T2-weighted images were carried out for both the lumbar and the cervical spine. Characteristic findings of iNPH on MRI are known to include disproportionately enlarged subarachnoid space hydrocephalus (DESH) [2]. DESH consists of ventriculomegaly, tight high convexity, and enlarged subarachnoid space. Each of these components was categorized into marked, fair, or none. Patients classified as DESH were marked for all three components. Patients classified as incomplete DESH had one fair and two marked categories among the three components. Patients with other classifications were considered non-DESH [13]. CISS findings from this study are reported elsewhere [14].

Tap test

For the TT, 30 ml of CSF were removed via a lumbar tap. Quantitative assessments of gait and cognition were performed before the lumbar tap, on day 1 (within 24 h of the tap), and on day 4. Fifty-seven patients were assessed within 24 h (18–24 h) to fit with the time schedules of rehabilitation staff and 4 patients were assessed within 3 h after the CSF removal.

Physiotherapists examined patients quantitatively using the TUG (s), the 10Ti (s), and the 10St (steps). On the TUG, the examination was performed in the rehabilitation room and physiotherapists measured time while a patient rises from an arm chair, walks 3 m, turns, walks back and sits down again, with maximum speed [15]. Assessments were done twice for each measure and the faster time or fewer steps were adopted. For the 10Ti and 10St, the patient was also requested to walk with maximal speed. The Mini-Mental State Examination and the Frontal Assessment Battery were carried out by speech therapists. Measured values, changes in measured values from baseline, and percent changes were compared between day 1 and day 4 groups for statistical significance (Table 1).

Shunt surgery

Shunt surgery, consisting of either a ventriculoperitoneal (VP) shunt (n = 44) [2] or a lumboperitoneal (LP) shunt (n = 17) [16], was performed in all patients within one month after the TT. Selection of the type of shunt was based on the presence or absence of severe lumbar or cervical canal stenosis, the patient's preference, and the surgeon's preference. The Codman Hakim programmable valve with Siphonguard or Medtronic Strata NSC system, were used. The outcome was assessed 3 months after the shunt surgery using the gait domain of the Japanese iNPH GS by the senior author (MI) at the outpatient clinic. The outcome at 3 months was chosen to

Table 1 Clinical summary of patients

Contents	Early assessment	Delayed assessment
Number of patients	61	51
Age[a]	76.9 ± 6.0	76.6 ± 5.5
Male preponderance[b]	73.8	70.6
Gait/cognition/urination[b]	100/80.3/73.8	100/82.3/76.4
Onset of gait disturbance <1 year/improved at 1 year	32/24	26/20
MRI of DESH/incomplete DESH/non-DESH[b]	55.7/23.0/21.3	60.8/17.6/21.6
Gait improvement on tap test[b]	91.8	96.1
Number of VP shunt/LP shunt	44/17	39/12
Improvement of gait at 3 months[b]	73.8	76.5%

Patients with early assessment on day 1 after CSF removal and delayed assessment on day 4 were subjected in study. Patients whom support was necessary for assessment of gait were not included in this study. The clinical characteristics were comparable among the two groups

DESH disproportionately enlarged subarachnoid-space by MRI, *VP* ventriculoperitoneal, *LP* lumboperitoneal

[a] Years: mean ± standard deviation

[b] Percentages

largely reflect the results of surgery, whereas if delayed for 6 months or 1 year the outcome could have been confounded by further modifications of comorbidity and nursing care. Improvement of gait at three months was defined as a one-point-or-larger improvement on the GS [11].

Statistical analyses

For the analysis of the means of continuous data, we used the Wilcoxon signed-rank test to perform nonparametric statistics. Comparisons of percentages of categorical data were performed using the Chi square test. Comparisons among the three groups (Baseline, Day1 and Day4) were performed using repeat measures analysis of variance (ANOVA) with Bonferroni post hoc comparison. Diagnostic accuracy of each variable was calculated using area under the curve (AUC), sensitivity, specificity, and cutoff levels obtained using receiver operating characteristic (ROC) curves. The significance level was set at 0.05. All statistical analyses were performed using the open-source software R (version 3.0.1; R Foundation for Statistical Computing, Vienna, Austria; http://www.R-project.org). ROC analyses were performed using the package program pROC (version 1.8) [17].

Results

Clinical background data are summarized in Table 1. Early assessment on day 1 after TT was performed in 61 patients with a mean age of 76.9 years. Delayed assessment on day 4 was performed in 51 patients with a mean age was 76.6 years. Gender, symptoms, MRI findings, and positive response on the TT were comparable between the groups with or without delayed assessment and no statistical differences were noted.

Positive response rates in gait which was defined as improvements of 10% or more over baseline in the TUG, the 10Ti, and the 10St on day 1 and day 4 are depicted in Fig. 1. Positive response rates on day 4 were equal to or higher in the three measures compared to day 1, with statistical significance in the 10St test. In the TUG and the 10Ti tests, repeat measures ANOVA analysis of the measured values at baseline and on days 1 and 4 revealed a statistically significant difference (Fig. 2). Post hoc analysis revealed significantly reduced times between baseline and day 1 and between baseline and day 4 in the TUG and 10Ti tests (Fig. 2). No statistical differences were noted in the 10St test.

The ROC curves of the three measures on days 1 and 4 are depicted for changes in the measured values (Fig. 3, left) and their percent changes (Fig. 3, right). AUC values were computed using the ROC analyses. The measured change and the percent change of TUG on day 1 both had higher AUCs. The AUC, sensitivity, specificity, and cutoff values are tabulated in Table 2. Each measure has a different sensitivity and specificity and a different AUC.

Among these measures, the percent change in the TUG on day 1 had the highest AUC value (0.808) and a sensitivity of 78.8% and a specificity of 80.0%. The cut-off value for the TUG was 11.3%. Although this AUC value was significantly different from most variables of 10St, no statistical differences were noted between the variables of the TUG and the 10Ti. The second highest AUC (0.770) was noted for the change in the measured value of the TUG on day 1. The TUG on day 1 had a sensitivity of 76.6%, a specificity of 75.0%, and a cutoff value of 2.0 s. Overall, the sensitivity of the TT ranged from 34.1 to 78.3%, while its specificity ranged from 50.0 to 93.8%

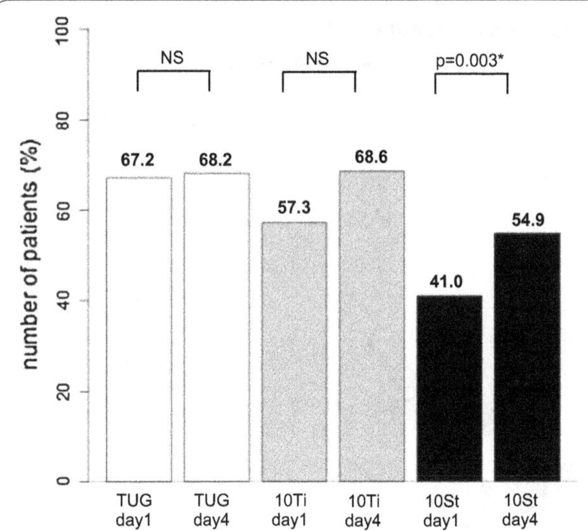

Fig. 1 Number of patients showing a positive response to the three tests on days 1 and 4 after the tap test. The percentage of positive responses was comparable between day 1 and day 4 for the timed up and go (TUG) and the 10-m walk in time (10Ti) tests but significantly higher for the 10-m walk in step (10St) test at day 4. The number of patients was 61 on day 1 and 51 on day 4

(Table 2). Thus, the TT tended to have a relatively low sensitivity and a high specificity. The variables on day 4 tended to have high specificities of around 90%, although their sensitivities were low. Among these variables, the 10Ti had fairly high AUCs of above 0.7. When a positive response was defined as positive in any one of the three assessment measures, the sensitivities became very high but specificities became low and their AUCs did not exceed the AUC of the TUG on day 1 (Fig. 4).

Discussion

Improvement of gait is the most frequent and useful finding after surgical treatment of iNPH. TT is a popular method to predict and assess shunt effectiveness and is not very invasive. Regarding the diagnostic accuracy of the TT, the specificity has been reported to be high with low sensitivity [4–6], although high sensitivity was also reported [7]. In our previous cooperative study of iNPH, named SINPHONI, the gait domain had a high specificity of 80% and a relatively low sensitivity of 51.3% [8]. We have often observed delayed improvement in gait after CSF removal. This observation led us to study the clinical significance of delayed assessment for the prediction of shunt effectiveness. Recently, Schniepp et al. reported a delayed improvement over 3 days after CSF removal [10]. Thus, the timing of assessment after CSF removal is an important issue in the tap test. In this study, delayed assessment was performed on day 4. The positive response rate on day 4 was equal to or higher in three measures than on day 1. The TUG and the 10Ti had statistically significant reductions in time both on day 1 and on day 4. Multiple ROC curve analyses indicated that the percent change of the TUG on day 1 had the highest AUC value, 0.808, which is a fairly high value. The TUG had a good balance between sensitivity and specificity. The second highest AUC of 0.770 was noted in the change of the measured value in the TUG on day 1. Most of measures on day 4 had fairly high AUCs, but they did not exceed the percent change of the TUG on day 1. We also examined the possibility of a high AUC if any of the three measures was positive. Any measure that was positive on day 1 had a fairly high AUC value. However, none were superior to the percent change of the TUG on day 1.

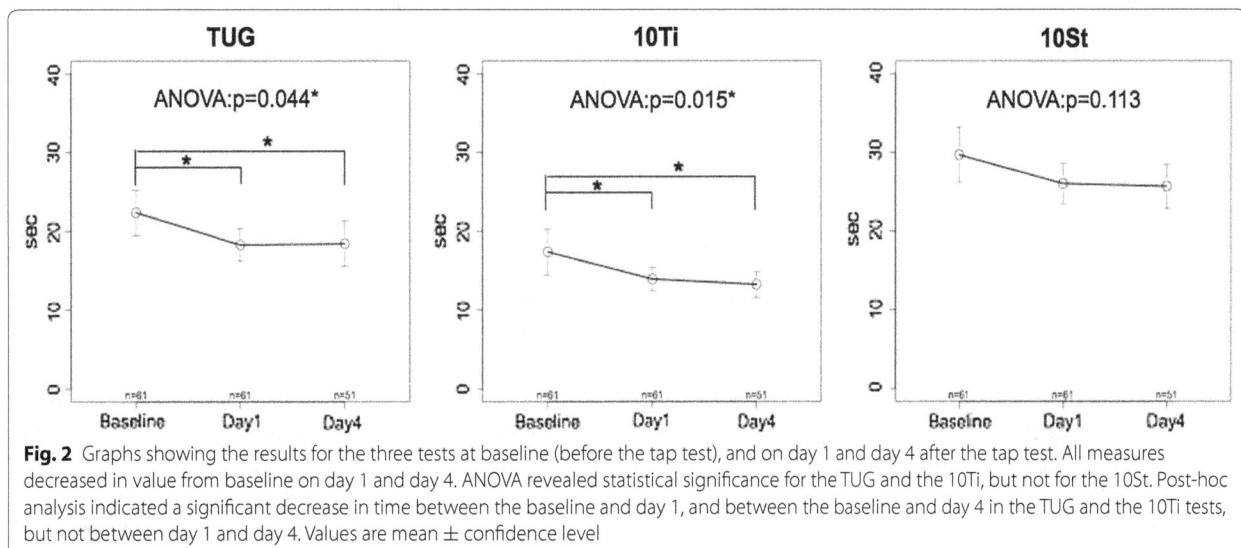

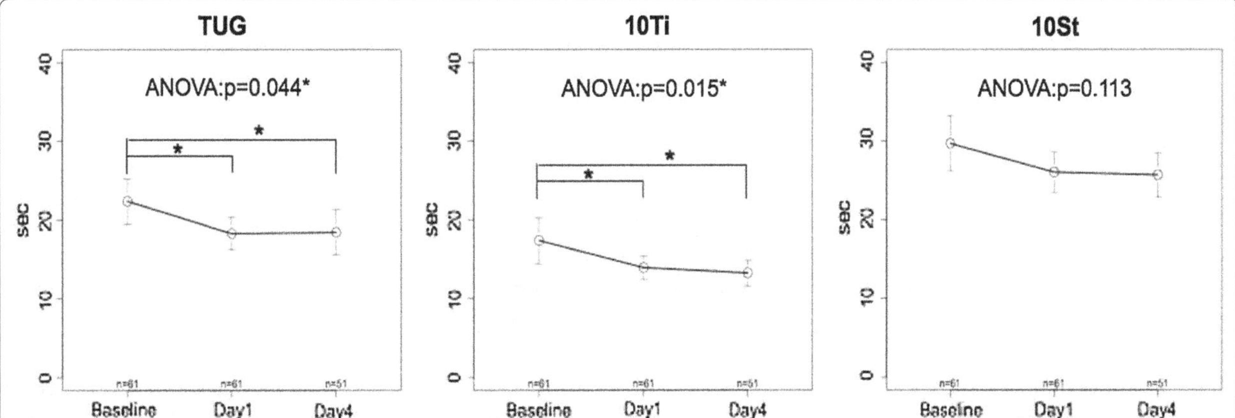

Fig. 2 Graphs showing the results for the three tests at baseline (before the tap test), and on day 1 and day 4 after the tap test. All measures decreased in value from baseline on day 1 and day 4. ANOVA revealed statistical significance for the TUG and the 10Ti, but not for the 10St. Post-hoc analysis indicated a significant decrease in time between the baseline and day 1, and between the baseline and day 4 in the TUG and the 10Ti tests, but not between day 1 and day 4. Values are mean ± confidence level

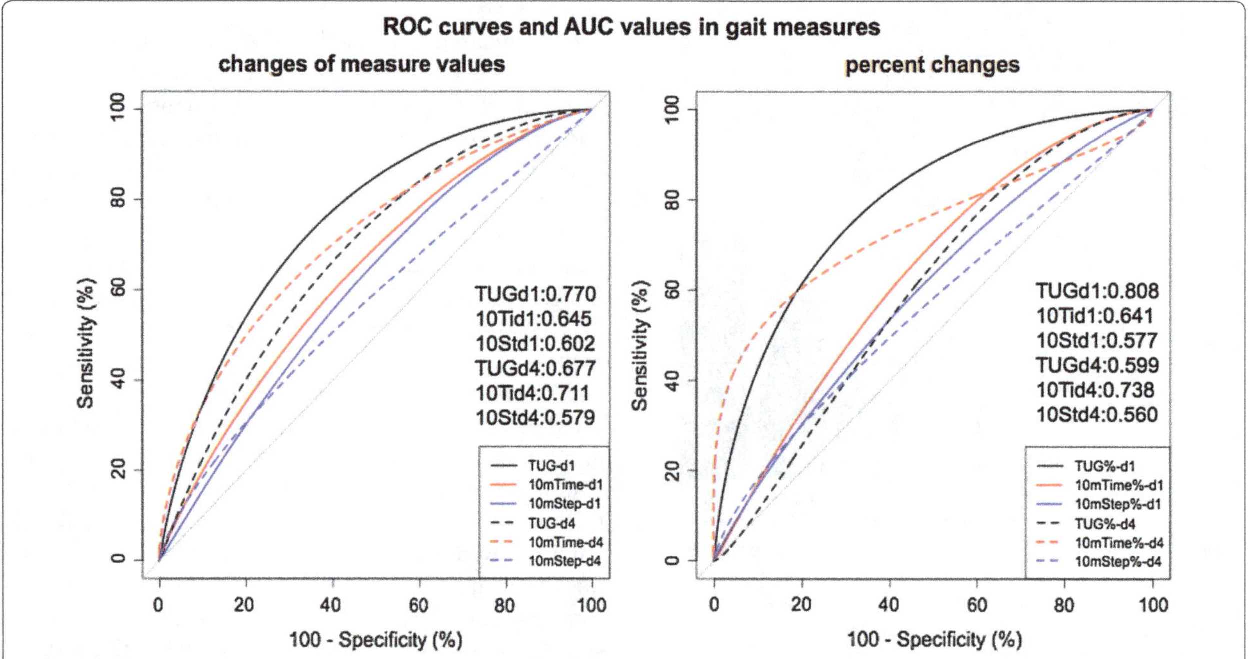

Fig. 3 Receiver operating characteristic (ROC) curves and area under the curve (AUC) values on day 1 (*solid lines*) and day 4 (*dotted lines*). ROC curves for changes of measured values from baseline are left and ROC curves for percent changes are on the right. The AUC for TUG on day 1 was highest for both ROC curves

Table 2 Receiver operating curve analysis

Examination day	Measures (change in time or step number from baseline)	AUC	p	Sensitivity (%)	Specificity (%)	Cutoff
Day 1 (N = 63)	TUG (s)	0.770	0.249	76.6	75.0	2.0
	10Ti (s)	0.645	0.102	63.8	68.8	0.8
	10St (step)	0.602	0.027*	36.1	93.8	4.5
Day 4 (N = 52)	TUG (s)	0.677	0.283	43.9	90.9	5.0
	10Ti (s)	0.711	0.383	63.4	81.2	2.3
	10St (step)	0.579	0.053	34.1	90.0	5.5
Examination day	**Measures (change in percentage from baseline)**	**AUC**	**p**	**Sensitivity (%)**	**Specificity (%)**	**Cutoff (%)**
Day 1 (N = 63)	TUG (%)	0.808	–	78.3	80.0	11.3
	10Ti (%)	0.641	0.193	63.0	66.6	9.4
	10St (%)	0.577	0.016*	41.3	86.7	13.6
Day 4 (N = 52)	TUG (%)	0.599	0.109	73.2	50.0	10.0
	10Ti (%)	0.738	0.483	63.4	90.0	15.8
	10St (%)	0.560	0.036*	41.5	80.0	17.0

ROC curve analysis showed the AUCs, sensitivities, specificities and cutoff values. The percent change from baseline of AUC on day 1 was regarded as a control and compared with other variables. Note the TUG on day 1, both for change in time and change in percentage, showed the highest AUC

Statistical differences were noted in most of 10Sts (*), but not in other variables of the TUG and the 10Ti

Thus, the TUG on day 1, either as a percent change or as a change in the measured value, was shown to be useful for predicting shunt effectiveness.

In this study, most of the assessments on day 4 had high specificities around 90%. High specificity indicates that the number of false positive cases is small, which is favorable from the standpoint of recommendation for surgery. Similarly, high sensitivity indicates that the number of false negative cases is small, which is favorable for selecting candidates from the general population.

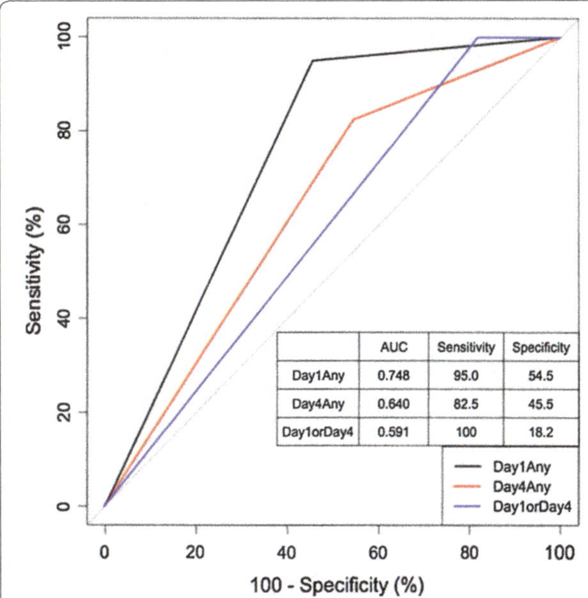

Fig. 4 Positive response in any of three assessment measures. Positive response in any of three assessment measures on day1 (*black line*), day 4 (*red line*) or either day 1 or day 4 (*blue line*) showed high sensitivity but their specificities were low

In this context, the day 4 study is still useful if a positive response is noted. This is because of the high specificity of the test on day 4.

The second issue to consider is the modality of the examination of gait. The 3-m TUG and the 10-m walk are popular choices. Stoltz et al. reported increased velocity due to an enlarged stride length after the removal of 30 ml of CSF [18]. In this study, gait was simply assessed using time and step number. A decrease in the time and an increased velocity was confirmed using the TUG and the 10Ti. However, the decrease in the number of steps on the 10St was not confirmed. Instrumented walkway assessments could provide more objective information. Williams et al. reported that velocity, double support time, and cadence improve significantly after CSF drainage in patients with iNPH in assessments using an instrumented walkway [19]. Schniepp et al. also reported an increase in walking speed in various tasks performed on the walkway [10]. They noted maximal improvements of dual task paradigms on days 2 and 3, and recommend that assessments of gait be performed on day 2 or day 3.

In this study, a positive response in quantitative measures was defined as 10% improvement from the baseline according to the proposal of Japanese iNPH guidelines. This proposal is based on clinical experience. In this study, the cut-off values in TUG, 10 m walk in time and in step on day 1 were close to 10%. Thus, present study reveals that the guidelines' proposal is appropriate for gait.

Third issue that we investigated is the assessment of improvement. Change of gait after CSF removal is usually assessed using various kinds of qualitative grading scales, such as Kiefer's scale [20] and the Japan iNPH grading scale [7]. The scores obtained using these scales may be different depending on the individual examiner. Assessment of the baseline state may vary, and assessment of changes after the interventions may be more variable. As a result, the reproducibility of these scales may be low. Furthermore, the qualitative scores obtained are difficult to compare among the different grading systems. We have observed differences in the scores as determined by physicians vs. physiotherapists, even when using the same grading scale [21]. The former tended to place more emphasis on changes in symptoms, while the latter emphasized changes in daily activities. Quantitative measures are more reliable and can be compared between reports. However, measured values may only represent a part of the patient's disability.

This study has several limitations. This is a retrospective study in a single third-referral hospital. The outcome was assessed by a neurosurgeon using the qualitative scale of the Japan iNPH GS. The improvement rate of 76.9% may be relatively low. This is assessed using a subjective score and may cause some bias in ROC curve analyses. Scores on the iNPH GS after the TT may be different when assessed by different examiners. To overcome these problems, well-designed grading scales to assess the degree of severity and subsequent changes with high inter-rater agreement are necessary. The instrumental walkway may provide more information regarding gait changes. This study did not include cognitive data. Cognition may be associated with gait improvement, as reported by Allali et al. [22]. We tried the dual-task walk in some patients, but no consistent findings were noted. Further study is necessary to obtain a high prediction rate for shunt effectiveness.

Conclusions

To improve the diagnostic performance of the CSF TT, early and delayed assessments in gait were performed after the removal of 30 ml of CSF from patients with suspected iNPH. Quantitative data from the TUG, the 10Ti, and the 10St were obtained before CSF removal and on day 1 and day 4 after CSF removal. The gait outcome was assessed 3 months after CSF shunt surgery. ROC curve analysis indicated that the highest AUC value (0.808) was observed for the percent change in the TUG on day 1. The TUG on day 1 showed the highest diagnostic accuracy with the sensitivity of 78.8% and the specificity of 80%, and the cutoff value was 11.3%. Delayed assessment on day 4 was not superior to that on day 1. Thus, the TUG on day 1 is useful as a simple quantitative measure for predicting shunt effectiveness.

Abbreviations
ANOVA: analysis of variance; AUC: area under the curve; CISS: constructive interference in steady state; CSF: cerebrospinal fluid; DESH: disproportionately enlarged subarachnoid-space hydrocephalus; GS: grading scale; iNPH: idiopathic normal pressure hydrocephalus; LP: lumboperitoneal shunt; MRI: magnetic resonance imaging; ROC: receiver operating characteristic; TT: tap test; TUG: timed up and go test; VP: ventriculoperitoneal shunt; 10Ti: 10-m walk in time; 10St: 10-m walk in step.

Authors' contributions
MI carried out patient data collection, statistical analysis, and drafted the manuscript. YS carried out patient data collection and statistical analysis. KY participated in the coordination of the study. All authors read and approved the final manuscript.

Author details
[1] Rakuwa Villa Ilios, 186 Jyrakumawari-nishimachi, Nakagyouku, Kyoto 604-8402, Japan. [2] Normal Pressure Hydrocephalus Center, Rakuwakai Otowa Hospital, 2 Chinjicho, Yamashinaku, Otowa, Kyoto 607-8062, Japan. [3] Department of Neurosurgery, Rakuwakai Otowa Hospital, 2 Chinjicho, Yamashinaku, Otowa, Kyoto 607-8062, Japan.

Acknowledgements
The authors would like to thank the patients and the staffs at the Rehabilitation Center at Rakuwakai Otowa Hospital.

Competing interests
MI receives honoraria for lecturing by Codman, Johnson and Johnson, and Medtronic Japan. SY receives honoraria for lecturing by Codman and Johnson and Johnson. KY has no competing interests.

Funding
This study was supported by a Health and Labor Sciences Research Grant for Research on Intractable Diseases, Ministry of Health, Labor and Welfare. The sponsors were not involved in the study design, in the collection, analysis, or interpretation data; in the writing of the report; or in the decision to submit the paper for publication.

References

1. Hakim S, Adams RD. The special clinical problems of symptomatic hydrocephalus with normal cerebrospinal fluid pressure: observations on cerebrospinal fluid dynamics. J Neurol Sci. 1965;2:302–27.
2. Hashimoto M, Ishikawa M, Mori E, Kuwana N. For the study of idiopathic normal pressure hydrocephalus on neurological improvement (SINPHONI) group. Diagnosis of idiopathic normal pressure hydrocephalus is supported by MRI-based scheme: a prospective study. Cerebrospinal Fluid Res. 2010;7:18. doi:10.1186/1743-8454-7-S1-S18.
3. Wikkelsø C, Andersson H, Blomstrand C, Lindqvist G. The clinical effect of lumbar puncture in normal pressure hydrocephalus. J Neurol Neurosurg Psychiatry. 1982;45:64–9. doi:10.1136/jnnp.45.1.64.
4. Haan J, Thomeer RT. Predictive value of temporary external lumbar drainage in normal pressure hydrocephalus. Neurosurgery. 1988;22:388–91.
5. Walchenbach R, Geiger E, Thomeer RT, Vanneste JA. The value of temporary external lumbar CSF drainage in predicting the outcome of shunting on normal pressure hydrocephalus. J Neurol Neurosurg Psychiatry. 2002;72:503–6.
6. Damasceno BP, Carelli EF, Honorato DC, Facure JJ. The predictive value of cerebrospinal fluid tap-test in normal pressure hydrocephalus. Arq Neuropsiquiatr. 1997;55:179–85.
7. Wikkelsø C, Hellström P, Klinge PM, Tans JT. European iNPH Multicentre Study Group. The European iNPH Multicenter Study on the predictive values of resistance to CSF outflow and the CSF Tap Test in patients with idiopathic normal pressure hydrocephalus. J Neurol Neurosurg Psychiat. 2013;84:562–8.
8. Ishikawa M, Hashimoto M, Mori E, Kuwana M, Hiroaki Kazui H. The value of the cerebrospinal fluid tap test for predicting shunt effectiveness in idiopathic normal pressure hydrocephalus. Fluids Barriers CNS. 2012;9(1):1. doi:10.1186/2045-8118-9-1.
9. Virhammar J, Cesarini KG, Laurell K. The CSF tap test in normal pressure hydrocephalus: evaluation time, reliability and the influence of pain. Eur J Neurol. 2011. doi:10.1111/j.1468-1331,2011.03486.x.
10. Schniepp R, Trabold R, Romagna A, Akrami F, Hesselbarth K, Wuehr M, Peraud P, Brandt T, Dieterich M, Jahn K. Walking assessment after lumbar puncture in normal-pressure hydrocephalus: a delayed improvement over 3 days. J Neurosurg. 2016. doi:10.3171/2015.12.jns151663.
11. Mori E, Ishikawa M, Kato T, Kazui H, Miyake H, Miyajima M, Nakajima M, Hashimoto M, Kuriyama N, Tokuda T, Ishii K, Kaijima M, Hirata Y, Saito M, Arai H. Japanese Society of normal pressure hydrocephalus: guidelines for management of idiopathic normal pressure hydrocephalus: second edition. Neurol Med Chir (Tokyo). 2012;52(11):775–809.
12. Kubo Y, Kazui H, Yoshida T, Kito Y, Kimura N, Tokunaga H, Ogino A, Miyake H, Ishikawa M, Takeda M. Validation of grading scale for evaluating symptoms of idiopathic normal-pressure hydrocephalus. Dement Geriatr Cogn Disord. 2008;25:37–45.
13. Ishikawa M, Oowaki H, Takezawa M, Takenaka T, Yamada S, Yamamoto K, Okamoto S. Disproportionately enlarged subarachnoid space hydrocephalus in idiopathic normal-pressure hydrocephalus and its implication in pathogenesis. Intracranial pressure and brain monitoring XV. Berlin: Springer; 2016. p. 287–90.
14. Ishikawa M, Yamada S, Yamamoto K. Three-dimensional observation of Virchow-Robin spaces in the basal ganglia and white matter and their relevance to idiopathic normal pressure hydrocephalus. Fluids Barriers CNS. 2015;26(12):15. doi:10.1186/s12987-015-0010-1.
15. Podsiadlo D, Richardson S. The timed 'Up & Go': a test of basic functional mobility for frail elderly persons. J Am Geriatr Soc. 1991;39(2):142–8.
16. Kazui H, Miyajima M, Mori E, Ishikawa M. on behalf of the SINPHONI-2 Investigators* Lumboperitoneal shunt surgery for idiopathic normal pressure hydrocephalus (SINPHONI-2): an open-label randomised trial. Lancet Neurol. 2015;14:585–94.
17. Robin X, Turck N, Hainard A, Tiberti N, Lisacek F, Sanchez J and Müller M. pROC: an open-source package for R and S+ to analyze and compare ROC curves. BMC Bioinform. 2011. doi: 10.1186/1471-2105-12-77. http://www.biomedcentral.com/1471-2105/12/77/.
18. Stolze H, Kuhtz-Buschbeck J, Drucke H, Johnk K, Diercks C, Mehdom HM, Illert M, Deuschl G. Gait analysis in idiopathic normal pressure hydrocephalus–which parameters respond to the CSF tap test? Clin Neurophysol. 2000;111:1678–86.
19. Williams MA, Thomas G, de Lateur B, Imteyaz H, Rose JG, Shore WS, Kharkar S, Rigamonti D. Objective assessment of gait in normal-pressure hydrocephalus. Am J Phys Med Rehabil. 2008;87(1):39–45.
20. Kiefer M, Eymann R, Komenda Y, Steudel WI. A grading system for chronic hydrocephalus. Zentralbl Neurochir. 2003;64:109–15 **(Ger)**.
21. Ishikawa M. Comparison of various assessment measures on shunt effectiveness in idiopathic normal pressure hydrocephalus. Presented at the first meeting of the European Academy of Neurology in Copenhagen; 2014.
22. Allali G, Leidet M, Beauchet O, Herrmann FR, Assal F, Armand S. Dual-task related gait changes after CSF taping: a new way to identify idiopathic normal pressure hydrocephalus. J Neuroeng Rehabil. 2013;10:117. doi:10.1186/1743-0003-10-117.

15

Characterization of cardiac- and respiratory-driven cerebrospinal fluid motion based on asynchronous phase-contrast magnetic resonance imaging in volunteers

Ken Takizawa[1], Mitsunori Matsumae[1*], Saeko Sunohara[2], Satoshi Yatsushiro[2] and Kagayaki Kuroda[2]

Abstract

Background: A classification of cardiac- and respiratory-driven components of cerebrospinal fluid (CSF) motion has been demonstrated using echo planar imaging and time-spatial labeling inversion pulse techniques of magnetic resonance imaging (MRI). However, quantitative characterization of the two motion components has not been performed to date. Thus, in this study, the velocities and displacements of the waveforms of the two motions were quantitatively evaluated based on an asynchronous two-dimensional (2D) phase-contrast (PC) method followed by frequency component analysis.

Methods: The effects of respiration and cardiac pulsation on CSF motion were investigated in 7 healthy subjects under guided respiration using asynchronous 2D-PC 3-T MRI. The respiratory and cardiac components in the foramen magnum and aqueduct were separated, and their respective fractions of velocity and amount of displacement were compared.

Results: For velocity in the Sylvian aqueduct and foramen magnum, the fraction attributable to the cardiac component was significantly greater than that of the respiratory component throughout the respiratory cycle. As for displacement, the fraction of the respiratory component was significantly greater than that of the cardiac component in the aqueduct regardless of the respiratory cycle and in the foramen magnum in the 6- and 10-s respiratory cycles. There was no significant difference between the fractions in the 16-s respiratory cycle in the foramen magnum.

Conclusions: To separate cardiac- and respiratory-driven CSF motions, asynchronous 2D-PC MRI was performed under respiratory guidance. For velocity, the cardiac component was greater than the respiratory component. In contrast, for the amount of displacement, the respiratory component was greater.

Keywords: Cerebrospinal fluid, Magnetic resonance imaging, Fluid dynamics, Phase-contrast image, Quantitative analysis

Background

Intracranial cerebrospinal fluid (CSF) motion changes with cardiac and respiratory rhythms [1]. In clinical practice, most clinicians accept that the motion of the CSF has two elements, a fast movement synchronized with the heartbeat and a somewhat slower movement synchronized with respiratory movements, on the basis of observations of the fluid surface during surgery or CSF drainage. When discussing the physiological role of CSF, analyzing its motion in terms of its separate cardiac and respiratory components is valuable for elucidating the pathologies of diseases that cause abnormal movement of the CSF, such as hydrocephalus. Magnetic resonance imaging (MRI) provides a noninvasive technique for studying CSF dynamics in human subjects [2–6].

*Correspondence: mike@is.icc.u-tokai.ac.jp
[1] Department of Neurosurgery, Tokai University School of Medicine, 143 Shimokasuya, Isehara, Kanagawa 2591193, Japan
Full list of author information is available at the end of the article

Numerous researchers have investigated cardiac modulation of CSF using various MRI techniques [2, 6, 7]. On the other hand, only a few studies of the modulation of CSF motion induced by respiration have been performed [8–10]. To visualize the cardiac- and respiratory-driven CSF motions separately, Yamada et al. [8] used a spin-labeling technique called time-spatial labeling inversion pulse (Time-SLIP). Chen used the simultaneous multi-slice (SMS) echo planar imaging (EPI) technique [11] based on MRI. A new approach using frequency analysis has recently also come into use. Yatsushiro et al. [12] used the 2-dimensional phase-contrast (2D-PC) technique to classify intracranial CSF motion into cardiac and respiratory components and expressed these by means of correlation mapping.

We consider that quantitative analysis of velocity and displacement, the integral of velocity over time, is required to ascertain the dynamics of CSF motion as water, and this study was conceived on the assumption that quantitative analysis of CSF motion by 2D-PC, a development building on previous techniques, is appropriate for this purpose. To separate the cardiac and respiratory components of CSF motion, the asynchronous real-time 2D-PC technique was used in seven healthy volunteers under controlled respiration. The velocity and the amount of displacement of the cardiac and respiratory components of CSF motion were quantified. The velocity and displacement were then compared in each respiratory cycle, and the effects of respiratory and cardiac components on CSF motion were quantitatively investigated.

Methods

Our institutional review board approved this research. All volunteers were examined after providing appropriate informed consent, consistent with the terms of approval from the institutional review board of our institution.

Asynchronous 2D-PC technique under controlled respiration was performed in 7 healthy volunteers (6 male and 1 female) aged 21–31 years. The respiratory cycle was set to 6, 10, and 16 s, to cover the range of the normal respiratory cycle. Volunteers were requested to control their respiration according to audio guidance for inhalation and exhalation timing. To monitor respiration, a bellows-type pressure sensor was placed around the abdomen of the subject, and an electrocardiogram (ECG) was monitored to identify the frequency distribution of individual cardiac motion. Asynchronous 2D-PC steady-state-free precession (SSFP) was performed on a 3-T MR scanner with the following conditions: flow encode direction foot–head (FH); data points 256; repetition time (TR) 6.0 ms; echo time (TE) 3.9 ms; flip angle (FA) 10°; field of view (FOV) 28 × 28 cm^2; velocity encoding (VENC) 10 cm/s; acquisition matrix 89 × 128 (half-Fourier); reconstruction matrix 256 × 256; and slice thickness 7 mm. These conditions yielded a frame rate of 4.6 images/s (temporal resolution of 217 ms). The total duration of data acquisition for each subject was 55 s. After obtaining the color-coded velocity vector images, rough outlines of the ROI were specified around the Sylvian aqueduct and the foramen of Monro. The partial volume effect arising from the relatively large voxel size (approximately 2 mm) used in the present experiment made a simple threshold-based segmentation of the T_2-weighted image difficult. To segment the CSF regions on the images with a reduced partial volume effect and to apply these images to the velocity and pressure images as masks for the quantitative analyses, a novel segmentation technique, called spatial-based fuzzy clustering, was applied. The details of this technique are explained elsewhere [13].

The waveform in the individual voxels was separated into respiratory and cardiac components based on frequency range, and the maximum velocity was determined for the respective components. The technical details of the procedure were explained in our previous study [12, 14].

The ratio of the individual velocity of the respiratory or cardiac component to the sum of the velocities of the respiratory and cardiac components was calculated for both velocity and displacement. The results of the above calculations for the cerebral aqueduct and the foramen magnum were compared statistically. Equation 1 shows the formula for the calculation of the fraction, F_r, of the velocity of the respiratory component to the sum of the velocities for the respiratory and cardiac components.

$$F_{\mathrm{r}} = \frac{v_{\mathrm{r}}}{v_{\mathrm{r}} + v_{\mathrm{c}}} \tag{1}$$

where v_r is the respiratory component of the velocity, while v_c is the cardiac component.

The mean CSF displacement of each component in the cranial and caudal directions was calculated from the velocity waveform based on the following equation,

$$D = \frac{1}{N}\sum_{n=1}^{N}\left(\Delta t \sum_{m=1}^{M} v(m \cdot \Delta t)\right) \tag{2}$$

where $v(m\cdot \Delta t)$ is the velocity at the mth time point of the observation with a sampling period of Δt, and M is the number of time points in the cranial or caudal direction. For example, when the velocity was positive, its direction was regarded as cranial, and the number of corresponding data points was set to M. N is the number of voxels in a region of interest (ROI) for the displacement measurement. Fractions of cardiac- and respiratory-induced displacements were calculated in a similar manner with equation [1], but separately for the cranial and caudal directions.

The Kolmogorov–Smirnov test and the Mann–Whitney U test were used to compare the respiratory and cardiac components of the velocity and the amount of displacement.

Results

Figure 1b presents a CSF velocity waveform obtained with a 6-s respiratory cycle by the asynchronous time-resolved 2D-PC technique at region of interest (ROI) #1 placed at the foramen magnum, as depicted in Fig. 1a. Summary of the velocities and displacement of the respiratory and cardiac components of the CSF at the Sylvian aqueduct and the foramen magnum are shown in Tables 1, 2. The fractions of the respiratory and cardiac components of the CSF velocity at the Sylvian aqueduct are shown in Fig. 2. The cardiac component was significantly greater than the respiratory component ($p = 0.002$) regardless of the respiratory period. A similar plot for the fractions at the foramen magnum is shown in Fig. 3. In results for both the Sylvian aqueduct and the foramen magnum, the cardiac component was significantly greater than the respiratory component ($p = 0.002$) throughout the three different respiratory cycles. There was no significant difference between the

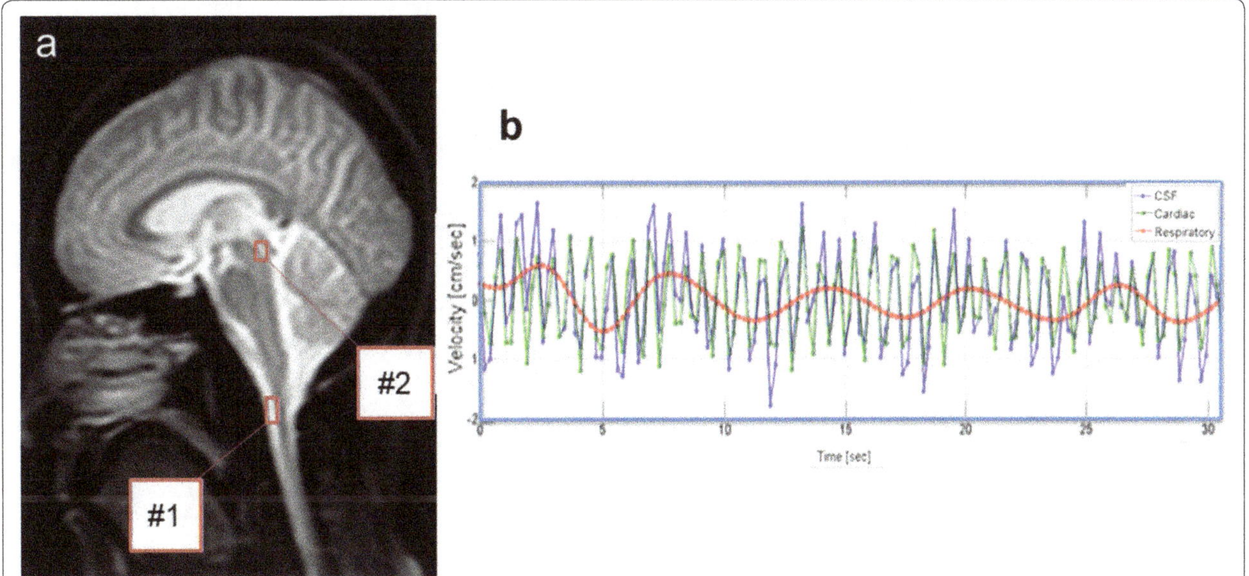

Fig. 1 A T_2-weighted image (**a**) of a healthy subject with 2 ROIs (red rectangles) placed in the foramen magnum (#1) and the Sylvian aqueduct (#2). The temporal changes of the total velocity wave of the CSF, and separated the cardiac and respiratory velocity components at ROI #1 are shown in (**b**)

Table 1 Summary of the cardiac- and respiratory-driven CSF velocities (cm/s) in the cranial and caudal directions for the three different respiratory periods

Respiratory period (s)	Cranial		Caudal	
	Cardiac	Respiratory	Cardiac	Respiratory
Sylvian aqueduct				
6	0.216 ± 0.049	0.109 ± 0.025	−0.219 ± 0.058	−0.121 ± 0.020
10	0.209 ± 0.061	0.119 ± 0.016	−0.212 ± 0.052	−0.137 ± 0.028
16	0.201 ± 0.041	0.110 ± 0.031	−0.205 ± 0.045	−0.131 ± 0.033
Foramen magnum				
6	0.948 ± 0.431	0.384 ± 0.194	−0.976 ± 0.466	−0.348 ± 0.232
10	1.003 ± 0.534	0.359 ± 0.178	−1.028 ± 0.511	−0.301 ± 0.095
16	1.008 ± 0.540	0.246 ± 0.095	−1.008 ± 0.489	−0.275 ± 0.117

Velocity (cm/s) in the aqueduct and foramen magnum

Values are shown as mean ± standard deviation

Table 2 Summary of the cardiac- and respiratory-driven CSF displacements (cm) in the cranial and caudal directions for the three different respiratory periods

Respiratory period (s)	Cranial		Caudal	
	Cardiac	Respiratory	Cardiac	Respiratory
Sylvian aqueduct				
6	0.051 ± 0.022	0.124 ± 0.023	−0.049 ± 0.019	−0.121 ± 0.024
10	0.054 ± 0.027	0.138 ± 0.043	−0.052 ± 0.023	−0.140 ± 0.052
16	0.054 ± 0.025	0.147 ± 0.054	−0.053 ± 0.024	−0.156 ± 0.058
Foramen magnum				
6	0.319 ± 0.154	0.505 ± 0.314	−0.313 ± 0.147	−0.489 ± 0.325
10	0.334 ± 0.169	0.614 ± 0.355	−0.331 ± 0.169	−0.670 ± 0.362
16	0.308 ± 0.133	0.501 ± 0.281	−0.308 ± 0.132	−0.572 ± 0.424

Displacement (cm) in the aqueduct and foramen magnum

Values are shown as mean ± standard deviation

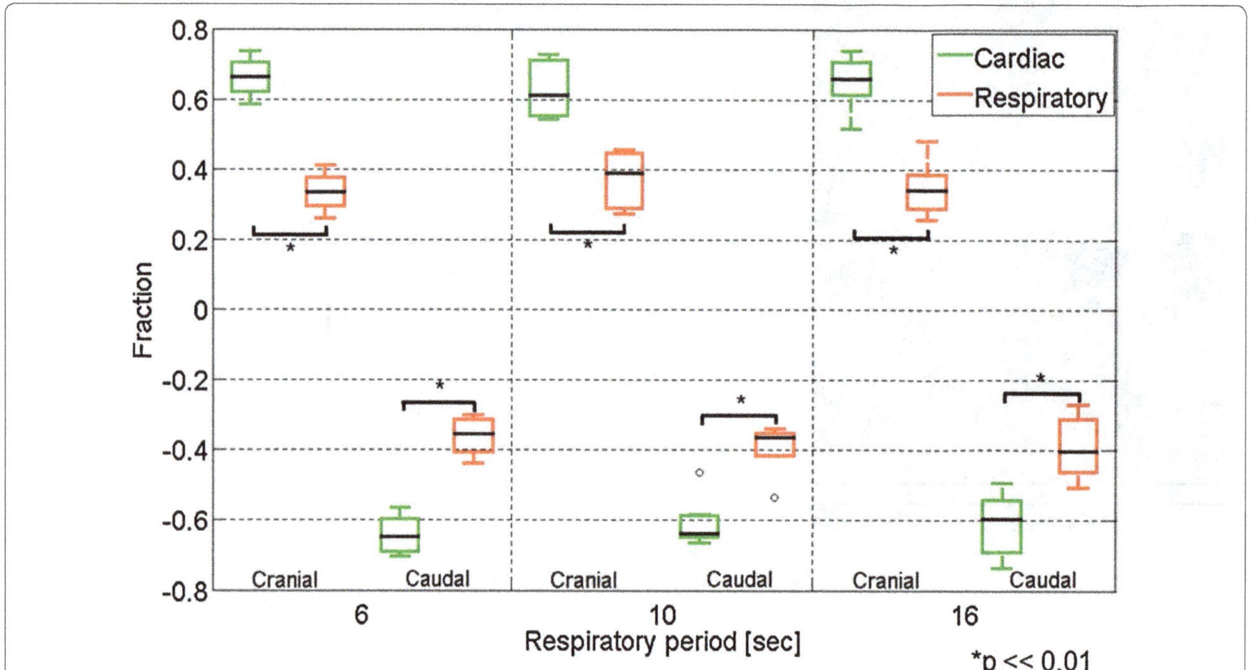

Fig. 2 Box plots of the fractions of the respiratory and cardiac components of the CSF velocity in the three different respiratory cycles (6, 10, and 16 s) at the aqueduct. The cranial and caudal directions are plotted separately. Outlying values are indicated by "o"

fractions of the different respiratory periods for both the respiratory and cardiac components.

The fraction of the displacement of the CSF for the respiratory and cardiac components at the Sylvian aqueduct is shown in Fig. 4. Throughout the respiratory cycle, the respiratory component was significantly greater than the cardiac component ($p = 0.002$). No significant difference was found between the fractions of the different respiratory periods. A similar plot for the displacement fraction at the foramen magnum is shown in Fig. 5. In this region, the displacement fraction of the respiratory component was significantly greater than that of the cardiac component in the respiratory cycle at 6 and 10 s ($p = 0.02$). However, no significant difference was observed at 16 s ($p = 0.85$). Significant differences between the respiratory cycles of 6 and 16 s were observed in both the respiratory and cardiac components ($p = 0.004$). No differences were observed in the other respiratory cycles.

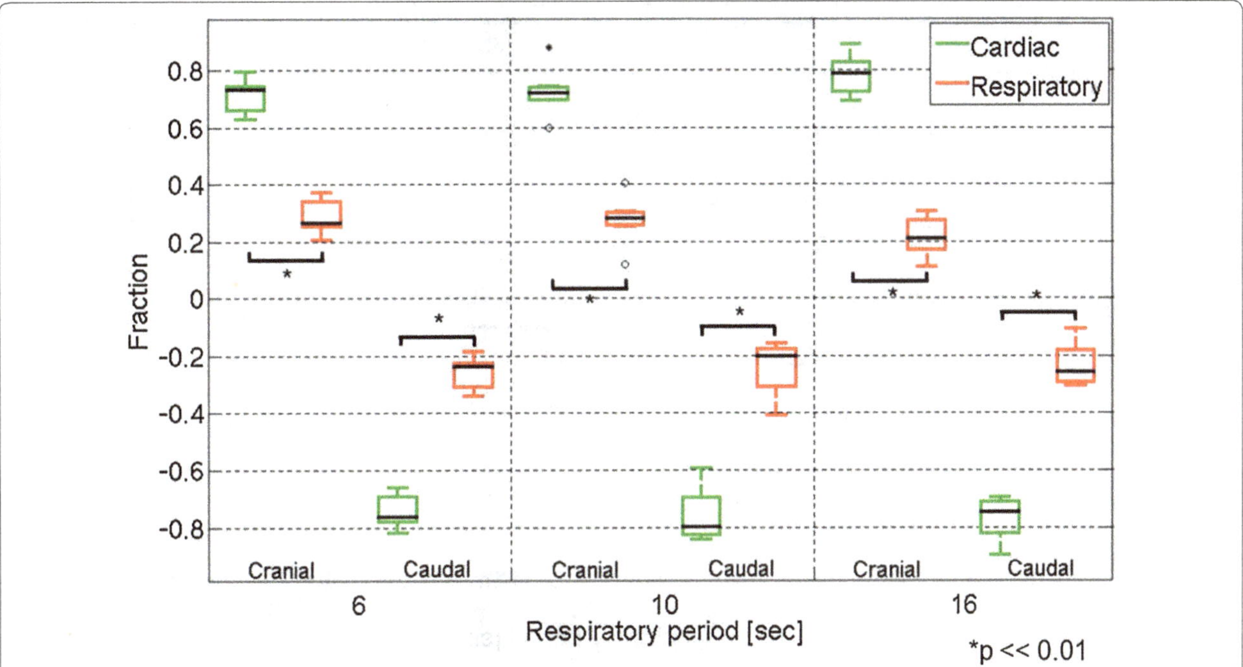

Fig. 3 Similar box plots of the fractions of the CSF velocity components as Fig. 2 but at the foramen magnum. Outlying values are indicated by "o", and far-outlying values are indicated by an asterisk

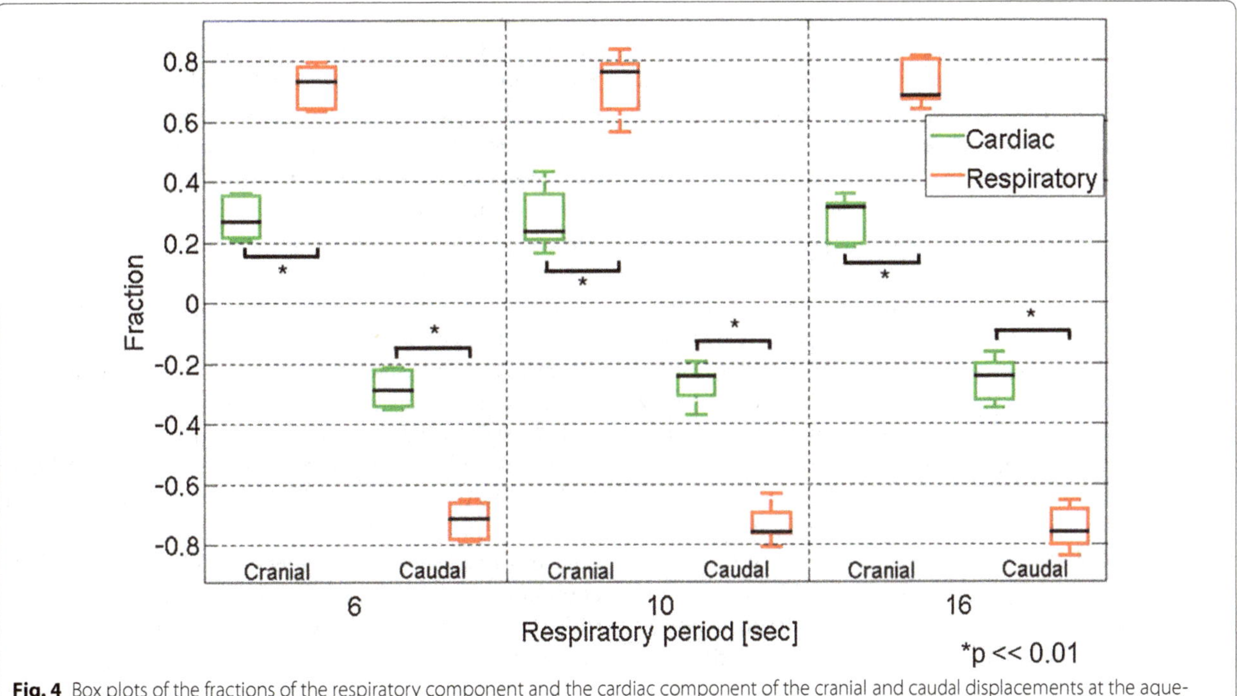

Fig. 4 Box plots of the fractions of the respiratory component and the cardiac component of the cranial and caudal displacements at the aqueduct. The cranial and caudal directions are plotted separately

Discussion

To understand the driving force of CSF motion, researchers have investigated animals and humans using a variety of techniques [1]. Many concluded that CSF pulsations are mainly arterial in origin. On the other hand, CSF flow changes due to respiration have been the subject of

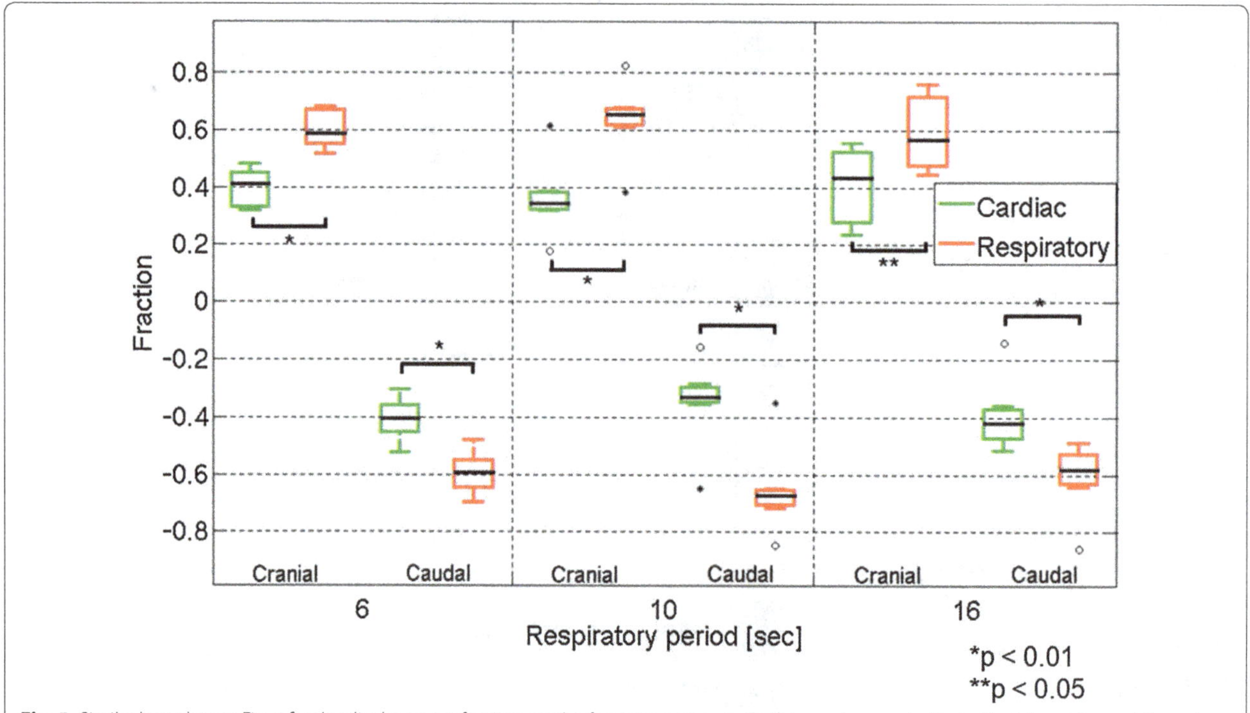

Fig. 5 Similar box plots as Fig. 4 for the displacement fractions at the foramen magnum. Outlying values are indicated by "o", and far-outlying values are indicated by an asterisk

only a few MRI studies. However, some researchers have investigated the effects of respiratory motion on CSF flow using MRI techniques [8, 10, 11, 15]. Beckett et al. [15] used simultaneous multi-slice (SMS) velocity imaging to investigate spinal and brain CSF motion. They reported that the CSF motion in the spine and brain is modulated not only by cardiac motion, but also by respiratory motion. Chen et al. [11] used SMS EPI technique under respiratory guidance to measure respiratory- and cardiac-modulated CSF velocity and direction. They concluded that, during the inspiratory phase, there is upward (inferior to superior) CSF movement into the cranial cavity and lateral ventricles, with a reversal of direction in the expiratory phase. Yamada et al. [8] investigated the effect of respiration on CSF movement by using a non-contrast Time-SLIP technique with balanced steady-state-free precession (bSSFP) readout. Their results demonstrated that a substantially greater amount of CSF movement occurs with deep respiration than with cardiac pulsations. Later, Dreha-Kulaczewski et al. [10] concluded that inspiration is the major regulator of CSF motion. Dreha-Kulaczewski et al. [10] used a highly under-sampled radial gradient–echo sequence with image reconstruction by regularized nonlinear inversion (NLINV) for observing the effect of respiratory on the CSF motion. Since signal intensity modulation due to the inflow effect was used in their work, separated and direct quantification for the CSF velocities due to the cardiac pulsation and respiration were not performed. In the recent publication, Yildiz et al. [9] used very similar technique with our present work to quantify and characterize the cardiac and respiratory-induced CSF motions at the level of the foramen magnum. Assessment of intracranial CSF motions was, however, not made in their work. Thus we believe our present work is adding new insights concerning on the cardiac and respiratory-induced CSF motions in the intracranial space. In the present study, we differentiated the cardiac and respiratory components to evaluate CSF motion. One of the simplest ways to separate cardiac and respiratory motions is to understand frequency analysis. Sunohara et al. [14] developed a method using 2D-PC to analyze the driving force of CSF in terms of power and frequency mapping and successfully analyzed the cardiac and respiratory components of CSF motion, albeit obtaining their images from volunteers engaged in controlled respiration. Our frequency technique was taken further for quantitative analysis of CSF motion related to cardiac and respiratory components. The mathematical algorithm for separating the cardiac and respiratory components of the CSF motion is described in our previous work [12]. Shortly, Fourier transformation was applied to the time series of the obtained velocity data at each voxel. The components of CSF motion were extracted from the frequency spectrum by selecting the particular frequency bands corresponding to the cardiac and respiratory frequencies. In this particular work, the frequency band for the cardiac component was set as 1.0–1.6 Hz, while that for the respiratorion was 0.018–0.3 Hz.

In the present study, CSF motion was separated into respiratory and cardiac components. The amount of CSF displacement was found to be larger in the respiratory component than in the cardiac component in both cranial and caudal directions. Simultaneously, while the cardiac component showed a smaller displacement, the velocity was higher compared to the respiratory component. In other words, the movement of CSF due to the cardiac component was rapid and small, and that due to the respiratory component was slow and large. These results are consistent with those of the visual analysis of CSF reported by Yamada et al. [8] demonstrating that the influence of the respiratory component on the amount of displacement per unit of time was greater than that of the cardiac component. These findings provide quantitative values for results that will be readily understandable to clinicians who have observed the rapid, short-period, powerful CSF motion synchronized with the heartbeat and the slowly pulsing, long-period CSF motion in clinical practice. The difference in the displacement was significant ($p < 0.001$) and clear in the Sylvian aqueduct for all respiratory periods. The difference became slightly less clear in the foramen magnum, particularly for longer respiratory periods ($p < 0.05$ for the 16-s cycle). This may be attributed to the fact that the respiratory process tended to be unstable in the longer period (16 s), and, thus, the individual variation among the volunteers became larger than that in the shorter period.

Time-SLIP enables changes in spin to be visualized. This approximates the results for displacement shown in the present study, showing that CSF moves long distances in accordance with respiratory variations. In the present results, the velocity indicated the rapid movement of CSF with a short period associated with the heartbeat. To summarize CSF motion on the basis of these results, although CSF moves fast as it spreads around the vessels with the heartbeat, it moves over comparatively long distances in accordance with the slower movements of breathing, and this fast movement and movement over long distances may be responsible for physical exchanges in the brain and spinal cord.

However, the physical quantity measured in the present study is the displacement calculated by integrating the CSF velocity in the cranial or caudal direction, unlike the spin traveling distance, which the spin-labeling technique measures. Another important point is that the temporal resolution for data sampling (217 ms/frame) was not high enough to sample the cardiac-driven motion. Assuming a heart rate of 1 Hz, only 4–5 points can cover a cycle of cardiac-driven CSF motion resulting in a lack of waveform sampling accuracy, although the present technique is a quantitative measurement based on the 2D-PC technique, which can measure the fluid velocity with 10% accuracy [16].

Conclusions

In this study the asynchronous 2D-PC method was used under respiratory guidance, which also enabled the evaluation of the respiratory movement element. This was done by performing 2D-PC scanning continuously without a trigger in order to evaluate the slow, long-period motion of CSF and then carrying out quantitative analysis. The feature of the PC method in combining the time element with velocity and direction makes it possible to observe the complex motion of the CSF, providing the next step forward in elucidating the physiological functions of the CSF in vivo. The cardiac-related CSF motion is predominant over the respiratory-related motion, which maintains CSF pressure in the CSF cavity. However, the CSF moves a long distance, as shown by our analysis of displacement. The displacement of CSF in different cavities is important to exchange substances between the parenchyma and the CSF space. During surgery, neurosurgeons frequently see powerful short-range cardiac-related CSF waves and long range, large-wave rhythmical pulsations related to the ventilator. Furthermore, at the tip of external ventricular drainage, clinicians always see the short-range, short-distance CSF pulsation and the long-range, long-distance CSF pulsation, and this alternate CSF pulsation can be identified using the present technique non-invasively. Our final goal was to identify the pathogenesis of CSF circulatory disturbances, as in hydrocephalus and Alzheimer dementia. Using quantitative analysis, we were able to differentiate the subgroup of disease or do a pre- and post-treatment analysis. One of the limitations is that the present MR technique is vulnerable to changes in the position of the human body. Such a position change makes the CSF motion more complex, resulting in failure to assess the association between human movements and CSF motion in daily life.

Abbreviations

CSF: cerebrospinal fluid; Time-SLIP: time-spatial labeling inversion pulse; MRI: magnetic resonance imaging; 2D: 2-dimensional; PC: phase-contrast; 2D-PC: 2-dimensional phase-contrast; EEG: electrocardiogram; SSFP: steady-state-free precession; FH: foot-head; TR: repetition time; TE: echo time; FA: flip angle; FOV: field of view; VENC: velocity encoding; ROI: region of interest; SMS: simultaneous multi-slice; EPI: echo planar imaging; bSSFP: balanced steady-state-free precession.

Authors' contributions

KT, SY, and SS carried out volunteers' data collection, statistical analysis, and drafted the manuscript. KT, MM, and KK drafted the manuscript. KK participated in the coordination of the study. All authors read and approved the final manuscript.

Author details

[1] Department of Neurosurgery, Tokai University School of Medicine, 143 Shimokasuya, Isehara, Kanagawa 2591193, Japan. [2] Course of Science and Technology, Graduate School of Science and Technology, Tokai University, 4-1-1 Kitakaname, Hiratsuka, Kanagawa 2591292, Japan.

Acknowledgements

The authors are grateful to Mr. Nao Kajiwara, Department of Radiology, Tokai University School of Medicine for his technical assistance with MR imaging.

Competing interests

Kagayaki Kuroda is an employee of Bioview Inc. Other the authors declare that they have no competing interests.

Funding

This study was supported in part by the Research and Study Project of Tokai University Educational System General Research Organization, and Health and Labor Sciences Research grants from the Japanese government for research on rare and intractable disease. The authors have no financial competing or any interest with any commercial product used in this study or any substantial relationship with an entity that may impact or benefit from the conclusions of this research.

References

1. Matsumae M, Sato O, Hirayama A, Hayashi N, Takizawa K, Atsumi H, Sorimachi T. Research into the physiology of cerebrospinal fluid reaches a new horizon: intimate exchange between cerebrospinal fluid and interstitial fluid may contribute to maintenance of homeostasis in the central nervous system. Neurol Med Chir (Tokyo). 2016;56:416–41.
2. Matsumae M, Hirayama A, Atsumi H, Yatsushiro S, Kuroda K. Velocity and pressure gradients of cerebrospinal fluid assessed with magnetic resonance imaging. J Neurosurg. 2014;120:218–27.
3. Atsumi H, Matsumae M, Hirayama A, Kuroda K. Measurements of intracranial pressure and compliance index using 1.5-T clinical MRI machine. Tokai J Exp Clin Med. 2014;39:34–43.
4. Yatsushiro S, Hirayama A, Matsumae M, Kuroda K. Visualization of pulsatile CSF motion separated by membrane-like structure based on four-dimensional phase-contrast (4D-PC) velocity mapping. Conf Proc IEEE Eng Med Biol Soc. 2013;2013:6470–3.
5. Horie T, Kajihara N, Matsumae M, Obara M, Hayashi N, Hirayama A, Takizawa K, Takahara T, Yatsushiro S, Kuroda K. Magnetic resonance imaging technique for visualization of irregular cerebrospinal fluid motion in the ventricular system and subarachnoid space. World Neurosurg. 2017;97:523–31.
6. Hayashi N, Matsumae M, Yatsushiro S, Hirayama A, Abdullah A, Kuroda K. Quantitative analysis of cerebrospinal fluid pressure gradients in healthy volunteers and patients with normal pressure hydrocephalus. Neurol Med Chir (Tokyo). 2015;55:657–62.
7. Hirayama A, Matsumae M, Yatsushiro S, Abdulla A, Atsumi H, Kuroda K. Visualization of pulsatile csf motion around membrane-like structures with both 4D velocity mapping and time-slip technique. Magn Reson Med Sci. 2015;14:263–73.
8. Yamada S, Miyazaki M, Yamashita Y, Ouyang C, Yui M, Nakahashi M, Shimizu S, Aoki I, Morohoshi Y, McComb JG. Influence of respiration on cerebrospinal fluid movement using magnetic resonance spin labeling. Fluids Barriers CNS. 2013;10:36.
9. Yildiz S, Thyagaraj S, Jin N, Zhong X, Heidari Pahlavian S, Martin BA, Loth F, Oshinski J, Sabra KG. Quantifying the influence of respiration and cardiac pulsations on cerebrospinal fluid dynamics using real-time phase-contrast MRI. J Magn Reson Imaging. 2017;46:431–9.
10. Dreha-Kulaczewski S, Joseph AA, Merboldt KD, Ludwig HC, Gartner J, Frahm J. Inspiration is the major regulator of human CSF flow. J Neurosci. 2015;35:2485–91.
11. Chen L, Beckett A, Verma A, Feinberg DA. Dynamics of respiratory and cardiac CSF motion revealed with real-time simultaneous multi-slice EPI velocity phase contrast imaging. Neuroimage. 2015;122:281–7.
12. Yatsushiro S, Sunohara S, Takizawa K, Matsumae M, Kajihara N, Kuroda K. Characterization of cardiac- and respiratory-driven cerebrospinal fluid motions using correlation mapping with asynchronous 2-dimensional phase contrast technique. Conf Proc IEEE Eng Med Biol Soc. 2016;2016:3867–70.
13. Abdullah A, Hirayama A, Yatsushiro S, Matsumae M, Kuroda K. Cerebrospinal fluid image segmentation using spatial fuzzy clustering method with improved evolutionary expectation maximization. Conf Proc IEEE Eng Med Biol Soc. 2013;2013:3359–62.
14. Sunohara S, Yatsushiro S, Takizawa K, Matsumae M, Kajihara N, Kuroda K. Investigation of driving forces of cerebrospinal fluid motion by power and frequency mapping based on asynchronous phase contrast technique. Conf Proc IEEE Eng Med Biol Soc. 2016;2016:1232–5.
15. Beckett A, Chen L, Verma A, Feinberg DA. Velocity phase imaging with simultaneous multi-slice EPI reveals respiration driven motion in spinal CSF. Proc Intl Soc Mag Reson Med. 2015;23:4445.
16. Tang C, Blatter DD, Parker DL. Accuracy of phase-contrast flow measurements in the presence of partial-volume effects. J Magn Reson Imaging. 1993;3:377–85.

16

Immunohistochemical and in situ hybridization study of urate transporters GLUT9/URATv1, ABCG2, and URAT1 in the murine brain

Naoko H. Tomioka[1*], Yoshifuru Tamura[2], Tappei Takada[3], Shigeru Shibata[2], Hiroshi Suzuki[3], Shunya Uchida[2] and Makoto Hosoyamada[1*]

Abstract

Background: Uric acid (UA) is known to exert neuroprotective effects in the brain. However, the mechanism of UA regulation in the brain is not well characterized. In our previous study, we described that the mouse urate transporter URAT1 is localized to the cilia and apical surface of ventricular ependymal cells. To further strengthen the hypothesis that UA is transported transcellularly at the ependymal cells, we aimed to assess the distribution of other UA transporters in the murine brain.

Methods: Immunostaining and highly-sensitive in situ hybridization was used to assess the distribution of UA transporters: GLUT9/URATv1, ABCG2, and URAT1.

Results: Immunostaining for GLUT9 was observed in ependymal cells, neurons, and brain capillaries. Immunostaining for ABCG2 was observed in the choroid plexus epithelium and brain capillaries, but not in ependymal cells. These results were validated by in situ hybridization.

Conclusions: We propose that given their specific expression patterns in ependymal, choroid plexus epithelial, and brain capillary endothelial cells in this study, UA may be transported by these UA transporters in the murine brain. This may provide a novel strategy for targeted neuroprotection.

Background

Uric acid (UA) exerts a neuroprotective effect due to its antioxidant property, and epidemiological and experimental evidence suggests that UA plays an important role in the development or progression of neurodegenerative disorders [1]. For instance, higher serum UA is associated with the decreased incidence and slower progression of Parkinson's disease (PD) [2]. Moreover, recent studies indicate that UA transporter genes, which control the transport of UA in the kidney and extra renal tissues, and thus affect serum UA levels, are also associated with the risk and age at onset of PD [3–6]. In rodent models of PD, elevated UA levels attenuated behavioral and neurodegenerative deficits [7, 8]. Urate-elevating clinical trials are currently underway in patients with the early stages of PD. An oral administration of inosine, a precursor of UA, can elevate UA levels in serum and cerebrospinal fluid (CSF), with a persistent elevation of plasma antioxidant capacity [9, 10]. Further, CSF UA is inversely correlated with the clinical progression of PD, albeit to a lesser extent than serum UA [11]. However, the molecular mechanism as to how the UA in blood reaches the brain parenchyma and affects neuronal viability remains unclear.

We previously demonstrated that URAT1, which is a urate transporter responsible for urate reabsorption in the kidney [12], is localized to cilia and the apical surface of ventricular ependymal cells in the murine brain [13]. Ependymal cells form a single-layer of epithelial cells which line the surface of the cerebral ventricles. Although the lateral ventricular

*Correspondence: nhtomioka@pharm.teikyo-u.ac.jp; hosoyamd@pharm.teikyo-u.ac.jp

[1] Department of Human Physiology and Pathology, Faculty of Pharma-Sciences, Teikyo University, 2-11-1 Kaga, Itabashi-ku, Tokyo 173-8605, Japan

Full list of author information is available at the end of the article

CSF-brain interface does not usually act as a barrier due to the lack of tight junctions and may allow passive molecular exchange, immunoreactivity of tight junction proteins has been demonstrated in the ependymal cells of specific regions of the third and fourth ventricles [14–17]. Therefore, alternative carrier-mediated transport systems may exist at the ependymal layer in addition to slow paracellular diffusion. For example, a recent study indicates that the glutamate transporter EAAT1, which is localized on the apical membrane of the ependymal cell is involved in the removal of L-Glutamate from the CSF [18]. It is also known that proximal tubules which express functional UA transporters, are leaky epithelial cells [19]. In this regard, we hypothesized that ependymal URAT1 and other transporters may function as a UA transporter between the ventricular CSF and the interstitial fluid of the brain parenchyma.

To further strengthen the hypothesis that UA transport systems exist in ependymal cells, the aim of this study was to address if other UA transporters were also localized in those cells. In this study, we focused on two other UA transporters, GLUT9/URATv1 and ABCG2, which are known to regulate serum UA levels [20]. RT-PCR analyses showed that mRNA encoding the long isoform of GLUT9 is found both in the human and murine brain [21, 22]. Furthermore, GLUT9 is also expressed in cultured dopaminergic neurones and astroglial cells [23]. However, the spatial distribution of GLUT9 in the brain is still unknown. Further, while ABCG2 luminal localization in brain capillaries, and on murine choroid plexus epithelial cells has been previously described [24, 25], its localization on ependymal cells is still unknown.

Thus, the aim of this study was to investigate the distribution of GLUT9 and ABCG2 in the murine brain, particularly in ependymal cells. To do this, we performed immunostaining and highly-sensitive in situ hybridization analyses of the murine brain.

Methods

Animals

A total of seven male C57BL/6J mice (Sankyo Laboratories, Tokyo, Japan), a male Abcg2-knockout (KO) mouse (FVB.129P2-Abcg2, Taconic Farms, Hudson, NY), and a littermate wild-type (WT) mouse were used in this study. Mice were maintained in 12 h light and dark cycles, with free access to food and water. All animal experiments were carried out in accordance with the guidelines for animal experimentation in Teikyo University and the University of Tokyo, and the project was approved by the local committee.

Tissue section preparation

To prepare fixed, frozen sections, mice were anesthetized by pentobarbital injection (50 mg/kg, i.p.) and perfused intracardially with HEPES buffer (30 mM HEPES, 100 mM NaCl, 2 mM $CaCl_2$, pH 7.4), followed by 4% paraformaldehyde (PFA) in HEPES buffer. Brains were then removed and post-fixed for 3 h at 4 °C in the same fixative. The post-fixed brains were cut coronally and cryoprotected in 15% sucrose (wt/vol) in PBS for 48 h at 4 °C, embedded in Tissue-Tek OCT compound (Sakura Finetek Japan, Tokyo, Japan), and frozen on dry ice. Sections were cut at 12 μm for immunostaining.

To prepare paraffin sections, anesthetized mice were perfused intracardially with methacarn fixative (methanol:chloroform:acetic acid = 6:3:1). Brains were removed, cut coronally, and post-fixed 2 h at 4 °C in the same fixative. For paraffin embedding, tissues were dehydrated in a graded series of alcohols, cleared with Hemo-De (a Xylene substitutive, FALMA, Tokyo, Japan), embedded in Paraplast Plus (Sigma, St. Louis, MO, USA), and sectioned at 4 μm.

To prepare unfixed, fresh frozen sections for immunostaining, mice were killed by cervical dislocation and the brains were removed and frozen on dry ice. Sections were cut at 20 μm on a cryostat. To prepare paraffin sections for in situ hybridization, the anesthetized mouse was perfused intracardially with PBS, followed by 4% PFA in PBS. Brains were removed and cut coronally, post-fixed overnight (i.e. for at least 16 h), at 4 °C in 4% PFA in PBT (PBS containing 0.1% Tween 20). After rinsing in PBT, tissues were dehydrated in a graded series of ethanol in PBT, cleared with Hemo-De, embedded in Paraplast Plus and sectioned at 5 μm.

Immunostaining for brain sections

For immunofluorescence staining of cryostat sections, sections were autoclaved in 10 mM citrate buffer, pH 6.0, for 5 min at 105 °C for antigen retrieval, and incubated in blocking solution (PBS containing 10% normal goat serum and 0.1% Triton X-100) for 1 h at room temperature (22–25 °C). The sections were then subsequently incubated with primary antibodies overnight at 4 °C and with Alexa 488- or Alexa 594-conjugated secondary antibodies (Molecular Probes, Tokyo, Japan) for 1 h at room temperature. Slides were mounted with Vectashield containing DAPI (Vector Laboratories, Burlingame, CA, USA).

Paraffin sections were deparaffinized with Hemo-De and rehydrated prior to staining. For immunohistochemistry, sections were further incubated in 0.3% H_2O_2/methanol solution for 10 min to block the endogenous peroxidase activity. Sections were then incubated for 1 h at room temperature in blocking solution, which consisted of 5% normal goat serum and 0.1% Triton X-100, followed by an overnight-incubation at 4 °C with primary antibodies diluted in blocking solution. Detection was performed with EnVision™ + Systems and DAB+, Liquid (Dako Japan, Tokyo, Japan). Sections were counterstained with Mayer's hematoxylin (Wako, Tokyo, Japan). Immunofluorescence staining of the rehydrated sections was performed using the protocol outlined above for cryostat sections, but without the antigen retrieval. For immunofluorescence staining of fresh frozen sections, sections was fixed in methanol (−20 °C, 30 min) and acetone (4 °C, 10 min), incubated with blocking buffer, primary, and fluorescently-labelled secondary antibodies. The following primary antibodies were used in this study: anti-GLUT9 (NBP1-05054, Novus Biologicals, 1/500 or 1/1000 dilution for immunofluorescence staining, 1/5000 dilution for immunohistochemistry); anti-acetylated-α-tubulin (6-11B-1, Sigma, 1:500); anti-NeuN (A60, Millipore, 1/500); anti-P Glycoprotein (C219, GeneTax, 1/200); anti-BCRP/ABCG2 (BXP-9, Abcam, 1/100). For antigen absorption experiment, GLUT9 peptide (NBP1-05054PEP, Novus Biologicals) was used at a concentration of 100 μg/ml.

In situ hybridization

In situ hybridization was performed using ViewRNA™ ISH Tissue 2-Plex assay (Affymetrix, Tokyo, Japan) according to the manufacturer's protocol. Paraffin sections were deparaffinized with Hemo-De, boiled in pretreatment solution for 10 min, and digested with protease for 10 min. Sections were then hybridized with ViewRNA probes (Mouse Slc22a12, Type 6; Mouse Slc2a9, Type 1: Mouse Abcg2, Type 1). Bound probes were amplified by hybridization with preamplifier and amplifier mix solutions. Sections were incubated with Label Probe 6-alkaline phosphatase (AP) solution and Fast Blue substrate. Subsequently, sections were incubated with Label Probe 1-AP Type 1 solution and Fast Red substrate. Finally, the sections were counterstained with Gill's hematoxylin and cover-slipped with Ultramount Permanent Mounting Medium (Dako Japan, Tokyo, Japan).

Image acquisition

DAB-stained sections were scanned with a NanoZoomer 2.0-HT slide scanner (Hamamatsu Photonics, Hamamatsu, Japan). For immunofluorescence experiments, single-plane images were captured using a Nikon A1 confocal microscope (Nikon, Tokyo, Japan) with identical settings. In situ hybridization, fluorescence, and bright field images were also acquired with the Nikon A1 confocal microscope. The Fast Blue and Fast Red signals were observed using Alexa 750 and Cy3 filter sets, respectively.

Results

Immunofluorescence staining of GLUT9 in PFA-fixed murine brain sections

To determine whether GLUT9 is localized in ependymal cells, we first performed immunostaining analysis using a rabbit polyclonal anti-GLUT9 antibody on PFA-fixed murine brain frozen sections. Distinct GLUT9 immunoreactivity in the ependymal cells of the dorsal third ventricle, and weaker staining in the brain parenchyma region were detected (Fig. 1a). The specificity of anti-GLUT9 antibody was verified by antigen absorption test (Fig. 1b). Higher magnification imaging revealed that GLUT9 was not localized to the nucleus or the cilia, visualized using anti-acetylated-α-tubulin, suggesting an intracellular and plasma membrane localization (Fig. 1c, d). To identify the cell type of GLUT9-positive cells in the brain parenchyma, we performed double immunostaining for GLUT9 and NeuN (neuronal marker; Fig. 1e–g). All GLUT9-positive cells in the parenchyma co-localized with NeuN, suggesting that GLUT9 is also present in neurons.

GLUT9 immunoreactivity is detected in ependymal cells of all ventricles

Next, we observed the distribution of GLUT9 in other ventricles using PFA-fixed, frozen coronal sections at different levels. In addition to the ependymal cells of dorsal third ventricle (Figs. 1a, 2c), GLUT9 immunoreactivity was detected in ependymal cells of all ventricles including the lateral, ventral third, and fourth ventricles, and the aqueduct (Fig. 2a, b, d–f). GLUT9 was also prominent in tanycytes, which are specialized ependymal cells that line the floor of the ventral third ventricle, and in its long processes that extend into the parenchyma (Fig. 2d). No immunostaining was detected in the choroid plexus (Fig. 2b, c, f).

Immunohistochemistry and immunofluorescence staining of GLUT9 in a methacarn-fixed murine brain

Next, we performed immunostaining analysis using methacarn-fixed tissue. Similar to the results obtained from PFA-fixed tissue, GLUT9 immunoreactivity was detected in ependymal cells (Fig. 3a). In addition, capillary-like structures were also immunopositive for GLUT9 in the brain parenchyma, including the cortical region (Fig. 3a, c). No staining was detected with antigen-preabsorbed antibody (Fig. 3b). To investigate the distribution of GLUT9 in the brain capillary endothelium, we conducted double-immunostaining with anti-GLUT9 and anti-P-glycoprotein (P-gp) antibody, which is a luminal marker (Fig. 3d–f). GLUT9 co-localized with P-gp (Fig. 3f), indicating that GLUT9 possibly localizes to the luminal membrane of the brain capillary endothelium.

Immunofluorescence staining of ABCG2 in methanol/acetone-fixed and methacarn-fixed murine brain

Immunohistochemistry of ABCG2 was done on fresh, frozen sections of the wild type (Fig. 4a) and Abcg2 KO (Fig. 4b) mice, which were post-fixed with methanol and

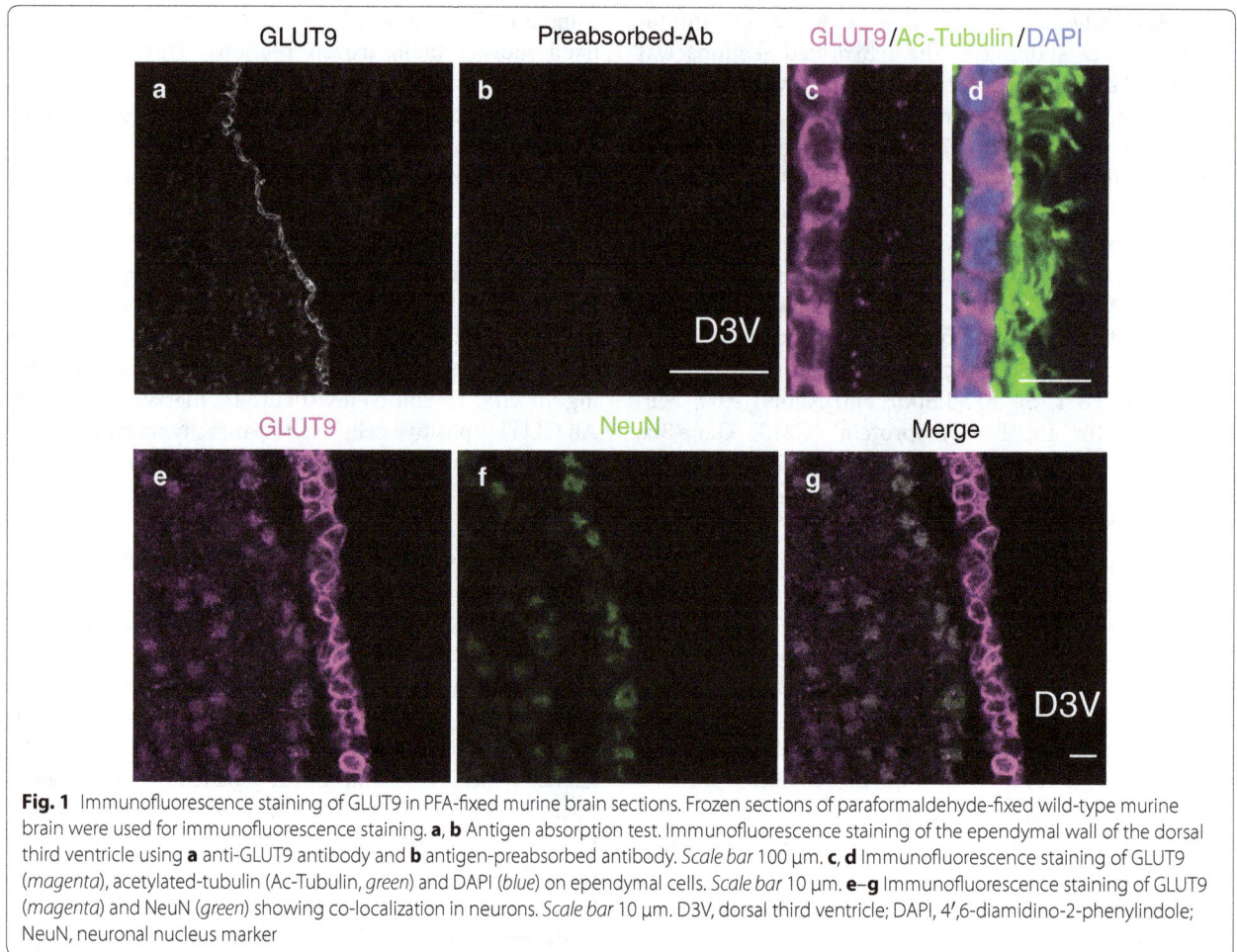

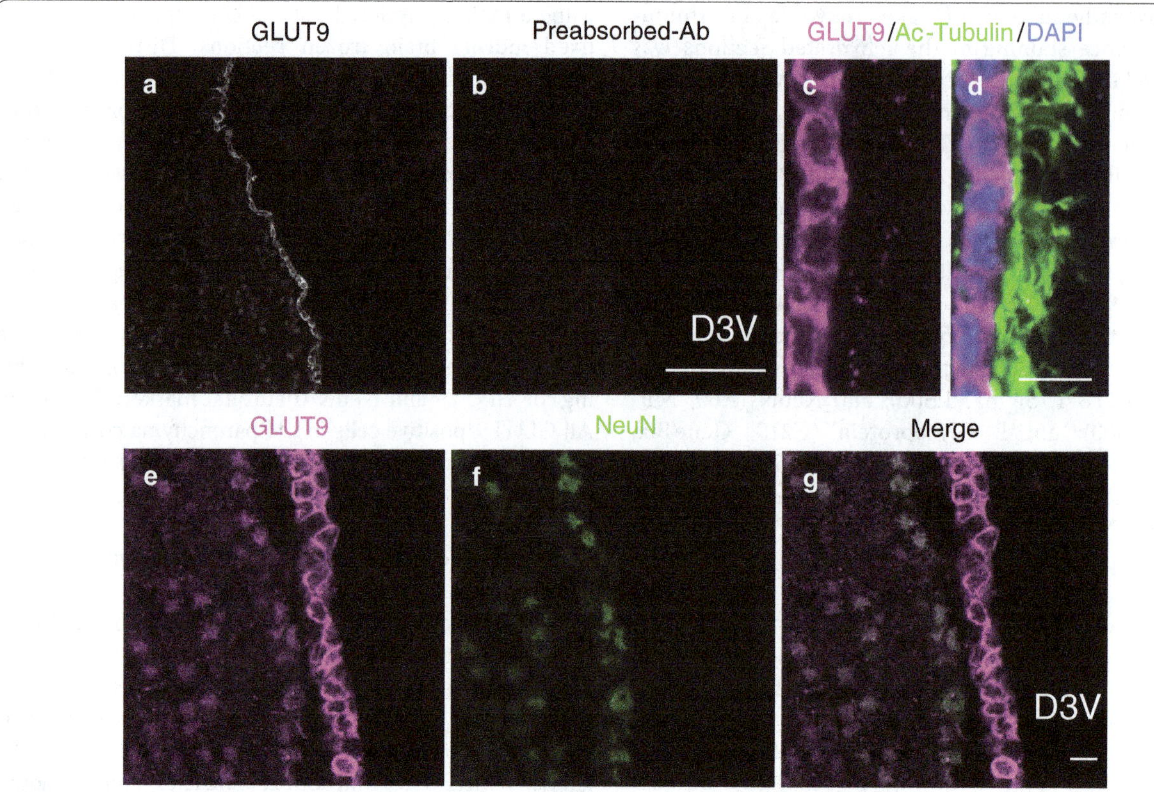

Fig. 1 Immunofluorescence staining of GLUT9 in PFA-fixed murine brain sections. Frozen sections of paraformaldehyde-fixed wild-type murine brain were used for immunofluorescence staining. **a**, **b** Antigen absorption test. Immunofluorescence staining of the ependymal wall of the dorsal third ventricle using **a** anti-GLUT9 antibody and **b** antigen-preabsorbed antibody. *Scale bar* 100 µm. **c**, **d** Immunofluorescence staining of GLUT9 (*magenta*), acetylated-tubulin (Ac-Tubulin, *green*) and DAPI (*blue*) on ependymal cells. *Scale bar* 10 µm. **e–g** Immunofluorescence staining of GLUT9 (*magenta*) and NeuN (*green*) showing co-localization in neurons. *Scale bar* 10 µm. D3V, dorsal third ventricle; DAPI, 4′,6-diamidino-2-phenylindole; NeuN, neuronal nucleus marker

acetone. ABCG2 immunoreactivity on the luminal membrane of the capillary endothelium and the CSF side of the choroid plexus epithelial cells has been previously reported [25]. Using a different antibody, we also demonstrated a similar distribution of ABCG2 in the capillary endothelium and choroid plexus epithelial cells (Fig. 4a). These immunoreactivity patterns were not observed in sections from the Abcg2 KO mouse (Fig. 4b), demonstrating antibody specificity. ABCG2 immunoreactivity was not detected in ependymal cells (Fig. 4c). Using paraffin sections from methacarn-fixed brain, we observed the colocalization of ABCG2 and GLUT9 on the capillary endothelium (Fig. 4d–f).

Localization of mRNA of urate transporters in the murine brain by fluorescence in situ hybridization

The distribution of urate transporters in the murine brain was further verified by a highly-sensitive in situ hybridization system using *Slc22a12* (URAT1), *Slc2a9* (GLUT9), and *Abcg2* probes. In accordance with our previous URAT1 immunostaining results, where URAT1 was distributed in ependymal cells [13], *Slc22a12* mRNA was expressed in the ependymal cells (Fig. 5a). Weaker signals were observed in choroid plexus and brain parenchyma where the protein localization was not confirmed (Fig. 5a). *Slc2a9* mRNA was expressed broadly in ependymal cells, the choroid plexus, and brain parenchyma (Fig. 5b). *Abcg2* mRNA was expressed in choroid plexus epithelial cells and weakly in brain parenchyma, but not in ependymal cells (Fig. 5c). These results establish the validity of immunostaining results, which revealed the distribution of URAT1 and GLUT9 in ependymal cells, and of ABCG2 in the choroid plexus.

Discussion

In the current study, we showed that GLUT9 is expressed in ependymal cells, neurons, and brain capillaries, while ABCG2 is expressed in choroid plexus epithelium and brain capillaries, but not in ependymal cells. Taken together with our previous findings that URAT1 is localized at the CSF side of the ependymal cells, we speculate that UA may be transported via transporters expressed

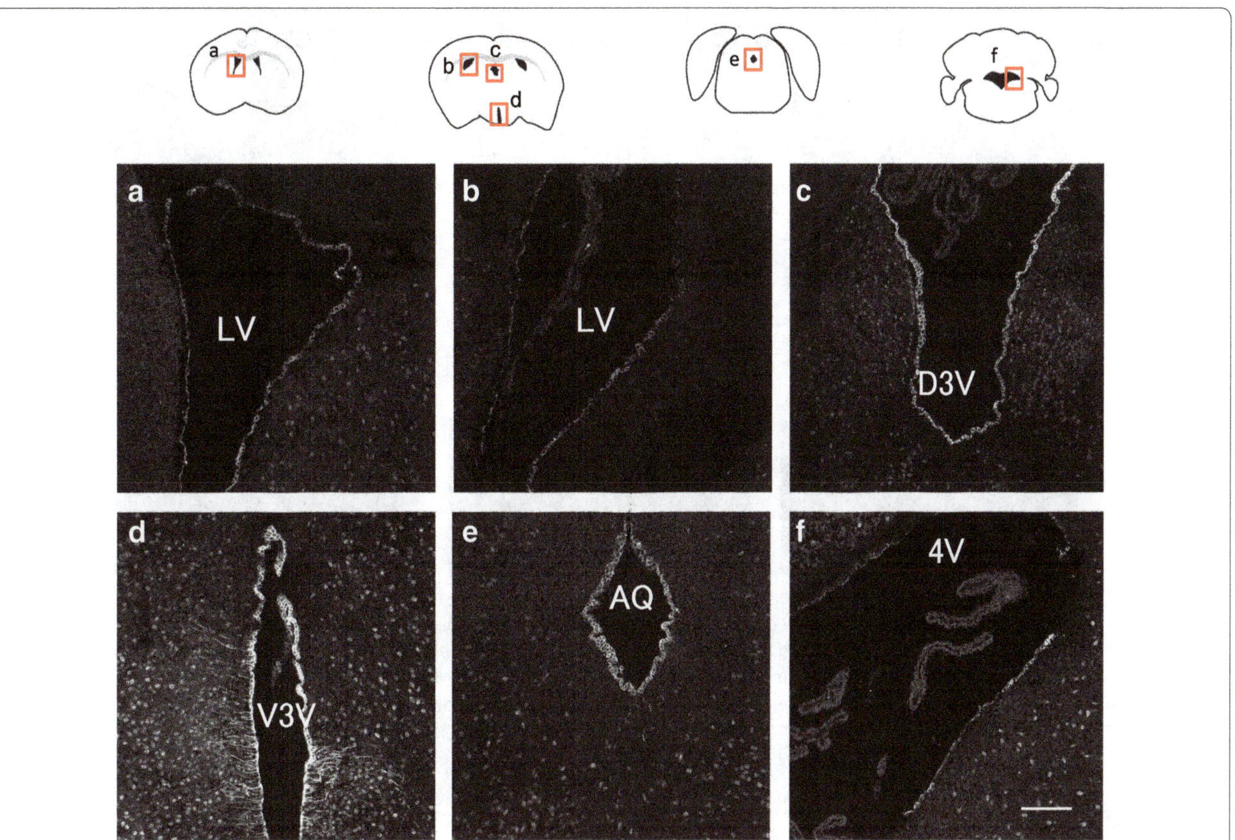

Fig. 2 GLUT9/URATv1 immunoreactivity is detected in ependymal cells of all ventricles. Frozen sections of paraformaldehyde-fixed wild-type murine brain were used for immunofluorescence staining. The *red squares* in the diagrams indicate the region shown in each image. **a–f** GLUT9 staining of coronal sections. **b–d** Images were obtained from the same section. *Scale bar* 100 μm. LV, lateral ventricle; V3V, ventral third ventricle; AQ, aqueduct; 4V, fourth ventricle

at the cells which form the boundary between brain, CSF and blood.

While the immunoreactivity of GLUT9 in the ependymal cells was consistently observed in our experiments, its immunoreactivity in neurons or brain capillaries was dependent on fixation or antigen retrieval conditions. The difference in the immunostaining pattern may be caused by antigen masking or degradation. The preservation of antigenicity can be affected by fixation methods and may vary among tissues. Methacarn fixation is a non-cross-linking organic solvent, which has been shown to improve immunoreactivity, in comparison to aldehyde-based fixatives, against particular antigens [26]. The neuronal expression of GLUT9 is feasible, since its expression in cultured dopaminergic neurons has been previously demonstrated using western blot [23]. Two isoforms of GLUT9, which differ in the amino terminus, are known to exist in the human and mouse. The long isoform of human GLUT9 is expressed at the basolateral membrane of proximal tubules of human kidney, whereas the short isoform is expressed at the apical membrane of the collecting duct [21, 27]. In contrast, mouse GLUT9 is reportedly expressed both in the apical and basolateral membranes of distal convoluted tubules of the murine kidney and enterocytes of the murine jejunum, albeit with no information about its isoform-specific localization [22, 28, 29]. Since the current study did not reveal the exclusive plasma membrane localization compared to our previous finding of apical localization of URAT1 [13], further work including electron microscopy analysis is required to determine if GLUT9 is specifically localized in the apical and/or basolateral membrane of ependymal cells and neuronal somatic membranes. Unknown mechanisms, such as a stimulus-dependent translocation to the plasma membrane like the insulin-dependent GLUT4 translocation may exist [30]. Surprisingly, we found that methacarn fixation alone showed the localization of GLUT9 on brain capillary endothelial cells. This result supports RT-PCR findings that GLUT9 mRNA is detected in bEnd.3 cells (a murine brain endothelial cell line) [31, 32].

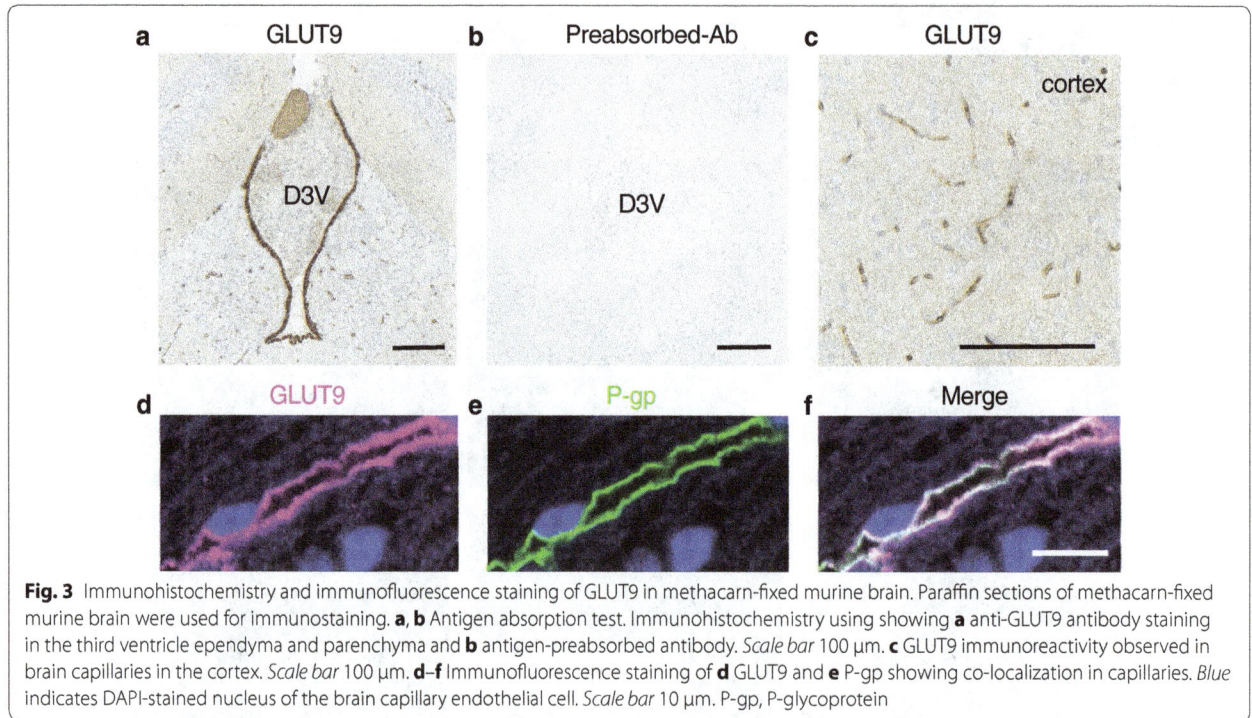

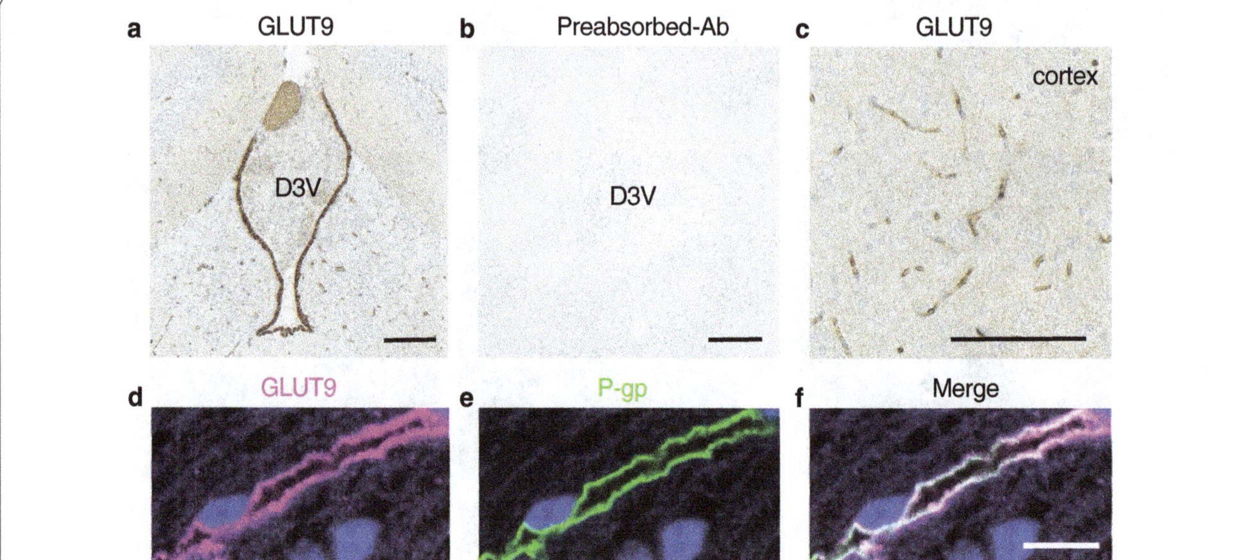

Fig. 3 Immunohistochemistry and immunofluorescence staining of GLUT9 in methacarn-fixed murine brain. Paraffin sections of methacarn-fixed murine brain were used for immunostaining. **a**, **b** Antigen absorption test. Immunohistochemistry using showing **a** anti-GLUT9 antibody staining in the third ventricle ependyma and parenchyma and **b** antigen-preabsorbed antibody. *Scale bar* 100 μm. **c** GLUT9 immunoreactivity observed in brain capillaries in the cortex. *Scale bar* 100 μm. **d–f** Immunofluorescence staining of **d** GLUT9 and **e** P-gp showing co-localization in capillaries. *Blue* indicates DAPI-stained nucleus of the brain capillary endothelial cell. *Scale bar* 10 μm. P-gp, P-glycoprotein

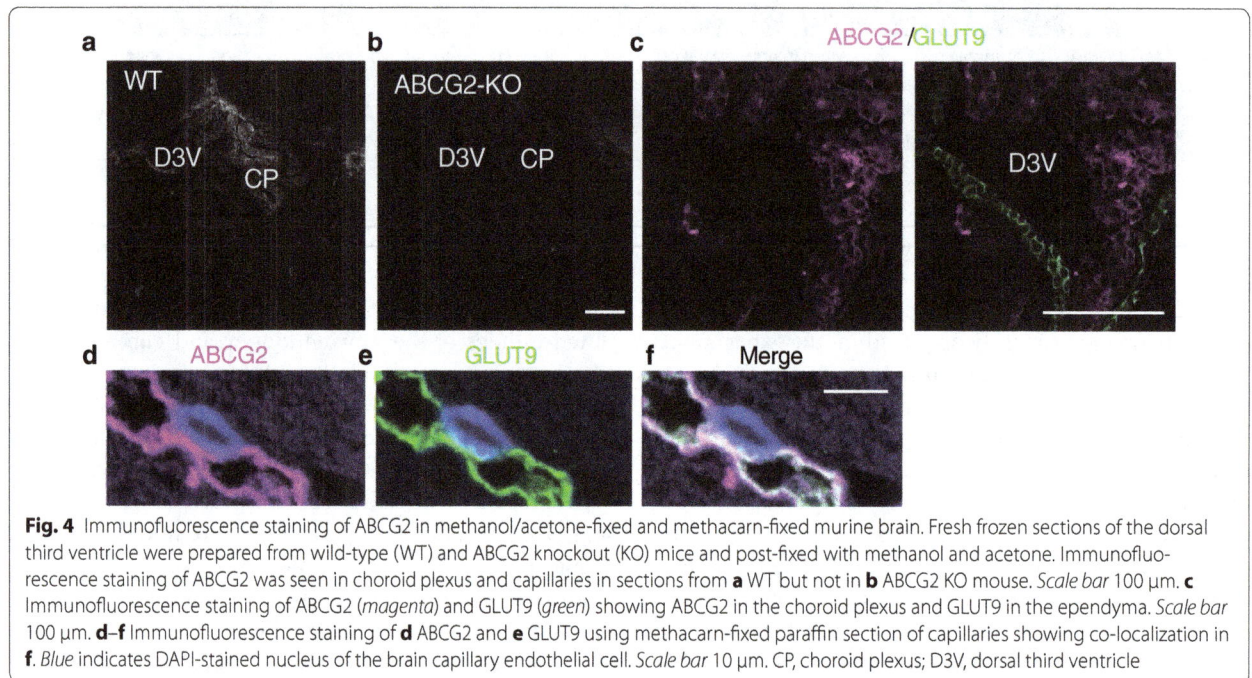

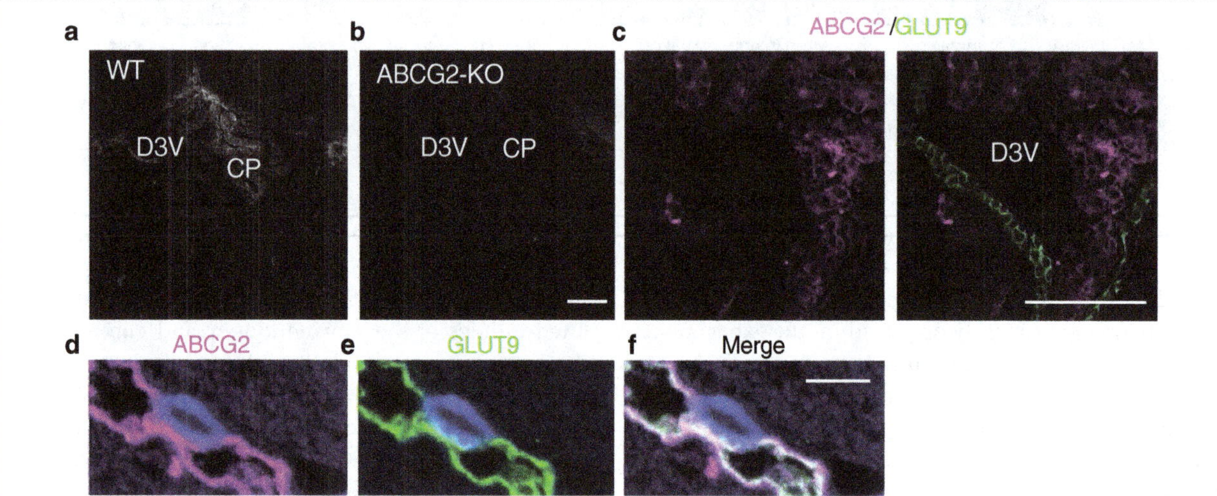

Fig. 4 Immunofluorescence staining of ABCG2 in methanol/acetone-fixed and methacarn-fixed murine brain. Fresh frozen sections of the dorsal third ventricle were prepared from wild-type (WT) and ABCG2 knockout (KO) mice and post-fixed with methanol and acetone. Immunofluorescence staining of ABCG2 was seen in choroid plexus and capillaries in sections from **a** WT but not in **b** ABCG2 KO mouse. *Scale bar* 100 μm. **c** Immunofluorescence staining of ABCG2 (*magenta*) and GLUT9 (*green*) showing ABCG2 in the choroid plexus and GLUT9 in the ependyma. *Scale bar* 100 μm. **d–f** Immunofluorescence staining of **d** ABCG2 and **e** GLUT9 using methacarn-fixed paraffin section of capillaries showing co-localization in **f**. *Blue* indicates DAPI-stained nucleus of the brain capillary endothelial cell. *Scale bar* 10 μm. CP, choroid plexus; D3V, dorsal third ventricle

The protein expression of URAT1 and GLUT9, but not ABCG2, in the ependymal cells was also validated by the use of highly-sensitive in situ hybridization. Similarly, the expression of ABCG2 in choroid plexus cells was also confirmed. *Slc2a9* and *Abcg2* mRNA distribution in the brain parenchyma may correspond to the protein localization in neurons and brain capillary endothelial cells. Conversely, *Slc22a12* mRNA signals were observed in the choroid plexus and the brain parenchyma, and *Slc2a9* mRNA signals were observed in the choroid

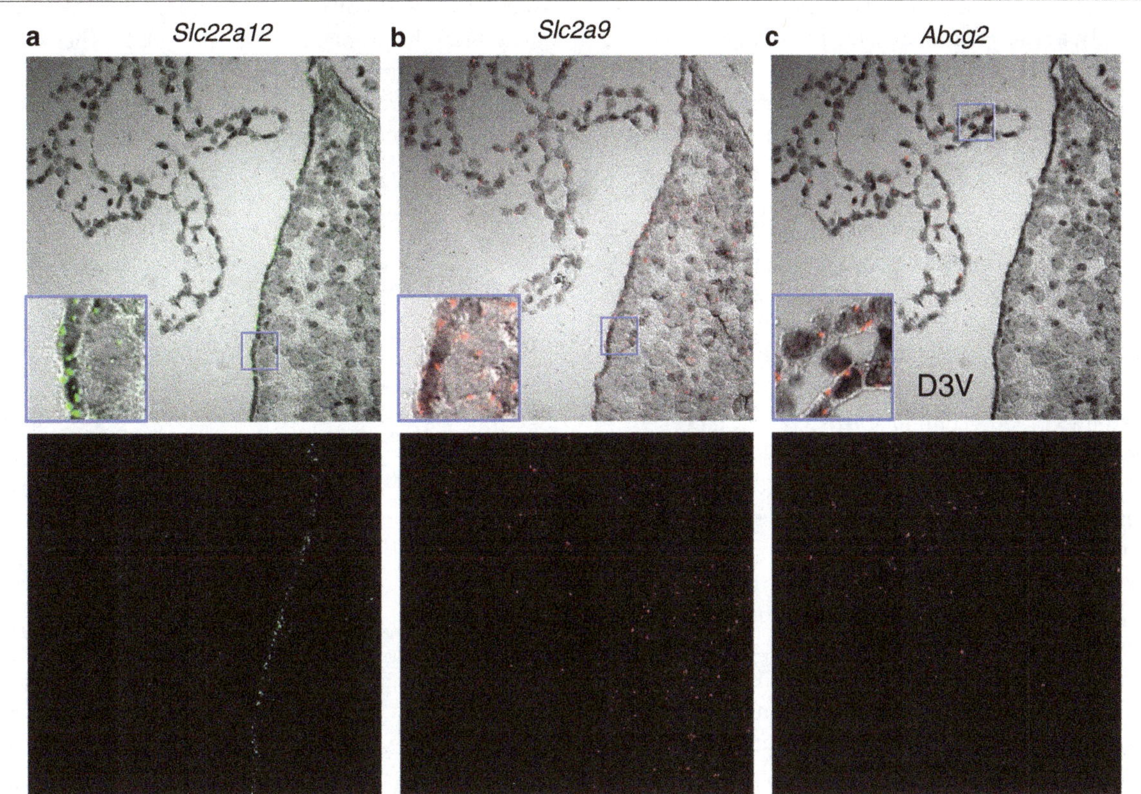

Fig. 5 Localization of mRNA of urate transporters in murine brain by fluorescence in situ hybridization. **a–c** Merged bright field and fluorescence images are seen in the *upper panels*, while the *lower panels* show the fluorescence images alone. *Green dots* show Fast Blue signal observed with the Alexa 750 filter set, while the red dots show Fast Red signal observed with the Cy3 filter set. mRNA probes: Slc22a12 (URAT1), Slc2a9 (GLUT9), Abcg2 (ABCG2). Slc22a12 is expressed largely in the ependyma and less in the parenchyma, Slc2a9 is expressed in the ependyma and parenchyma and Abcg2 in the choroid plexus epithelium

plexus, which is inconsistent with the immunostaining results. Immunoblotting analysis in earlier studies has reported that URAT1 was detected in the murine choroid plexus, brain capillaries, cultured dopaminergic neurons, and astrocytes [23, 33]. Our previous study exhibited weak immunostaining in the choroid plexus and the brain parenchyma, both in wild type and URAT1 KO mice, indicating the possibility of non-specific staining [13]. The discrepancy between the immunostaining and in situ hybridization data of GLUT9 (*Slc2a9*) and URAT1 (*Slc22a12*) could be considered that the mRNA is not translated to protein or that the translated protein is unstable. Alternatively, other optimum fixative conditions for immunostaining may be needed.

Specific localization of UA transporters in the murine brain could be involved in the transport of UA derived from blood or by intracellular purine metabolism. Considering the correlation between blood and CSF UA levels [34], we suppose that brain interstitial UA could be mainly provided by CSF, which originates from blood at the choroid plexus. The endothelial cells of the choroid plexus are fenestrated and tight junctions of choroid plexus epithelial cells constitute the blood-CSF barrier [35]. Our group and others have demonstrated that ABCG2 is localized at the apical membrane of choroid plexus epithelial cells [25], raising the possibility that UA may be partly secreted by ABCG2 into the ventricular CSF. An unidentified UA transporter at the blood side may be involved in the uptake of blood UA into the choroid plexus epithelial cells. CSF flows through the ventricles, enters into the subarachnoid space, and is reabsorbed into the blood or reaches lymphatic drainage [36]. During the ventricular circulation, UA in the CSF could be transported into ependymal cells by URAT1 located at the apical membrane of ependymal cells [13]. Since it has been reported that ependymal cells express xanthine oxidase, which converts hypoxanthine to xanthine and xanthine to uric acid [37], metabolized UA in the ependymal cells could also be the transport target. If GLUT9 is localized at the basolateral membrane, then it is likely to contribute to the transport of UA from ependymal cells to brain parenchyma. CSF-derived UA could increase the regional UA concentration near the ventricle, for example in the striatum near the lateral ventricles. Conversely, apically-localized GLUT9 could transport UA from ependymal cells to the ventricular CSF. It has been demonstrated that ATP-binding cassette transporters ABCG2 and MRP4/ABCC4 that transport UA are localized to luminal membrane of endothelial cells [20, 25, 38]. At the abluminal membrane, OAT3, which can function as a urate/dicarboxylate exchanger, is present [39, 40]. In addition to these transporters, we revealed that GLUT9 also exists at the capillary endothelial cells, albeit its luminal/abluminal distribution should be further investigated by electron microscopy analysis. We postulate that at the blood–brain barrier, UA in the capillary endothelial cell is excreted into blood via luminal ABCG2 and GLUT9 may also be involved in the UA transport at this site.

In the present paper, we have mainly discussed about the possible role of brain GLUT9 and ABCG2 regarding the transport activity of UA [41–43]. However, association with other candidate substrates of the transporters needs to be taken into consideration. Initially, GLUT9 was shown to be a high-affinity, low-capacity glucose and fructose transporter [44]. Other GLUT transporters are also expressed in the brain [45] and among them, GLUT1 is highly expressed in both the luminal and abluminal membranes of the endothelial cells and predominantly involved in the glucose transport into the brain [46, 47]. Whether the brain UA transporters are actually involved in the UA transport at the ependymal cells, choroid plexus epithelial cells and brain capillary endothelial cells and the effect of competitive substrates should be ascertained in future studies including the direct measurement of local UA at the cellular level.

It has recently been reported that genetic variants of *SLC2A9* (GLUT9) and *ABCG2*, which influence the serum level of UA, can modify susceptibility to PD [3, 5, 6]. Further, an elevated/reduced UA level in serum correlates closely with an elevated/reduced UA level in the brain [34]. Moreover, the dysfunction of regional UA transport in the brain may have additional effects on the level of UA in the brain. GLUT9 dysfunction in the ependymal cells may reduce the UA supply for brain parenchyma. ABCG2 dysfunction in the brain capillary endothelial cells may inhibit UA excretion into blood and maintain the brain parenchyma UA level. Since multiple UA transporters exist on the luminal side of endothelial cells, further investigation is required to reveal the main driver of UA transport.

Conclusions

In this study, we propose that UA in the brain could be transported by UA transporters, which show specific expression patterns in ependymal, choroid plexus epithelial and brain capillary endothelial cells. Thus far, the importance of UA in the brain as an antioxidant has been widely discussed however, the dynamics of UA transport in the brain has remained unexplored. Further clarification of the regulatory mechanism of the level of UA in the central nervous system would be helpful for the realization of targeted neuroprotective therapy.

Abbreviations

CSF: cerebrospinal fluid; KO: knockout; PD: Parkinson's disease; PFA: paraformaldehyde; UA: uric acid; WT: wild-type.

Authors' contributions

NHT and MH conceived, designed the study and wrote the paper. NHT performed the immunohistochemical and in situ hybridization studies. TT and HS participated in the study with ABCG2 KO mouse. YT, SS and SU participated in the design of the immunohistochemical study. All authors read and approved the final manuscript.

Author details

[1] Department of Human Physiology and Pathology, Faculty of Pharma-Sciences, Teikyo University, 2-11-1 Kaga, Itabashi-ku, Tokyo 173-8605, Japan. [2] Department of Internal Medicine, Teikyo University School of Medicine, Teikyo University, 2-11-1 Kaga, Itabashi-ku, Tokyo 173-8605, Japan. [3] Department of Pharmacy, The University of Tokyo Hospital, Faculty of Medicine, The University of Tokyo, 7-3-1 Hongo, Bunkyo-ku, Tokyo 113-8655, Japan.

Acknowledgements

The authors thank Yui Ishiyama, Chiemi Shigetomi, Natsumi Hasebe and Seiha Katabami for technical assistance.

Competing interests

The authors declare that they have no competing interests.

Funding

This work was in part supported by Grant-in-Aid for Research Activity Start-up from Japan Society of the Promotion of Science (JSPS) (Grant No. 26893275) and the Gout Research Foundation of Japan.

References

1. Kutzing MK, Firestein BL. Altered uric acid levels and disease states. J Pharmacol Exp Ther. 2008;324:1–7.
2. Chen X, Wu G, Schwarzschild MA. Urate in Parkinson's disease: more than a biomarker? Curr Neurol Neurosci Rep. 2012;12:367–75.
3. Matsuo H, Tomiyama H, Satake W, Chiba T, Onoue H, Kawamura Y, Nakayama A, Shimizu S, Sakiyama M, Funayama M, Nishioka K, Shimizu T, Kaida K, Kamakura K, Toda T, Hattori N, Shinomiya N. ABCG2 variant has opposing effects on onset ages of Parkinson's disease and gout. Ann Clin Transl Neurol. 2015;2:302–6.
4. Simon KC, Eberly S, Gao X, Oakes D, Tanner CM, Shoulson I, Fahn S, Schwarzschild MA, Ascherio A, Parkinson Study G. Mendelian randomization of serum urate and parkinson disease progression. Ann Neurol. 2014;76:862–8.
5. Facheris MF, Hicks AA, Minelli C, Hagenah JM, Kostic V, Campbell S, Hayward C, Volpato CB, Pattaro C, Vitart V, Wright A, Campbell H, Klein C, Pramstaller PP. Variation in the uric acid transporter gene SLC2A9 and its association with AAO of Parkinson's disease. J Mol Neurosci. 2011;43:246–50.

6. Gonzalez-Aramburu I, Sanchez-Juan P, Jesus S, Gorostidi A, Fernandez-Juan E, Carrillo F, Sierra M, Gomez-Garre P, Caceres-Redondo MT, Berciano J, Ruiz-Martinez J, Combarros O, Mir P, Infante J. Genetic variability related to serum uric acid concentration and risk of Parkinson's disease. Mov Disord. 2013;28:1737–40.
7. Chen X, Burdett TC, Desjardins CA, Logan R, Cipriani S, Xu Y, Schwarzschild MA. Disrupted and transgenic urate oxidase alter urate and dopaminergic neurodegeneration. Proc Natl Acad Sci USA. 2013;110:300–5.
8. Gong L, Zhang QL, Zhang N, Hua WY, Huang YX, Di PW, Huang T, Xu XS, Liu CF, Hu LF, Luo WF. Neuroprotection by urate on 6-OHDA-lesioned rat model of Parkinson's disease: linking to Akt/GSK3beta signaling pathway. J Neurochem. 2012;123:876–85.
9. Parkinson Study Group S-PDI, Schwarzschild MA, Ascherio A, Beal MF, Cudkowicz ME, Curhan GC, Hare JM, Hooper DC, Kieburtz KD, Macklin EA, Oakes D, Rudolph A, Shoulson I, Tennis MK, Espay AJ, Gartner M, Hung A, Bwala G, Lenehan R, Encarnacion E, Ainslie M, Castillo R, Togasaki D, Barles G, Friedman JH, Niles L, Carter JH, Murray M, Goetz CG, Jaglin J, et al. Inosine to increase serum and cerebrospinal fluid urate in Parkinson disease: a randomized clinical trial. JAMA Neurol. 2014;71:141–50.
10. Bhattacharyya S, Bakshi R, Logan R, Ascherio A, Macklin EA, Schwarzschild MA. Oral inosine persistently elevates plasma antioxidant capacity in Parkinson's disease. Mov Disord. 2016;31:417–21.
11. Ascherio A, LeWitt PA, Xu K, Eberly S, Watts A, Matson WR, Marras C, Kieburtz K, Rudolph A, Bogdanov MB, Schwid SR, Tennis M, Tanner CM, Beal MF, Lang AE, Oakes D, Fahn S, Shoulson I, Schwarzschild MA, Parkinson Study Group DI. Urate as a predictor of the rate of clinical decline in Parkinson disease. Arch Neurol. 2009;66:1460–8.
12. Enomoto A, Kimura H, Chairoungdua A, Shigeta Y, Jutabha P, Cha SH, Hosoyamada M, Takeda M, Sekine T, Igarashi T, Matsuo H, Kikuchi Y, Oda T, Ichida K, Hosoya T, Shimokata K, Niwa T, Kanai Y, Endou H. Molecular identification of a renal urate anion exchanger that regulates blood urate levels. Nature. 2002;417:447–52.
13. Tomioka NH, Nakamura M, Doshi M, Deguchi Y, Ichida K, Morisaki T, Hosoyamada M. Ependymal cells of the mouse brain express urate transporter 1 (URAT1). Fluids Barriers CNS. 2013;10:31.
14. Jimenez AJ, Dominguez-Pinos MD, Guerra MM, Fernandez-Llebrez P, Perez-Figares JM. Structure and function of the ependymal barrier and diseases associated with ependyma disruption. Tissue Barriers. 2014;2:e28426.
15. Johanson C, Stopa E, McMillan P, Roth D, Funk J, Krinke G. The distributional nexus of choroid plexus to cerebrospinal fluid, ependyma and brain: toxicologic/pathologic phenomena, periventricular destabilization, and lesion spread. Toxicol Pathol. 2011;39:186–212.
16. Mullier A, Bouret SG, Prevot V, Dehouck B. Differential distribution of tight junction proteins suggests a role for tanycytes in blood-hypothalamus barrier regulation in the adult mouse brain. J Comp Neurol. 2010;518:943–62.
17. Petrov T, Howarth AG, Krukoff TL, Stevenson BR. Distribution of the tight junction-associated protein ZO-1 in circumventricular organs of the CNS. Brain Res Mol Brain Res. 1994;21:235–46.
18. Akanuma S, Sakurai T, Tachikawa M, Kubo Y, Hosoya K. Transporter-mediated L-glutamate elimination from cerebrospinal fluid: possible involvement of excitatory amino acid transporters expressed in ependymal cells and choroid plexus epithelial cells. Fluids Barriers CNS. 2015;12:11.
19. Gunzel D, Yu AS. Claudins and the modulation of tight junction permeability. Physiol Rev. 2013;93:525–69.
20. Mandal AK, Mount DB. The molecular physiology of uric acid homeostasis. Annu Rev Physiol. 2015;77:323–45.
21. Augustin R, Carayannopoulos MO, Dowd LO, Phay JE, Moley JF, Moley KH. Identification and characterization of human glucose transporter-like protein-9 (GLUT9): alternative splicing alters trafficking. J Biol Chem. 2004;279:16229–36.
22. Keembiyehetty C, Augustin R, Carayannopoulos MO, Steer S, Manolescu A, Cheeseman CI, Moley KH. Mouse glucose transporter 9 splice variants are expressed in adult liver and kidney and are up-regulated in diabetes. Mol Endocrinol. 2006;20:686–97.
23. Cipriani S, Desjardins CA, Burdett TC, Xu Y, Xu K, Schwarzschild MA. Protection of dopaminergic cells by urate requires its accumulation in astrocytes. J Neurochem. 2012;123:172–81.
24. Cooray HC, Blackmore CG, Maskell L, Barrand MA. Localisation of breast cancer resistance protein in microvessel endothelium of human brain. Neuroreport. 2002;13:2059–63.
25. Tachikawa M, Watanabe M, Hori S, Fukaya M, Ohtsuki S, Asashima T, Terasaki T. Distinct spatio-temporal expression of ABCA and ABCG transporters in the developing and adult mouse brain. J Neurochem. 2005;95:294–304.
26. Mitchell D, Ibrahim S, Gusterson BA. Improved immunohistochemical localization of tissue antigens using modified methacarn fixation. J Histochem Cytochem. 1985;33:491–5.
27. Kimura T, Takahashi M, Yan K, Sakurai H. Expression of SLC2A9 isoforms in the kidney and their localization in polarized epithelial cells. Plos ONE. 2014;9:e84996.
28. Preitner F, Bonny O, Laverriere A, Rotman S, Firsov D, Da Costa A, Metref S, Thorens B. Glut9 is a major regulator of urate homeostasis and its genetic inactivation induces hyperuricosuria and urate nephropathy. Proc Natl Acad Sci USA. 2009;106:15501–6.
29. DeBosch BJ, Kluth O, Fujiwara H, Schurmann A, Moley K. Early-onset metabolic syndrome in mice lacking the intestinal uric acid transporter SLC2A9. Nat Commun. 2014;5:4642.
30. Leto D, Saltiel AR. Regulation of glucose transport by insulin: traffic control of GLUT4. Nat Rev Mol Cell Biol. 2012;13:383–96.
31. Cura AJ, Carruthers A. Acute modulation of sugar transport in brain capillary endothelial cell cultures during activation of the metabolic stress pathway. J Biol Chem. 2010;285:15430–9.
32. Sugihara S, Hisatome I, Kuwabara M, Niwa K, Maharani N, Kato M, Ogino K, Hamada T, Ninomiya H, Higashi Y, Ichida K, Yamamoto K. Depletion of uric acid due to SLC22A12 (URAT1) loss-of-function mutation causes endothelial dysfunction in hypouricemia. Circ J. 2015;79:1125–32.
33. Imaoka T, Kusuhara H, Adachi-Akahane S, Hasegawa M, Morita N, Endou H, Sugiyama Y. The renal-specific transporter mediates facilitative transport of organic anions at the brush border membrane of mouse renal tubules. J Am Soc Nephrol. 2004;15:2012–22.
34. Bowman GL, Shannon J, Frei B, Kaye JA, Quinn JF. Uric acid as a CNS antioxidant. J Alzheimers Dis. 2010;19:1331–6.
35. Wolburg H, Paulus W. Choroid plexus: biology and pathology. Acta Neuropathol. 2010;119:75–88.
36. Brinker T, Stopa E, Morrison J, Klinge P. A new look at cerebrospinal fluid circulation. Fluids Barriers CNS. 2014;11:10.
37. Moriwaki Y, Yamamoto T, Yamaguchi K, Takahashi S, Higashino K. Immunohistochemical localization of aldehyde and xanthine oxidase in rat tissues using polyclonal antibodies. Histochem Cell Biol. 1996;105:71–9.
38. Leggas M, Adachi M, Scheffer GL, Sun D, Wielinga P, Du G, Mercer KE, Zhuang Y, Panetta JC, Johnston B, Scheper RJ, Stewart CF, Schuetz JD. Mrp4 confers resistance to topotecan and protects the brain from chemotherapy. Mol Cell Biol. 2004;24:7612–21.
39. Sweet DH, Chan LM, Walden R, Yang XP, Miller DS, Pritchard JB. Organic anion transporter 3 (Slc22a8) is a dicarboxylate exchanger indirectly coupled to the Na+ gradient. Am J Physiol Renal Physiol. 2003;284:F763–9.
40. Bakhiya A, Bahn A, Burckhardt G, Wolff N. Human organic anion transporter 3 (hOAT3) can operate as an exchanger and mediate secretory urate flux. Cell Physiol Biochem. 2003;13:249–56.
41. Anzai N, Ichida K, Jutabha P, Kimura T, Babu E, Jin CJ, Srivastava S, Kitamura K, Hisatome I, Endou H, Sakurai H. Plasma urate level is directly regulated by a voltage-driven urate efflux transporter URATv1 (SLC2A9) in humans. J Biol Chem. 2008;283:26834–8.
42. Woodward OM, Kottgen A, Coresh J, Boerwinkle E, Guggino WB, Kottgen M. Identification of a urate transporter, ABCG2, with a common functional polymorphism causing gout. Proc Natl Acad Sci USA. 2009;106:10338–42.
43. Matsuo H, Takada T, Ichida K, Nakamura T, Nakayama A, Ikebuchi Y, Ito K, Kusanagi Y, Chiba T, Tadokoro S, Takada Y, Oikawa Y, Inoue H, Suzuki K, Okada R, Nishiyama J, Domoto H, Watanabe S, Fujita M, Morimoto Y, Naito M, Nishio K, Hishida A, Wakai K, Asai Y, Niwa K, Kamakura K, Nonoyama S, Sakurai Y, Hosoya T, et al. Common defects of ABCG2, a high-capacity urate exporter, cause gout: a function-based genetic analysis in a Japanese population. Sci Transl Med. 2009;1:5ra11.
44. Doblado M, Moley KH. Facilitative glucose transporter 9, a unique hexose and urate transporter. Am J Physiol Endocrinol Metab. 2009;297:E831–5.

45. Castro MA, Beltran FA, Brauchi S, Concha II. A metabolic switch in brain: glucose and lactate metabolism modulation by ascorbic acid. J Neurochem. 2009;110:423–40.
46. Klepper J, Voit T. Facilitated glucose transporter protein type 1 (GLUT1) deficiency syndrome: impaired glucose transport into brain—a review. Eur J Pediatr. 2002;161:295–304.
47. De Vivo DC, Trifiletti RR, Jacobson RI, Ronen GM, Behmand RA, Harik SI. Defective glucose transport across the blood-brain barrier as a cause of persistent hypoglycorrhachia, seizures, and developmental delay. N Engl J Med. 1991;325:703–9.

Modeling and rescue of defective blood–brain barrier function of induced brain microvascular endothelial cells from childhood cerebral adrenoleukodystrophy patients

Catherine A. A. Lee[1†], Hannah S. Seo[2†], Anibal G. Armien[3], Frank S. Bates[2], Jakub Tolar[4*‡] and Samira M. Azarin[2*‡]

Abstract

Background: X-linked adrenoleukodystrophy (X-ALD) is caused by mutations in the *ABCD1* gene. 40% of X-ALD patients will convert to the deadly childhood cerebral form (ccALD) characterized by increased permeability of the brain endothelium that constitutes the blood–brain barrier (BBB). Mutation information and molecular markers investigated to date are not predictive of conversion. Prior reports have focused on toxic metabolic byproducts and reactive oxygen species as instigators of cerebral inflammation and subsequent immune cell invasion leading to BBB breakdown. This study focuses on the BBB itself and evaluates differences in brain endothelium integrity using cells from ccALD patients and wild-type (WT) controls.

Methods: The blood–brain barrier of ccALD patients and WT controls was modeled using directed differentiation of induced pluripotent stem cells (iPSCs) into induced brain microvascular endothelial cells (iBMECs). Immunocytochemistry and PCR confirmed characteristic expression of brain microvascular endothelial cell (BMEC) markers. Barrier properties of iBMECs were measured via trans-endothelial electrical resistance (TEER), sodium fluorescein permeability, and frayed junction analysis. Electron microscopy and RNA-seq were used to further characterize disease-specific differences. Oil-Red-O staining was used to quantify differences in lipid accumulation. To evaluate whether treatment with block copolymers of poly(ethylene oxide) and poly(propylene oxide) (PEO–PPO) could mitigate defective properties, ccALD-iBMECs were treated with PEO–PPO block copolymers and their barrier properties and lipid accumulation levels were quantified.

Results: iBMECs from patients with ccALD had significantly decreased TEER ($2592 \pm 110\ \Omega\ cm^2$) compared to WT controls ($5001 \pm 172\ \Omega\ cm^2$). They also accumulated lipid droplets to a greater extent than WT-iBMECs. Upon treatment with a PEO–PPO diblock copolymer during the differentiation process, an increase in TEER and a reduction in lipid accumulation were observed for the polymer treated ccALD-iBMECs compared to untreated controls.

Conclusions: The finding that BBB integrity is decreased in ccALD and can be rescued with block copolymers opens the door for the discovery of BBB-specific molecular markers that can indicate the onset of ccALD and has therapeutic implications for preventing the conversion to ccALD.

*Correspondence: tolar003@umn.edu; azarin@umn.edu
†Catherine A. A. Lee and Hannah S. Seo contributed equally to this work
‡Jakub Tolar and Samira M. Azarin contributed equally to senior authorship
[2] Department of Chemical Engineering and Materials Science, University of Minnesota, Minneapolis, MN 55455, USA
[4] Department of Pediatrics, University of Minnesota, Minneapolis, MN 55455, USA
Full list of author information is available at the end of the article

Keywords: Adrenoleukodystrophy, In vitro human blood–brain barrier (BBB) model, Brain microvascular endothelial cells, Trans-endothelial electrical resistance, Human induced pluripotent stem cells (hiPSC), Amphiphilic block copolymers

Background

The molecular mechanisms responsible for the onset and progression of childhood cerebral adrenoleukodystrophy (ccALD) remain poorly understood. ccALD is one form of X-linked adrenoleukodystrophy (X-ALD), an inherited metabolic storage disorder affecting 1 in 17,000 individuals [1]. X-ALD is caused by mutations in the *ABCD1* gene which codes for the ABCD1 protein [2]. ABCD1 is a peroxisomal transporter protein responsible for transporting very long-chain fatty acids (VLCFAs) from the cytosol into the peroxisome for subsequent beta-oxidation [3, 4]. Mutation type and location are not predictive of phenotype, as the same *ABCD1* mutation can lead to clinically distinct phenotypes [5–9]. A more frequent and less severe phenotype, adrenomyeloneuropathy (AMN), presents with demyelination in the long tracts of the spinal cord and progressive axonopathy, usually around the third or fourth decade of life. Heterozygous females will develop similar symptoms by age 60 [10–12]. ccALD, the most rapidly progressing phenotype, occurs in boys ages 2–12 and is characterized by sudden inflammatory demyelination in the brain and death within a few years [13, 14]. ccALD affects about 40% of males with an *ABCD1* mutation [15, 16]. MRI observation of gadolinium enhancement in the brain remains the only method to detect this progression [17–21]. Infections or head trauma have been described as initiators of the conversion from AMN to ccALD, but typically no extrinsic factor can be identified [22–24]. Current treatment for ccALD includes hematopoietic cell transplant (HCT), but this must be performed at the earliest stages of the disease [12, 14, 25, 26].

Much attention has focused on VLCFAs in the search for alternative treatments. While the accumulation of VLCFAs appears to directly contribute to symptoms of AMN, how VLCFAs contribute to the onset or progression of ccALD is unclear [27, 28]. VLCFAs accumulate in many tissue types in X-ALD patients, but this accumulation is not predictive of clinical phenotype [29, 30]. Furthermore, dietary regimens or treatments aimed at reducing the accumulation of VLCFAs (e.g. "Lorenzo's oil") cannot prevent ccALD onset [31–33], just as immunosuppression cannot prevent the cerebral inflammation seen during ccALD progression [34, 35]. Other biomarkers have been investigated for their potential correlation with ccALD conversion including mitochondrial defects, AMP-activated protein kinases, reactive oxygen species (ROS), and oxidative stress [15, 36–40]. Antioxidant activity levels of superoxide dismutase in blood plasma have been found to decrease prior to and during cerebral diagnosis [41]. Treatment with the antioxidant *N*-acetyl-L-cysteine improves survival of patients with advanced ccALD undergoing HCT [42], and oxidative stress levels decrease in patients after HCT [43]. A clinical trial testing a cocktail of antioxidants on patients with AMN has recently been completed though the results have yet to be published [44]. Identification at the molecular level of defects underlying the rapid BBB breakdown seen in ccALD would enable the development of strategies aimed at preventing the onset and progression of ccALD.

The initial blood–brain barrier (BBB) breakdown is thought to be mediated by immune cells (specifically T-cells and to some extent B-cells) translocating from the blood into the brain [45, 46]. Until recently, however, little attention has been paid to the brain endothelium constituting the BBB [47]. X-ALD lacks a suitable mouse model to study the BBB, as mice lacking ABCD1 only develop symptoms of AMN [48]. A human model of the BBB is difficult to obtain, as primary cells isolated from human brain biopsies are not readily available and tend to de-differentiate upon removal from the in vivo microenvironment [49]. Additionally, immortalized BMEC cell lines display poor barrier properties [50, 51]. To address these challenges, a system that enables modeling of the BBB through directed differentiation of human induced pluripotent stem cells (hiPSCs) into induced brain microvascular endothelial cells (iBMECs) was recently developed [52–55]. iBMECs from this system are readily renewable and have been shown to recapitulate important BMEC properties such as junctional protein expression, formation of a tight barrier with physiologically relevant trans-endothelial electrical resistance (TEER) ($\sim 5000\ \Omega\ cm^2$), and multidrug resistance protein efflux activity [54]. This system has been used to model the BBB of other neurological diseases such as Huntington's [56] and to model bacterial interaction with the BBB [57]. Use of this system provides a unique opportunity to study the BBB of ccALD patients and to ask whether there are differences in barrier function compared to WT controls.

Additionally, this same system can be used to investigate potential therapeutic interventions to improve defects in barrier function. We hypothesized that treatment of diseased iBMECs with block copolymers of poly(ethylene oxide) (PEO) and poly(propylene oxide)

(PPO) may improve barrier function. PEO–PPO–PEO triblock copolymers, called poloxamers or Pluronics, are widely used in biomedical applications due to their biocompatibility and amphiphilicity [58, 59]. Poloxamer 188 (P188; number average molar mass = 8.4 kg/mol and 80 wt% PEO) is approved for human use in certain applications [60] and has been demonstrated to provide cell membrane stabilization for a panoply of cell and tissue types under various stresses. P188 has been shown to be effective in ameliorating the effects of electropermeabilized skeletal muscle cells in rats [61], skeletal muscle cell necrosis [62, 63], dystrophic heart failure in mice [64], mechanical stress of dystrophic skeletal muscle in mice [65], damaged neuron-like cells in vitro [66, 67], injured primary neurons [68], and acute injury to the BBB in vivo [69–71]. Moreover, we recently found that a diblock analog of P188, a PEO–PPO diblock copolymer with one-half the composition and size of P188, can also protect model lipid membranes [72]. PEO–PPO diblock copolymers offer an opportunity to tune the end group on the PPO block, which recent work suggests to be an important molecular parameter in the ability of a PEO–PPO copolymer to confer protection [73]. A systematic in vitro screening of PEO–PPO diblock copolymers identified the polymer $E_{182}P_{16}\underline{t}$ (number average molar mass = 9 kg/mol and 90 wt% PEO; numerical subscripts indicate number of repeat units), which has a hydrophobic *tert*-butyl ($\underline{t}$) end group on the PPO block, to be the most efficacious in stabilizing myoblasts under hypo-osmotic stress and isotonic recovery [74]. Thus, in addition to the commonly used Poloxamer 188, we hypothesized that $E_{182}P_{16}\underline{t}$ could also improve iBMEC function.

In this study, we used a previously established directed differentiation protocol to derive iBMECs from WT- and ccALD-iPSCs. This enabled us to model the BBB of ccALD patients and to examine potential differences in barrier function specific to ccALD. P188 and a PEO–PPO$\underline{t}$ diblock copolymer, $E_{182}P_{16}\underline{t}$, were investigated for their potential to improve BMEC integrity. Testing of these two copolymers with this BBB model is a new avenue of investigation for X-ALD. Improvements in barrier function produced by amphiphilic block copolymers have implications for translation into a treatment for preventing the onset of ccALD by improving the BBB integrity of X-ALD patients. Translating the results from this study has the potential to reduce the number of individuals with X-ALD who develop deadly and rapidly progressive ccALD.

Methods

Derivation and culture of hiPSCs

Normal and ccALD iPSC lines (see Additional file 1: Table S1) were used [75, 76]. Cell lines were reprogrammed using retroviral gene delivery using the reprogramming factors OCT4, SOX2, KLF4, and c-MYC (Addgene) (WT1, WT2, ccALD1, ccALD2, ccALD3) or obtained from American Type Culture Collection (ATCC) (WT3 = ACS-1024). Cells were derived from somatic cells on irradiated MEF cultures and transferred to Matrigel (Corning) and E8 Medium (Thermo Fisher Scientific) or TeSR-E8 (STEMCELL Technologies) for additional feeder-free expansion and maintenance. All cell lines tested negative for Mycoplasma contamination via a MycoAlert™ Mycoplasma Detection Kit (Lonza). With the exception of the cell line obtained from ATCC, all cell lines were authenticated using genetic fingerprinting and were also found to be karyotypically normal.

hiPSC differentiation to iBMECs

hiPSCs were differentiated according to Stebbins et al. [52]. On Day 8, cells were subcultured at a ratio of 1 well of a 6-well plate to 3 wells of a 12-well plate, 6 wells of a 24-well plate, Transwell filters (12 mm), or 11.4 wells of a μ-slide. When the cells reached confluence 48 h after subculture (Day 10), cells were utilized for permeability, efflux transporter, immunocytochemistry, RT-PCR, RNA-seq, and Oil-Red-O staining experiments using endothelial cell (EC) medium: human endothelial serum free medium (Thermo Fisher Scientific) with 1% platelet-poor plasma derived serum (Biomedical Technologies).

Immunocytochemistry

iBMECs were subcultured onto μ-slides (Ibidi). 48 h post-subculture, cells were fixed in ice-cold 100% methanol (MilliporeSigma). Fixed iBMECs were blocked for 1 h at room temperature in a blocking buffer of PBS containing 10% normal goat serum (Thermo Fisher Scientific). Cells were incubated with primary antibodies diluted in blocking buffer overnight at 4 °C. After 3 washes with PBS for a minimum of 5 min per wash, cells were incubated with secondary antibody for 1 h in the dark at room temperature (see Additional file 1: Tables S2, S3). Cells were subsequently washed with PBS three times for a minimum of 5 min per wash and incubated with 4′,6-diamidino-2-pheny-lindoldihydrochloride (DAPI; Thermo Fisher Scientific) for 5 min to label nuclei. Cells were washed once with PBS for 5 min before imaging with an EVOS FL Auto Cell Imaging microscope.

RT-PCR

Cells were differentiated as described above and detached with trypsin. Total RNA was extracted using an RNeasy Mini Kit (Qiagen) following the manufacturer's protocol and quantified using a NanoDrop® ND-1000. cDNA was generated from 1 μg of RNA using Omniscript reverse-transcriptase (Qiagen) and oligo-dT primers (Thermo

Fisher Scientific). RT-PCR was performed using the GoTaq Green Master Mix (Promega) and PrimePCR primer sets (Bio-Rad) (see Additional file 1: Table S4). Glyceraldehyde-3-phosphate dehydrogenase (GAPDH) was used as the housekeeping gene. Gel electrophoresis of RT-PCR products with a 2% agarose gel was used to analyze transcript amplification.

Trans-endothelial electrical resistance

iBMECs were seeded onto Transwell filters. TEER was measured daily starting 24 h after subculture utilizing the EVOM2 voltohmmeter with STX3 chopstick electrodes (World Precision Instruments). TEER was measured on an empty Transwell filter coated with collagen and fibronectin, and this value was subtracted from the TEER of the cell monolayer each time. TEER values were normalized by the surface area of the Transwell filter.

Sodium fluorescein permeability

iBMECs were seeded onto Transwell filters. An empty Transwell filter coated with collagen and fibronectin was utilized to measure the permeability of the membrane. After a complete medium change, the cells were incubated at 37 °C for 1.5 h. TEER was measured before and after the medium change to confirm monolayer equilibration. Medium from the apical chamber was aspirated and replaced with EC medium containing 10 μM sodium fluorescein (MilliporeSigma). Every 30 min for 2 h, 150 μL aliquots were extracted from the basolateral chamber and replaced with 150 μL of fresh medium. At 2 h, a 150 μL sample was extracted from the apical chamber and then fluorescence was measured on a BioTek Synergy H1 multi-mode microplate reader at excitation of 485 nm and emission of 530 nm. Calculation of sodium fluorescein permeability was done following Stebbins et al. [52].

Rhodamine 123 accumulation

Accumulation of rhodamine 123, a P-glycoprotein (P-gp) substrate, was measured in the absence and presence of a P-gp inhibitor cyclosporin A to quantify P-gp efflux potential. iBMECs were seeded onto 24-well plates. Cells were pre-incubated with or without 10 μM cyclosporin A (MilliporeSigma) in HBSS (Thermo Fisher Scientific) for 1 h at 37 °C. Next, all cells were incubated with 10 μM rhodamine 123 (MilliporeSigma) in HBSS for 2 h at 37 °C. Following the incubation steps, cells were lysed using RIPA buffer (MilliporeSigma) and fluorescence was measured on a BioTek Synergy H1 multi-mode microplate reader at excitation of 485 nm and emission of 530 nm. Unlysed cells from a parallel setup were dissociated with Accutase (Thermo Fisher Scientific) and counted using the Countess II to normalize the fluorescence on a per cell basis.

Analysis of tight junction continuity

For quantitative analysis of iBMEC integrity, the percentage of cells expressing frayed tight junctions was counted using iBMECs immunolabeled for occludin. Cells were defined as having frayed tight junctions if any cell–cell contact point appeared discontinuous. A blinded analysis in which three different people each counted 15 separate frames and 12,530 total junctions was used to obtain a percentage of frayed tight junctions for both the ccALD- and WT-iBMECs.

Electron microscopy

iBMECs were seeded onto 6-well plates. Two days after subculture, the cells were fixed with 1 mL of 2.5% glutaraldehyde (Electron Microscopy Sciences) in 0.1 M sodium cacodylate for 1 h at room temperature. Using cell lifters to detach the cells while preserving cell–cell junctions, cells were collected in microcentrifuge tubes and stored in fresh fixative solution for pelleting via centrifugation. Following 3 washes with 0.1 M sodium cacodylate buffer, cells were post-fixed with 1% osmium tetroxide (Electron Microscopy Sciences). Cells were dehydrated in acetone and subsequently embedded with Embed 812 resin (Electron Microscopy Sciences). A Leica UC6 Ultramicrotome (Leica Microsystems) was used to section the embedded samples. A JEM 1400 Plus transmission electron microscope (JEOL LTD) and AMT Capture Engine Version 7.00 (Advanced Microscopy Techniques Corp.) were used to analyze and image the samples.

RNA-sequencing

Cells were differentiated as described above and detached with trypsin. Total RNA was isolated from WT- and ccALD-iBMECs using an RNeasy Mini Kit (Qiagen) following the manufacturer's protocol. RNA with a RNA Integrity Number (RIN) score > 8 was used for library generation with the TruSeq Stranded mRNA Sample Preparation kit (Illumina). Paired-end 150 bp length reads were generated using an Illumina MiniSeq. Low quality bases were trimmed using Trimmomatic (enabled with the optional "--qualitycontrol" option and a 3 bp sliding-window trimming from the 3′ end requiring minimum Q16). The remaining reads were mapped to hg19 using Tophat2. The featureCounts program in the R SubRead package was used to generate a transcript abundance file for input into the R package edgeR to identify differentially expressed genes. Ingenuity Pathway Analysis [77] was used for network analysis and gene ontology [78, 79] for pathway analysis.

Oil-Red-O staining and image analysis

iBMECs were seeded onto 12-well plates. Cells were fixed with 10% formalin for 20 min, subsequently dehydrated with 60% isopropanol, and incubated with Oil-Red-O (MilliporeSigma) for 10 min before being washed 4 times with deionized water. Images were captured using a Nikon Eclipse TS100 inverted light microscope connected to a Unitron Microscopes Lumenera® Cameras AU-310-CMOS Infinity 1 camera. To measure the abundance of lipid droplets from the Oil-Red-O stained images, a custom MATLAB script was used to quantify the number and intensity of red pixels. Red pixels were defined on the HSV (hue, saturation, value) scale as having hue between 0.833 and 0.073, saturation between 0.300–1, and value between 0 and 1. The MATLAB Color Thresholder tool was used to mask as black any pixels not defined as red. Average intensity was measured by summing the value in the red channel of the RGB scale for each pixel, while the average number of pixels was calculated as the total number of red pixels.

Diblock copolymer synthesis

$E_{182}P_{16}\underline{t}$ diblock copolymer was synthesized via ring-opening anionic polymerization following established techniques necessary for air and water free environments described elsewhere [72, 80, 81] with alumina column-dried tetrahydrofuran (THF) as the solvent. The PPO block was first synthesized at room temperature by initiation with potassium *tert*-butoxide (MilliporeSigma) in the presence of 18-crown-6 ether (MilliporeSigma) [82–84]. The reaction was carried out for 48 h, after which the reaction was terminated with excess acidic methanol (1:10 w/w% hydrochloric acid/methanol) to give *tert*-butoxy-terminated PPO chains. The PPO homopolymer was purified by iterative filtration, solvent removal, and dissolution in fresh THF. Subsequently, the hydroxyl terminated PPO was reinitiated with potassium naphthalenide, reacted with ethylene oxide for 20 h, and then terminated with excess acidic methanol. The resulting diblock copolymer was purified by iterative filtration, solvent removal, and dissolution in fresh THF. The final product was retrieved upon an additional purification step via dialysis.

Polymer characterization

P188 (MilliporeSigma) and $E_{182}P_{16}\underline{t}$ were characterized via proton nuclear magnetic resonance spectroscopy (Bruker AX-400; deuterated chloroform as solvent) to determine compositions and/or number average molecular weight by end-group analysis. A size exclusion chromatograph (Waters) with a refractive index detector was used to obtain dispersity of the polymers. THF was utilized as the solvent, and the chromatograph was calibrated with polystyrene standards. The weight percent of PEO and dispersity of P188 were found to be 80 wt% and 1.06, respectively (number average molecular weight of P188 was provided by the manufacturer to be 8400 g/mol). The weight percent of PEO, number average molecular weight, and dispersity of $E_{182}P_{16}\underline{t}$ were determined to be 90 wt%, 8900 g/mol, and 1.07, respectively (see Additional file 1: Figure S1).

Polymer treatment

Working solutions of polymers were prepared by dissolving P188 and $E_{182}P_{16}\underline{t}$ in 1X DPBS without magnesium or calcium (Thermo Fisher Scientific) to a concentration of 12 mM and sterilized via filtration. For polymer treatment during development, the polymers were added to the culture on Day 3 of the differentiation protocol. The polymer working solutions were diluted to a concentration of 0.5 mM or 1 mM in the culture medium, and the resulting solution was added to the culture during standard medium change. The control received medium with DPBS such that all conditions had the same volume of DPBS in the medium. After 24 h, the medium was changed in accordance with the differentiation protocol, effectively removing any excess polymers. On Day 8, the iBMECs were subcultured onto Transwells for TEER measurements or 12-well plates for Oil-Red-O staining. For polymer treatment post-differentiation, iBMECs were subcultured onto Transwells on Day 8; on Day 9, a small aliquot of the P188 or $E_{182}P_{16}\underline{t}$ working solutions was added to the apical chamber such that the final concentration of polymers in the apical chamber was 1 mM. A corresponding volume of DPBS was added to the control cells.

Statistical analysis

Data are presented as mean ± standard error (SEM) with n defined in figure legends. *p*-values were determined using an unpaired Student's *t*-test. Statistical analysis was performed using GraphPad Prism.

Results

Directed differentiation of WT- and ccALD-iPSCs into iBMECs

A previously published protocol [52] was used to direct the differentiation of iPSCs into iBMECs from three clinically confirmed cases of ccALD and three WT controls. Immunofluorescence and RT-PCR demonstrated that both patient and control iBMECs expressed the requisite endothelial markers PECAM-1 and VE-cadherin (*CDH5*), the tight junction markers claudin-5 and occludin, and the BBB markers P-glycoprotein and GLUT-1 (*SLC2A1*) (Fig. 1a, b) (see Additional file 1: Figure S2). Since expression of *ABCB1*, which encodes the

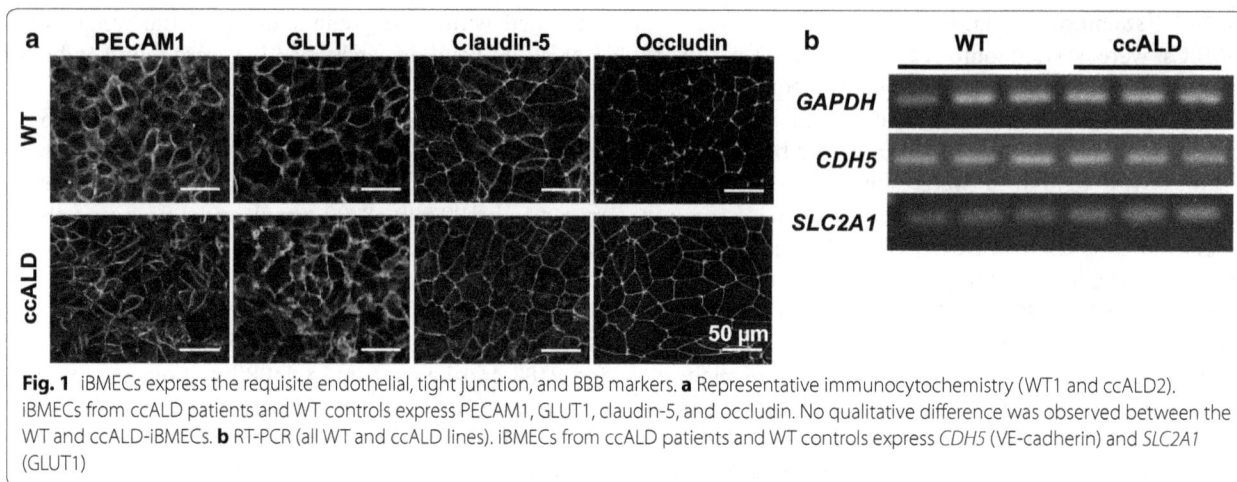

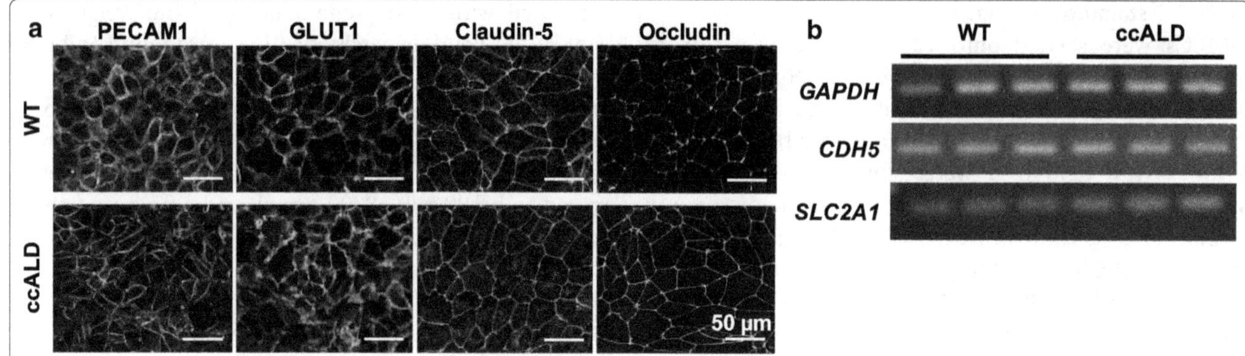

Fig. 1 iBMECs express the requisite endothelial, tight junction, and BBB markers. **a** Representative immunocytochemistry (WT1 and ccALD2). iBMECs from ccALD patients and WT controls express PECAM1, GLUT1, claudin-5, and occludin. No qualitative difference was observed between the WT and ccALD-iBMECs. **b** RT-PCR (all WT and ccALD lines). iBMECs from ccALD patients and WT controls express *CDH5* (VE-cadherin) and *SLC2A1* (GLUT1)

BMEC-specific efflux transporter P-gp, was decreased for one of the ccALD-iBMEC lines (see Additional file 1: Figure S3a), we employed a rhodamine 123 accumulation assay to check the P-gp efflux potential of the ccALD-iBMECs (see Additional file 1: Figure S3b). Normalized accumulation after inhibiting P-gp with cyclosporin A (CsA) was lower for the same iBMEC line in which we noticed the decreased *ABCB1* expression (102.7 ± 2.3) compared to the other ccALD-iBMEC lines (152.7 ± 23.4 and 167.1 ± 19.0) as well as the WT-iBMECs lines (258.2 ± 16.2, 220.8 ± 26.4, and 204.7 ± 20.2).

ccALD-iBMECs have impaired barrier properties

To investigate functional differences between the ccALD- and WT-iBMECs, we used trans-endothelial electrical resistance (TEER) to measure the barrier integrity of the iBMECs on Days 1–4 following subculture onto Transwell filters. At all days measured, we found a statistically significant difference ($p < 0.0001$) in TEER between the ccALD- and WT-iBMECs (peak TEER on Day 2 of measurement: $2592 \pm 110\ \Omega\ cm^2$ compared to $5001 \pm 172\ \Omega\ cm^2$ for the ccALD-iBMECs and WT-iBMECs, respectively) (Fig. 2a) (see Additional file 1: Figure S4 for TEER measurements for individual cell lines). Additionally, permeability of sodium fluorescein was measured to be $1.85 \pm 0.19 \times 10^{-5}$ cm/min for the ccALD-iBMECs and $1.50 \pm 0.31 \times 10^{-5}$ cm/min for the WT-iBMECs (Fig. 2b). The difference in permeability is not statistically significant despite the substantial difference ($\sim 2400\ \Omega\ cm^2$) in TEER between the WT- and ccALD-iBMECs; however, our results are consistent with previous studies that report sodium fluorescein permeability values on the order of 10^{-5} cm/min for BMECs with TEER greater than $2000\ \Omega\ cm^2$ [52, 53, 85, 86] and with reports that demonstrate that small molecule passive permeability does not correlate strongly with TEER above certain TEER thresholds [86–89]. To examine potential differences in tight junction organization, we employed a frayed junction analysis. The ccALD-iBMECs had more frayed junctions ($p < 0.01$) compared to the WT-iBMECs ($37 \pm 3\%$ versus $25 \pm 3\%$) (Fig. 2c, d). Overall, iBMECs from ccALD patients appear to form a less intact cellular barrier that permits increased passive transport of ions as well as small molecules. This defect in barrier integrity may result from mislocalization of tight junction proteins between cells.

Lipid droplets accumulate in ccALD-iBMECs

To assess any structural differences between the ccALD-iBMECs and WT controls, we performed transmission electron microscopy (TEM) of ccALD- and WT-iBMECs using cross-sections of fixed and pelleted cells. Numerous and large lipid droplets were present in the ccALD-iBMECs, with fewer and smaller lipid droplets in the WT-iBMECs (Fig. 3a) (see Additional file 1: Figure S5). To quantify the abundance of lipid droplets in the iBMECs, Oil-Red-O staining was used. This histological stain is specific to neutral lipids and does not stain the polarized phospholipids of the cell membrane [90]. Lipid droplets are stained bright red, and image analysis can be used to quantify either the amount (total number of red pixels) or intensity (redness of the red pixels) of red in micrographs. Quantification of the lipid deposition in ccALD- and WT-iBMECs revealed a significant increase ($p < 0.005$) in lipid abundance in the ccALD-iBMECs compared to the WT-iBMECs (Fig. 3b, c). The average intensity of red pixels in images of Oil-Red-O stained WT-iBMECs was calculated to be $1.8 \pm 0.5 \times 10^6$ compared to $5.4 \pm 1.0 \times 10^6$ for the ccALD-iBMECs. The average number of red pixels was calculated to be $1.1 \pm 0.2 \times 10^4$ for the WT-iBMECs and $2.8 \pm 0.4 \times 10^4$ for the ccALD-iBMECs (Fig. 3c). Very few lipid droplets

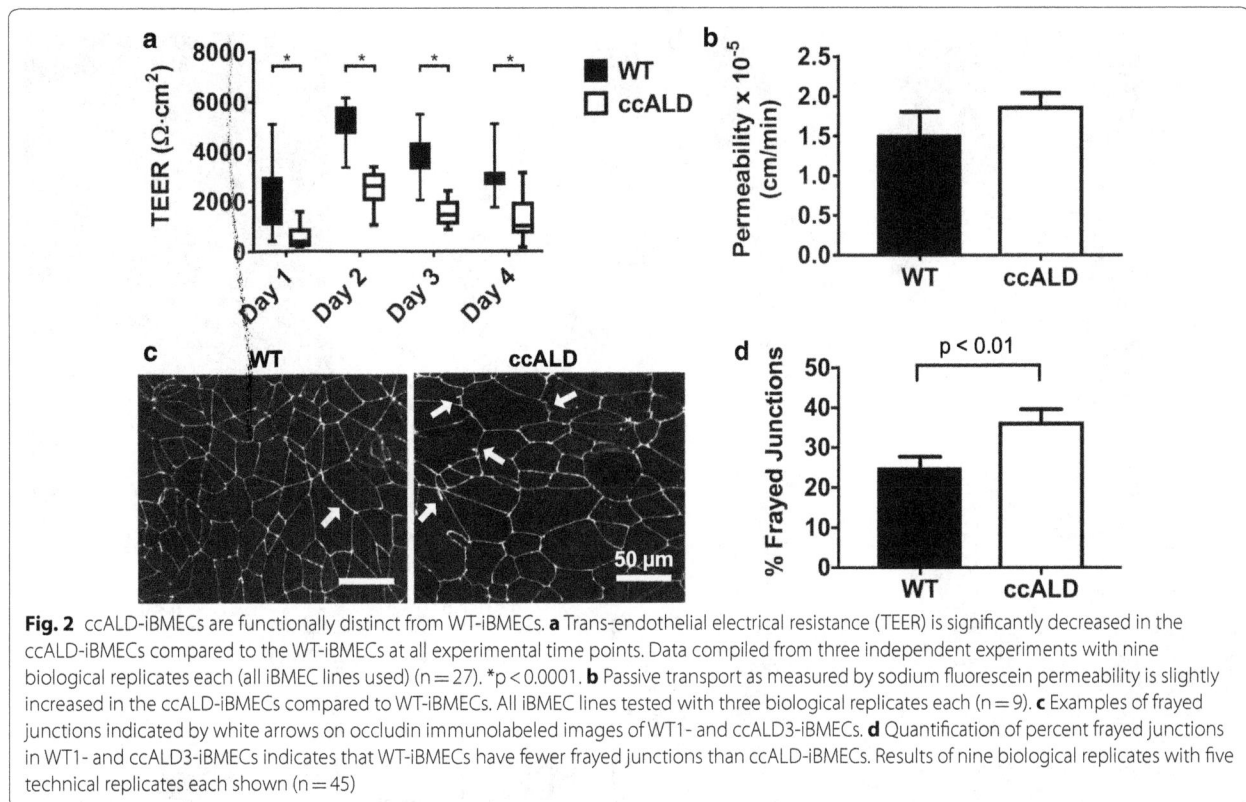

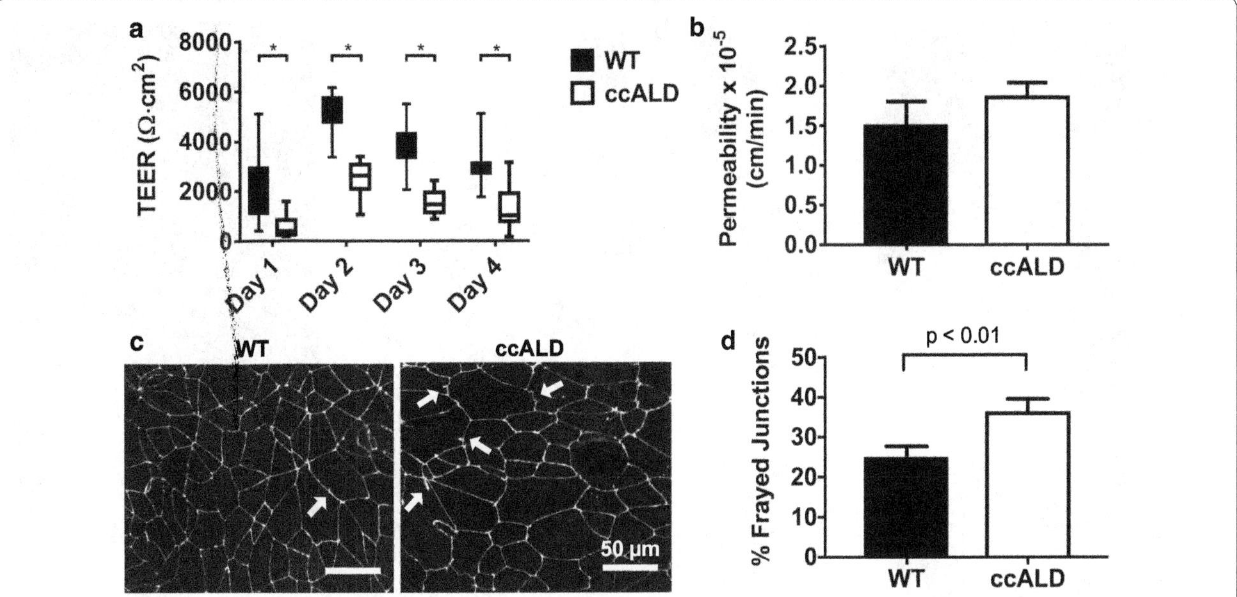

Fig. 2 ccALD-iBMECs are functionally distinct from WT-iBMECs. **a** Trans-endothelial electrical resistance (TEER) is significantly decreased in the ccALD-iBMECs compared to the WT-iBMECs at all experimental time points. Data compiled from three independent experiments with nine biological replicates each (all iBMEC lines used) ($n = 27$). $^*p < 0.0001$. **b** Passive transport as measured by sodium fluorescein permeability is slightly increased in the ccALD-iBMECs compared to WT-iBMECs. All iBMEC lines tested with three biological replicates each ($n = 9$). **c** Examples of frayed junctions indicated by white arrows on occludin immunolabeled images of WT1- and ccALD3-iBMECs. **d** Quantification of percent frayed junctions in WT1- and ccALD3-iBMECs indicates that WT-iBMECs have fewer frayed junctions than ccALD-iBMECs. Results of nine biological replicates with five technical replicates each shown ($n = 45$)

were seen in the iPSCs and no statistical difference was observed between the ccALD-iPSCs and WT-iPSCs in the number of red pixels (22 ± 8 and 35 ± 11, respectively) or the intensity of red pixels ($4.2 \pm 2 \times 10^3$ and $6.4 \pm 2 \times 10^3$, respectively) (see Additional file 1: Figure S6). VLCFA accumulation was not observed in the ccALD-iBMECs via TEM. The presence of an increased amount of lipid droplets in the ccALD-iBMECs compared to the WT-iBMECs that arises upon differentiation (i.e. is not present during the iPSC stage) is a difference that potentially contributes to the decreased barrier integrity of the ccALD-iBMECs.

Transcriptome analysis indicates differences in Type I interferon activation and lipid metabolism pathways

To further characterize differences between ccALD- and WT-iBMECs and to elucidate potential mechanisms for the decreased barrier integrity seen in the ccALD-iBMECs, we performed RNA-sequencing of three replicate differentiations for each of our ccALD- and WT-iBMEC lines. Principal component analysis (PCA) separated the WT-iBMECs from the ccALD-iBMECs along the first principal component (Fig. 4a). Hierarchical clustering of differentially expressed genes (DEGs) (2× fold change, false-discovery rate (FDR) < 0.05) and samples revealed a cluster of genes that were decreased in the ccALD-iBMECs involving the attachment of cells to each other including intracellular attachment between membrane regions (gene ontology (GO): 0022610), while Type I interferon-activated signaling (GO: 0060337) and insulin-like growth factor receptor signaling (GO: 0043568) pathways were increased in the ccALD-iBMECs (Fig. 4b). We used Ingenuity Pathway Analysis (IPA) to query upstream regulators of our DEGs. IPA builds a graph-based network from gene expression data and uses this information to predict upstream regulators. The z-score (calculated as the number of standard deviations from the mean of a normal distribution of activity edges using this graph-based network) represents the magnitude of bias in gene regulation that predicts the activity of specific upstream regulators. This analysis revealed upstream regulators involving TGFβ1 signaling, Type I interferon response, and other immune signaling signatures highly activated in the ccALD-iBMECs (IFNG, LPS, TNF, and TGFβ1 z-scores of 5.5, 7.6, 5.6, and 4.6 respectively) (Fig. 4c). GO analysis was performed on genes differentially expressed between the ccALD- and WT-iBMECs. This analysis calculates a p-value based on enrichment of genes in a particular GO annotation ($-\log_{10}$(p-value) reported as enrichment score for upregulated genes, $\log_{10}$(p-value) reported as enrichment score for downregulated genes). GO analysis on genes upregulated

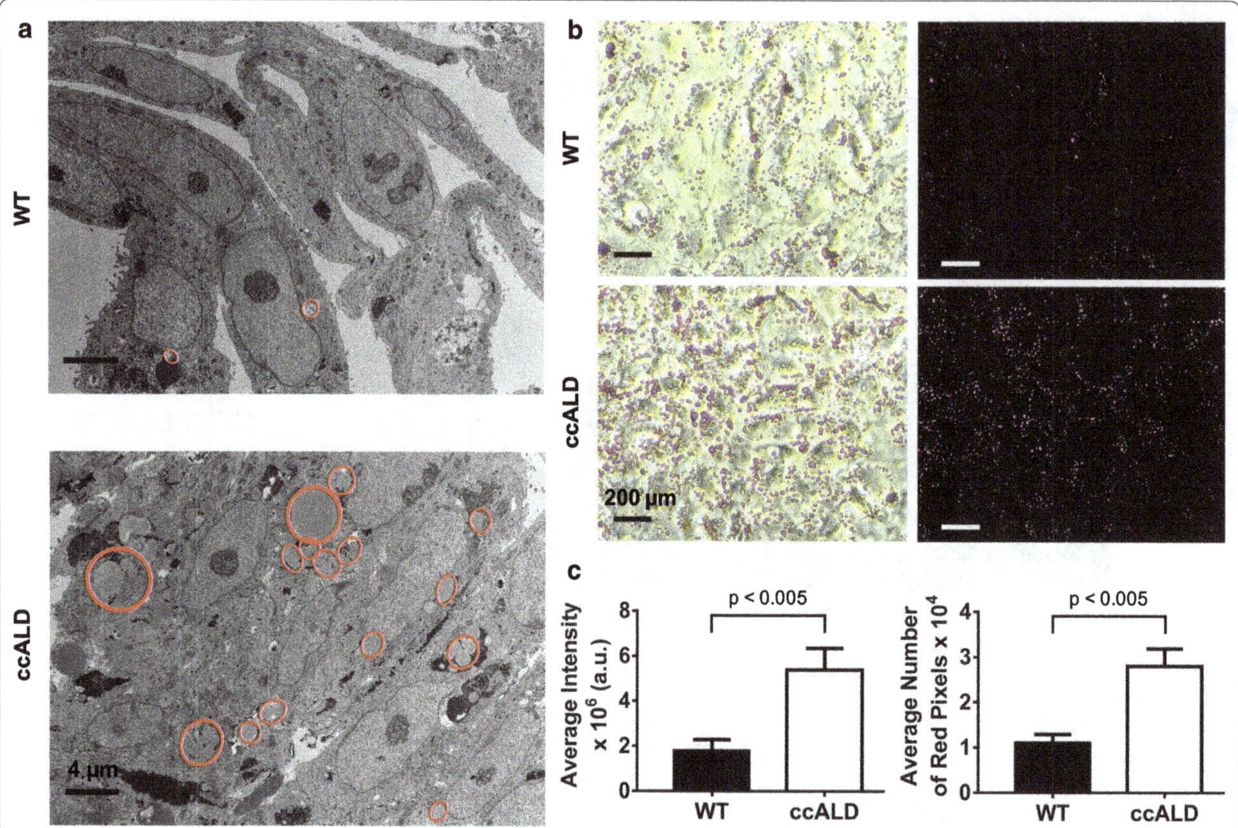

Fig. 3 ccALD-iBMECs accumulate more lipid droplets than WT-iBMECs. **a** Comparison of transmission electron micrographs of WT1- and ccALD3-iBMECs show increased lipid droplet accumulation in ccALD-iBMECs. Lipid droplets outlined in red. **b** Representative images of Oil-Red-O stained WT3 and ccALD1-iBMECs. Raw images on left and masked images on right. **c** Quantification of intensity and number of red pixels in images of Oil-Red-O stained iBMECs indicate increased lipid droplet accumulation in ccALD-iBMECs compared to WT-iBMECs. Oil-Red-O staining images of all iBMEC lines were used for quantification using three biological replicates for each cell line ($n = 9$)

(increased activity) in ccALD-iBMECs indicated an increase in Type I interferon signaling (enrichment score 8.45) and response to lipid pathways (enrichment score 4.34). GO analysis on genes downregulated (decreased activity) in ccALD-iBMECs indicated a decrease in transmembrane and ion transport (enrichment scores − 1.58 and − 3.5, respectively) (Fig. 4d). The lipid pathway upregulation is consistent with both the primary ccALD phenotype and our TEM results, while Type I interferon signaling and other inflammatory pathways are secondary and could have many sources.

Block copolymers reverse impaired barrier integrity and mitigate lipid accumulation

We next investigated whether polymer treatment could rescue the impaired barrier integrity of the ccALD-iBMECs. ccALD-iBMECs were treated with 1 mM of P188 or $E_{182}P_{16}\underline{t}$ at the end of the differentiation protocol (Day 9) or during development (Day 3) (see Fig. 5a for chemical structures of the polymers). Day 3 was chosen because the cells begin to express endothelial cell markers at this time point [55]. Polymer treatment with either P188 or $E_{182}P_{16}\underline{t}$ at the end of the differentiation protocol showed minimal effect on ccALD-iBMEC TEER (see Additional file 1: Figure S7a). However, we saw a significant effect ($p < 0.05$) when the ccALD-iBMECs were treated with the diblock copolymer ($E_{182}P_{16}\underline{t}$) during development. The maximum TEER of the ccALD-iBMECs treated with $E_{182}P_{16}\underline{t}$ was $3316 \pm 246\ \Omega\ cm^2$. This was higher than both the untreated and P188 treated ccALD-iBMECs (2409 ± 254 and $2162 \pm 260\ \Omega\ cm^2$, respectively; Fig. 5b). The effect of dosage was investigated by treating the ccALD-iBMECs with 0.5 or 1 mM $E_{182}P_{16}\underline{t}$ on Day 3 of the differentiation protocol, and we observed a larger increase in TEER compared to the control when treated with 1 mM $E_{182}P_{16}\underline{t}$ than with 0.5 mM $E_{182}P_{16}\underline{t}$ (see Additional file 1: Figure S7b). Notably, the barrier function of the WT-iBMECs was unaffected by polymer treatment as the TEER of the untreated WT-iBMECs ($3074 \pm 127\ \Omega\ cm^2$) was not significantly different than that of WT-iBMECs treated with P188 ($2998 \pm 50\ \Omega\ cm^2$) or $E_{182}P_{16}\underline{t}$ ($3165 \pm 95\ \Omega\ cm^2$).

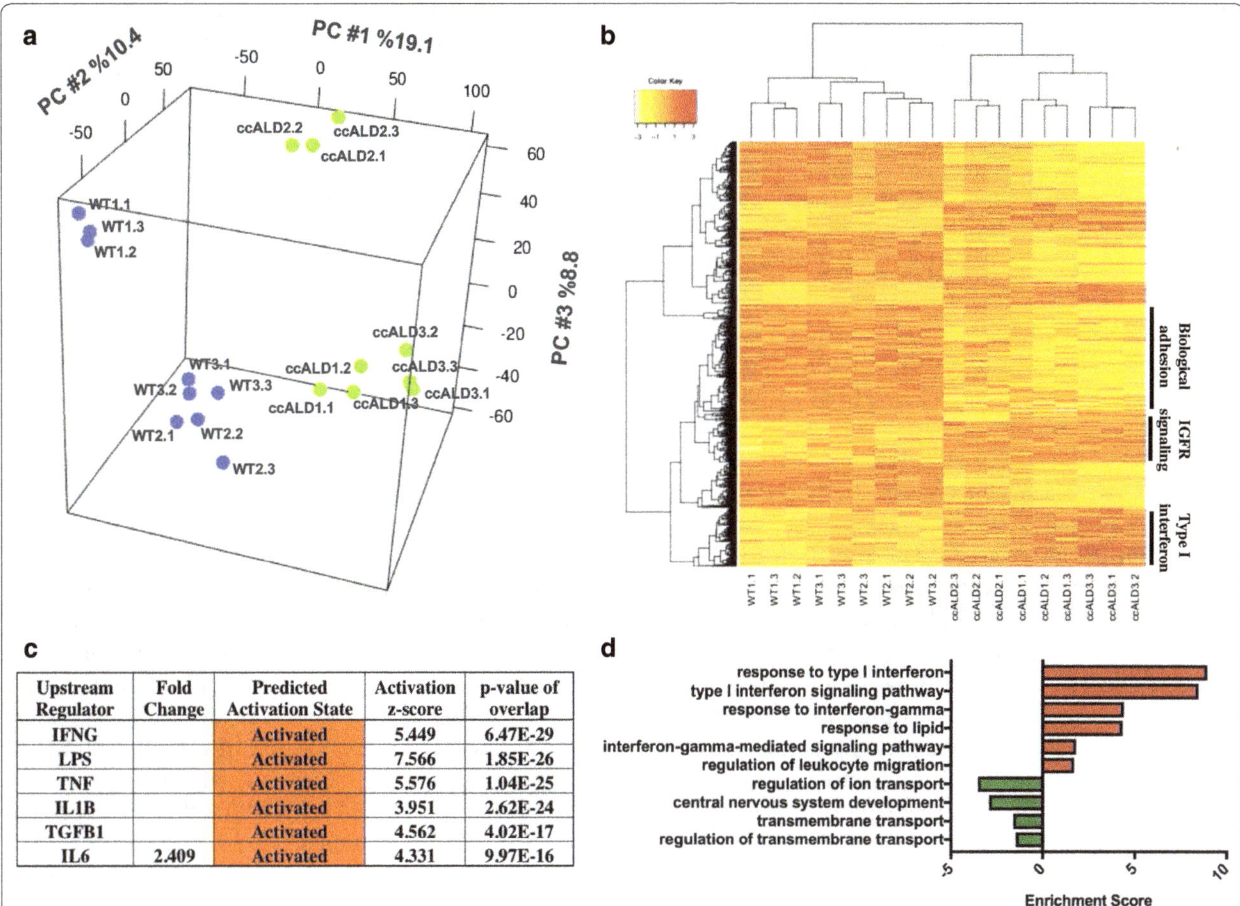

Upstream Regulator	Fold Change	Predicted Activation State	Activation z-score	p-value of overlap
IFNG		Activated	5.449	6.47E-29
LPS		Activated	7.566	1.85E-26
TNF		Activated	5.576	1.04E-25
IL1B		Activated	3.951	2.62E-24
TGFB1		Activated	4.562	4.02E-17
IL6	2.409	Activated	4.331	9.97E-16

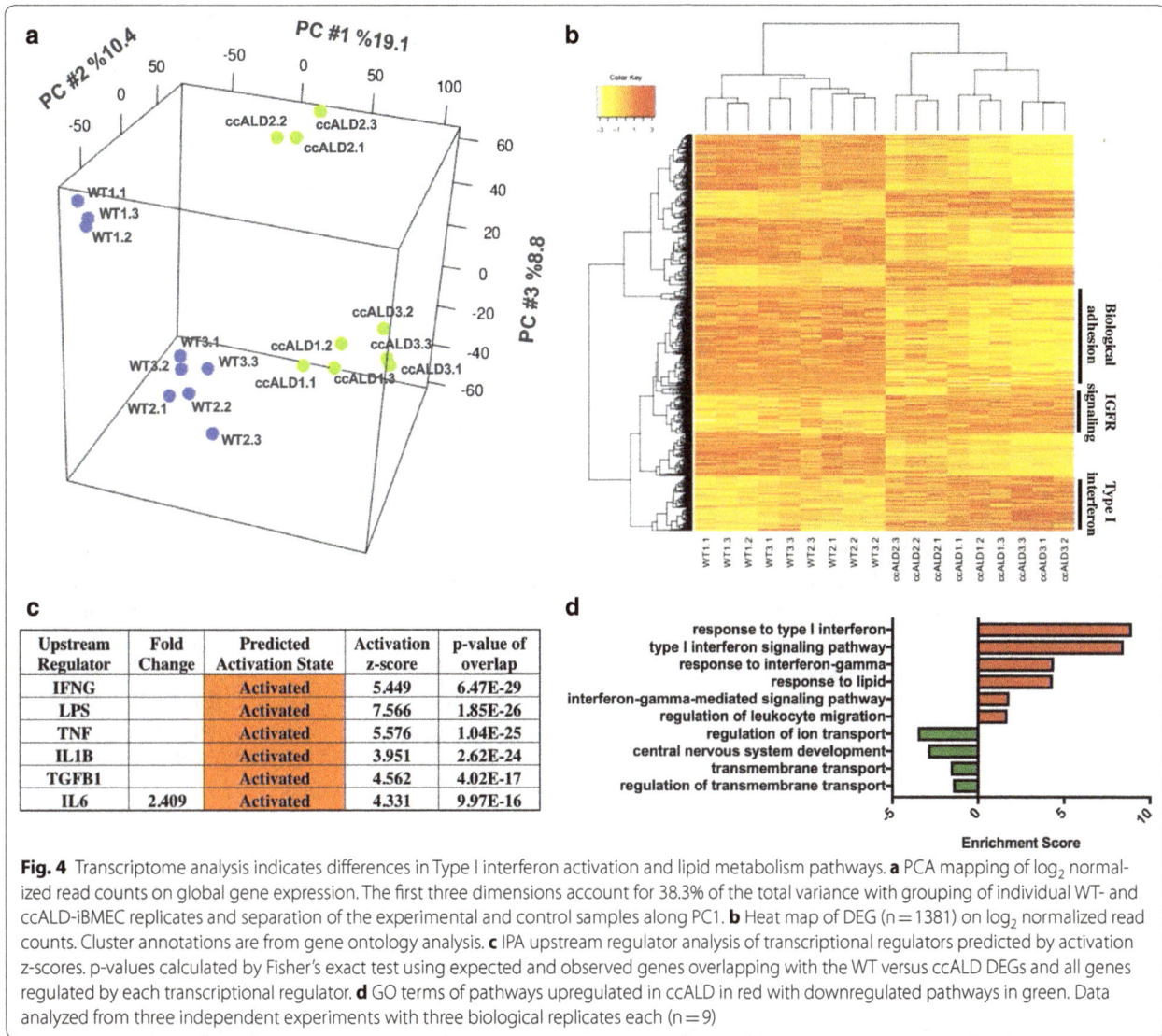

Fig. 4 Transcriptome analysis indicates differences in Type I interferon activation and lipid metabolism pathways. **a** PCA mapping of $\log_2$ normalized read counts on global gene expression. The first three dimensions account for 38.3% of the total variance with grouping of individual WT- and ccALD-iBMEC replicates and separation of the experimental and control samples along PC1. **b** Heat map of DEG (n = 1381) on $\log_2$ normalized read counts. Cluster annotations are from gene ontology analysis. **c** IPA upstream regulator analysis of transcriptional regulators predicted by activation z-scores. p-values calculated by Fisher's exact test using expected and observed genes overlapping with the WT versus ccALD DEGs and all genes regulated by each transcriptional regulator. **d** GO terms of pathways upregulated in ccALD in red with downregulated pathways in green. Data analyzed from three independent experiments with three biological replicates each (n = 9)

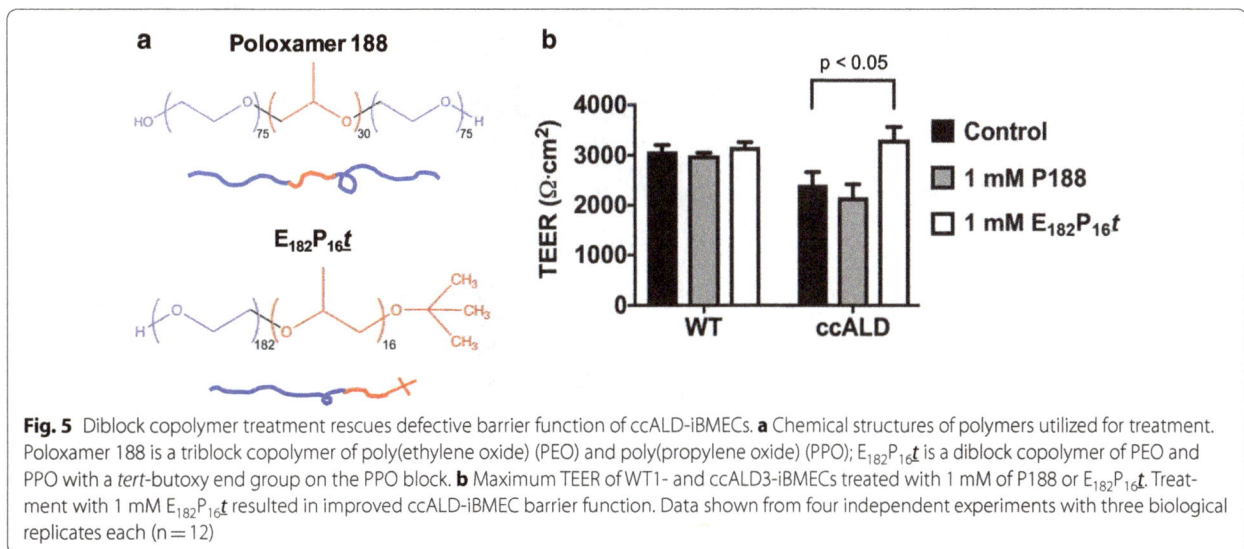

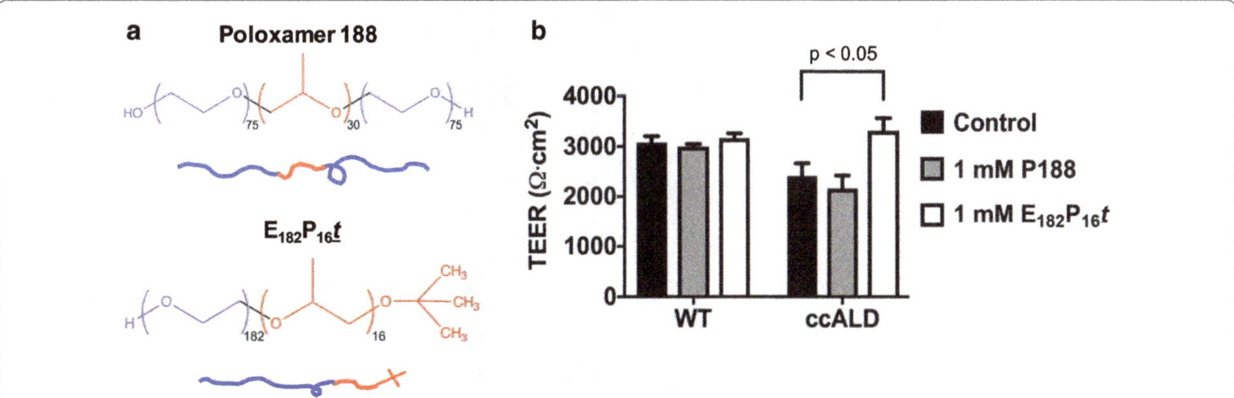

Fig. 5 Diblock copolymer treatment rescues defective barrier function of ccALD-iBMECs. **a** Chemical structures of polymers utilized for treatment. Poloxamer 188 is a triblock copolymer of poly(ethylene oxide) (PEO) and poly(propylene oxide) (PPO); $E_{182}P_{16}t$ is a diblock copolymer of PEO and PPO with a *tert*-butoxy end group on the PPO block. **b** Maximum TEER of WT1- and ccALD3-iBMECs treated with 1 mM of P188 or $E_{182}P_{16}t$. Treatment with 1 mM $E_{182}P_{16}t$ resulted in improved ccALD-iBMEC barrier function. Data shown from four independent experiments with three biological replicates each (n = 12)

Additionally, lipid droplet accumulation was decreased in ccALD-iBMECs treated with 1 mM $E_{182}P_{16}\underline{t}$ during development (Fig. 6). Quantification of Oil-Red-O staining images indicated a statistically significant ($p < 0.05$) decrease in ccALD-iBMECs treated with 1 mM $E_{182}P_{16}\underline{t}$ when compared to untreated ccALD-iBMECs. The average intensity of red pixels in images of Oil-Red-O stained ccALD-iBMECs treated with 1 mM $E_{182}P_{16}\underline{t}$ was $10.9 \pm 1 \times 10^6$ compared to $14.8 \pm 1 \times 10^6$ for the control. The average number of red pixels was calculated to be $4.9 \pm 0.5 \times 10^4$ for ccALD-iBMECs treated with 1 mM $E_{182}P_{16}\underline{t}$ and $6.7 \pm 0.5 \times 10^4$ for the control.

Discussion

Our model of the BBB demonstrating that the barrier function is defective and lipid droplets accumulate in iBMECs from patients with ccALD opens the door to new therapeutic avenues aimed at maintaining the integrity of the BBB and preventing the onset of ccALD. In the present work, our findings indicate a significant improvement in barrier function and a decrease in lipid droplet accumulation when ccALD-iBMECs are treated during differentiation with a diblock copolymer with a hydrophobic *tert*-butoxy end group ($E_{182}P_{16}\underline{t}$). No effect was seen when the ccALD-iBMECs were treated at the same time with P188 or when the ccALD-iBMECs were treated post differentiation with either polymer. Treatment of WT-iBMECs with either polymer during development did not improve barrier function. Response of the ccALD-iBMECs but not the WT-iBMECs to polymer treatment further highlights that there are fundamental differences between the ccALD- and WT-iBMECs.

Overall, our study demonstrates that one of the intrinsic defects in ccALD is with the integrity of the BMECs that constitute the BBB. These findings are in line with the study by Musolino et al. [47] in which they knocked down *ABCD1* in BMECs and saw mislocalization of the tight junction protein claudin-5. The presence of frayed or discontinuous junctions and its relation to barrier function has been noted in other systems as well. In an in vitro epithelium model, an induced opening of the barrier for drug delivery purposes was marked by both morphological changes in the connectivity of zonula occluden tight junction proteins and a decrease in TEER [91]. In our study of the brain endothelium, we went beyond qualitative observations of tight junction proteins and quantified the integrity of the barrier formed by the WT- and ccALD-iBMECs using TEER. By this metric, we found that the barrier integrity of the ccALD-iBMECs was decreased compared to WT-iBMECs. Musolino et al. also observed an increase in TGFβ1 expression connected to the mislocalization of claudin-5. Interestingly, our transcriptome analysis also indicated increased TGFβ1 activity in the ccALD-iBMECs that could be contributing to the decreased barrier function. With ccALD, in contrast to other demyelinating disorders such as

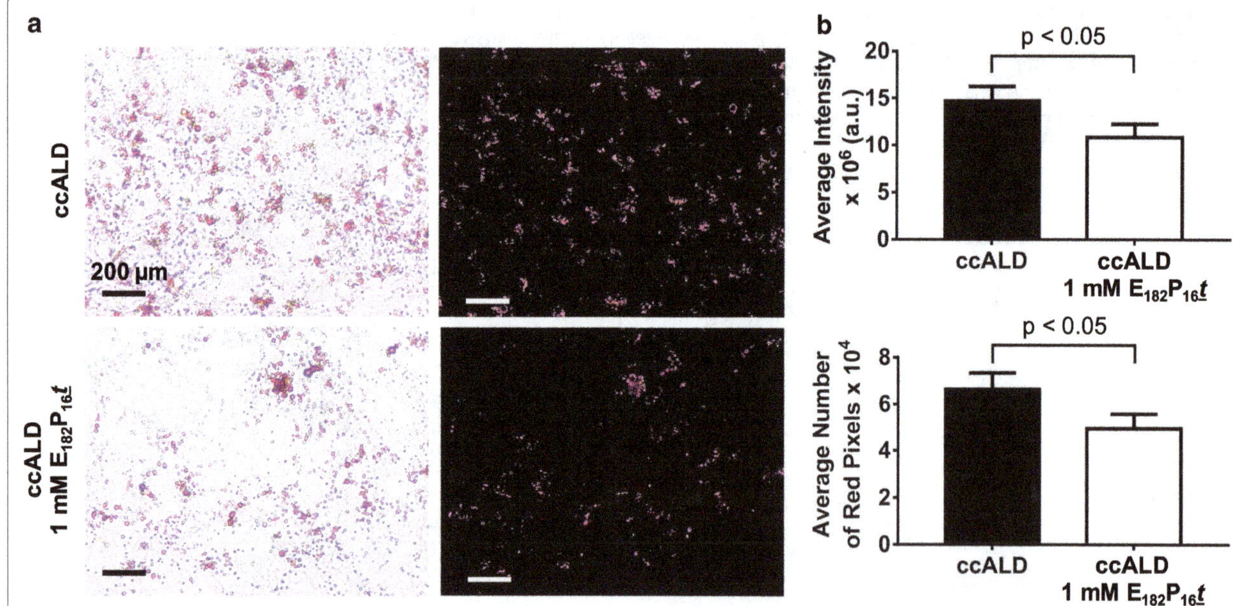

Fig. 6 Diblock copolymer treatment decreases lipid droplet accumulation in ccALD-iBMECs. **a** Representative Oil-Red-O staining of untreated control ccALD3-iBMECs and 1 mM $E_{182}P_{16}\underline{t}$ treated ccALD3-iBMECs during development. Raw images shown on left and masked images on right. **b** Quantification of intensity and number of red pixels in Oil-Red-O stained images indicates decreased lipid droplet accumulation in ccALD-iBMECs treated with 1 mM $E_{182}P_{16}\underline{t}$ during development. Six biological replicates used for quantification ($n = 6$)

multiple sclerosis, demyelination is thought to precede BBB breakdown. Thus, it is possible that an initial subtle loss in the ability of the BBB to restrict passive transport, as seen with the ccALD-iBMECs in our study, could cause immune cell infiltration and leakage that accelerates demyelination in a feedback loop that eventually results in complete BBB breakdown [29]. In this context, increased matrix metalloproteinases in the cerebral spinal fluid of ccALD patients could also be contributing to further breakdown of the BBB [38, 47]. Inherent decreased BBB integrity could also begin to explain why head trauma can initiate the onset of ccALD. The lack of genotype–phenotype correlation is not explained by our model; however, our finding of an inherent decrease in BMEC integrity in ccALD individuals could direct the search for additional environmental or genetic factors specific to the BBB that begin to explain why only a subset of individuals with an *ABCD1* mutation progress to ccALD.

While we did not observe by TEM the classic crystalline aggregates first observed in the adrenal cortex, testis, and white matter of ccALD patients, our finding of increased accumulation of non-pathological lipid droplets in ccALD-iBMECs is novel and warrants further investigation [92–94]. A study by Schluter et al. [95] showed that VLCFAs can trigger insulin desensitization characterized by oxidative stress and alteration of adipocytokine signaling pathways and chronic inflammation, culminating in changes similar to metabolic syndrome. Increased insulin-like growth factor receptor signaling in the ccALD-iBMECs indicated by our transcriptome analysis further hints at metabolic dysfunction as a factor contributing to the ccALD phenotype. Another study by van de Beek et al. [96] showed that exposure of X-ALD fibroblasts to VLCFAs resulted in endoplasmic reticulum stress correlated with an increase in lipid droplet deposition. Both studies suggest that VLCFA accumulation would precede lipid droplet accumulation. A key question that then arises is whether lipid droplet accumulation contributes to the decreased BBB integrity in the ccALD-iBMECs and whether targeting non-VLCFA lipids would have therapeutic relevance in that it could potentially rescue the decrease in BBB integrity of ccALD patients.

Using this system to model the BBB, we achieved physiological levels of TEER. One limitation of our study, however, is that we only investigated one cell type, BMECs. Adding other cell types involved in the neurovascular unit such as pericytes, astrocytes, and neurons to our model could further inform ccALD-specific defects of the BBB. Nevertheless, the differences we found modeling the BBB using iBMECs were significant. These differences included a decrease in barrier integrity as well as an increase in lipid accumulation. Both of these findings represent potential biomarkers for brain endothelium health of X-ALD patients and provide a new direction in the search for molecular markers that indicate ccALD onset. Combining the findings from the results of this study with antioxidant therapy currently in clinical trials could provide a much-needed alternative treatment for patients with AMN at risk of converting to ccALD.

With our BBB model, we investigated whether amphiphilic block copolymers can improve defects in barrier function as such polymers have been reported to be able to improve function of many cell and tissue types under various injuries. The application of the diblock copolymer $E_{182}P_{16}\underline{t}$ in addition to the widely used P188 was inspired by recent work within our group, which revealed $E_{182}P_{16}\underline{t}$ to be the most efficacious in stabilizing damaged myoblasts in vitro [74]. It is interesting and crucial to note that this enhanced efficacy of $E_{182}P_{16}\underline{t}$ compared to P188 is consistent with the results of Kim et al. although the cell types and form of damage are vastly different [74]. This raises many questions as to how the polymers interact with the cell and what cellular responses this interaction promotes. At present, the fundamental mechanism of interaction between the PEO–PPO diblock and triblock copolymers and the plasma membrane is far from conclusive. Lee et al. speculate that poloxamers insert partially or fully into the membrane after initially adsorbing onto the lipid bilayer depending on the hydrophobicity of the polymer and the incubation time [97, 98]. Enhanced efficacy with the presence of an additional hydrophobic *tert*-butoxy end group on the PPO block provides evidence for the "anchor and chain" mechanism, which proposes that the additional hydrophobic unit at the end of the PPO block provides an anchor in the lipid bilayer, resulting in more efficacious stabilization of the block copolymer in the lipid membrane [73, 74]. The aforementioned studies focus on the polymer interaction with the plasma membrane for stabilization, but the results of our work showing the decrease in lipid accumulation in ccALD-iBMECs upon treatment with $E_{182}P_{16}\underline{t}$ suggest a more complex cellular response that has yet to be fully explored.

As the breadth of applications continues to expand, there is a pressing need to elucidate the amphiphilic block copolymer-cell interaction mechanism in order to translate this action into a therapeutic solution. To this end, the in vitro disease model presented in this work could provide a platform for studying the mechanism of PEO–PPO block copolymer mediated recovery of cellular function. Furthermore, while most researchers have focused solely on P188, there is potential for the design of the polymer to further improve efficacy in restoring function to damaged cells as demonstrated in this work.

Elucidating the mechanism of BMEC interaction with the PEO–PPO diblock copolymer will not only engender insight as to how the polymer restores function of ccALD-iBMECs but may also provide a deeper knowledge as to how the BBBs of ccALD patients are damaged compared to healthy individuals.

At present, there is no suitable in vivo model for X-ALD [48]. Nevertheless, as functional in vivo models are developed, the work presented here has the potential to be translated to in vivo studies. Treatment of ccALD-iBMECs with either P188 or $E_{182}P_{16}\underline{t}$ at the end of the differentiation protocol yielded a slight but non-significant increase in TEER. However, efficacy of polymer treatment at a later stage might be improved upon optimization of pharmacodynamics and pharmacokinetic variables. Furthermore, the superior efficacy of treatment with $E_{182}P_{16}\underline{t}$ when added earlier in the iBMEC differentiation process compared to at the end of the differentiation process suggests that the treatment could be applied at an early stage of BBB development to inhibit the onset and progression of ccALD.

Thus, clinical application might mean using the polymer as a preventative therapy, which requires pre-symptomatic diagnosis of X-ALD. Fortunately, high throughput screening of X-ALD is feasible and reliably identifies affected males [99]. Furthermore, in 2016 the US Department of Health and Human Services recommended that X-ALD be added to the recommended uniform screening panel for state newborn screening programs [100]. Testing of the 4 million infants born each year in the US is predicted to identify around 143 newborns with an *ABCD1* mutation. Early detection will lead to more timely intervention in the form of hematopoietic cell transplant (HCT), which is only advantageous in the early stages of the disease because cerebral inflammation can progress up to 18 months after transplant [25, 101]. Pioneering clinical trials involving the use of Lenti-D for autologous HCT are taking place at several centers around the US and promise to further reduce severe outcomes associated with allogeneic transplants (such as graft-versus-host disease) and to circumvent issues with finding HLA matched donors (currently, cord blood grafts are used when a suitable donor cannot be found) [102–104]. For those displaying neurological symptoms or MRI abnormalities indicating ccALD onset, the current standard of care for HCT involves fully myoablative chemotherapy, a highly toxic procedure. If a treatment that prevents the onset of ccALD were available, a newborn identified as having an *ABCD1* mutation given this treatment may never show symptoms of ccALD conversion and would not need to undergo HCT. In this study, we have shown that amphiphilic block copolymers are one such treatment with the potential to prevent the onset of ccALD and reduce the number of patients needing to undergo HCT.

Conclusion

Modeling the BBB of ccALD patients using iPSC-derived BMECs indicates that ccALD patients form a less intact BBB. These results open the door for the discovery of brain endothelium-specific molecular markers indicative of the onset of ccALD and for the development of treatment strategies targeted at the brain endothelium that could reduce the number of X-ALD patients who progress to ccALD. One such treatment strategy that we have shown can rescue defective ccALD-iBMECs barrier integrity is PEO–PPO block copolymers. These results have therapeutic implications for preventing the onset of ccALD.

Abbreviations

X-ALD: X-linked adrenoleukodystrophy; ccALD: childhood cerebral adrenoleukodystrophy; BBB: blood–brain barrier; ROS: reactive oxygen species; WT: wild-type; iPSCs: induced pluripotent stem cells; iBMECs: induced brain microvascular endothelial cells; BMECs: brain microvascular endothelial cells; TEER: trans-endothelial electrical resistance; VLCFA: very long chain fatty acids; AMN: adrenomyeloneuropathy; HCT: hematopoietic cell transplant; hiPSCs: human induced pluripotent stem cells; PEO: poly(ethylene oxide); PPO: poly(propylene oxide); P188: Poloxamer 188; EC: endothelial cell; RIN: RNA Integrity Number; THF: tetrahydrofuran; P-gp: P-glycoprotein; CsA: cyclosporin A; TEM: transmission electron microscopy; PCA: principal component analysis; DEG: differentially expressed gene; FDR: false-discovery rate; GO: gene ontology; IPA: Ingenuity Pathway Analysis.

Authors' contributions

JT and SMA designed the research. CAAL and HSS performed the research. AGA conducted the transmission electron microscopy and contributed to its interpretation. FSB provided essential guidance. CAAL and HSS analyzed the data. CAAL, HSS, AGA, FSB, JT and SMA wrote and edited the manuscript. All authors read and approved the final manuscript.

Author details

[1] Department of Genetics and Cell Development, University of Minnesota, Minneapolis, MN 55455, USA. [2] Department of Chemical Engineering and Materials Science, University of Minnesota, Minneapolis, MN 55455, USA. [3] Ultrastructural Pathology Unit, Veterinary Diagnostic Laboratory, College of Veterinary Medicine, University of Minnesota, St. Paul, MN 55108, USA. [4] Department of Pediatrics, University of Minnesota, Minneapolis, MN 55455, USA.

Acknowledgements

The authors would like to thank Dean Muldoon at the Veterinary Diagnostic Lab for preparing the EM samples, John Garbe and Dr. Juan Abrahante from the University of Minnesota Informatics Institute for assistance with the RNA-seq data processing and analysis, LeAnn Oseth and Paula Haffner from the University of Minnesota Cytogenomics Laboratory for genetic fingerprinting and karyotyping, and Dr. Mihee Kim for aid in preparing the polymer samples. Additionally, the authors would like to thank Abby Silbaugh, Hope Leslie, and Faith Leslie for assistance with the frayed junction analysis, Valencia Owens for assistance with the iPSC and iBMEC cell culture, and Anna Xue for assistance with the sodium fluorescein permeability assay and iPSC and iBMEC cell culture. The authors would also like to thank the University of Minnesota Genomics Center for quality control of the NGS libraries used in this study as well as Nancy Morgan and Susan Julson for administrative support.

Competing interests

The authors declare that they have no competing interests.

Funding

Research reported in this study was supported by the University of Minnesota and NHLBI R01AR063070. C.A.A.L was supported by NIH T32 GM113846. H.S.S. is a recipient of the NSF Graduate Research fellowship (Grant Number #00039202).

References

1. Bezman L, Moser AB, Raymond GV, Rinaldo P, Watkins PA, Smith KD, et al. Adrenoleukodystrophy: incidence, new mutation rate, and results of extended family screening. Ann Neurol. 2001;49:512–7.
2. Douar AM, Mosser J, Sarde CO, Lopez J, Mandel JL, Aubourg P. X-linked adrenoleukodystrophy gene: identification of a candidate gene by positional cloning. Biomed Pharmacother. 1994;48:215–8.
3. Aubourg P, Mosser J, Douar AM, Sarde CO, Lopez J, Mandel JL. Adrenoleukodystrophy gene: unexpected homology to a protein involved in peroxisome biogenesis. Biochimie. 1993;75:293–302.
4. Mosser J, Douar AM, Sarde CO, Kioschis P, Feil R, Moser H, et al. Putative X-linked adrenoleukodystrophy gene shares unexpected homology with ABC transporters. Nature. 1993;361:726–30.
5. Korenke GC, Fuchs S, Krasemann E, Doerr HG, Wilichowski E, Hunneman DH, et al. Cerebral adrenoleukodystrophy (ALD) in only one of monozygotic twins with an identical ALD genotype. Ann Neurol. 1996;40:254–7.
6. Kok F, Neumann S, Sarde CO, Zheng S, Wu KH, Wei HM, et al. Mutational analysis of patients with X-linked adrenoleukodystrophy. Hum Mutat. 1995;6:104–15.
7. Moser HW. Adrenoleukodystrophy. Curr Opin Neurol. 1995;8:221–6.
8. Sobue G, Ueno-Natsukari I, Okamoto H, Connell TA, Aizawa I, Mizoguchi K, et al. Phenotypic heterogeneity of an adult form of adrenoleukodystrophy in monozygotic twins. Ann Neurol. 1994;36:912–5.
9. Martin JJ, Dompas B, Ceuterick C, Jacobs K. Adrenomyeloneuropathy and adrenoleukodystrophy in two brothers. Eur Neurol. 1980;19:281–7.
10. Moser HW, Mahmood A, Raymond GV. X-linked adrenoleukodystrophy. Nat Clin Pract Neurol. 2007;3:140–51.
11. Moser HW, Raymond GV, Dubey P. Adrenoleukodystrophy: new approaches to a neurodegenerative disease. JAMA. 2005;294:3131–4.
12. Moser H, Dubey P, Fatemi A. Progress in X-linked adrenoleukodystrophy. Curr Opin Neurol. 2004;17:263–9.
13. Chu ML, Sala DA, Weiner HL. Intrathecal baclofen in X-linked adrenoleukodystrophy. Pediatr Neurol. 2001;24:156–8.
14. Shapiro E, Krivit W, Lockman L, Jambaqué I, Peters C, Cowan M, et al. Long-term effect of bone-marrow transplantation for childhood-onset cerebral X-linked adrenoleukodystrophy. Lancet (London, England). 2000;356:713–8.
15. Drover VA. Adrenoleukodystrophy: recent advances in treatment and disease etiology. Future Lipidol. 2009;4:205–13.
16. Wilken B, Dechent P, Brockmann K, Finsterbusch J, Baumann M, Ebell W, et al. Quantitative proton magnetic resonance spectroscopy of children with adrenoleukodystrophy before and after hematopoietic stem cell transplantation. Neuropediatrics. 2003;34:237–46.
17. Miller WP, Mantovani LF, Muzic J, Rykken JB, Gawande RS, Lund TC, et al. Intensity of MRI gadolinium enhancement in cerebral adrenoleukodystrophy: a biomarker for inflammation and predictor of outcome following transplantation in higher risk patients. AJNR Am J Neuroradiol. 2016;37:367–72.
18. Musolino PL, Rapalino O, Caruso P, Caviness VS, Eichler FS. Hypoperfusion predicts lesion progression in cerebral X-linked adrenoleukodystrophy. Brain. 2012;135(Pt 9):2676–83.
19. Ratai E, Kok T, Wiggins C, Wiggins G, Grant E, Gagoski B, et al. Seven-tesla proton magnetic resonance spectroscopic imaging in adult X-linked adrenoleukodystrophy. Arch Neurol. 2008;65:1488–94.
20. Eichler F, Van Haren K. Immune response in leukodystrophies. Pediatr Neurol. 2007;37:235–44.
21. Eichler FS, Itoh R, Barker PB, Mori S, Garrett ES, van Zijl PCM, et al. Proton MR spectroscopic and diffusion tensor brain MR imaging in X-linked adrenoleukodystrophy: initial experience. Radiology. 2002;225:245–52.
22. Budhram A, Pandey SK. Activation of cerebral X-linked adrenoleukodystrophy after head trauma. Can J Neurol Sci. 2017;44:597–8.
23. Raymond GV, Seidman R, Monteith TS, Kolodny E, Sathe S, Mahmood A, et al. Head trauma can initiate the onset of adreno-leukodystrophy. J Neurol Sci. 2010;290:70–4.
24. Wilkinson IA, Hopkins IJ, Pollard AC. Can head injury influence the site of demyelination in adrenoleukodystrophy? Dev Med Child Neurol. 1987;29:797–800.
25. Turk BR, Moser AB, Fatemi A. Therapeutic strategies in adrenoleukodystrophy. Wien Med Wochenschr. 2017;167:219–26.
26. Miller WP, Rothman SM, Nascene D, Kivisto T, DeFor TE, Ziegler RS, et al. Outcomes after allogeneic hematopoietic cell transplantation for childhood cerebral adrenoleukodystrophy: the largest single-institution cohort report. Blood. 2011;118:1971–8.
27. Wiesinger C, Eichler FS, Berger J. The genetic landscape of X-linked adrenoleukodystrophy: inheritance, mutations, modifier genes, and diagnosis. Appl Clin Genet. 2015;8:109–21.
28. Ferrer I, Aubourg P, Pujol A. General aspects and neuropathology of X-linked adrenoleukodystrophy. Brain Pathol. 2010;20:817–30.
29. Aubourg P. Cerebral adrenoleukodystrophy: a demyelinating disease that leaves the door wide open. Brain. 2015;138(Pt 11):3133–6.
30. Forss-Petter S, Werner H, Berger J, Lassmann H, Molzer B, Schwab MH, et al. Targeted inactivation of the X-linked adrenoleukodystrophy gene in mice. J Neurosci Res. 1997;50:829–43.
31. Fourcade S, Ferrer I, Pujol A. Oxidative stress, mitochondrial and proteostasis malfunction in adrenoleukodystrophy: a paradigm for axonal degeneration. Free Radic Biol Med. 2015;88:18–29.
32. van Geel BM, Assies J, Haverkort EB, Koelman JH, Verbeeten B, Wanders RJ, et al. Progression of abnormalities in adrenomyeloneuropathy and neurologically asymptomatic X-linked adrenoleukodystrophy despite treatment with "Lorenzo's oil". J Neurol Neurosurg Psychiatry. 1999;67:290–9.
33. Aubourg P, Adamsbaum C, Lavallard-Rousseau MC, Rocchiccioli F, Cartier N, Jambaqué I, et al. A two-year trial of oleic and erucic acids ("Lorenzo's oil") as treatment for adrenomyeloneuropathy. N Engl J Med. 1993;329:745–52.
34. Horvath GA, Eichler F, Poskitt K, Stockler-Ipsiroglu S. Failure of repeated cyclophosphamide pulse therapy in childhood cerebral X-linked adrenoleukodystrophy. Neuropediatrics. 2012;43:48–52.
35. Korenke GC, Christen HJ, Kruse B, Hunneman DH, Hanefeld F. Progression of X-linked adrenoleukodystrophy under interferon-beta therapy. J Inherit Metab Dis. 1997;20:59–66.
36. Marchetti DP, Donida B, da Rosa HT, Manini PR, Moura DJ, Saffi J, et al. Protective effect of antioxidants on DNA damage in leukocytes from X-linked adrenoleukodystrophy patients. Int J Dev Neurosci. 2015;43:8–15.
37. Singh J, Giri S. Loss of AMP-activated protein kinase in X-linked adrenoleukodystrophy patient-derived fibroblasts and lymphocytes. Biochem Biophys Res Commun. 2014;445:126–31.
38. Thibert KA, Raymond GV, Nascene DR, Miller WP, Tolar J, Orchard PJ, et al. Cerebrospinal fluid matrix metalloproteinases are elevated in cerebral adrenoleukodystrophy and correlate with MRI severity and neurologic dysfunction. PLoS ONE. 2012;7:e50430.
39. Fourcade S, López-Erauskin J, Galino J, Duval C, Naudi A, Jove M, et al. Early oxidative damage underlying neurodegeneration in X-adrenoleukodystrophy. Hum Mol Genet. 2008;17:1762–73.

40. Deon M, Sitta A, Barschak AG, Coelho DM, Pigatto M, Schmitt GO, et al. Induction of lipid peroxidation and decrease of antioxidant defenses in symptomatic and asymptomatic patients with X-linked adrenoleukodystrophy. Int J Dev Neurosci. 2007;25:441–4.
41. Turk BR, Theisen BE, Nemeth CL, Marx JS, Shi X, Rosen M, et al. Antioxidant capacity and superoxide dismutase activity in adrenoleukodystrophy. JAMA Neurol. 2017;74:519.
42. Tolar J, Orchard PJ, Bjoraker KJ, Ziegler RS, Shapiro EG, Charnas L. *N*-acetyl-L-cysteine improves outcome of advanced cerebral adrenoleukodystrophy. Bone Marrow Transplant. 2007;39:211–5. https://doi.org/10.1038/sj.bmt.1705571.
43. Rockenbach FJ, Deon M, Marchese DP, Manfredini V, Mescka C, Ribas GS, et al. The effect of bone marrow transplantation on oxidative stress in X-linked adrenoleukodystrophy. Mol Genet Metab. 2012;106:231–6.
44. ClinicalTrials.gov [Internet]. Bethesda (MD): National Library of Medicine (US). 1993 Jan 01. Identifier NCT01495260. A clinical trial for AMN: validation of biomarkers of oxidative stress. Efficacy and safety of a mixture of antioxidants; 2017. Available from: https://clinicaltrials.gov/ct2/show/NCT01495260.
45. Berger J, Forss-Petter S, Eichler FS. Pathophysiology of X-linked adrenoleukodystrophy. Biochimie. 2014;98:135–42.
46. Ito M, Blumberg BM, Mock DJ, Goodman AD, Moser AB, Moser HW, et al. Potential environmental and host participants in the early white matter lesion of adreno-leukodystrophy: morphologic evidence for CD8 cytotoxic T cells, cytolysis of oligodendrocytes, and CD1-mediated lipid antigen presentation. J Neuropathol Exp Neurol. 2001;60:1004–19.
47. Musolino PL, Gong Y, Snyder JMT, Jimenez S, Lok J, Lo EH, et al. Brain endothelial dysfunction in cerebral adrenoleukodystrophy. Brain. 2015;138:3206–20.
48. Lu JF, Lawler AM, Watkins PA, Powers JM, Moser AB, Moser HW, et al. A mouse model for X-linked adrenoleukodystrophy. Proc Natl Acad Sci USA. 1997;94:9366–71.
49. Bernas MJ, Cardoso FL, Daley SK, Weinand ME, Campos AR, Ferreira AJG, et al. Establishment of primary cultures of human brain microvascular endothelial cells to provide an in vitro cellular model of the blood–brain barrier. Nat Protoc. 2010;5:1265–72.
50. Helms HC, Abbott NJ, Burek M, Cecchelli R, Couraud P-O, Deli MA, et al. In vitro models of the blood–brain barrier: an overview of commonly used brain endothelial cell culture models and guidelines for their use. J Cereb Blood Flow Metab. 2016. https://doi.org/10.1177/0271678X16630991.
51. Weksler BB, Subileau EA, Perrière N, Charneau P, Holloway K, Leveque M, et al. Blood–brain barrier-specific properties of a human adult brain endothelial cell line. FASEB J. 2005. https://doi.org/10.1096/fj.04-3458fje.
52. Stebbins MJ, Wilson HK, Canfield SG, Qian T, Palecek SP, Shusta EV. Differentiation and characterization of human pluripotent stem cell-derived brain microvascular endothelial cells. Methods. 2016;101:93–102. https://doi.org/10.1016/j.ymeth.2015.10.016.
53. Wilson HK, Canfield SG, Hjortness MK, Palecek SP, Shusta EV. Exploring the effects of cell seeding density on the differentiation of human pluripotent stem cells to brain microvascular endothelial cells. Fluids Barriers CNS. 2015;12:13. https://doi.org/10.1186/s12987-015-0007-9.
54. Lippmann ES, Al-Ahmad A, Azarin SM, Palecek SP, Shusta EV. A retinoic acid-enhanced, multicellular human blood–brain barrier model derived from stem cell sources. Sci Rep. 2014;4:4160. https://doi.org/10.1038/srep04160.
55. Lippmann ES, Azarin SM, Kay JE, Nessler RA, Wilson HK, Al-ahmad A, et al. Derivation of blood–brain barrier endothelial cells from human pluripotent stem cells. Nat Biotechnol. 2012;30:783.
56. Lim RG, Quan C, Reyes-Ortiz AM, Lutz SE, Kedaigle AJ, Gipson TA, et al. Huntington's disease iPSC-derived brain microvascular endothelial cells reveal WNT-mediated angiogenic and blood–brain barrier deficits. Cell Rep. 2017;19:1365–77. https://doi.org/10.1016/j.celrep.2017.04.021.
57. Kim BJ, Bee OB, McDonagh MA, Stebbins MJ, Palecek SP, Doran KS, et al. Modeling group B Streptococcus and blood–brain barrier interaction by using induced pluripotent stem cell-derived brain endothelial Cells. mSphere. 2017;2:e00398-17.
58. Schmolka IR. Physical basis for poloxamer interactions. Ann NY Acad Sci. 1994;720:92–7. https://doi.org/10.1111/j.1749-6632.1994.tb30437.x.
59. Schmolka IR. A review of block polymer surfactants. J Am Oil Chem Soc. 1977;54:110–6. https://doi.org/10.1007/BF02894385.
60. Moloughney JG, Weisleder N. Poloxamer 188 (P188) as a membrane resealing reagent in biomedical applications. Recent Pat Biotechnol. 2012;6:200–11.
61. Lee RC, River LP, Pan F, Ji L, Wollmann RL. Surfactant-induced sealing of electropermeabilized skeletal muscle membranes in vivo. Proc Natl Acad Sci USA. 1992;89:4524–8.
62. Wong SW, Yao Y, Hong Y, Ma Z, Kok SHL, Sun S, et al. Preventive effects of Poloxamer 188 on muscle cell damage mechanics under oxidative stress. Ann Biomed Eng. 2017;45(4):1083–92. https://doi.org/10.1007/s10439-016-1733-0
63. Greenebaum B, Blossfield K, Hannig J, Carrillo CS, Beckett MA, Weichselbaum RR, et al. Poloxamer 188 prevents acute necrosis of adult skeletal muscle cells following high-dose irradiation. Burns. 2004;30:539–47. https://doi.org/10.1016/j.burns.2004.02.009.
64. Yasuda S, Townsend D, Michele DE, Favre EG, Day SM, Metzger JM. Dystrophic heart failure blocked by membrane sealant poloxamer. Nature. 2005;436:1025–9. https://doi.org/10.1038/nature03844.
65. Houang EM, Haman KJ, Filareto A, Perlingeiro RC, Bates FS, Lowe DA, et al. Membrane-stabilizing copolymers confer marked protection to dystrophic skeletal muscle in vivo. Mol Ther Methods Clin Dev. 2015;2:15042. https://doi.org/10.1038/mtm.2015.42.
66. Bao H, Yang X, Zhuang Y, Huang Y, Wang T, Zhang M, et al. The effects of Poloxamer 188 on the autophagy induced by traumatic brain injury. Neurosci Lett. 2016;634:7–12. https://doi.org/10.1016/j.neulet.2016.09.052.
67. Serbest G, Horwitz J, Barbee K. The effect of poloxamer-188 on neuronal cell recovery from mechanical injury. J Neurotrauma. 2005;22:119–32. https://doi.org/10.1089/neu.2005.22.119.
68. Luo C-L, Chen X-P, Li L-L, Li Q-Q, Li B-X, Xue A-M, et al. Poloxamer 188 attenuates in vitro traumatic brain injury-induced mitochondrial and lysosomal membrane permeabilization damage in cultured primary neurons. J Neurotrauma. 2012;30:597–607. https://doi.org/10.1089/neu.2012.2425.
69. Wang T, Chen X, Wang Z, Zhang M, Meng H, Gao Y, et al. Poloxamer-188 can attenuate blood–brain barrier damage to exert neuroprotective effect in mice intracerebral hemorrhage model. J Mol Neurosci. 2014;55:240–50. https://doi.org/10.1007/s12031-014-0313-8.
70. Gu JH, Ge J. Bin, Li M, Xu HD, Wu F, Qin ZH. Poloxamer 188 protects neurons against ischemia/reperfusion injury through preserving integrity of cell membranes and blood brain barrier. PLoS ONE. 2013;8:e61641.
71. Bao H-J, Wang T, Zhang M-Y, Liu R, Dai D-K, Wang Y-Q, et al. Poloxamer-188 attenuates TBI-induced blood–brain barrier damage leading to decreased brain edema and reduced cellular death. Neurochem Res. 2012;37:2856–67. https://doi.org/10.1007/s11064-012-0880-4.
72. Haman K. Development of model diblock copolymer surfactants for mechanistic investigations of cell membrane stabilization. Ph.D. thesis, University of Minnesota; 2015.
73. Houang EM, Haman KJ, Kim M, Zhang W, Lowe DA, Sham YY, et al. Chemical end group modified diblock copolymers elucidate anchor and chain mechanism of membrane stabilization. Mol Pharm. 2017;14:2333–9.
74. Kim M, Haman KJ, Houang EM, Zhang W, Yannopoulos D, Metzger JM, et al. PEO–PPO diblock copolymers protect myoblasts from hypo-osmotic stress in vitro dependent on copolymer size, composition, and architecture. Biomacromolecules. 2017. https://doi.org/10.1021/acs.biomac.7b00419.
75. Lindborg BA, Brekke JH, Vegoe AL, Ulrich CB, Haider KT, Subramaniam S, et al. Rapid induction of cerebral organoids from human induced pluripotent stem cells using a chemically defined hydrogel and defined cell culture medium. Stem Cells Transl Med. 2016;5:970–9.
76. Tolar J, Xia L, Riddle MJ, Lees CJ, Eide CR, McElmurry RT, et al. Induced pluripotent stem cells from individuals with recessive dystrophic epidermolysis bullosa. J Invest Dermatol. 2011;131:848–56.
77. Krämer A, Green J, Pollard J, Tugendreich S. Causal analysis approaches in Ingenuity Pathway Analysis. Bioinformatics. 2014;30:523–30.
78. The Gene Ontology Consortium. Expansion of the gene ontology knowledgebase and resources. Nucleic Acids Res. 2017;45:D331–8.

79. Ashburner M, Ball CA, Blake JA, Botstein D, Butler H, Cherry JM, et al. Gene ontology: tool for the unification of biology. The Gene Ontology Consortium. Nat Genet. 2000;25:25–9.
80. Hillmyer MA, Bates FS. Synthesis and characterization of model polyalkane–poly(ethylene oxide) block copolymers. Macromolecules. 1996;29:6994–7002. https://doi.org/10.1021/ma960774t.
81. Ndoni S, Papadakis CM, Bates FS, Almdal K. Laboratory-scale setup for anionic polymerization under inert atmosphere. Rev Sci Instrum. 1995;66:1090.
82. Ding J, Heatley F, Price C, Booth C. Use of crown ether in the anionic polymerization of propylene oxide—2. Molecular weight and molecular weight distribution. Eur Polym J. 1991;27:895–9. https://doi.org/10.1016/0014-3057(91)90029-N.
83. Ding J, Attwood D, Price C, Booth C. Use of crown ether in the anionic polymerization of propylene oxide—3. Preparation and micellization of diblock-copoly(oxypropylene/oxyethylene). Eur Polym J. 1991;27:901–5. https://doi.org/10.1016/0014-3057(91)90030-R.
84. Ding J, Price C, Booth C. Use of crown ether in the anionic polymerization of propylene oxide—1. Rate of polymerization. Eur Polym J. 1991;27:891–4. https://doi.org/10.1016/0014-3057(91)90028-M.
85. Hollmann EK, Bailey AK, Potharazu AV, Neely MD, Bowman AB, Lippmann ES. Accelerated differentiation of human induced pluripotent stem cells to blood–brain barrier endothelial cells. Fluids Barriers CNS. 2017;14:1–13.
86. Mantle JL, Min L, Lee KH. Minimum transendothelial electrical resistance thresholds for the study of small and large molecule drug transport in a human in vitro blood–brain barrier model. Mol Pharm. 2016;13:4191–8.
87. Deli MA, Abrahám CS, Kataoka Y, Niwa M. Permeability studies on in vitro blood–brain barrier models: physiology, pathology, and pharmacology. Cell Mol Neurobiol. 2005;25:59–127.
88. Gaillard PJ, De Boer AG. Relationship between permeability status of the blood–brain barrier and in vitro permeability coefficient of a drug. Eur J Pharm Sci. 2000;12:95–102.
89. Madara JL. Regulation of the movement of solutes across tight junctions. Annu Rev Physiol. 1998;60:143–59. https://doi.org/10.1146/annurev.physiol.60.1.143.
90. Mehlem A, Hagberg CE, Muhl L, Eriksson U, Falkevall A. Imaging of neutral lipids by oil red O for analyzing the metabolic status in health and disease. Nat Protoc. 2013;8:1149–54.
91. Kam KR, Walsh LA, Bock SM, Koval M, Fischer KE, Ross RF, et al. Nanostructure-mediated transport of biologics across epithelial tissue: enhancing permeability via nanotopography. Nano Lett. 2013;13:164–71.
92. Powell H, Tindall R, Schultz P, Paa D, O'Brien J, Lampert P. Adrenoleukodystrophy. Electron microscopic findings. Arch Neurol. 1975;32:250–60.
93. Powers JM, Schaumburg HH. Adreno-leukodystrophy (sex-linked Schilder's disease). A pathogenetic hypothesis based on ultrastructural lesions in adrenal cortex, peripheral nerve and testis. Am J Pathol. 1974;76:481–91.
94. Schaumburg HH, Richardson EP, Johnson PC, Cohen RB, Powers JM, Raine CS. Schilder's disease. Sex-linked recessive transmission with specific adrenal changes. Arch Neurol. 1972;27:458–60.
95. Schluter A, Espinosa L, Fourcade S, Galino J, Lopez E, Ilieva E, et al. Functional genomic analysis unravels a metabolic-inflammatory interplay in adrenoleukodystrophy. Hum Mol Genet. 2012;21:1062–77.
96. van de Beek M-C, Ofman R, Dijkstra I, Wijburg F, Engelen M, Wanders R, et al. Lipid-induced endoplasmic reticulum stress in X-linked adrenoleukodystrophy. Biochim Biophys Acta. 2017;1863:2255–65.
97. Cheng C-Y, Wang J-Y, Kausik R, Lee KYC, Han S. Nature of Interactions between PEO–PPO–PEO triblock copolymers and lipid membranes: (II) role of hydration dynamics revealed by dynamic nuclear polarization. Biomacromolecules. 2012;13:2624–33. https://doi.org/10.1021/bm300848c.
98. Wang J-Y, Marks J, Lee KYC. Nature of interactions between PEO–PPO–PEO triblock copolymers and lipid membranes: (I) effect of polymer hydrophobicity on its ability to protect liposomes from peroxidation. Biomacromolecules. 2012;13:2616–23. https://doi.org/10.1021/bm300847x.
99. Theda C, Gibbons K, Defor TE, Donohue PK, Golden WC, Kline AD, et al. Newborn screening for X-linked adrenoleukodystrophy: further evidence high throughput screening is feasible. Mol Genet Metab. 2014;111:55–7.
100. Kemper AR, Brosco J, Comeau AM, Green NS, Grosse SD, Jones E, et al. Newborn screening for X-linked adrenoleukodystrophy: evidence summary and advisory committee recommendation. Genet Med. 2017;19(1):121–6. https://doi.org/10.1038/gim.2016.68.
101. Weber FD, Wiesinger C, Forss-Petter S, Regelsberger G, Einwich A, Weber WHA, et al. X-linked adrenoleukodystrophy: very long-chain fatty acid metabolism is severely impaired in monocytes but not in lymphocytes. Hum Mol Genet. 2014;23:2542–50.
102. Eichler F, Duncan C, Musolino PL, Orchard PJ, De Oliveira S, Thrasher AJ, et al. Hematopoietic stem-cell gene therapy for cerebral adrenoleukodystrophy. N Engl J Med. 2017;377:1630–8.
103. Orchard PJ, Tolar J. Transplant outcomes in leukodystrophies. Semin Hematol. 2010;47:70–8.
104. Cartier N, Hacein-Bey-Abina S, Bartholomae CC, Veres G, Schmidt M, Kutschera I, et al. Hematopoietic stem cell gene therapy with a lentiviral vector in X-linked adrenoleukodystrophy. Science. 2009;326:818–23.

18

A perfused human blood–brain barrier on-a-chip for high-throughput assessment of barrier function and antibody transport

Nienke R. Wevers[1,2*], Dhanesh G. Kasi[1], Taylor Gray[3], Karlijn J. Wilschut[1], Benjamin Smith[3], Remko van Vught[1], Fumitaka Shimizu[4], Yasuteru Sano[4], Takashi Kanda[4], Graham Marsh[3], Sebastiaan J. Trietsch[1], Paul Vulto[1], Henriëtte L. Lanz[1†] and Birgit Obermeier[3†]

Abstract

Background: Receptor-mediated transcytosis is one of the major routes for drug delivery of large molecules into the brain. The aim of this study was to develop a novel model of the human blood–brain barrier (BBB) in a high-throughput microfluidic device. This model can be used to assess passage of large biopharmaceuticals, such as therapeutic antibodies, across the BBB.

Methods: The model comprises human cell lines of brain endothelial cells, astrocytes, and pericytes in a two-lane or three-lane microfluidic platform that harbors 96 or 40 chips, respectively, in a 384-well plate format. In each chip, a perfused vessel of brain endothelial cells was grown against an extracellular matrix gel, which was patterned by means of surface tension techniques. Astrocytes and pericytes were added on the other side of the gel to complete the BBB on-a-chip model. Barrier function of the model was studied using fluorescent barrier integrity assays. To test antibody transcytosis, the lumen of the model's endothelial vessel was perfused with an anti-transferrin receptor antibody or with a control antibody. The levels of antibody that penetrated to the basal compartment were quantified using a mesoscale discovery assay.

Results: The perfused BBB on-a-chip model shows presence of adherens and tight junctions and severely limits the passage of a 20 kDa FITC-dextran dye. Penetration of the antibody targeting the human transferrin receptor (MEM-189) was markedly higher than penetration of the control antibody (apparent permeability of 2.9×10^{-5} versus 1.6×10^{-5} cm/min, respectively).

Conclusions: We demonstrate successful integration of a human BBB microfluidic model in a high-throughput plate-based format that can be used for drug screening purposes. This in vitro model shows sufficient barrier function to study the passage of large molecules and is sensitive to differences in antibody penetration, which could support discovery and engineering of BBB-shuttle technologies.

Keywords: Blood–brain barrier, Microfluidics, Organ-on-a-chip, BBB, Antibody transcytosis

*Correspondence: n.wevers@mimetas.com
†Henriëtte L. Lanz and Birgit Obermeier contributed equally to this work
[1] Mimetas BV, J.H. Oortweg 19, 2333 CH Leiden, The Netherlands
Full list of author information is available at the end of the article

Background

The blood–brain barrier (BBB) ensures a homeostatic environment for the central nervous system (CNS) and is essential for healthy brain functioning. The BBB comprises specialized endothelial cells and supporting cells, such as astrocytes and pericytes. Due to a combination of specific transport mechanisms and the presence of adherens junctions and tight junctions, the BBB controls passage of compounds into the brain [1–5]. This way, the BBB protects the brain from many harmful substances that circulate in the blood. However, the BBB's barrier properties also complicate the treatment of CNS disorders, as many small- and large-molecule pharmaceuticals are restricted from entering the brain in quantities that are large enough to elicit a therapeutic response [6]. It is therefore necessary to develop improved drug delivery strategies that enable efficient delivery of biopharmaceuticals to the brain.

The BBB employs specialized transporter systems to allow essential nutrients to enter the brain. The transport system that is most attractive to deliver large-molecule drugs into the brain is receptor-mediated transcytosis (RMT). In RMT, a ligand (or antibody) binds a receptor on the luminal surface of a brain endothelial cell, after which it undergoes internalization via endocytosis and is trafficked to the abluminal side, where it can be released and gain access to the brain parenchyma. Harnessing this process for therapeutic drug delivery is compelling, as it could allow for selective transport into the CNS in a non-invasive manner, without disruption of the BBB [7, 8]. Several studies have demonstrated increased CNS exposure to therapeutic antibodies by combining them with RMT targeting antibodies against the transferrin receptor, insulin receptor, low-density lipoprotein receptor-related proteins 1 and 2, and the large neutral amino acid transporter 1 [9–11]. However, challenges exist in optimizing antibody properties (such as affinity, valency, bispecific format, and Fc receptor engagement) to effectively and safely traffic across the brain endothelium [12–16]. Improved in vitro models that enable further research of the cellular and molecular mechanisms underlying transcytosis at the BBB are needed to improve these CNS drug delivery technologies [14, 17, 18].

While in vivo models can be used to study an intact BBB in its physiological environment, the complexity involved in deciphering whole-organism drug distribution and the lower throughput of these studies limits their use in screening for BBB-penetrant antibodies. For this reason, in vivo research in the field is complemented by simpler and faster in vitro models, such as the Transwell method [19–22] and several on-a-chip systems [23–29]. Although the field of in vitro BBB modelling has tremendously progressed in recent years, there is a need for a model that combines fast, high-throughput readouts with physiologically relevant conditions, such as flow, co-culture, and the absence of artificial membranes.

In this manuscript, we show the development of an in vitro model of the human BBB in a high-throughput microfluidic platform. The platform allows patterning of extracellular matrix gel by means of surface tension. A blood vessel is grown adjacent to that gel and a third channel is used to insert astrocytes and pericytes. The system is free of artificial membranes, accommodates fluid flow through the blood vessels, and allows fluid-phase sampling of molecules that penetrate the endothelial and matrix layers. Using two different antibodies, we show that the model is sensitive to differences in antibody penetration of brain endothelial cells. The model may support further discovery of antibody BBB-shuttle technologies.

Methods

Cell culture

Cell lines of brain endothelial cells, pericytes, and astrocytes were provided by Yamaguchi University, Japan, and originate from the following human primary cell sources: human brain microvascular endothelial cells (TY10 cell line) were isolated from normal brain tissue from a patient with meningioma. Human brain pericytes (hBPCT cell line) were derived from brain tissue of a patient that died from a heart attack. Human astrocytes (hAst cell line) were generated from human primary astrocytes distributed by Lonza (Basel, Switzerland). All three cell types were immortalized with retroviral vectors harboring a SV40 large T antigen gene that is engineered to drive proliferation at 33 °C [30–34] and have been used to model the BBB in previous studies [35–38]. Cells were cultured at 33 °C, 5% CO_2 to allow optimal cell expansion in T75 flasks (734-2705, Corning, NY, USA), which were pre-coated with 50 µg/mL collagen-I (Cultrex 3D collagen-I Rat Tail, 5 mg/mL, 3447-020-01, AMSbio, Abingdon, UK) in 1% acetic acid (A6283, Sigma, St. Louis, MO, USA) in water. TY10 cells were used between passage 17–25 and cultured in ScienCell endothelial cell medium (#1001, Sciencell, Carlsbad, CA, USA). The hAst cells were used between passage 7–12 and cultured in ScienCell astrocyte medium (#1018, Sciencell). The hBPCT cells were used between passage 14–25 and cultured in ScienCell pericyte medium (#1012, Sciencell). Cells were routinely tested for mycoplasma contamination and found negative.

Culture of TY10 microvessels in the two-lane OrganoPlate

Two-lane OrganoPlates (Mimetas BV, the Netherlands) with 400 µm × 220 µm (w × h) channels were employed. Phaseguides had dimensions of 100 µm × 55 µm (w × h) and 2 µL of gel composed of 4 mg/mL collagen-I (Cultrex 3D collagen-I Rat Tail, 5 mg/mL, 3447-020-01, AMSbio), 100 mM HEPES (15630-122, Thermo Fisher, Waltham, MA, USA) and 3.7 mg/mL $NaHCO_3$ (S5761, Sigma) was dispensed in the gel inlet and the OrganoPlate was incubated for 15 min at 33 °C. After plate incubation, 25 µL of PBS was added to the gel inlet to prevent the gel from drying out. A TY10 cell suspension of 1.5×10^7 cells/mL was prepared and 2 µL was seeded in the medium inlet. 50 µL of medium was added to the medium inlet and PBS was aspirated from the gel inlet. The plate was incubated on the side for 3 h in the incubator to allow the cells to sediment against the collagen-I gel and attach. After incubation, 50 µL of medium was added to the medium outlet. The OrganoPlate was placed on an interval rocker switching between a +7° and −7° inclination every 8 min (Mimetas Rocker Mini, Mimetas BV), allowing bidirectional flow. Cells were cultured at 33 °C (and 5% CO_2) to allow full cell coverage of the ECM gel. Medium was refreshed every 2–3 days. A schematic representation of all steps is shown in Additional file 1. The following media were used to assess their influence on barrier function: ScienCell endothelial cell medium (#1001, Sciencell), Cell Biologics endothelial cell medium (#H1168, Cell Biologics, Chicago, IL, USA), MV2 medium (C-22121, Bioconnect, Huissen, the Netherlands), and EBM-2 medium (cc-3156, Lonza).

BBB co-culture in the three-lane OrganoPlate

OrganoPlate BBB co-culture was performed using three-lane OrganoPlates with 400 µm × 220 µm (w × h) channels (Mimetas BV). Phaseguides had dimensions of 100 µm × 55 µm (w × h). To establish a BBB co-culture, a collagen-I gel was dispensed in the gel inlet of the chips and filled the middle channel. TY10 cells were seeded and cultured in the top channel as described in the previous section. After 3 days, 2 µL of a 7×10^6 cells/mL cell suspension of hAst and hBPCT cells (1:3 ratio) was seeded in the bottom channel. The plate was incubated on the side for 1.5 h to allow the hAst and hBPCT cells to attach to the collagen-I gel. After incubation, fresh Sciencell astrocyte medium is added to the inlet and outlets of the top channel (50 µL in each), after which perfusion is reinstated by placing the plate on the rocker platform. During the entire culture period, only the top channel, which contains the TY10 microvessel, is perfused to allow optimal endothelial barrier strength. Medium was refreshed every 2–3 days. Assays were performed at day 7. A schematic representation of all steps is shown in Additional file 2.

For the images shown in Fig. 3f, g, hBPCT cells were labeled with Calcein red™ AM (21900, AAT Bioquest, Sunnyvale, CA, USA) and hAst cells were labeled with green-fluorescent calcein-AM (C3099, Thermo Fisher) before seeding in the OrganoPlate.

Immunocytochemistry

Cultures in the OrganoPlate were fixed with 100% methanol (−20 °C, 494437, Sigma) and permeabilized with 0.3% Triton X-100 (T8787, Sigma). Cells were incubated with blocking solution (2% FCS, 2% bovine serum albumin (BSA, A2153, Sigma), 0.1% Tween-20 (P9416, Sigma)) for 45 min. Primary antibody was incubated for 1–2 h, after which secondary antibody was incubated for 30 min. The following antibodies were used: anti-claudin-5 (35-2500, Thermo Fisher), anti-VE-cadherin (ab33168, Abcam), anti-PECAM-1 (M0823, Dako), goat anti-rabbit AlexaFluor 488 (A11008, Thermo Fisher), goat anti-rabbit AlexaFluor 555 (A21428, Thermo Fisher), goat anti-mouse AlexaFluor 488 (A11001, Thermo Fisher), goat anti-mouse AlexaFluor 555 (A21422, Thermo Fisher), and donkey anti-mouse AlexaFluor 647 (A31571, Thermo Fisher). Nuclei were stained using Hoechst (H3570, Thermo Fisher). All steps were performed at room temperature (RT). Cells were imaged with ImageXpress Micro XLS and Micro XLS-C HCI Systems (Molecular Devices, San Jose, CA, USA).

TY10 cells grown in a collagen-I coated 24-well glass bottom plate (P24-0-N, Cellvis, Mountain View, CA, USA) were fixed with 4% paraformaldehyde (50-980-487, Thermo Fisher) for 10 min and incubated with primary antibody against the human transferrin receptor (A11130, Thermo Fisher) for 3 h, followed by 1 h incubation with goat anti-mouse Alexa Fluor 488 (A11001, Thermo Fisher). Nuclei were stained with Hoechst and cells were imaged using a Zeiss LSM 710 Confocal Microscope (Zeiss, Oberkochen, Germany).

Barrier integrity assay

Chips were washed with culture medium (25 µL on all inlets and outlets, 1 × 5 min) to ensure proper flow profiles during the subsequent barrier integrity assay. Next, all medium was aspirated from the chips and 20 µL of medium without fluorescent compound was added to the basal side of the chips (for the two-lane OrganoPlate this is the gel inlet, for the three-lane OrganoPlate these are the gel inlets and outlets and bottom medium inlets and outlets). Medium containing 0.1 mg/mL FITC-dextran (20 kDa, FD20S, Sigma) was added to the top channel, which contained the TY10 microvessel (40 µL on inlet, 30 µL on outlet) and image acquisition was started. Leakage of the fluorescent molecule from the lumen of the microvessel into the adjacent gel channel was automatically imaged using an ImageXpress XLS Micro HCI system (molecular devices). The ratio between the fluorescent signal in the basal and apical region of the tube was analyzed using FiJi [39]. Graphs were plotted using GraphPad Prism 6 (GraphPad Software, San Diego, CA, USA).

Analysis of cell surface binding of anti-hTfR MEM-189

TY10 cells were cultured to confluency and lifted with accutase for 1 h. 2.5×10^5 cells/mL were mixed with antibody in PBS with 0.5% BSA and incubated for 1 h at 4 °C. Cells were washed 3× and incubated with 3 µg/mL PE-goat anti-mIgG (115-116-146, Jackson ImmunoResearch, Cambridgeshire, UK) for 1 h at 4 °C, then washed and fixed with 1% paraformaldehyde for 10 min at RT. Cell fluorescence intensity was analyzed by flow cytometry (FACSCalibur, BD Biosciences, Franklin Lakes, NJ, USA) and data was analyzed in FlowJo v10 (FlowJo LLC, Ashland, OR, USA) and GraphPad Prism software.

Antibody transcytosis assay

Anti-human transferrin receptor mouse monoclonal antibody MEM-189 mIgG1 (MA1-21562, Thermo Fisher, 10 × 0.1 mg) was dialyzed into pyrogen free PBS to remove the azide in the supplied storage solution. For negative control, an anti-Hen egg lysozyme (anti-HEL) antibody (F10.6.6, Genbank AF110316 VH and AY277254.1 VL) was expressed as a mouse IgG1 antibody in CHO cells and purified by recombinant protein A Sepharose (GE) affinity chromatography and size exclusion chromatography (superdex 200).

Chips were washed once with medium to ensure proper flow profiles (as described for the barrier integrity assay). Next, medium was aspirated from the chips, after which 20 µL of fresh medium without antibody was added to the gel inlets and outlets and the bottom medium inlets and outlets. A total of 70 µL of antibody dilution (1.25 µM in medium) was added to the top channel and the OrganoPlate was incubated on the rocker platform in the incubator for 1 h after which basal samples were taken, which consisted of the full contents of the gel inlet and outlet and bottom medium inlet and outlet.

Analysis of antibody contents in basal samples

A Meso Scale Discovery (MSD) platform based quantitative immunoassay was used to determine the concentration of antibodies in basal samples collected from the OrganoPlate. Multi-Array 96-well MSD high-binding plates (L15XB-3/L11XB-3, Meso Scale Discovery, Rockville, MD, USA) were coated overnight at 4 °C with 5 µg/mL capturing agent AffiniPure goat anti-mouse IgG, Fcγ fragment specific (115-005-071, Jackson ImmunoResearch). Plates were blocked (1% BSA in PBS) for 2 h, after which 100 µL/well standards (generated from 1.25 µM antibody stock dilutions) or samples were added to the plate and incubated for 1.5–2 h. Plates were incubated with 100 µL/well 0.25 µg/mL primary detection agent Biotin-SP-conjugated AffiniPure goat-anti-mouse IgG (115-005-071, Jackson ImmunoResearch) for 45 min, followed by 100 µL/well 0.75 µg/mL secondary detection agent MSD Sulfo-TAG StreptAvidin (R32AD-1, Meso Scale Discovery) for 30 min. Between each step, the plates were washed 4× with wash buffer (PBST: 1× PBS with 0.05% Tween-20, 28352, Thermo Fisher). Immediately before MSD read, 2× Read Buffer (MSD Read Buffer T (4×), R92TD-2, diluted 1:2 in diH_2O) was added to the plates. Plates were read on a MSD Quick-Plex SQ 120 in automatic read mode, then a Sigmoidal, 4PL, X = log(concentration) interpolation was used to determine antibody concentration in GraphPad Prism 7.02 (GraphPad Software). The apparent permeability (P_{app}) of both antibodies was determined using the following formula: $P_{app} = [\Delta C_{receiver}/\Delta t] \times [V_{receiver}/(A_{barrier} \times C_{donor,\ initial})]$, in which $\Delta C_{receiver}/\Delta t$ is the change in antibody concentration in the receiving compartment over time, $V_{receiver}$ is the volume of the receiving compartment, $A_{barrier}$ is the surface area of the barrier, and $C_{donor,\ initial}$ is the initial antibody concentration of the donor compartment.

Results

Perfused microvessels of TY10 brain endothelial cells in the two-lane OrganoPlate

The two-lane OrganoPlate (see Fig. 1a, b) allows parallel culture of 96 miniaturized tissues on microfluidic tissue chips [40–42]. In each chip, a microvessel of brain endothelial cells was grown under perfusion against an extracellular matrix gel (see Fig. 1c–e and Additional file 1). A 3D reconstruction of a TY10 microvessel stained with ActinRed is shown in Fig. 1e and demonstrates that a vessel-like structure of endothelial cells has formed. Immunostaining was performed to assess the expression of key BBB adherens junction and tight junction proteins (see Fig. 1f–h). TY10 microvessels showed expression of vascular endothelial cadherin (VE-cadherin), platelet endothelial cell adhesion molecule 1 (PECAM-1), and claudin-5 at the cell–cell contacts as expected. The expression and interendothelial localization of these markers are indicative of barrier formation [2, 43].

Assessment of barrier function in TY10 brain endothelial microvessels

The barrier function of TY10 microvessels grown in the OrganoPlate was assessed using a fluorescent barrier integrity assay. TY10 microvessels were perfused with a 20 kDa FITC-dextran dye, which has a hydrodynamic radius slightly smaller than a folded IgG antibody (3 nm [44] versus 5–6 nm [45], respectively). Leakage of the dye from the microvessel into the adjacent gel channel

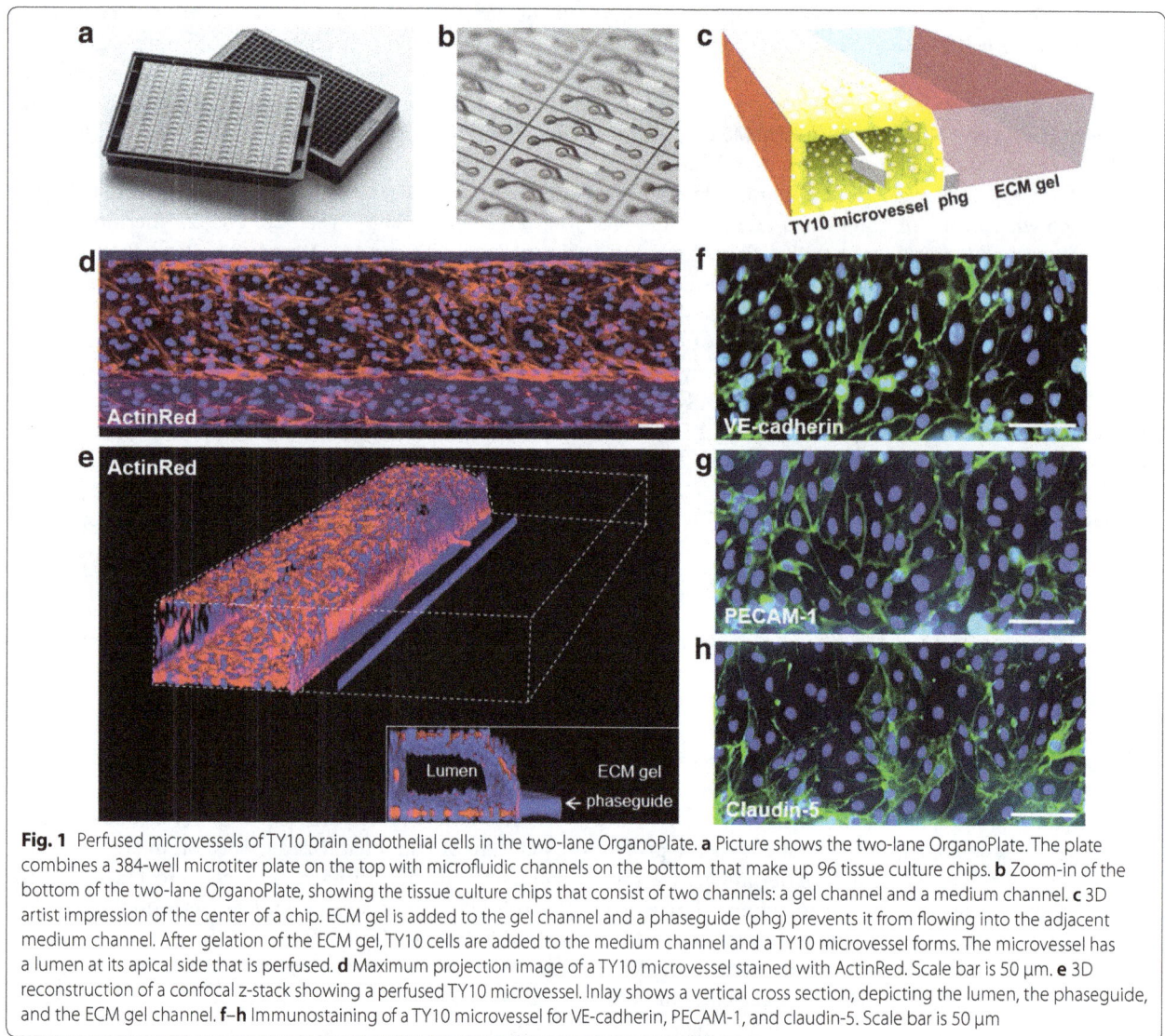

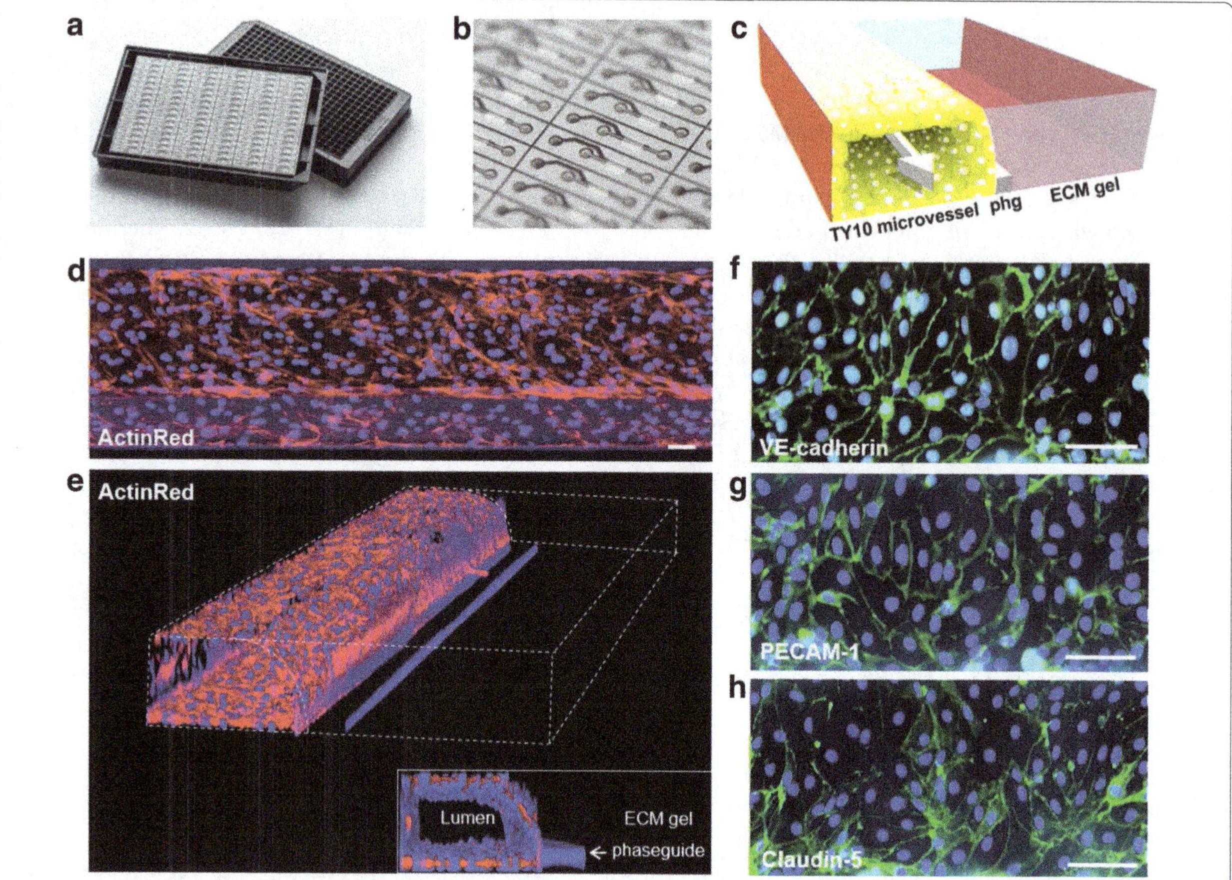

Fig. 1 Perfused microvessels of TY10 brain endothelial cells in the two-lane OrganoPlate. **a** Picture shows the two-lane OrganoPlate. The plate combines a 384-well microtiter plate on the top with microfluidic channels on the bottom that make up 96 tissue culture chips. **b** Zoom-in of the bottom of the two-lane OrganoPlate, showing the tissue culture chips that consist of two channels: a gel channel and a medium channel. **c** 3D artist impression of the center of a chip. ECM gel is added to the gel channel and a phaseguide (phg) prevents it from flowing into the adjacent medium channel. After gelation of the ECM gel, TY10 cells are added to the medium channel and a TY10 microvessel forms. The microvessel has a lumen at its apical side that is perfused. **d** Maximum projection image of a TY10 microvessel stained with ActinRed. Scale bar is 50 µm. **e** 3D reconstruction of a confocal z-stack showing a perfused TY10 microvessel. Inlay shows a vertical cross section, depicting the lumen, the phaseguide, and the ECM gel channel. **f–h** Immunostaining of a TY10 microvessel for VE-cadherin, PECAM-1, and claudin-5. Scale bar is 50 µm

was assessed by acquisition of fluorescent images over time (see Fig. 2a). In a chip containing a leak-tight TY10 microvessel, all fluorescent dye is retained within the vessel (see Fig. 2b, top image). In a cell-free control chip, the fluorescent dye can freely diffuse into the adjacent gel channel (see Fig. 2b, middle image).

(See figure on next page.)

Fig. 2 Assessment of barrier function in TY10 brain endothelial microvessels. **a** Schematic representation of the barrier integrity assay. A perfused TY10 microvessel is grown against an ECM gel. A fluorescent dye is added to the medium inlets and outlets and perfused through the lumen of the microvessel. In case of a leaktight vessel, all dye is retained in the vessel. In case of a leaky vessel, the dye leaks into the adjacent gel channel. **b** Fluorescent dye distribution for a TY10 microvessel (top image) and a cell-free control (middle image) during a barrier integrity assay (FITC-dextran, 20 kDa, t = 30 min). To quantify leakage of the fluorescent dye in a chip, the fluorescence intensity measured in the medium channel and the gel channel ($Fluo_{Med}$ and $Fluo_{Gel}$, respectively) are measured over time (bottom image). **c** For each condition the ratio between the fluorescence signals measured in the two channels is plotted over time. In case of a leaktight TY10 microvessel, the ratio $Fluo_{Gel}/Fluo_{Med}$ is constant, resulting in a flat horizontal line. In case of a leaky microvessel or a cell-free control, the fluorescence signal measured in the gel channel increases over time, resulting in an increase in the ratio $Fluo_{Gel}/Fluo_{Med}$. **d** TY10 microvessels were grown under perfusion or static conditions for 7 days, after which barrier integrity assays (for FITC-dextran, 20 kDa) were performed. n = 6 for TY10 microvessels, n = 2 for cell-free controls. Error bars show standard deviation of the mean. **e** Assessment of barrier function (for FITC-dextran, 20 kDa) of TY10 microvessels cultured under perfusion for 7 days in various commercially available cell culture media. n = 7 for all conditions. Error bars show standard deviation of the mean

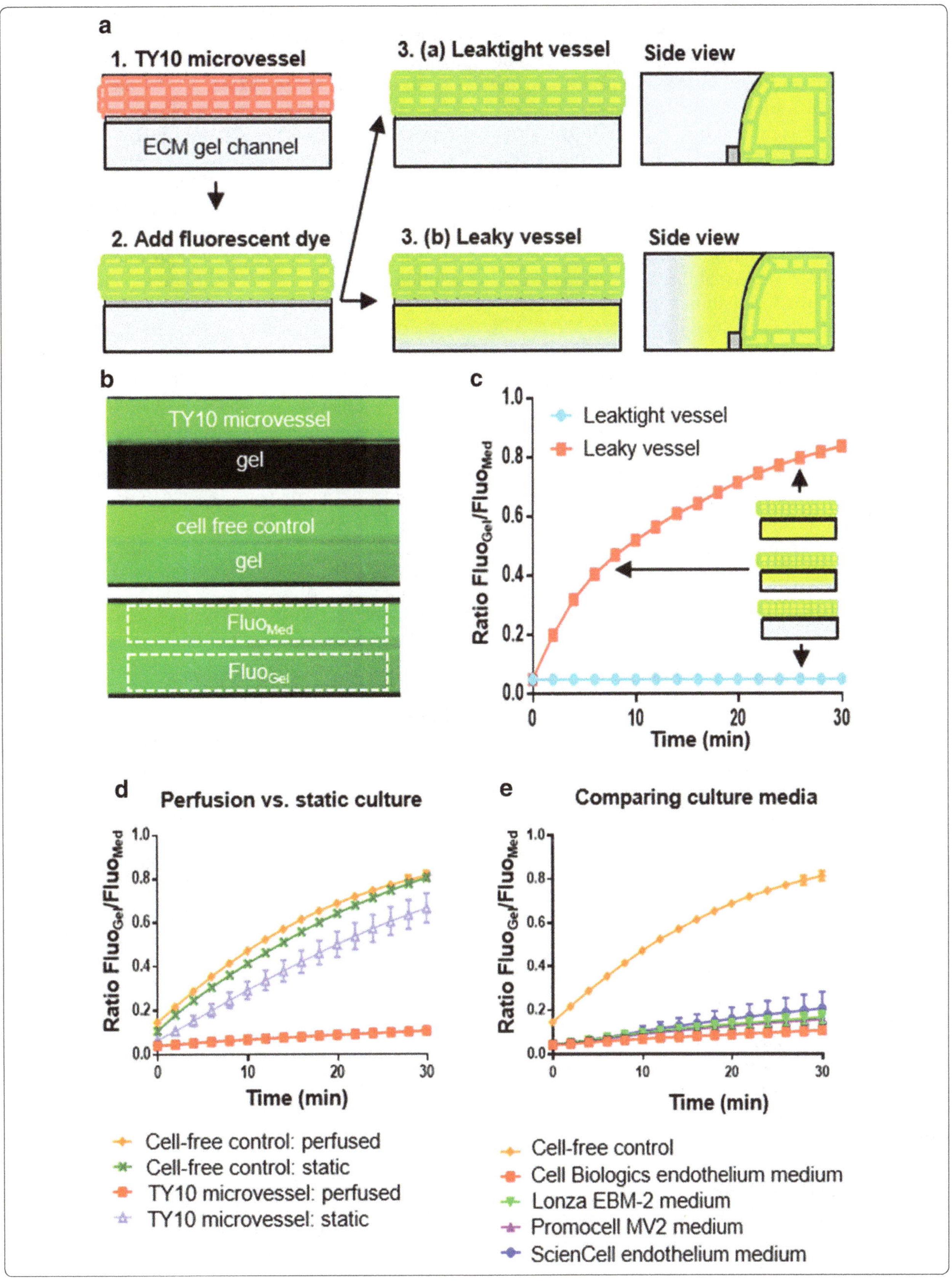
a
1. TY10 microvessel
ECM gel channel
2. Add fluorescent dye
3. (a) Leaktight vessel
Side view
3. (b) Leaky vessel
Side view
b
TY10 microvessel
gel
cell free control
gel
$Fluo_{Med}$
$Fluo_{Gel}$
c
Leaktight vessel
Leaky vessel
Ratio $Fluo_{Gel}/Fluo_{Med}$
Time (min)
d
Perfusion vs. static culture
Ratio $Fluo_{Gel}/Fluo_{Med}$
Time (min)
Cell-free control: perfused
Cell-free control: static
TY10 microvessel: perfused
TY10 microvessel: static
e
Comparing culture media
Ratio $Fluo_{Gel}/Fluo_{Med}$
Time (min)
Cell-free control
Cell Biologics endothelium medium
Lonza EBM-2 medium
Promocell MV2 medium
ScienCell endothelium medium

To quantify leakage of the fluorescent dye, areas were selected automatically for each chip to compare over time (see Fig. 2b, bottom image). The ratio of the fluorescence signal measured in the gel channel and the medium channel is plotted over time as an average of all chips within a condition (see Fig. 2c). In chips that contain a tight cellular barrier, this ratio remains constant, as all dye is retained in the microvessel that is grown in the medium channel. In leaky vessels and cell-free controls, the ratio increases over time, as dye leaks into the gel channel. We compared barrier integrity of TY10 microvessels cultured under static conditions to microvessels cultured under perfusion (by passive leveling using an interval rocker). TY10 cells cultured under perfusion show much tighter barrier formation (Fig. 2d) resulting from increased proliferation and elevated expression and improved localization of junctional proteins (see Additional file 3). In addition, we assessed four different commercially available endothelial cell culture media and found that for this specific type of brain microvascular endothelial cell, the endothelial cell medium from Cell Biologics was optimal for barrier formation (see Fig. 2e).

BBB co-cultures of brain endothelium, astrocytes, and pericytes in the three-lane OrganoPlate

While endothelial cells make up the brain's vasculature, other cell types, such as astrocytes and pericytes, are also part of the BBB and help maintain barrier function. A three-lane OrganoPlate [46] (see Fig. 3a, b) was employed to establish a BBB co-culture of TY10 brain endothelial cells with hAst and hBPCT cells (see Fig. 3c, f, g and Additional file 2). A barrier integrity assay (see Fig. 3h) was performed to determine barrier function in TY10 monocultures (Fig. 3d) and BBB co-cultures (Fig. 3e) at different time points during culture. Both TY10 monocultures and BBB co-cultures successfully retained, to a great extent, a 20 kDa FITC-dextran dye in the endothelial microvessel at days 5, 7, and 9 as is apparent by the marginal increase in the ratio of fluorescence signal measured in the gel channel and the medium channel over time (see Fig. 3i). This barrier integrity assay is useful in identifying optimal culture conditions and timing for which to perform antibody transcytosis assays and showed minimal passive permeability of molecules that are similar in size to antibodies.

Assessment of antibody transcytosis across the BBB

Two different antibodies were used to assess their passage across our human in vitro BBB-on-a-chip. The first was MEM-189, an antibody that binds the human transferrin receptor (hTfR), which is expressed by TY10 endothelial cells (see Additional file 4a) and has been reported to undergo RMT [47]. Flow cytometry analysis showed that anti-hTfR MEM-189 bound to TY10 cells and that binding was not blocked by 25 μg/mL transferrin [$EC_{50} = 0.44 \pm 0.09$ nM (−Tf); 0.5 ± 0.1 nM (+Tf)], see Additional file 4b). The second antibody, anti-hen egg lysozyme (anti-HEL), does not bind a target on human cells and served as a negative control [48]. Both antibodies showed the expected molecular weight, heavy-light chain composition, and size in solution for properly folded antibodies. The antibodies were perfused through the lumen of BBB co-cultures in the three-lane OrganoPlate for 1 h, after which samples were collected from the basal side of the chips (see Fig. 4a). Antibody concentrations in basal samples were determined using MesoScale Discovery® MULTI-ARRAY® technology and the apparent permeability (P_{app}) was calculated. Similar basal concentrations of both antibodies were measured in samples taken from chips without a TY10 microvessel, indicating that when no barrier is present, both antibodies diffuse through the gel to an equal extent (see Fig. 4b). However, in BBB co-cultures, passage of antibody MEM-189 was markedly higher than passage of the control antibody (2.9×10^{-5} versus 1.6×10^{-5} cm/min, respectively) (see Fig. 4b).

Discussion

This study describes a significant advancement in the development of a novel BBB model that incorporates human brain endothelial cells, astrocytes, and pericytes in a high-throughput microfluidic platform that can be used for screening purposes. The cells used in this model are immortalized and thus their phenotype may differ from cells of the BBB in living organisms. Therefore, results obtained in this model may not directly apply to patients. However, the TY10 brain endothelial cell line used in this study has been shown to express relevant junctional markers and transporters, independent of the passage number [31]. Although primary brain endothelial cells offer an interesting alternative, they are difficult to obtain reliably from human donors and have been described to rapidly dedifferentiate and lose their BBB characteristics after removal from the in vivo environment, resulting in decreased expression of essential BBB modulators and impaired barrier function [49, 50]. In recent years, tremendous progress has been made in the generation of induced pluripotent stem cell (iPSC)-derived brain endothelial cells. These cells have been shown to express relevant junctional proteins and transporters, respond well to cues from supporting cell types

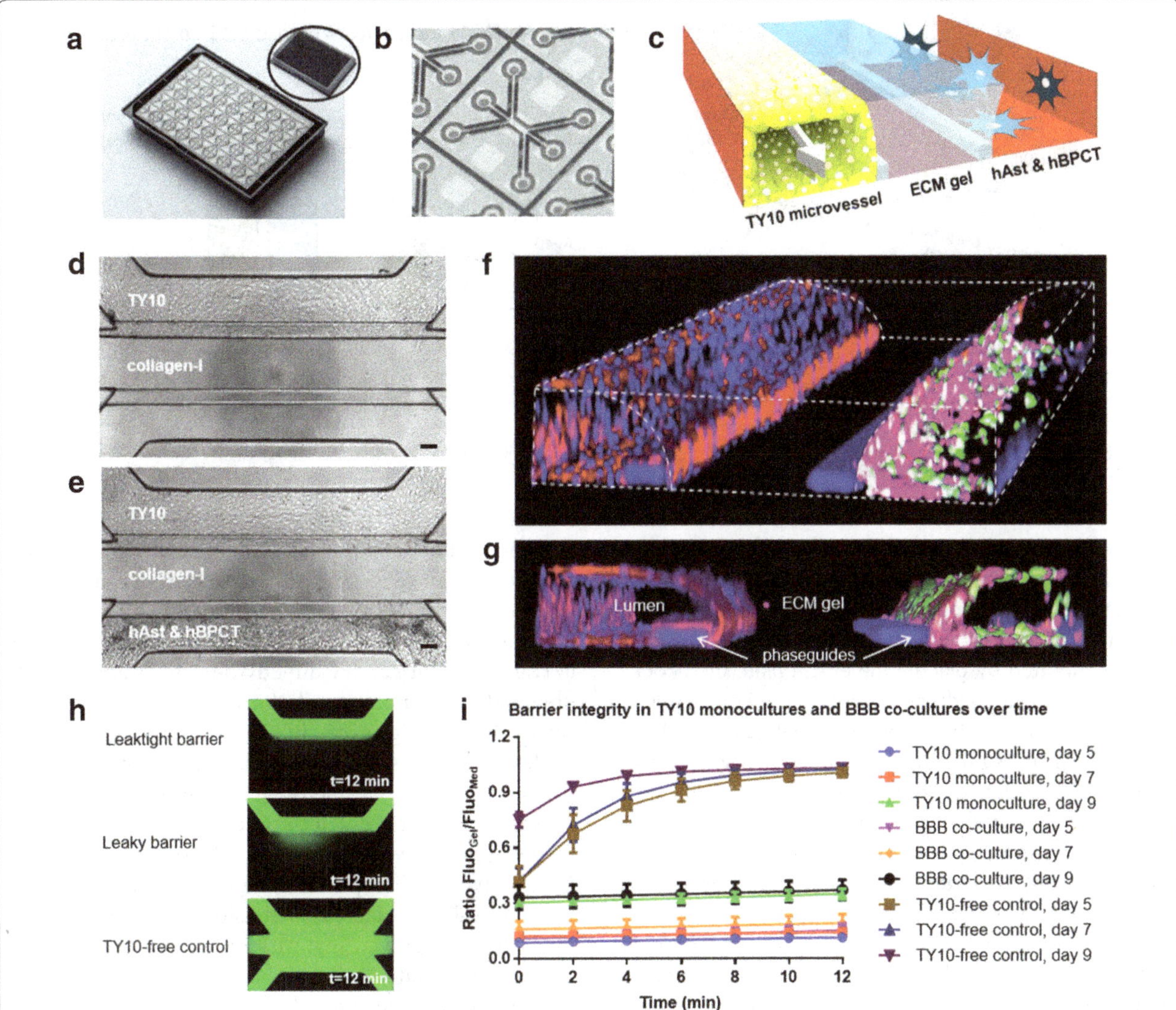

Fig. 3 BBB co-cultures of brain endothelium, astrocytes, and pericytes in the three-lane OrganoPlate. **a** Picture shows the three-lane OrganoPlate. The plate combines a 384-well microtiter plate on the top with microfluidic channels on the bottom that make up 40 tissue culture chips. **b** Zoom-in of the bottom of the three-lane OrganoPlate, showing one tissue culture chip that consists of three channels. **c** 3D artist impression of the center of a chip. ECM gel is added to the gel channel and two phaseguides (white rims) prevent it from flowing into the adjacent medium channels. After gelation of the ECM gel, TY10 cells are added to one of the medium channels and allowed to form a vessel structure. The microvessel has a lumen at its apical side that is perfused. Next, astrocytes (hAst cells) and pericytes (hBPCT cells) are added to the other medium channel to establish a BBB co-culture. **d, e** Phase contrast images of a TY10 monoculture (top image) and a BBB co-culture (bottom image) in the three-lane OrganoPlate, day 7. Scale bar is 100 µm. **f, g** 3D reconstruction of a confocal z-stack showing the organization of the three cell types in a BBB co-culture. The hAst and hBPCT cells were labeled with green-fluorescent calcein-AM and calcein red™ AM, respectively, here depicted in the colors green and magenta. Tight junctions of the TY10 microvessel are shown by a PECAM-1 staining (red). **h** Images acquired of chips with a leaktight barrier (top), a leaky barrier (middle), or TY10-free control (gel with hAst and hBPCT, bottom) during a barrier integrity assay (for FITC-dextran, 20 kDa, t = 12 min). **i** Assessment of barrier function (for FITC-dextran, 20 kDa) at different time points for TY10 monocultures and BBB co-cultures cultured under perfusion in the three-lane OrganoPlate. n = 3 for TY10-free controls and TY10 monocultures and n = 6 for BBB co-cultures. Error bars show standard deviation of the mean

such as astrocytes and pericytes, and display in vivo-like barrier properties [51–55]. In addition, a recent report showed that iPSC-derived brain endothelial cells could be used to study antibody transcytosis across the BBB [55]. The combination of our high-throughput, membrane-free, perfused platform with the ongoing advancements in iPSC-derived cell types may potentially bring about highly relevant BBB models in the future.

In contrast to the standard 2D Transwell approach [19, 56–58], the OrganoPlate supports perfused culture

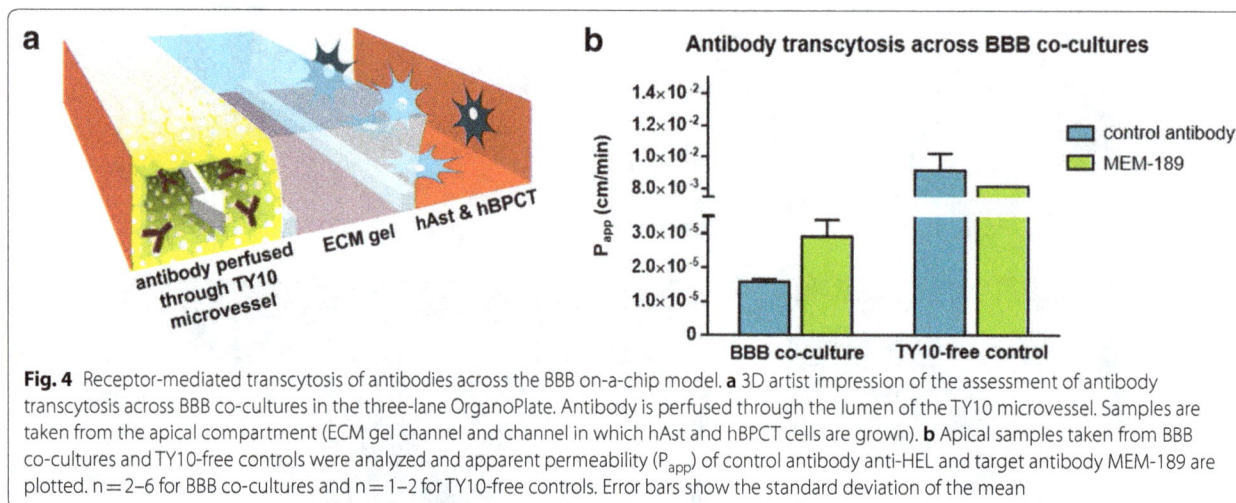

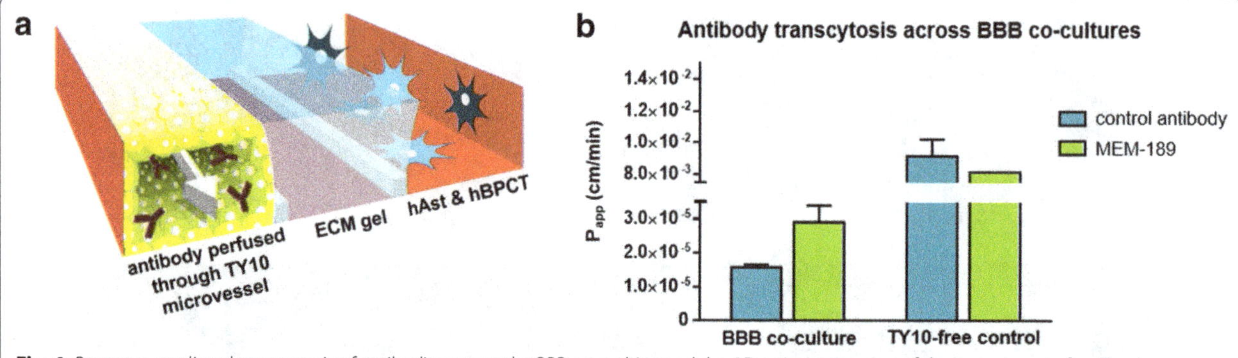

Fig. 4 Receptor-mediated transcytosis of antibodies across the BBB on-a-chip model. **a** 3D artist impression of the assessment of antibody transcytosis across BBB co-cultures in the three-lane OrganoPlate. Antibody is perfused through the lumen of the TY10 microvessel. Samples are taken from the apical compartment (ECM gel channel and channel in which hAst and hBPCT cells are grown). **b** Apical samples taken from BBB co-cultures and TY10-free controls were analyzed and apparent permeability (P_{app}) of control antibody anti-HEL and target antibody MEM-189 are plotted. n = 2–6 for BBB co-cultures and n = 1–2 for TY10-free controls. Error bars show the standard deviation of the mean

of brain endothelial cells, which was shown to be essential for proper lumen formation, proper expression and localization of junctional proteins, and improved barrier function (see Fig. 2d and Additional file 3). Perfusion is generated by placing the entire plate on a rocker platform, allowing medium to flow from medium inlet to outlet and back, creating a bidirectional flow. Fluid flow is controlled by regulating the inclination angle and the interval with which the rocker platform switches sides. Although direct in vivo measurements of shear stress in BBB vessels and venules of different diameters are lacking, it is likely that the shear stress established in our model (~ 1.2 dyne/cm^2) is low compared to the shear stress experienced by vessels of similar diameter and curvature in vivo [59, 60]. Several reports have described improved barrier function of brain endothelial cells as a result of increased shear stress due to an upregulation in junctional proteins [61–63]. Interestingly, other studies did not find increased expression of junctional proteins, but report that brain endothelial cells exhibit a unique response to shear stress compared to endothelium in different organs. Unlike other endothelial cell types, brain endothelial cells did not elongate or align in response to shear stress, a phenotype that may be associated with the BBB's unique properties [64, 65]. The setup used in this study bypasses the need for pumps and intricate tubing systems, which are often associated with microfluidic culture systems, and improves the user-friendliness and throughput of the method.

Comparison of barrier integrity in different culture platforms is challenging, as the properties of the platform itself often influence the measured outcome and are difficult to properly correct for. Among these properties are the presence or lack of a membrane, the pore size of the membrane, the volumes used for the assay, the presence of flow, and the nature of the read-out. Standard measures such as a barrier's transelectrical endothelial resistance (TEER) or a compound's P_{app} can be used to compare results obtained within the same platform, i.e. a Transwell, but cannot directly be compared to results obtained in other culture platforms. The observation that the BBB on-a-chip successfully limits the passage of molecules of similar size as antibodies shows that sufficient barrier function is established to investigate antibody passage. In addition, Trietsch et al. [46] have reported higher sensitivity in detection of compound-induced CaCo-2 barrier disruption in the OrganoPlate compared to Transwell. The increased sensitivity was expected to result from improved maturity of the culture as well as a decreased dead volume and higher surface-to-volume ratio in the OrganoPlate.

Many microfluidic systems employ polydimethylsiloxane (PDMS) because of its optical properties and ease of use in the fabrication process. However, PDMS has several limitations in organ-on-a-chip applications. The intrinsic hydrophobicity of the material impedes cell adhesion and can cause non-specific absorption of proteins and hydrophobic analytes. Although several methods are available to reduce PDMS hydrophobicity and fouling problems, the most successful method requires a complex process that is difficult to incorporate for large scale production [66, 67]. The OrganoPlate employs optical quality (170 μm) glass and polymers that are biocompatible and low compound-absorbing and does not include an artificial membrane. Furthermore, the collagen gel does not significantly restrict passage of antibody into the basal compartment, which was demonstrated by the observation that antibody P_{app} increased > 500-fold when the endothelial cells were omitted from the model (Fig. 4b). Together, the low level passive permeability of the brain endothelial cell layer, minimal absorption, and the ease of antibody sampling from the basal compartment could support sensitive and high-throughput screening of antibody transcytosis in this BBB on-a-chip.

The human transferrin receptor is of special interest for drug targeting to the brain due to its expression on brain endothelial cells and potential to support receptor mediated transcytosis [9, 12, 68, 69]. In this study, we observed an approximately two-fold higher passage of MEM-189, an antibody targeting the hTfR receptor, across our BBB model compared to a control antibody. The P_{app} value we measured for the non-binding control antibody agrees well with those reported recently in other in vitro human BBB models [55, 70]. The passage of this murine IgG control antibody could in theory result from Fc receptor mediated transport through the neonatal Fc receptor (FcRn), which is expressed at the BBB. However, since murine IgG1 antibodies show very little binding to the human FcRn [71] and FcRn likely does not result in BBB transcytosis [72], the passage of this antibody is most likely the result of paracellular flux or non-receptor mediated endocytic flux (i.e. micropinocytosis). The enhanced permeability of the MEM-189 antibody is consistent with previous reports [47] and could result from active transport mediated by the transferrin receptor. This bivalent antibody has high affinity for hTfR and thus is not optimized for high transport, as has been shown for other anti-TfR BBB shuttles [9, 12, 15]. As a large portion of endocytosed TfR has been shown to remain in the endothelial cells instead of undergoing transcytosis, it is likely that a relatively large quantity of endocytosed MEM-189 remains within the endothelial cells [73]. However, Sade et al. [47] have shown that binding of MEM-189 to the TfR is pH-dependent, which may support transcytosis via release from the TfR in the endosomal environment and could contribute to its observed transcytosis. The assay developed in this study is sensitive to differences in antibody passage across the BBB model and holds potential to be applied in larger screens for discovery of CNS-penetrant antibodies. The addition of neurons to the model may add an extra layer of complexity that brings about possibilities for modelling the full neurovascular unit and studying the passage of molecules across the BBB as well as the effects of these molecules on neuronal function.

Conclusion

In summary, the model described here is the first perfused BBB-on-a-chip culture system that is compatible with standard laboratory equipment and allows throughput to an extent that is necessary for drug screening. Moreover, co-culture complexity is easily expanded as shown by the addition of pericytes and astrocytes. This model could support further discovery and engineering of antibody BBB-shuttle technologies.

Additional files

Additional file 1. Endothelial microvessel seeding in the two-lane OrganoPlate. (**a**) Schematic representation of one chip of a two-lane OrganoPlate. (**b**) An ECM gel is seeded in the gel channel, after which endothelial cells are seeded in the medium channel. (**c**) Endothelial cells attach to the ECM gel and perfusion is started by placing the OrganoPlate on a rocker platform. (**d**) A microvessel of endothelial cells is formed. (**e–g**) Cross sectional view of steps described in **b–d**.

Additional file 2. BBB co-culture seeding in the three-lane OrganoPlate®. (**a**) Schematic representation of one chip of a three-lane OrganoPlate. (**b**) ECM gel is seeded in the middle gel of the chip, after which endothelial cells (TY10) are seeded in the top channel. (**c**) Endothelial cells attach to the ECM and perfusion is started by placing the plate on a rocking platform. (**d**) A microvessel of endothelial cells forms in the top channel, against the ECM gel. (**e**) Astrocytes (hAst) and pericytes (hBPCTs) are seeded in the bottom channel. (**f**) hAst and hBPCT cells attach and a BBB co-culture is established. (**g–k**) Cross sectional view of steps described in **b–f**.

Additional file 3. Comparing perfused and static culture of TY10 microvessels. (**a**, **b**) Phase contrast images of TY10 microvessels grown in the two-lane OrganoPlate under perfused or static conditions (day 7). Scale bar is 100 µm. (**c**) Microvessels grown under perfused or static conditions were fixed and nuclei were stained with Hoechst. The average number of nuclei was counted in both conditions and normalized to the perfused condition. $n=6$, Student's t-test $p<0.05$. (**d–f**) Immunofluorescent staining of TY10 microvessels grown under perfusion for adherens and tight junction markers VE-cadherin, claudin-5, and PECAM-1. (**g–i**) Immunofluorescent staining of TY10 microvessels grown static for adherens and tight junction markers VE-cadherin, claudin-5, and PECAM-1. Scale bar is 100 µm.

Additional file 4. Characterization of the human transferrin receptor in TY10 endothelial cells. (**a**) Immunofluorescent staining of the hTfR in TY10 endothelial cells. Scale bar is 50 µm. (**b**) Flow cytometry analysis of cell surface binding of anti-TfR MEM-189 to TY10 endothelial cells in the presence and absence of transferrin (25 µg/mL), $EC_{50}=0.44 \pm 0.09$ nM (−Tf); 0.5 ± 0.1 nM (+Tf).

Abbreviations

BBB: blood–brain barrier; CNS: central nervous system; FcRn: neonatal Fc receptor; FCS: fetal calf serum; hAst: human astrocyte cell line; hBPCT: human brain pericyte cell line; HEL: hen egg lysozyme; HEPES: 4-(2-hydroxyethyl)-1-piperazineethanesulfonic acid; hTfR: human transferrin receptor; iPSC: induced pluripotent stem cell; MEM-189: anti-transferrin receptor antibody; PBS: phosphate buffered saline; PDMS: polydimethylsiloxane; PECAM-1: platelet endothelial cell adhesion molecule 1; RMT: receptor-mediated transcytosis; TEER: transendothelial electrical resistance; TY10 cell line: human brain endothelial cell line; VE-cadherin: vascular endothelial cadherin.

Authors' contributions

Authors NRW, BS, RV, GM, and BO designed the study. Authors NRW, DGK, TG, and BS performed experiments and data analysis. Authors KJW, SJT, PV, HLL, and BO supervised the research. Authors FS, YS, and TK developed the cells and advised on cell culture procedures. Authors NRW, DGK, TG, BS, HLL, and BO wrote the paper. All authors read and approved the final manuscript.

Author details

[1] Mimetas BV, J.H. Oortweg 19, 2333 CH Leiden, The Netherlands. [2] Department of Cell and Chemical Biology, Leiden University Medical Centre, Einthovenweg 20, 2333 ZC Leiden, The Netherlands. [3] Biogen, 225 Binney Street, Cambridge, MA 02142, USA. [4] Yamaguchi University Graduate School of Medicine, Minamikogushi, Ube, Yamaguchi 7558505, Japan.

Acknowledgements
The authors thank Dr. Thomas Cameron for his scientific input and Fang Qian for his help with reagent preparation and advice on MSD analysis.

Competing interests
This study was funded by Biogen. Authors T.G., B.S., G.M., and B.O. are employees and shareholders of Biogen. Authors N.W., D.K., K.W., R.V., H.L., S.T. and P.V. are employees of MIMETAS and S.T. and P.V. are shareholders of that same company. The OrganoPlate® is a registered trademark of MIMETAS BV.

Funding
This work was partly supported by the CoSTREAM consortium, which has received funding from the European Union's Horizon 2020 research and innovation program under grant agreement No 667375, and the ADAPTED consortium, which has received funding from the Innovative Medicines Initiative 2 Joint Undertaking under grant agreement No 115975. This Joint Undertaking receives support from the European Union's Horizon 2020 research and innovation program and the European Federation of Pharmaceutical Industries and Associations.

References

1. Abbott NJ, Patabendige AAK, Dolman DEM, Yusof SR, Begley DJ. Structure and function of the blood–brain barrier. Neurobiol Dis. 2010;37:13–25.
2. Wolburg H, Lippoldt A. Tight junctions of the blood–brain barrier: development, composition and regulation. Vasc Pharmacol. 2002;38:323–37.
3. Daneman R. The blood–brain barrier in health and disease. Ann Neurol. 2012;72:648–72.
4. Obermeier B, Daneman R, Ransohoff RM. Development, maintenance and disruption of the blood–brain barrier. Nat Med. 2013;19:1584–96.
5. Wevers NR, de Vries HE. Morphogens and blood–brain barrier function in health and disease. Tissue Barriers. 2016;4:e1090524.
6. Pardridge WM. Drug transport across the blood–brain barrier. J Cereb Blood Flow Metab. 2012;32:1959–72.
7. Pardridge WM. Drug and gene delivery to the brain: the vascular route. Neuron. 2002;36:555–8.
8. Freskgård PO, Urich E. Antibody therapies in CNS diseases. Neuropharmacology. 2017;120:38–55.
9. Niewoehner J, Bohrmann B, Collin L, et al. Increased brain penetration and potency of a therapeutic antibody using a monovalent molecular shuttle. Neuron. 2014;81:49–60.
10. Webster CI, Caram-Salas N, Haqqani AS, et al. Brain penetration, target engagement, and disposition of the blood–brain barrier-crossing bispecific antibody antagonist of metabotropic glutamate receptor type 1. FASEB J. 2016;30:1927–40.
11. Zuchero YJY, Chen X, Bien-Ly N, et al. Discovery of novel blood–brain barrier targets to enhance brain uptake of therapeutic antibodies. Neuron. 2016;89:70–82.
12. Yu YJ, Zhang Y, Kenrick M, et al. Boosting brain uptake of a therapeutic antibody by reducing its affinity for a transcytosis target. Sci Transl Med. 2011;3:84ra44.
13. Couch JA, Yu YJ, Zhang Y, et al. Addressing safety liabilities of TfR bispecific antibodies that cross the blood–brain barrier. Sci Transl Med. 2013;5:183ra57.
14. Haqqani AS, Delaney CE, Brunette E, et al. Endosomal trafficking regulates receptor-mediated transcytosis of antibodies across the blood brain barrier. J Cereb Blood Flow Metab. 2018;38:727–40.
15. Thom G, Hatcher J, Hearn A, et al. Isolation of blood–brain barrier-crossing antibodies from a phage display library by competitive elution and their ability to penetrate the central nervous system. MAbs. 2018;10:304–14.
16. Weber F, Bohrmann B, Niewoehner J, et al. Brain shuttle antibody for Alzheimer's disease with attenuated peripheral effector function due to an inverted binding mode. Cell Rep. 2018;22:149–62.
17. Ben-Zvi A, Lacoste B, Kur E, et al. Mfsd2a is critical for the formation and function of the blood–brain barrier. Nature. 2014;509:507–11.
18. Villaseñor R, Ozmen L, Messaddeq N, et al. Trafficking of endogenous immunoglobulins by endothelial cells at the blood–brain barrier. Sci Rep. 2016;6:25658.
19. Abbott NJ, Hughes CC, Revest PA, Greenwood J. Development and characterisation of a rat brain capillary endothelial culture: towards an in vitro blood–brain barrier. J Cell Sci. 1992;103(Pt 1):23–37.
20. Biegel D, Pachter JS. Growth of brain microvessel endothelial cells on collagen gels: applications to the study of blood–brain barrier physiology and CNS inflammation. In Vitro Cell Dev Biol Anim. 1994;30:581–8.
21. Gardner TW, Lieth E, Khin SA, et al. Astrocytes increase barrier properties and ZO-1 expression in retinal vascular endothelial cells. Invest Ophthalmol Vis Sci. 1997;38:2423–7.
22. He Y, Yao Y, Tsirka SE, Cao Y. Cell-culture models of the blood–brain barrier. Stroke. 2014;45:2514–26.
23. Wolff A, Antfolk M, Brodin B, Tenje M. In vitro blood–brain barrier models—an overview of established models and new microfluidic approaches. J Pharm Sci. 2015;104:2727–46.
24. van der Helm MW, van der Meer AD, Eijkel JCT, van den Berg A, Segerink LI. Microfluidic organ-on-chip technology for blood–brain barrier research. Tissue Barriers. 2016;4:e1142493.
25. Reichel A, Begley DJ, Abbott NJ. An overview of in vitro techniques for blood–brain barrier studies. Methods Mol Med. 2003;89:307–24.
26. van der Meer AD, Orlova VV, ten Dijke P, van den Berg A, Mummery CL. Three-dimensional co-cultures of human endothelial cells and embryonic stem cell-derived pericytes inside a microfluidic device. Lab Chip. 2013;13:3562.
27. Prabhakarpandian B, Shen MC, Nichols JB, et al. SyM-BBB: a microfluidic blood brain barrier model. Lab Chip. 2013;13:1093.
28. Herland A, Van Der Meer AD, FitzGerald EA, Park TE, Sleeboom JJF, Ingber DE. Distinct contributions of astrocytes and pericytes to neuroinflammation identified in a 3D human blood–brain barrier on a chip. PLoS ONE. 2016;11:1–21.
29. Bang S, Lee SR, Ko J, et al. A low permeability microfluidic blood–brain barrier platform with direct contact between perfusable vascular network and astrocytes. Sci Rep. 2017;7:1–10.
30. Sano Y, Shimizu F, Abe M, et al. Establishment of a new conditionally immortalized human brain microvascular endothelial cell line retaining an in vivo blood–brain barrier function. J Cell Physiol. 2010;225:519–28.
31. Sano Y, Kashiwamura Y, Abe M, et al. Stable human brain microvascular endothelial cell line retaining its barrier-specific nature independent of the passage number. Clin Exp Neuroimmunol. 2013;4:92–103.
32. Shimizu F, Sano Y, Tominaga O, Maeda T, Abe M, Kanda T. Advanced glycation end-products disrupt the blood–brain barrier by stimulating the release of transforming growth factor-β by pericytes and vascular endothelial growth factor and matrix metalloproteinase-2 by endothelial cells in vitro. Neurobiol Aging. 2013;34:1902–12.
33. Haruki H, Sano Y, Shimizu F, et al. NMO sera down-regulate AQP4 in human astrocyte and induce cytotoxicity independent of complement. J Neurol Sci. 2013;331:136–44.
34. Shimizu F, Sano Y, Abe M, et al. Peripheral nerve pericytes modify the blood-nerve barrier function and tight junctional molecules through the secretion of various soluble factors. J Cell Physiol. 2011;226:255–66.
35. Takeshita Y, Obermeier B, Cotleur A, Sano Y, Kanda T, Ransohoff RM. An in vitro blood–brain barrier model combining shear stress and endothelial cell/astrocyte co-culture. J Neurosci Methods. 2014;232:165–72.
36. Spampinato SF, Obermeier B, Cotleur A, et al. Sphingosine 1 plhosphate at the blood brain barrier: can the modulation of S1P receptor 1 influence the response of endothelial cells and astrocytes to inflammatory stimuli? PLoS ONE. 2015;10:e0133392.
37. Takeshita Y, Obermeier B, Cotleur AC, et al. Effects of neuromyelitis optica-IgG at the blood–brain barrier in vitro. Neurol Neuroimmunol Neuroinflamm. 2017;4:e311.
38. Shimizu F, Schaller KL, Owens GP, et al. Glucose-regulated protein 78 autoantibody associates with blood–brain barrier disruption in neuromyelitis optica. Sci Transl Med. 2017;9:eaai9111.
39. Schindelin J, Arganda-Carreras I, Frise E, et al. Fiji: an open-source platform for biological-image analysis. Nat Methods. 2012;9:676–82.

40. Trietsch SJ, Israëls GD, Joore J, Hankemeier T, Vulto P. Microfluidic titer plate for stratified 3D cell culture. Lab Chip. 2013;13:3548–54.
41. Wevers NR, van Vught R, Wilschut KJ, et al. High-throughput compound evaluation on 3D networks of neurons and glia in a microfluidic platform. Sci Rep. 2016;6:38856.
42. van Duinen V, van den Heuvel A, Trietsch SJ, et al. 96 perfusable blood vessels to study vascular permeability in vitro. Sci Rep. 2017;7:18071.
43. Tietz S, Engelhardt B. Brain barriers: crosstalk between complex tight junctions and adherens junctions. J Cell Biol. 2015;209:493–506.
44. Armstrong JK, Wenby RB, Meiselman HJ, Fisher TC. The hydrodynamic radii of macromolecules and their effect on red blood cell aggregation. Biophys J. 2004;87:4259–70.
45. Hawe A, Hulse WL, Jiskoot W, Forbes RT. Taylor dispersion analysis compared to dynamic light scattering for the size analysis of therapeutic peptides and proteins and their aggregates. Pharm Res. 2011;28:2302–10.
46. Trietsch SJ, Naumovska E, Kurek D, et al. Membrane-free culture and real-time barrier integrity assessment of perfused intestinal epithelium tubes. Nat Commun. 2017;8:262.
47. Sade H, Baumgartner C, Hugenmatter A, Moessner E, Freskgård P-O, Niewoehner J. A human blood–brain barrier transcytosis assay reveals antibody transcytosis influenced by pH-dependent receptor binding. PLoS ONE. 2014;9:e96340.
48. Goldbaum FA, Cauerhff A, Velikovsky CA, Llera AS, Riottot MM, Poljak RJ. Lack of significant differences in association rates and affinities of antibodies from short-term and long-term responses to hen egg lysozyme. J Immunol. 1999;162:6040–5.
49. Gumbleton M, Audus KL. Progress and limitations in the use of in vitro cell cultures to serve as a permeability screen for the blood–brain barrier. J Pharm Sci. 2001;90:1681–98.
50. Cho C-F, Wolfe JM, Fadzen CM, et al. Blood–brain-barrier spheroids as an in vitro screening platform for brain-penetrating agents. Nat Commun. 2017;8:15623.
51. Lippmann ES, Azarin SM, Kay JE, et al. Derivation of blood–brain barrier endothelial cells from human pluripotent stem cells. Nat Biotechnol. 2012;30:783–91.
52. Lippmann ES, Al-Ahmad A, Azarin SM, Palecek SP, Shusta EV. A retinoic acid-enhanced, multicellular human blood–brain barrier model derived from stem cell sources. Sci Rep. 2014;4:4160.
53. Katt ME, Linville RM, Mayo LN, Xu ZS, Searson PC. Functional brain-specific microvessels from iPSC-derived human brain microvascular endothelial cells: the role of matrix composition on monolayer formation. Fluids Barriers CNS. 2018;15:7.
54. Hollmann EK, Bailey AK, Potharazu AV, Neely MD, Bowman AB, Lippmann ES. Accelerated differentiation of human induced pluripotent stem cells to blood–brain barrier endothelial cells. Fluids Barriers CNS. 2017;14:9.
55. Ribecco-Lutkiewicz M, Sodja C, Haukenfrers J, et al. A novel human induced pluripotent stem cell blood–brain barrier model: applicability to study antibody-triggered receptor-mediated transcytosis. Sci Rep. 2018;8:1873.
56. Biegel D, Pachter JS. Growth of brain microvessel endothelial cells on collagen gels: applications to the study of blood–brain barrier physiology and CNS inflammation. In Vitro Cell Dev Biol Anim. 1994;30A:581–8.
57. Hopkins AM, DeSimone E, Chwalek K, Kaplan DL. 3D in vitro modeling of the central nervous system. Prog Neurobiol. 2015;125:1–25.
58. Naik P, Cucullo L. In vitro blood–brain barrier models: current and perspective technologies. J Pharm Sci. 2012;101:1337–54.
59. Dewey CF, Bussolari SR, Gimbrone MA, Davies PF. The dynamic response of vascular endothelial cells to fluid shear stress. J Biomech Eng. 1981;103:177.
60. Cucullo L, Hossain M, Tierney W, Janigro D. A new dynamic in vitro modular capillaries-venules modular system: cerebrovascular physiology in a box. BMC Neurosci. 2013;14:18.
61. Seebach J, Dieterich P, Luo F, et al. Endothelial barrier function under laminar fluid shear stress. Lab Invest. 2000;80:1819–31.
62. Siddharthan V, Kim YV, Liu S, Kim KS. Human astrocytes/astrocyte-conditioned medium and shear stress enhance the barrier properties of human brain microvascular endothelial cells. Brain Res. 2007;1147:39–50.
63. Cucullo L, Hossain M, Puvenna V, Marchi N, Janigro D. The role of shear stress in blood–brain barrier endothelial physiology. BMC Neurosci. 2011;12:40.
64. Reinitz A, DeStefano J, Ye M, Wong AD, Searson PC. Human brain microvascular endothelial cells resist elongation due to shear stress. Microvasc Res. 2015;99:8–18.
65. DeStefano JG, Xu ZS, Williams AJ, Yimam N, Searson PC. Effect of shear stress on iPSC-derived human brain microvascular endothelial cells (dhBMECs). Fluids Barriers CNS. 2017;14:20.
66. Zhang H, Chiao M. Anti-fouling coatings of poly(dimethylsiloxane) devices for biological and biomedical applications. J Med Biol Eng. 2015;35:143–55.
67. Wong I, Ho CM. Surface molecular property modifications for poly(dimethylsiloxane) (PDMS) based microfluidic devices. Microfluid Nanofluidics. 2009;7:291–306.
68. Jefferies WA, Brandon MR, Hunt SV, Williams AF, Gatter KC, Mason DY. Transferrin receptor on endothelium of brain capillaries. Nature. 1984;312:162–3.
69. Johnsen KB, Moos T. Revisiting nanoparticle technology for blood–brain barrier transport: unfolding at the endothelial gate improves the fate of transferrin receptor-targeted liposomes. J Control Release. 2016;222:32–46.
70. Farrington GK, Caram-Salas N, Haqqani AS, et al. A novel platform for engineering blood–brain barrier-crossing bispecific biologics. FASEB J. 2014;28:4764–78.
71. Ober RJ, Radu CG, Ghetie V, Ward ES. Differences in promiscuity for antibody-FcRn interactions across species: implications for therapeutic antibodies. Int Immunol. 2001;13:1551–9.
72. Garg A, Balthasar JP. Investigation of the Influence of FcRn on the distribution of IgG to the brain. AAPS J. 2009;11:553–7.
73. Moos T, Morgan EH. Restricted transport of anti-transferrin receptor antibody (OX26) through the blood–brain barrier in the rat. J Neurochem. 2001;79:119–29.

19

Is bulk flow plausible in perivascular, paravascular and paravenous channels?

Mohammad M. Faghih and M. Keith Sharp*

Abstract

Background: Transport of solutes has been observed in the spaces surrounding cerebral arteries and veins. Indeed, transport has been found in opposite directions in two different spaces around arteries. These findings have motivated hypotheses of bulk flow within these spaces. The glymphatic circulation hypothesis involves flow of cerebrospinal fluid from the cortical subarachnoid space to the parenchyma along the paraarterial (extramural, Virchow–Robin) space around arteries, and return flow to the cerebrospinal fluid (CSF) space via paravenous channels. The second hypothesis involves flow of interstitial fluid from the parenchyma to lymphatic vessels along basement membranes between arterial smooth muscle cells.

Methods: This article evaluates the plausibility of steady, pressure-driven flow in these channels with one-dimensional branching models.

Results: According to the models, the hydraulic resistance of arterial basement membranes is too large to accommodate estimated interstitial perfusion of the brain, unless the flow empties to lymphatic ducts after only several generations (still within the parenchyma). The estimated pressure drops required to drive paraarterial and paravenous flows of the same magnitude are not large, but paravenous flow back to the CSF space means that the total pressure difference driving both flows is limited to local pressure differences among the different CSF compartments, which are estimated to be small.

Conclusions: Periarterial flow and glymphatic circulation driven by steady pressure are both found to be implausible, given current estimates of anatomical and fluid dynamic parameters.

Keywords: Perivascular flow, Paravascular flow, Paravenous flow, Bulk flow, Brain clearance system, Glymphatic system

Background

Since the Virchow–Robin space was discovered, there has been disagreement about whether the fluid within is stagnant (as Robin [1] thought) or circulates (opinion held by Virchow [2]) [3]. The recent hypothesis of a "glymphatic" circulation, comprising convection of cerebrospinal fluid from the cortical subarachnoid space to the parenchyma via extramural paraarterial channels and return flow along veins [4], has revived this old question. Further complicating our understanding of flow and transport in this space is evidence of possible flow in the opposite direction within the walls of cerebral arteries, specifically within basement membranes between smooth muscle cell layers (the intramural perivascular space [5]). Motion retrograde to blood flow and to the propagation of the blood pressure pulse is counterintuitive, but a number of models have been developed as possible explanations [6–8]. What has to date not been evaluated, however, is the flow resistance of the full branching paravascular and perivascular networks. Simply put, if the hydraulic resistance of the network exceeds the capability of the available pressure difference to drive significant flow through it, then the steady pressure-driven flow hypothesis is disproven. In this paper, one-dimensional models are developed to test the plausibility of

*Correspondence: keith.sharp@louisville.edu
Biofluid Mechanics Laboratory, Department of Mechanical Engineering, University of Louisville, Louisville, KY 40292, USA

physiologically significant flow in the periarterial, paraarterial and paravenous trees. The anatomy of these spaces is first reviewed in section "Perivascular and paravascular anatomy", then evidence for solute transport within them and the potential driving mechanisms are outlined in the "Experimental observations of transport and potential mechanisms" section.

Perivascular and paravascular anatomy

The anatomy of the perivascular and paravascular channels is shown schematically in Fig. 1. Perivascular describes the basement membranes (about 100 nm thickness [9]) between smooth muscle cells (SMC), which occur in one layer around arterioles, and in 4–20 layers in larger arteries [10].

In the arteries, paravascular refers to the space outside the pia, but inside the astrocyte endfeet forming the glia limitans (Fig. 1). This channel has also been called the Virchow–Robin space [1, 2, 11]. The pial sheath is not found around veins in the parenchyma [12] thus the inner wall of the paravenous space may be the collagen layer between the endothelium and the glia limitans [12]. Interestingly, the space is rapidly and nearly completely closed by cortical spreading depression [13], which may be caused by astrocyte endfoot swelling [14]. This response may have implications for dysfunctions of this clearance pathway and suggests potential for its regulation.

Experimental observations of transport and potential mechanisms

Transport of molecules with immunological, metabolic and disease-related implications for the brain has been hypothesized in two different directions in the two different channels. First, clearance of amyloid-β suspended in parenchymal interstitial fluid has been hypothesized in the periarterial space [15, 16]. Second, inflow of cerebrospinal fluid from the cortical subarachnoid space to the parenchyma has been hypothesized in the paraarterial space, along with outflow back to the CSF space in the similar gap along cerebral veins (the "glymphatic" system) [17]. The small sizes of these channels make direct measurement of flow challenging, however, the appearance of tracers along the channels has been documented by a number of investigators (e.g., [4, 18]).

While simultaneous flows in opposite directions in the two different channels is theoretically possible [5], two conditions would need to be met. First, a wall with flow resistance greater than that in either channel must exist between the two channels to prevent mixing of the flows. The pia physically separates the two channels in the arteries, but it is unclear whether it has sufficient flow resistance to comprise a hydraulic barrier. Second, the mechanisms driving opposed flows must be identified. Opposed pressure gradients is a candidate mechanism. Since the two channels merge where the pia ends at the precapillaries, the same pressure prevails there. Therefore, opposed flows require pressures higher and

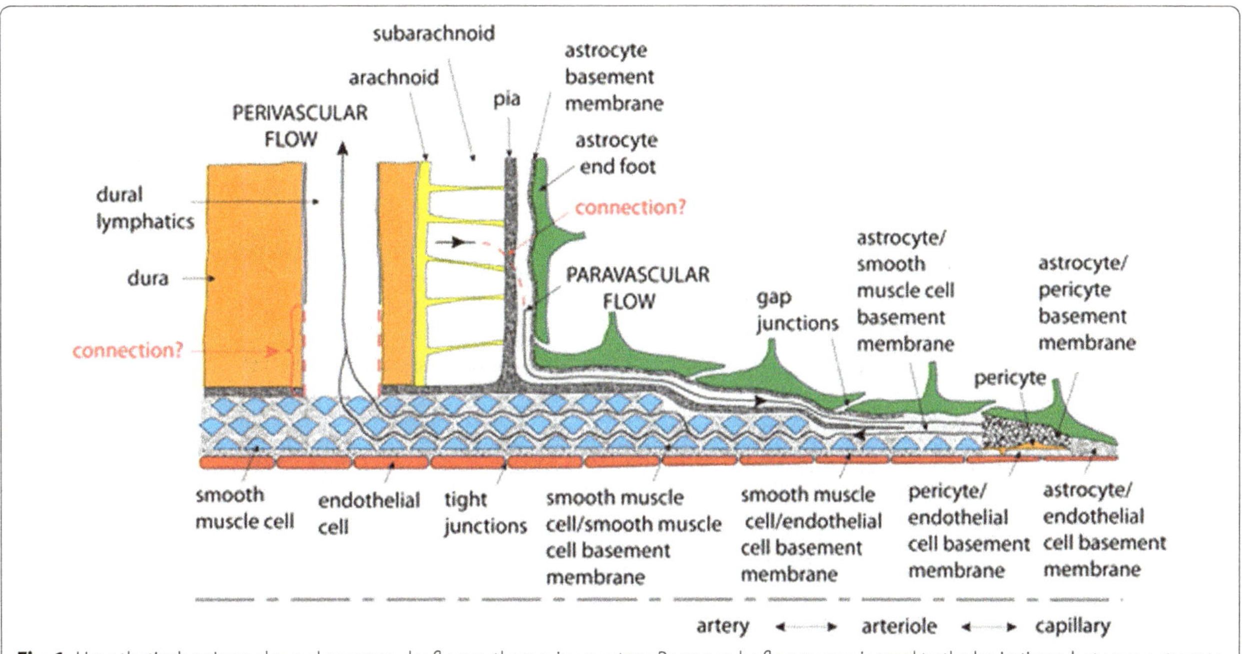

Fig. 1 Hypothetical perivascular and paravascular flow pathways in an artery. Paravascular flow moves inward to the brain tissue between astrocyte end feet and pia mater. Perivascular flow moves outward from the brain tissue in basement membranes between SMCs

lower than that in the precapillary channel in the paravascular and perivascular spaces surrounding the large arteries, respectively. If paraarterial flow originates in the subarachnoid space, and the periarterial flow empties into lymph vessels, then such pressure differences are possible. Paravenous flow back to the CSF space requires that a local pressure difference between CSF compartments, specifically the difference in pressure between the upstream compartment for paraarterial flow and the downstream compartment for paraarterial paravenous flow, is sufficient to drive both flows. The transmantle pressure difference (the difference in pressure between the lateral ventricles and the upper convexity of the subarachnoid space, the largest pressure difference among CSF compartments) is estimated to be no more than 0.03 mmHg [19].

Peristalsis caused by the blood pressure pulse would tend to create flow in the perivascular and paravascular channels in the direction of blood flow. Indeed, Bedussi et al. [20] used a thinned-skull cranial window to image microspheres oscillating at the heart beat frequency and advancing in the direction of blood flow within 20 μm of the surface branches of the middle cerebral artery. However, no evidence was observed of bulk flow into the parenchyma around the penetrating arteries nor clearance around the veins.

Identifying a mechanism for retrograde flow (in the direction opposite that of the blood flow) is essential to validating the periarterial clearance concept. Three hypothesized mechanisms include physical or chemical hinderance of the solute during forward flow, but not during reverse flow [6], flexible flow resistance elements that promote reverse flow [7] and incoherent reflection of waves in the inner and outer walls of the channel [8].

Tracer transport could alternatively be accomplished by molecular diffusion. However, for the relatively large molecules observed in previous experiments, diffusion alone is too slow to explain the rapid spreads observed. Shear-augmented dispersion by oscillatory flow without net bulk flow can increase transport [21]. This possibility was investigated by Sharp et al. [22], but found to be an unlikely explanation for the apparent transport observed in perivascular channels.

Arguably the simplest mechanism for causing bulk flow in the paraarterial space is a steady pressure difference between the subarachnoid space and the parenchyma. This pressure difference is small, about 1 mmHg or less [23, 24]. Two models have been developed of the flow through brain tissue [25, 26], but thus far, none have quantified the relationships between flow and pressure in the channels supplying and emptying the tissue. In this article, the potential for bulk flow within these channels is tested with mathematical models of the periarterial, paraarterial and paravenous trees.

Methods

Vascular tree models

In the following subsections, simplified models of periarterial, paraarterial and paravenous trees of annular cross section, through which amyloid-β and other tracers are assumed to flow, are explained.

Periarterial

For the periarterial space, the basement membrane between SMC layers was taken as 100 nm thick [9]. This gap between cells forms an irregular path along the vessel, but for simplicity was modeled as an annulus. Depending on the size of the artery, there may be from one layer in precapillaries [27] to 20 layers in large arteries, each forming basement membrane layers between adjacent layers of cells [10]. The hypothesis involves interstitial fluid entering the branching network at the precapillaries and exiting to the lymphatics, thus intracranial pressure prevails upstream and lymphatic pressure downstream.

A one-dimensional analytical solution was obtained that models the flow as steady Poiseuille flow through annular channels with rigid walls. The effect of the porous media in the channels was neglected, as was resistance in the bifurcations. The model consisted of a symmetrical tree from pre-capillaries to the main cerebral arteries.

While flow in the periarterial space is hypothesized to be in the opposite direction, the tree model will be described in the more conventional direction of luminal flow. Actual dimensions were used for large arteries (i.e., internal carotid arteries, vertebral artery, basilar artery, anterior, middle and posterior cerebral arteries), for which anatomic data are available (Table 1). The vertebral and internal carotid arteries were connected to the Circle of Willis and then to the middle, anterior and posterior cerebral arteries (Fig. 2). Murray's law of bifurcations was used to model the bores of the smaller

Table 1 Anatomical sizes of the large arteries (refer to Fig. 2 for definitions of abbreviations) [38, 39]

Artery	Length, mm	Diameter, mm
VA	125	2.5
ICA	142	3.6
BA	28	3.3
PCA1	13	2
PCA2	60	2
MCA	51	3
ACA1	20	2
ACA2	45	2

arteries (point D to point P in Fig. 2) [28, 29]. Murray's law equates the cube of a parent vessel's diameter to the sum of the cubes of the daughter vessels' diameters [30]. However, while the exponent in the original Murray's equation is 3, Cassot et al. [31] showed that the exponent should be modified to 3.67 for human cerebral arteries. The daughter vessels were assumed to have equal diameters. Therefore, the radius of the parent vessel is

$$r_p = \left(\frac{1}{2}\right)^{\frac{1}{3.67}} r_d \tag{1}$$

where r_d is the radius of the daughter vessels. Due to symmetry of the tree, the radius of vessels in a generation can be obtained in terms of the zeroth generation (i.e., largest vessel) by extending Eq. 1 as

$$r_i = \left(\frac{1}{2}\right)^{\frac{i}{3.67}} r_0 \; i = 0, 1, 2, \ldots. \tag{2}$$

The vessels MCA, ACA and PCA2 (Fig. 2) were considered to be the zeroth generation ($i=0$) of six subtrees. The length of each artery was related to its own radius, which with Eq. 2 is related to that of the zeroth generation [32, 33]

$$l_i = 20\, r_i = 20\left(\frac{1}{2}\right)^{\frac{i}{3.67}} r_0. \tag{3}$$

Starting from the diameters in Table 1, 30, 28 and 28 generations were required, including the zeroth generation, to reach precapillary diameters of 12.5, 12.2 and 12.2 µm as the final generations in the MCA, ACA and PCA2 subtrees, respectively [10, 34]. (The calculated precapillary diameters are different for each subtree since the zeroth generations have unique diameters.) Including four more generations as capillaries down to 4.7 µm in diameter [35, 36], the total number of capillaries in the model is 98 billion, which agrees with estimates in the literature [37].

The precapillaries, which have only one SMC layer, were nonetheless assumed to each have an annular flow channel of the same gap dimension as one basement membrane. A basement membrane layer was added to each generation of larger arteries up to a maximum of 20 annular channels (at generations 12, 10 and 10 for MCA,

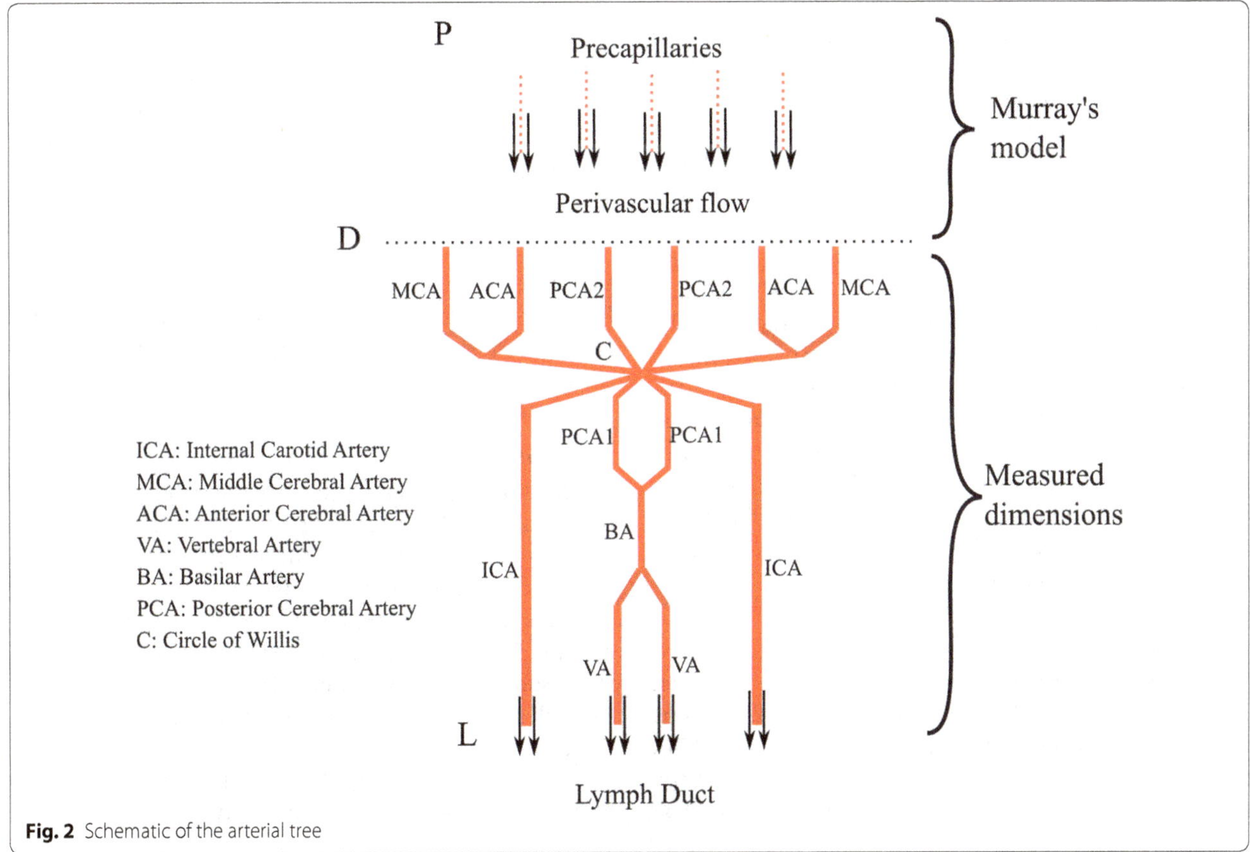

Fig. 2 Schematic of the arterial tree

ACA and PCA2, respectively). All larger generations were assigned 20 annular channels (21 SMC layers [27]).

Laminar flow resistance for the first annular space (closest to the lumen) at each generation was calculated for Poiseuille flow in an annular cross section [40]

$$R = \frac{8\mu}{\pi r^4}\left[\frac{l}{\left(k^{-4}-1\right) - \frac{\left(k^{-2}-1\right)^2}{Ln\left(k^{-1}\right)}}\right] \quad (4)$$

where R is the flow resistance, μ is the fluid viscosity, $k = r/(r+g)$ is the ratio of the inner radius to outer radius, g is the gap height of the annulus, and l is length of the arterial segment which is related to the radius of the segment by Eq. 3. As mentioned earlier, the thickness of a basement membrane was taken as $g = 100$ nm. For segments with more than one annular cross section, the same relation as Eq. 4 was used to calculate the flow resistance for annular layers other than the first one, with inner radius being $r + jg$, where $j = 1, 2, \ldots, J$ is the maximum number of annular layers in the generation.

Due to symmetry, the effective resistance of the arterial tree included identical, parallel subtrees representing MCA, ACA and PCA2 pairs.

Paraarterial

The model for the paraarterial space starts from the pial arteries (approximately 100 μm in diameter [41, 42]) in the subarachnoid space and ends at the precapillaries. To model this paraarterial part of the glymphatic system, the periarterial model was modified with different starting locations and annular spaces with different gaps. The modified model began at generations 18, 16 and 16 for MCA, ACA and PCA2 branches, respectively, where artery diameters were 100.16, 97.42 and 97.42 μm, respectively. The ratio of outer paraarterial radius to the lumen radius was assumed to be constant through the tree and equal to 1.12 [13] (about 12 μm gaps for the largest arteries of all three branches), except in the precapillaries where the annular gap was again assumed to be $g = 100$ nm [20]. Using this ratio (i.e., 1.12), the ratio of inner radius to outer radius in the paraarterial tree was calculated to be $k = 0.6652$. Flow resistance in each branch was calculated using Eq. 4.

Paravenous

The paravenous space begins at the postcapillaries just after the capillaries. The number of postcapillaries was taken to be the same as the number of precapillaries [34], but the diameter (20 μm) of postcapillaries was slightly larger [34, 43]. Taking the power in Murray's law as 3.54 for veins [31], after 10 generations the diameter of pial veins became 141.7 μm, which is in approximate agreement with observations [44, 45]. Equation 3 was again assumed to scale the length of veins, and Eq. 4 was used to calculate the flow resistance for the paravenous tree, except that $k = 0.94$, based on the ratio of paravenous to luminal area of 0.13 found for veins [13] (about a 18 μm gap for the pial veins).

Case conditions

The density and kinematic viscosity of interstitial and cerebrospinal fluid taken to be that of water at body temperature, $\rho = 993$ kg/m^3 and $\nu = 7 \times 10^{-7}$ m^2/s.

The resistance of the perivascular model was used to calculate the interstitial fluid perfusion that would result from a pressure drop of 14 mmHg, representing a typical difference between intracranial and lymphatic duct pressures [46]. These flow rates were compared to two different estimates of interstitial fluid perfusion. First, extrapolating from estimated interstitial fluid production in the rat brain of 0.1–0.3 μl/min/g [47, 48], flow rates in the human brain become 0.13–0.39 ml/min (assuming a mass of 1.3 kg). Second, since the brain receives about 15% of the total cardiac output [49], another estimate can be calculated as 15% of the lymphatic flow rate in the whole body of 1.4–2.1 ml/min [50, 51], which gives 0.21–0.32 ml/min. These estimates are in substantial agreement.

For the paraarterial model, the pressure difference necessary to drive the minimum flow rate of 0.13 ml/min from the cortical subarachnoid space to the parenchyma (and from parenchyma to CSF space for the paravenous model) was calculated.

Results

In this section, results of flow resistance for the periarterial, paraarterial and paravenous tree models, described above, are presented.

Periarterial flow

Periarterial resistance of the large arteries upstream of the Circle of Willis (between points L and C in Fig. 2) was calculated to be 2.13×10^8 mmHg/ml/min. Periarterial resistance from the Circle of Willis to the precapillaries (between points C and P) was equal to 1.4×10^8 mmHg/ml/min. Therefore, the total periarterial flow resistance is the sum of these two values, 3.53×10^8 mmHg/ml/min (the full cumulative resistance at the zeroth generation in Fig. 3).

For comparison, taking the typical pressure difference of 14 mmHg between the parenchyma and lymphatic

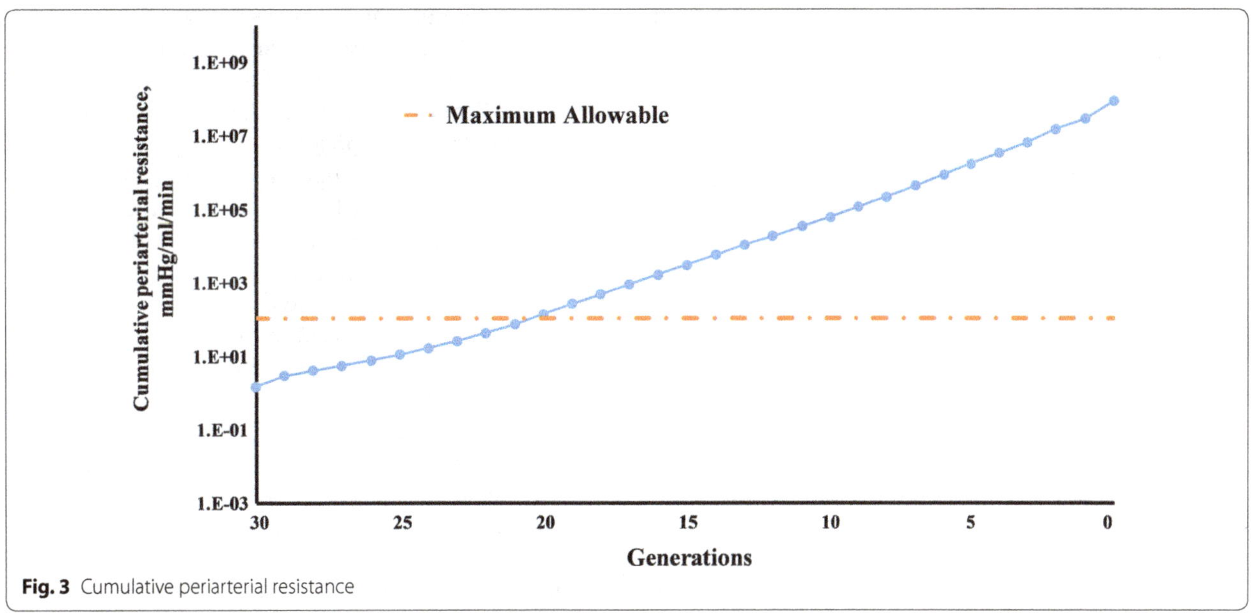

Fig. 3 Cumulative periarterial resistance

ducts and the lower limit of the range of interstitial fluid production of 0.13 ml/min gives a maximum flow resistance of 107.76 mmHg/ml/min to allow physiologic interstitial fluid clearance by the periarterial pathway (the dashed line in Fig. 3). To not exceed this maximum resistance, the flow would need to exit the periarterial tree to lymphatic ducts after no more than 10 generations (generations 30–21, Fig. 3). The diameters of the 21st generations are 56.83, 37.89 and 37.89 μm for MCA, ACA and PCA2 branches, which is still 3, 5 and 5 generations away from the pial arteries, respectively.

Paraarterial flow

The total resistance of the paraarterial model was calculated to be 1.14 mmHg/ml/min (Fig. 4). As can be seen in Fig. 4, the resistance of the paraarterial tree model is dominated by the small gaps in the precapillaries. If flow in the tree exits to the parenchyma earlier, then the resistance is about three orders of magnitude lower. Since the glymphatic circulation in the paraarterial space is hypothesized to originate in the cortical subarachnoid space and terminate in the parenchyma, a large pressure difference between the two ends is not expected. Therefore, the approach taken was to calculate the

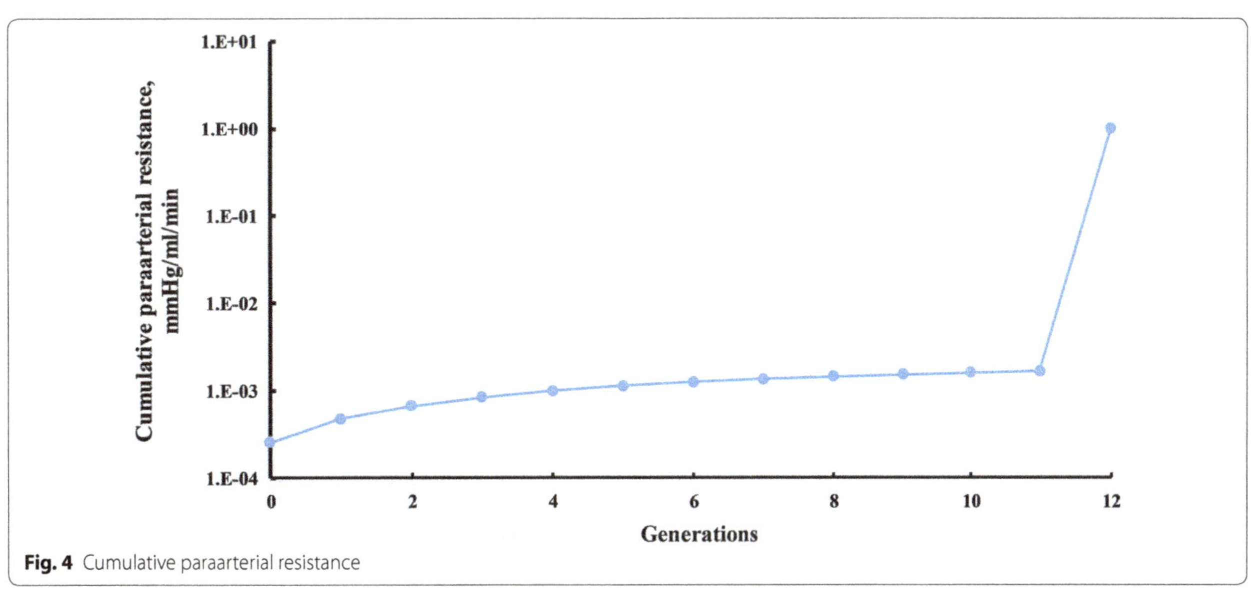

Fig. 4 Cumulative paraarterial resistance

pressure difference required to cause the lowest flow rate of 0.13 ml/min through the paraarterial tree. This lowest required pressure difference was 0.15 mmHg.

Paravenous flow

The total resistance of the paravenous tree was equal to 1.75×10^{-3} mmHg/ml/min, about three orders of magnitude smaller than that of the paraarterial tree (Fig. 5), which can be expected based on the larger gaps and larger vessel diameters compared to the paraarterial channels. A more consistent generation-to-generation increase in resistance is also evident. The required pressure difference to drive 0.13 ml/min of flow through the paravenous tree was calculated to be 0.00023 mmHg. If flow entered from the parenchyma later than the post capillaries, resistance would be even lower.

Discussion

The resistance of the full periarterial tree is approximately 4 million times too large to be a plausible pathway for steady, pressure-driven clearance. For 14 mmHg of pressure to drive 0.13 ml/min of flow, the periarterial tree would have to terminate at the 21st generation, which is still within the parenchyma.

Only 0.15 mmHg of pressure between the cortical subarachnoid space and the parenchyma is required to drive the same flow through the larger (larger annular gap) and shorter paraarterial tree. Such a pressure difference is not implausible, since it is within the range of estimates for this pressure difference [23, 24]. However, the hypothesized paravenous flow also terminates in the CSF space. Therefore, the total pressure difference driving both paraarterial and paravenous flows can be no greater than the transmantle pressure, which is estimated to be no greater than 0.03 mmHg [19]. The required paraarterial pressure difference alone being larger than this means that combined steady pressure-driven glymphatic flow along the entire length of both trees is unlikely.

If, however, flow exits the paraarterial tree before the precapillaries, the cumulative resistance of the paraarterial tree is 1.68×10^{-3} mmHg/ml/min. In this case, the pressure difference required to drive 0.13 ml/min of flow through both trees is 0.00045 mmHg, which is considerably less than the maximum transmantle pressure.

Because the cranium has low compliance, injections increase pressure in the space in which they occur. For instance, Iliff et al. [52] reported a 2.5 mmHg elevation of intracranial pressure during a 10 μl injection of tracer at a rate of 1 μl/min into the cisterna magna. According to the models in this work, this increase in pressure is significantly larger than that required to drive flow in the paravascular spaces. While some investigators have used smaller injection rates (e.g., Carare et al. [18] used injections of 0.5 μl over at least 2 min), observed transport may be in part an artifact of the location of injection.

On the other hand, the evidence for flow in these spaces is based on observation of the appearance of tracers in the channels some time after injection into the cerebrospinal fluid space or parenchyma. Therefore, solute, but not solvent, transport is a less stringent requirement to explain these observations. Shear-augmented dispersion [22] and streaming [53] are possible mechanisms that can cause tracer transport in the absence of net bulk flow in a particular direction.

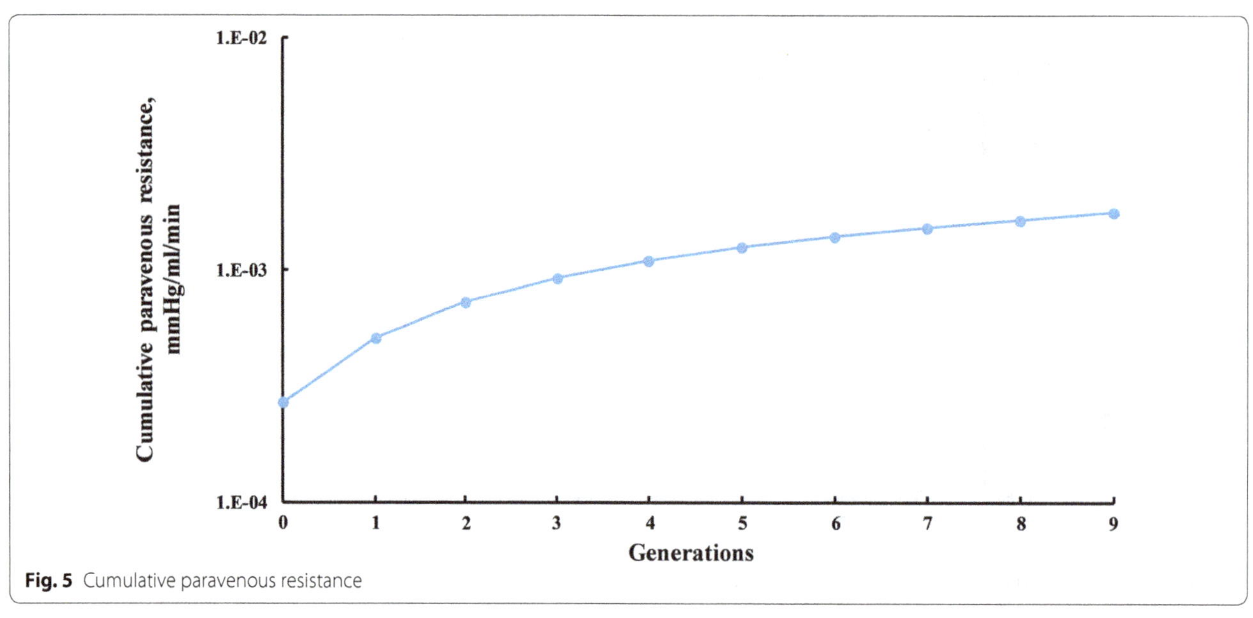

Fig. 5 Cumulative paravenous resistance

Limitations of the models include ignoring the tortuosity of the channels and the effects of branches and porous media, all of which would increase resistance, making it more difficult to explain hydraulically-driven flow in these channels.

A Darcy–Brinkman model can be used to estimate the influence of porous media. Using this model, the increase in resistance of the channel for large Darcy number *Da* scales with $Da^2/3$ [54]. For basement membranes with permeability of 1.432×10^{-18} m^2 [55], *Da* becomes 41.8 and resistance in the periarterial channels with porous media is 582 times higher than without porous media. The increase in resistance in the paravascular spaces depends on the gap dimension, with the largest increase occurring for the largest gap (surrounding the largest vessels). For a 12 μm gap around the largest arteries of the paraarterial tree and with an estimated permeability of 1.8×10^{-14} m^2 [56], *Da* becomes 44.7 and resistance in the largest paraarterial channels with porous media is 667 times higher. For a 18.4 μm gap around the pial veins of the paravenous tree and with the same estimated permeability, *Da* becomes 67.6 and resistance in the largest paravenous channels with porous media is 1567 times higher.

With porous media, the resistance of the periarterial tree becomes about 2 billion times too large to support the estimated physiologic flow. This result further reinforces the implausibility of pressure-driven flow in these channels.

Applying the resistance increases due to porous media estimated above to the entire paravascular trees, the required pressure differences become 99 and 0.36 mmHg for the paraarterial and paravenous trees, respectively. The necessary paravenous pressure difference is still small. The required paraarterial pressure difference, however, is beyond the range measured or theorized between the parenchyma and CSF spaces. To be limited to the transmantle pressure, flow would need to exit the pararterial tree earlier and enter the paravenous tree later. The total resistance of the two truncated trees could be no larger than 0.23 mmHg/ml/min for the transmantle pressure to drive 0.13 ml/min of flow. Maximum truncation would correspond to pial arteries only for the paraarterial tree and pial veins only for the paravenous tree. Without porous media, the resistances of the paraarterial channels surrounding the pial arteries and the paravenous channels surrounding the pial veins are 2.56×10^{-4} and 2.69×10^{-4} mmHg/ml/min, respectively (Figs. 4 and 5). With the Darcy numbers estimated above, the resistance of the paraarterial channels becomes 0.171 mmHg/ml/min, and that of the paravenous channels becomes 0.422 mmHg/ml/min. The combined resistance exceeds the transmantle pressure by a factor of 19.7. Though this rather large factor suggests that significant glymphatic circulation does not occur, the uncertainties of the accuracy of anatomical and kinematic variables involved in these estimates dictate caution regarding such a conclusion. If five estimates were in error by factors of 1.8 (say, roughly half the flow rate driven by twice the transmantle pressure in twice as many vessels with double the gap and double the permeability), then agreement would be obtained. This possibility highlights the need for in vivo measurements of these parameters.

Peristalsis represents an alternative mechanism for driving flows in these channels. The maximum peristaltic pressure that could possibly occur in the channels surrounding arteries can be estimated as the carotid artery pulse pressure of about 40 mmHg. This pressure is substantially higher than the 14 mmHg available for retrograde periarterial flow and the 0.03 mmHg transmantle pressure for paravascular flows. However, a confounding factor is that the wavelength of the blood pressure pulse (~ 10 m [57]) is much longer than the cerebral vessels. Under these conditions, arterial wall motion occurs nearly simultaneously along the entire channel, thus axial pressure gradients and the cycle-averaged flow in a particular direction that can be drive by them are small [25, 26]. Other contributing mechanisms in combination with wall motion are necessary to drive significant flow. (See, for instance, [6–8]. While the focus of these papers are on explaining retrograde flow in the periarterial space, similar, reversed mechanisms could promote forward flow in the paraarterial space.) Because venous pressure is less pulsatile, the potential for peristaltically-driven flow in the paravenous space is lower. With porous media, however, the estimated necessary pressure difference of 99 mmHg is double that available from the arterial pulse pressure. The additional resistance of porous media makes peristalsis a questionable driver of paraarterial flows even if another mechanism promotes forward flow.

Conclusions

Significant steady pressure-driven flow in the periarterial space is found to be unlikely, unless flow exits to the lymphatic circulation after only a few generations. An outlet to the lymphatic system at this early level has not been identified. With channel resistance increased by two orders of magnitude by porous media, steady pressure-driven flow becomes even less plausible.

A fundamental paradox of the glymphatic circulation is that cortical subarachnoid space pressure must be high to drive steady flow through paraarterial channels, but low pressure must prevail in the CSF space terminus downstream of the paravenous channels to draw flow through these channels. Even without porous media, the combined pressure difference required to drive flow through both trees exceeds the maximum transmantle pressure. With porous media, the necessary pressure is at least two orders of magnitude higher. Therefore, steady pressure-driven glymphatic flow through the entirety of both trees is also implausible. Predictions are less clear for flow through truncated trees. With porous media, the combined resistance of the paravascular spaces of just the pial arteries and veins also exceeds the transmantle pressure. However, the mismatch is small enough that uncertainties in parameter estimates limit confidence in a conclusion of implausibility of flow.

Although the blood pressure pulse wavelength is too long to allow peristalsis alone to drive these flows, the current results cannot rule out its importance in combination with another mechanism [6–8]. So far, these contributing mechanisms have not been confirmed by experiments, nor have the models been applied to branching networks of channels to determine the magnitude of total brain perfusion that could result. Both avenues of further investigation could yield valuable insights to explain the transport of tracers observed in experiments.

Abbreviations

ACA: anterior cerebral artery; MCA: middle cerebral artery; PCA: posterior cerebral artery; SMC: smooth muscle cells.

Authors' contributions

MKS conceived the research. MMF developed the model and performed the calculations. MMF and MKS analyzed the results and wrote the paper. Both authors read and approved the final manuscript.

Competing interests

The authors declare that they have no competing interests.

References

1. Robin C. Recherches sur quelques particularites de la structure des capillaires de l'encephale. J Physiol Homme Animaux. 1859;2:537–48.
2. Virchow R. Ueber die erweiterung kleinerer gefaesse. Arch Pathol Anat Physiol Klin Med. 1851;3:427–62.
3. Woollam DHM, Millen JW. The perivascular spaces of the mammalian central nervous system and their relation to the perineuronal and subarachnoid spaces. J Anat. 1955;89(193–200):191.
4. Iliff JJ, Wang M, Liao Y, Plogg BA, Peng W, Gundersen GA, Benveniste H, Vates GE, Deane R, Goldman SA, et al. A paravascular pathway facilitates CSF flow through the brain parenchyma and the clearance of interstitial solutes, including amyloid beta. Sci Transl Med. 2012;4:147ra111.
5. Hladky SB, Barrand MA. Mechanisms of fluid movement into, through and out of the brain: evaluation of the evidence. Fluids Barriers CNS. 2014;11:26.
6. Schley D, Carare-Nnadi R, Please CP, Perry VH, Weller RO. Mechanisms to explain the reverse perivascular transport of solutes out of the brain. J Theor Biol. 2006;238:962–74.
7. Sharp MK, Diem AK, Weller RO, Carare RO. Peristalsis with oscillating flow resistance: a mechanism for periarterial clearance of amyloid beta from the brain. Ann Biomed Eng. 2016;44:1553–65.
8. Coloma M, Schaffer JD, Carare RO, Chiarot PR, Huang P. Pulsations with reflected boundary waves: a hydrodynamic reverse transport mechanism for perivascular drainage in the brain. J Math Biol. 2016;73:469–90.
9. Yurchenco PD. Basement membranes cell scaffoldings and signaling platforms. Cold Spring Harb Perspect Biol. 2011;3:a004911.
10. Shiraishi T, Sakaki S, Uehara Y. Architecture of the medial smooth muscle of the arterial vessels in the normal human brain: a scanning electron-microscopic study. Scan Microsc. 1990;4:191–9.
11. Weed LH. The absorption of cerebrospinal fluid into the venous system. Am J Anat. 1923;31:191–221.
12. Zhang ET, Inman CB, Weller RO. Interrelationships of the pia mater and the perivascular (Virchow–Robin) spaces in the human cerebrum. J Anat. 1990;170:111–23.
13. Schain AJ, Melo-Carrillo A, Strassman AM, Burstein R. Cortical spreading depression closes paravascular space and impairs glymphatic flow: implications for migraine headache. J Neurosci. 2017;37:2904–15.
14. Tomita M, Tomita Y, Unekawa M, Toriumi H, Suzuki N. Oscillating neurocapillary coupling during cortical spreading depression as observed by tracking of FITC-labeled RBCs in single capillaries. Neuroimage. 2011;56:1001–10.
15. Hawkes CA, Jayakody N, Johnston DA, Bechmann I, Carare RO. Failure of perivascular drainage of beta-amyloid in cerebral amyloid angiopathy. Brain Pathol. 2014;24:396–403.
16. Weller RO, Djuanda E, Yow HY, Carare RO. Lymphatic drainage of the brain and the pathophysiology of neurological disease. Acta Neuropathol. 2009;117:1–14.
17. Jessen NA, Munk AS, Lundgaard I, Nedergaard M. The glymphatic system: a beginner's guide. Neurochem Res. 2015;40:2583–99.
18. Carare RO, Bernardes-Silva M, Newman TA, Page AM, Nicoll JA, Perry VH, Weller RO. Solutes, but not cells, drain from the brain parenchyma along basement membranes of capillaries and arteries: significance for cerebral amyloid angiopathy and neuroimmunology. Neuropathol Appl Neurobiol. 2008;34:131–44.
19. Sweetman B, Xenos M, Zitella L, Linninger AA. Three-dimensional computational prediction of cerebrospinal fluid flow in the human brain. Comput Biol Med. 2011;41:67–75.
20. Bedussi B, van der Wel NN, de Vos J, van Veen H, Siebes M, VanBavel E, Bakker EN. Paravascular channels, cisterns, and the subarachnoid space in the rat brain: a single compartment with preferential pathways. J Cereb Blood Flow Metab. 2017;37:1374–85.
21. Sharp MK, Kamm RD, Shapiro AH, Kimmel E, Karniadakis GE. Dispersion in a curved tube during oscillatory flow. J Fluid Mech. 1991;223:537–63.
22. Sharp MK, Darcy-Brinkman model of shearaugmented dispersion in cerebrovascular basement membranes and the spinal subarachnoid space. 2017 Cerebrospinal Fluid Dynamics Symposium, Atlanta, GA, 19–20 June 2017.
23. Penn RD, Linninger A. The physics of hydrocephalus. Pediatr Neurosurg. 2009;45:161–74.
24. Shahim K, Drezet JM, Martin BA, Momjian S. Ventricle equilibrium position in healthy and normal pressure hydrocephalus brains using an analytical model. J Biomech Eng. 2012;134:041007.
25. Asgari M, de Zelicourt D, Kurtcuoglu V. Glymphatic solute transport does not require bulk flow. Sci Rep. 2016;6:38635.
26. Jin BJ, Smith AJ, Verkman AS. Spatial model of convective solute transport in brain extracellular space does not support a "glymphatic" mechanism. J Gen Physiol. 2016;148:489–501.
27. Cipolla MJ. The cerebral circulation. San Rafael: Morgan & Claypool Life Sciences; 2010.
28. Mut F, Wright S, Ascoli GA, Cebral JR. Morphometric, geographic and territorial characterization of brain arterial trees. Int J Numer Methods Biomed Eng. 2014;30:755–66.

29. Moreau B, Mauroy B. Murray's law revisited: quémada's fluid model and fractal trees. J Rheol. 2015;59:1419–30.
30. Murray CD. The physiological principle of minimum work: i. The vascular system and the cost of blood volume. Proc Natl Acad Sci USA. 1926;12:207–14.
31. Cassot F, Lauwers F, Lorthois S, Puwanarajah P, Cances-Lauwers V, Duvernoy H. Branching patterns for arterioles and venules of the human cerebral cortex. Brain Res. 2010;1313:62–78.
32. Zamir M. On fractal properties of arterial trees. J Theor Biol. 1999;197:517–26.
33. Gabryś E, Rybaczuk M, Kędzia A. Fractal models of circulatory system. Symmetrical and asymmetrical approach comparison. Chaos Solitons Fractals. 2005;24:707–15.
34. Masamoto K, Hirase H, Yamada K. New horizons in neurovascular coupling a bridge between brain circulation and neural plasticity. Amsterdam: Elsevier; 2016.
35. Gaehtgens P. Flow of blood through narrow capillaries: rheological mechanisms determining capillary hematocrit and apparent viscosity. Biorheology. 1980;17:183–9.
36. Guyton AC, Hall JE. Human physiology and mechanisms of disease. Philadelphia: W.B. Saunders; 1997.
37. Pardridge WM. The blood-brain barrier: bottleneck in brain drug development. NeuroRx. 2005;2:3–14.
38. Kamath S. Observations on the length and diameter of vessels forming the circle of Willis. J Anat. 1981;133:419–23.
39. Cieslicki K. Experimental and numerical modeling in cerebral arteries. J Med Informat Technol. 2004;7:17–26.
40. Rosenhead L. Laminar boundary layers: An account of the development, structure and stability of laminar boundary layers in incompressible fluids, together with a description of the associated experimental techniques. New York: Dover; 1988.
41. Bevan JA, Dodge J, Walters CL, Wellman T, Bevan RD. Dimensions and wall force development capacity of human pial arteries from normotensives is not altered in obesity. Int J Obes Relat Metab Disord. 2001;25:756–8.
42. Moody DM, Bell MA, Challa VR. Features of the cerebral vascular pattern that predict vulnerability to perfusion or oxygenation deficiency: an anatomic study. Am J Neuroradiol. 1990;11:431–9.
43. Shepro D. Microvascular research: Biology and pathology. Amsterdam: Elsevier, Acad. Press; 2006.
44. Duvernoy HM. The human brain: surface, three-dimensional sectional anatomy with MRI and blood supply. Wien: Springer; 1999.
45. Duvernoy HM, Delon S, Vannson JL. Cortical blood vessels of the human brain. Brain Res Bull. 1981;7:519–79.
46. Rangel-Castillo L, Gopinath S, Robertson CS. Management of intracranial hypertension. Neurol Clin. 2008;26:521–41.
47. Abbott NJ. Evidence for bulk flow of brain interstitial fluid: significance for physiology and pathology. Neurochem Int. 2004;45:545–52.
48. Szentistvanyi I, Patlak CS, Ellis RA, Cserr HF. Drainage of interstitial fluid from different regions of rat brain. Am J Physiol. 1984;246:F835–44.
49. Meng L, Hou W, Chui J, Han R, Gelb AW. Cardiac output and cerebral blood flow: the integrated regulation of brain perfusion in adult humans. Anesthesiology. 2015;123:1198–208.
50. Yoffey JM, Courtice FC. Lymphatics, lymph and the lymphomyeloid complex. London: Academic Press Inc; 1970.
51. Orban BJ, Sicher H. Orban's oral histology and embryology. 5th ed. Saint Louis: C.V. Mosby Co.; 1962.
52. Iliff JJ, Wang M, Zeppenfeld DM, Venkataraman A, Plog BA, Liao Y, Deane R, Nedergaard M. Cerebral arterial pulsation drives paravascular CSF-interstitial fluid exchange in the murine brain. J Neurosci. 2013;33:18190–9.
53. Riley N. Steady streaming. Annu Rev Fluid Mech. 2001;33:43–65.
54. Liu H, Patil P, Narusawa U. On Darcy–Brinkman equation: viscous flow between two parallel plates packed with regular square arrays of cylinders. Entropy. 2007;9:118.
55. Tedgui A, Lever MJ. Filtration through damaged and undamaged rabbit thoracic aorta. Am J Physiol. 1984;247:H784–91.
56. Wang P, Olbricht WL. Fluid mechanics in the perivascular space. J Theor Biol. 2011;274:52–7.
57. Mitchell GF, van Buchem MA, Sigurdsson S, Gotal JD, Jonsdottir MK, Kjartansson O, Garcia M, Aspelund T, Harris TB, Gudnason V, Launer LJ. Arterial stiffness, pressure and flow pulsatility and brain structure and function: the age, gene/environment susceptibility-Reykjavik study. Brain. 2011;134:3398–407.

20

Extracellular vesicles: mediators and biomarkers of pathology along CNS barriers

Servio H. Ramirez[1,2,3*], Allison M. Andrews[1,3], Debayon Paul[4] and Joel S. Pachter[4*]

Abstract

Extracellular vesicles (EVs) are heterogeneous, nano-sized vesicles that are shed into the blood and other body fluids, which disperse a variety of bioactive molecules (e.g., protein, mRNA, miRNA, DNA and lipids) to cellular targets over long and short distances. EVs are thought to be produced by nearly every cell type, however this review will focus specifically on EVs that originate from cells at the interface of CNS barriers. Highlighted topics include, EV biogenesis, the production of EVs in response to neuroinflammation, role in intercellular communication and their utility as a therapeutic platform. In this review, novel concepts regarding the use of EVs as biomarkers for BBB status and as facilitators for immune neuroinvasion are also discussed. Future directions and prospective are covered along with important unanswered questions in the field of CNS endothelial EV biology.

Keywords: Brain endothelial cells, Blood brain barrier, Extracellular vesicles, Microvesicles, Exosomes, Neuroinflammation

Background

In the field of observation, chance favors only the prepared mind
Louis Pasteur

The observation by Chargaff and West in 1946, that a high-speed pellet derived from centrifuging blood contained factors that accelerated clotting of plasma—factors later recognized, in 1967, as bioactive vesicles and accorded the term "platelet dust" by Wolf [1]—has spawned a vast new field of biology with increasing ramifications in medicine and therapeutics. This advance would never have happened had early investigators not previously recognized the potential of "conditioned media" from cultured cells to impact growth and metabolism. It became clear that cell-derived factors released into extracellular fluid—both plasma and culture media—had nutritional value and powerful signaling potential. While many of these factors are simple organic solutes singularly secreted or transported, those of the platelet dust variety are complex, phospho-lipid, bilayer, plasma membranes that enclose cytoplasmic material and are shed from cells. Broad in derivation, composition, and activity, these membrane derivatives are now conventionally known as *extracellular vesicles*—more commonly referred to simply as EVs [2, 3].

As general reviews on EVs are vast, it is not the objective of this article to reiterate the already extensive literature on the well-recognized aspects of EV biogenesis and properties. Instead, given their burgeoning roles in neuroscience and neurology—including developmental biology [4, 5], neuroinflammation [6, 7], neuroinfection [8, 9], neurodegeneration [10, 11], brain tumors [12, 13], and psychiatric disease [14, 15]—the focus here is specifically on EVs that originate from and/or impact (CNS) barriers, and the prospects of EVs for diagnosis and treatment of neuroinflammatory/neurodegenerative diseases having CNS barrier involvement. However, where helpful in drawing certain analogies, references to EV activities along the peripheral vascular endothelium are included. And some general background in EVs is provided to aid

*Correspondence: servio.ramirez@temple.edu; pachter@uchc.edu
[1] Department of Pathology and Laboratory Medicine, The Lewis Katz School of Medicine at Temple University, 3500 N Broad St, Philadelphia, PA 19140, USA
[4] Department of Immunology, Blood-Brain Barrier Laboratory & Laser Capture Microdissection Core, UConn Health, 263 Farmington Ave., Farmington, CT 06070, USA
Full list of author information is available at the end of the article

in appreciating the roles of EVs in CNS barrier physiology, pathophysiology and therapy.

EVs are heterogeneous, nano-sized vesicles shed into blood and other body fluids by many cell types, which disperse a variety of bioactive molecules (e.g., protein, mRNA, miRNA, DNA and lipids) to cellular targets over long and short distances [16–19]. There are three EV subtypes conventionally recognized that are distinguished based on their respective size and route of biogenesis [3, 20, 21]. Two of these are released by live cells both constitutively and in response to stimulation, and are classified as *exosomes* (30–100 nm diameter) and *microvesicles* (100–1000 nm diameter (sometimes referred to as 'microparticles' [MPs]), though sometimes their respective sizes overlap (Fig. 1 and Table 1). Exosomes derive from in-budding of endosomes to form multi-vesicular bodies that fuse with the plasma membrane to release the membrane vesicles into the extracellular space. Microvesicles form by outward budding of the plasma membrane. A third subtype, *apoptotic bodies* (> 1000 nm), are released from dying cells and will not be a subject of this review. Besides originating via distinct processes, the varied subtype EVs—even from the same cell—carry different cargo within their membrane and luminal compartments and, a priori, execute different functions [22]. Recent evidence further suggests protein content of EVs might reflect the phenotype of the tissue of origin, such as the inflammatory state of the brain microvascular endothelium [23]. While all EVs tend to be highly enriched in tetraspanins, e.g., CD9, CD63, CD81, CD82 and CD151 [24], a consensus protein signature that faithfully distinguishes exosomes from microvesicles has not yet been realized. However, differential expression of proteins PDCC6IP and SDCB1 by exosomes, and ATP5A1, RACGAP1, and SEPT2 by microvesicles was observed in EVs released by cultured brain microvascular endothelial cells (BMECs)—which form the BBB—stimulated by the pro-inflammatory cytokine TNF-α [23] (Note: henceforth in this manuscript, in examples where brain endothelial cells are known to be specifically of microvessel origin, they will be referred to as BMEC; in other cases they will simply be noted as brain ECs). Exosomes from a human colon cancer cell line have further been shown to contain presumed "exosome marker proteins" Alix, TSG101, CD81 and CD63 not found in microvesicles isolated from culture supernatant of the same cells, while microvesicles showed selective enrichment of another 350 proteins [25]. And, there has also been report of unique miRNA sequences expressed by separate exosome and microvesicle populations isolated from blood of patients with clinically isolated syndrome (CSI), the first clinical evidence of CNS demyelination [26]. With refinements in isolation and characterization of EVs, there is expected to be growing awareness of additional unique markers for, and properties of, the different EV subtypes. These distinctions are likely to

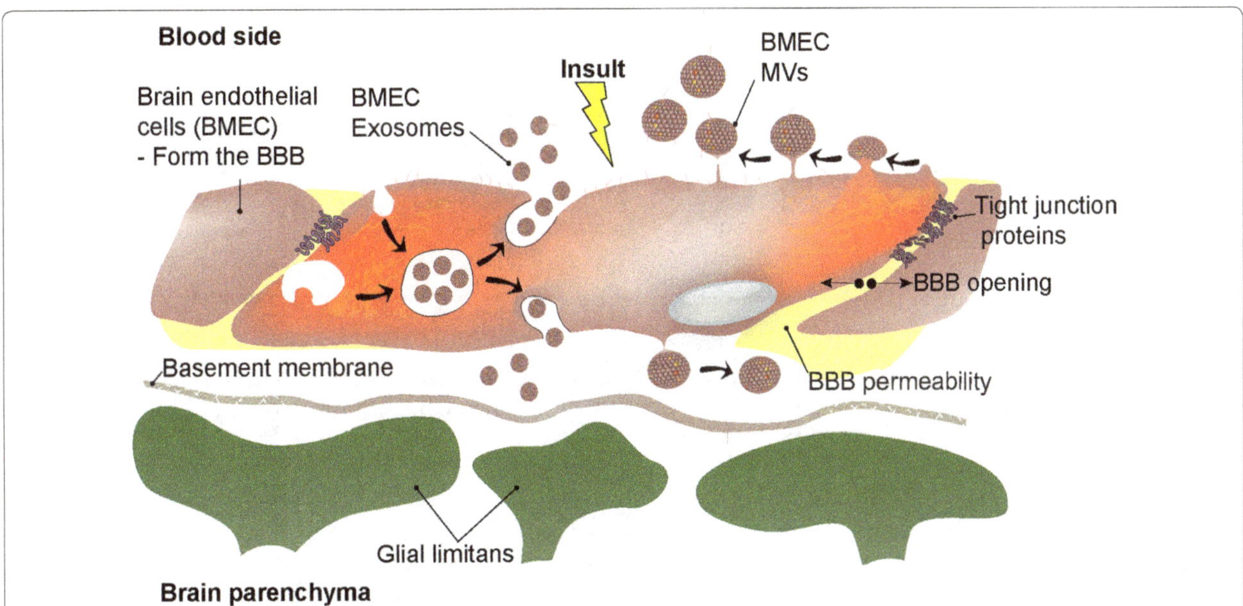

Fig. 1 Microvesicle (MV) and exosome biogenesis in brain endothelial cells. Upon inflammatory stimuli, brain endothelial cells respond by releasing MVs (microvesicles) and exosomes into the bloodstream and/or in theory perivascularly. For exosomes, stimuli lead to internalization and formation of early endosomes that invaginate to create multivesicular bodies (MVB). For MVs, the vesicle is formed from budding of the plasma membrane. Vesicles are then released either into the blood or the brain parenchyma (theorized)

hold significance for physiological and pathophysiological roles of EVs at CNS barriers, and enable EVs to be exploited therapeutically and also serve as biomarkers of disease.

There are several types of CNS barriers. Perhaps the most widely recognized is the blood–brain barrier (BBB), which lies at the level of parenchymal microvessels and is formed by a monolayer of specialized endothelial cells

Table 1 Markers, means of preparation, source (circulation or tissue culture), and assay of brain barrier-derived EVs according to subtype (exosomes or microvesicles)

TYPE	MARKERS	SIZE	ISOLATION	SOURCE	ASSAY	REF.
Microvesicles (MVs)	SEPT2 RACGAP1 ATP5A1 KIF23 CSE1L	150-300nm (TEM) 215-375nm (NTA)	Removal: 300*g*, 10 min, 4°C 2000*g*, 20 min, 4°C Pellet: 18000*g*, 45 min, 4°C	hCMEC/D3	Parallel reaction monitoring	[23]
	CLN-5	100-300nm (NTA)	Removal: 300*g*, 10 min, 4°C 2000g, 10 min, 4°C Pellet: Large MV 20000*g*, 30 min, 4°C Small MV 60000*g*, 30 min, 4°C	1. Primary-derived BMEC from eGFP-CLN-5 mice by immuno-bead selection 2. bEND3	FC, WB	[44]
	Occludin	100-300nm (cryo-EM)	Removal: 2000*g*, 20 min Polymer-based precipitation	1. Primary human BMECs 2. Murine plasma from animals with/without TBI	WB, FC, Cryo-EM	[60]
	CD31 CD42- CD62E CD54 (unknown EC origin from patient samples)		Pellet: 42000*g*, 15 min	1. Human cerebral microvascular EC (MVEC) 2. Serum from patients with/without MS	FC	[82]
	Annexin V CD105 ICAM-1 VCAM-1 MHC-I MHCII CD50 ICOSL		Removal: 1800*g*, 5 min Pellet: 18000*g*, 45 min	HBEC (Angio-proteomie Inc.), Mouse brain microvascular endothelial cells from C57BL/6 mice	FC	[91]
	Annexin V CD42b- CD31 (unknown EC origin from patient samples)		Removal: 3200*g*, 30 min 13000*g*, 10 min, Pellet: 18000*g*, 45 min	Serum from patients with/without MS	FC	[119]
	Annexin V CD41a- CD144 (unknown EC origin from patient samples)		Removal: 2600*g*, 15 min, 10°C 9900*g*, 5 min, 10°C Pellet: 17800*g*, 20 min x2	Serum from patients with/without Alzheimer's	FC	[122]
Exosomes	CD81 CD9 SDCB1 PDCD6IP	40-120nm (TEM) ~150nm (NTA)	Removal: 300*g*, 10 min, 4°C 2000*g*, 20 min, 4°C 18000*g*, 45 min, 4°C Pellet: 100000g, 120 min, 4°C	hCMEC/D3	Parallel reaction monitoring	[23]
	CLD-5	30-120nm (NTA)	Removal: 300*g*, 10 min, 4°C 2000*g*, 10 min, 4°C 20000*g*, 30 min, 4°C 60000*g*, 30 min, 4°C Pellet: 100000*g*, 60 min, 4°C	1. Primary-derived BMEC were obtained from eGFP-CLN-5 mice by immuno-bead selection 2. bEND3	WB	[44]
	Occludin	50nm (Cryo-EM)	Removal: 2000*g*, 20min Polymer-based precipitation	1. Primary human BMECs 2. Murine plasma from animals with/without TBI	Cryo-EM	[45]
	CD63	68nm, 600nm, 5000nm (DLS peaks, smallest assumed exosomes)	Polymer-based precipitation	Primary human brain microvascular endothelial cells	FL	[66]
	CD9 CD63 CD81	<150nm (SEM), 30-100nm (NanoC)	Removal: 2000*g*, 30min Polymer-based precipitation Pellet: 10000*g*, 60min	bEND.3	WB, ELISA	[178]
	CD63, CD9	95nm (NTA)	Removal: 3000*g*, 15min. Polymer-based precipitation	Rat brain microvascular endothelial cells	WB	[63]

Table 1 (continued)

TYPE	MARKERS	SIZE	ISOLATION	SOURCE	ASSAY	REF.
Unspecified/Undefined	N/A		Size exclusion (filtration at 0.22μm) Pellet: 120000*g*, 18Hr	Brain vascular endothelial cells (GP-8; ATCC)	No EV Characterization	[64]
	TSG101 Alix CD31 (Plasma, of unknown origin, CD31 assumed from cerebral vasculature)	80-200nm (TRPS, Izon Science Inc.)	Removal: 2700*g*, 10min Pellet: 120000*g*, 120min, 4°C	1. Murine brain vascular endothelial cells (bEND.3; ATCC) 2. C57BL/6 mice w/wo TBI	WB (Plasma)	[179]
	PKH26-positive labeling of vesicles, VEGFR-2 CD62E		Removal: 1000rpm, 10min, 4°C Pellet: 100000*g*, 90min, 4°C	Murine brain vascular endothelial cells (bEND.3, ATCC)	FC (EV counts measure, assumed MVs) DIC and IFA	[67]
	CD31 ICAM-1		Removal: 2000*g*, 20min Polymer-based precipitation	Primary human BMECs	WB	[45]
			Removal: 2000*g*, 20min, 4°C 10000g, 30min 4°C, Pellet: 100000g, 60min 4°C x 2	HCMEC/D3	Proteomics	[180]
	AnnexinV CD31 CD42b CD62E		Removal: 1500*g*, 15min, 13000*g*, 2min Labeled supernatant	Serum from healthy, acute stroke and at-risk patients for cardiovascular disease	FC (assumed MVs)	[115]
	E-selectin, ICAM-1, CD31 (unknown EC origin from patient samples)		Removal: 1500*g* for 20 min Labeled supernatant	Serum from patients with/without Alzheimer's	FC (assumed MVs)	[121]
	CD31, CD51, CD42- (unknown EC origin from patient samples)		Removal: 1500*g*, 15 min 13000*g*, 1 min Labeled supernatant 2. Removal: 160*g*, 10min 1500*g*, 10min Labeled supernatant	1. MVEC (Cell Systems) 2. Patient Plasma (Healthy, Thrombotic thrombocytopenic purpura)	FACS (assumed MVs)	[181]
	CD31 CD51 $CD42^-$ (unknown EC origin)		Removal: 500*g*, 6min Size exclusion (filtration at 0.1μm) Labeled supernatant	Serum from patients with/without MS (symptomatic and remission status)	FC (assumed MVs)	[87]
	AnnexinV $CD144^+$ $CD41a^-$ CD31 $CD41a^-$ $CD62E^+$ (unknown EC origin)		1500*g*, 10min, 4°C 2700*g*, 30min, 4 °C (labeled supernatant)	Serum from healthy and acute ischemic stroke patients	FC (assumed MVs)	[117]
	Alix, CD63 TSG101 CD81 LAMP-2	100nm (SEM)	Polymer-based precipitation	HBMECs (Cell Systems Inc.)	WB	[68]
	ICAM-1 endoglin VCAM-1		Removal: 1800*g*, 10min, 18000*g* x2 (~2min) Labeled supernatant	Mouse brain microvascular endothelial cells (B3 cell line)	FC	[114]

EV subtype is designated based on crude sedimentation properties (EVs sedimenting at < 100,000 × *g* are classified as microvesicles, while those sedimenting at ≥ 100,000 × *g* are classified as exosomes) or polymer-based precipitation (exosomes)

TEM transmission electron microscopy, *NTA* nanoparticle tracking analysis, *Cryo-EM* electron cryomicroscopy, *SEM* scanning electron microscopy, *DLS* dynamic light scattering, *DIC* differential interference contrast microscopy, *TRPS* tunable resistive pulse sensing, *FC* flow cytometry, *WB* western blot, *FL* fluorescence labeling, *MS* multiple sclerosis

characterized by high-resistance tight junctions (TJs) and subtended by the *glia limitans.* For the purposes of this review, we will consider the blood–spinal cord barrier in the same context as the BBB, though subtle differences between the two have been noted [27]. The blood–cerebrospinal barrier (BCSFB) is comprised of epithelial cells of the choroid plexus (localized in the brain ventricles) that separate blood–borne elements from the cerebrospinal fluid (CSF) [28]. A third type CNS barrier, the blood–leptomeningeal barrier (BLMB), is formed by a monolayer of endothelial cells of the microvessels coursing through the pia mater and overlying subarachnoid space (SAS), and may be considered another type of BCSFB [29]. The epithelioid pia matter, itself, has been suggested to act as yet an additional CNS barrier, regulating solute and cell traffic between the CSF in the SAS and the sub-pial parenchyma [30, 31]. While technically outside the CNS, there also exists a blood–retinal barrier (BRB), which consists of retinal pigment epithelial cells and retinal capillary endothelial cells each tightly connected by specialized junctional complexes similar to those found at the BBB [32]. This review will highlight known and prospective interactions of EVs with these different CNS barriers. The initial focus will be on the BBB and EVs derived from the microvascular endothelium comprising this barrier.

EVs in endothelial biology: inside and outside the CNS

What might be considered the earliest references to EVs from endothelial cells were described by Hamilton et al. [33] and Patel et al. [34]. These pioneering studies were then followed by a hiatus in endothelial EV research for nearly a decade. The revival of endothelial-EV research lead by Combes et al. [35] proceeded with a quickening pace and with focus on the potential for EVs as markers of cardiovascular damage. These studies mainly focused on the larger microvesicles, with many in the field commonly referring to them as "EMPs" or endothelial microparticles [36]. The study of endothelial-derived exosomes, however, has lagged behind until more recently.

Given the extensiveness of the vasculature, similarities and differences exist amongst its derivative branches. Nearly all endothelial cells are thought to express common "endothelial markers" such as PECAM-1 (CD31), von Willibrand factor (vWF), CD34, and CD144 [37–39]. The field of cardiovascular research has exploited this to define cardiovascular dysfunction and disease by the characterization of endothelial-derived EVs separately from other cell-derived EVs (i.e., immune cells, platelets). Due to the overlap in some protein expression, it is common to use a combination of markers, which includes multiple surface proteins such as adhesion molecules (PECAM-1, ICAM-1, E-selectin, VCAM-1, endoglin, MCAM), cadherins (i.e., VE-cadherin), and integrins [40–42]. Additionally, Annexin-V is also widely used because of known mechanisms of microvesicle release involving phosphatidylserine [43]. While analysis of endothelial EVs based on these common endothelial markers can give a picture of overall vascular health, it may also be possible to identify the health of a particular vascular network—for example, the cerebrovasculature. Combining general endothelial markers with specific vascular domain markers could potentially fine-tune our use of EVs. In the case of BMEC, there are a number of proteins and transporters that are highly enriched or brain specific [44, 45], and might be exploited to confirm a CNS microvascular origin for circulating EVs. For example, a recent study by Andrews et al. demonstrated the increased presence of the TJ protein, occludin, on EVs following TBI [45]. In another study circulating ECs were shown to carry a different TJ protein, claudin-5, in an animal model of MS [44]. Indeed, these studies show that detection of endothelial markers and of proteins highly expressed in the cerebrovasculature, could provide a means to interrogate the health of CNS endothelial barriers, such as those that form the BBB. However, as both occludin and CLN-5 are also expressed by peripheral endothelial cells, expression of these proteins alone is insufficient to confirm the CNS derivation of EVs. Co-expression of transporter proteins critical to BBB function might offer the best an option for specifically identifying BMEC-derived EVs. Interestingly, endothelial markers and barrier endothelium enriched proteins can be found on both forms of EVs. Given how much EVs could reveal about vascular health, future investigation in which EC-derived microvesicles versus exosomes are compared for differential release as a function of time could provide a snapshot of the respective relevance of each EV subtype in physiology and pathophysiology. It is likely that the kinetics of EC release may differ with other cell types due to their interface with the bloodstream, and their larger and flatter morphology (i.e., surface area) that could provide a higher membrane reserve than other cells.

Biogenesis and molecular composition of exosomes and microvesicles

Exosomes

As stated earlier, circulating endothelial EVs are elevated in conditions of vascular dysfunction, and their presence can be used as biosignatures of vascular pathology [46]. The change in endothelial status leading to the release of EVs may be reflective of maladaptive vascular tone, immune recruitment, and/or thrombosis [47]. Specifically, triggers that mediate EV release may involve either inflammatory cytokines, ROS, lipopolysaccharides, thrombin, hypoxia or aberrant shear stress or a combination thereof. Cellular insults subsequently can induce the release of exosomes and/or microvesicles. Because exosomes arise from within MVB, which in turn originate from the maturation process of intraluminal vesicles contained within early to late endosomes [48], exosomes will bear proteins characteristic of late endosomes such as CD63, LAMP1 and LAMP2. Importantly, the early endosomal proteins, Rab4 or Rab5, may also be found in exosomes, suggesting various routing mechanisms affecting vesicle exocytosis [49]. A key aspect in the formation of MVB is the involvement of the endosomal sorting complex required for transport (ESCRT) proteins (reviewed in [50]). These family of proteins form intracellular complexes comprised of: ESCRT-0, -I, -II, -III and the Vps4 complex. Cargo composition within exosomes is highly context dependent which is affected by the cell type, status of cell cycle, and exposure to environmental cues. However, in general the heterogeneity of the cargo is a mixture of genetic information (such as non-coding RNAs), proteins and lipids [50]. It is important to mention that although much is known about the molecular machinery involved in exosome biogenesis, much remains to be done to validate if the same processes apply to brain EC exosome production.

Microvesicles

Certain members of the endocytic pathway are recoverable in 10,000 x g pellets of cell-conditioned media from neuroblastoma cells, suggesting they are likewise involved in microvesicle formation, for example the ESCRT family of proteins Alix and TSG101. Recently, the ADP-ribosylation factor 6 (ARF6) has also been identified as important in mediating cytoskeletal changes that allows for microvesicle biogenesis. SCRT complexes are formed at the plasma membrane at areas of disrupted plasma membrane, which leads to the exposure of phosphatidylserine on the outer leaflet [51]. Recruitment and activation of flippase, floppase and scramblase mediate the final steps of the budding process [52]. The vertical packaging of cargo by microvesicles can include a milieu of bioactive agents that includes proteins, metabolites, DNA, mRNA, and miRNA (reviewed in [53]). The above processes of EV release appear to be universally involved in all cell types. However, similar to the need for comparative studies of exosome biogenesis between other cell types and brain ECs, the same can be said about microvesicle formation between brain ECs and other cell types.

EC-derived EVs: role in CNS pathology

Cell–cell communication (from brain ECs toward the brain parenchyma)

One of the main proposed functions of EVs is an involvement in cell-to-cell communication and signaling. Numerous reports have examined this intercellular signaling role in terms of both positive and negative effector function [54], although these studies concerned pathways operating outside the brain. Communication between the blood and the brain is critical due to the high metabolic demand of neurons and the need for the BBB to control trafficking of molecules and ions [55]. Consequently, EVs could potentially serve as a major mediator in these communications between the cells of the neurovascular unit (NVU).

As all cells of the NVU have the potential to communicate unidirectionally or bidirectionally among several cell types, this raises the question whether EVs have an exclusive target or engage in more promiscuous communications. A few studies have examined this in vitro and, from the scant results so far, we are beginning see a picture of cell specific cross-talk. Exosomes secreted from stimulated cortical neurons were shown to bind to and be endocytosed by only neurons. In contrast, neuroblastoma exosomes, which bind to neurons and glial cells indiscriminately, were only endocytosed by glial cells [56]. Furthermore, EVs released from metabolically labeled astrocytes/neurons were found in unlabeled endothelial cells, though this preferentially occurred with astrocyte-derived EVs [55].

The endothelium has long been known to secrete factors that act in a paracrine (acting on neighbors) as well as autocrine (acting on self) fashion. A priori, the use of EVs for endothelial communication seems logical. In paracrine, two forms of intercellular communications may be considered, direct and indirect. Direct communication occurs when ligands on the surface of EVs directly interact with receptors on the target cell. Whereas, indirect communication may be considered as a result of cargo proteins binding with cellular components of the target cell after EV internalization and decapsulation [57]. Moreover, since BMECs are also polarized cells, intercellular communication must also be considered within this context. Thus, the distinct luminal and abluminal protein expression, likely affecting the protein contents of EVs and their role in cell signaling. It also stands to reason, that cell polarization could affect protein cargo sorting and distribution—a key parameter to consider when performing studies in vitro [58]. A similar possibility could also result when using brain ECs under conditions of fluid flow and shear stress, since polarization is known to occur via mechanotransduction and could affect protein and gene expression during EV production [59]. Presently, no published studies have yet examined the impact of fluid dynamics on the release of EVs from the abluminal vs luminal endothelial surface of BMEC, and the cargo within these respective EV populations.

EVs released by ECs into the bloodstream have several potential targets including neighboring ECs, immune cells and downstream organ systems. Endothelial-derived EVs have been shown to affect the function of ECs from the same vascular bed [60–62]. Although these studies involve peripheral ECs, it would not be unexpected for brain ECs to also exhibit signaling changes in response to EC-derived vesicles. In fact, Kurachi et al. showed that EVs derived from various ECs (aortic, brain, umbilical) have similar effects on oligodendrocytes [63], which suggests potential similarities among EVs from different vascular beds in executing some actions. Although cross-talk between the vascular lineages has not been examined, it has been demonstrated by adoptive transfer of BMEC-derived EVs (in vivo) that these vesicles can have an effect on other organ systems such as the liver [64, 65].

Studying the fate and effect of endothelial EVs in the brain parenchyma remains more challenging than those appearing in the blood. However, several in vitro studies have begun examining the effects of brain EC-derived EVs on neighboring cells such as astrocytes, pericytes and oligodendrocytes. Due to their anatomical proximity within the NVU, astrocytes and pericytes are the most likely direct target of EVs released by BMECs. However, further investigations into the transport of vesicles in the extracellular space could reveal more direct contact with ECs without an intermediary cell. Recently, András et al. showed that BMEC-derived ECs treated with Aβ, triggered re-packaging of the Aβ in vesicles of various sizes [66]. This process was elevated in the context of exposure of cells to HIV particles, which induced the release of more EVs. Furthermore, these EVs were easily taken up by both astrocytes and pericytes—though analysis of resulting effects in the recipient cells was not pursued. The same group performed adoptive transfer experiments to investigate how the BBB may mediate Aβ trafficking into the brain in vivo. BMEC-derived EVs loaded with Aβ were seen to localize with the BBB and in the brain parenchyma [66]. Uptake of BMEC-derived-EVs by pericytes was also shown by Yamamoto et al. The results revealed that such EVs were produced in response to an LPS challenge and induced pericyte upregulation of VEGFB mRNA and protein expression [67]. The upregulation of VEGFB was suggested to mediate pathological angiogenesis and/or vascular leakage. Both of these studies examined vesicles from brain ECs under pro-inflammatory insults, which collectively reflect most studies on general EC vesicles produced under inflammatory conditions. In contrast, a few reports have shown positive effects of BMEC-derived EVs when produced under basal or non-inflammatory conditions [63, 68]. In the case of Kurachi et al., the authors examined the effect of basally produced BMEC-derived EVs that were then taken up by oligodendrocytes and inhibited apoptosis. Interestingly, this effect was not limited to BMEC-derived ECs, as EVs from other ECs (aortic, umbilical) also had a similar effect. Positive effects have also been seen from BMEC-derived EVs produced in response to TLR3 signaling. Li et al. showed these EVs contained antiviral factors that, when internalized by HIV infected macrophages, resulted in suppression of HIV reverse transcriptase activity [68]. Future studies will no doubt expand on our currently limited understanding of the positive and negative effects of EVs in the CNS.

EVs as facilitators of immune cell entry into the CNS

Endothelial EVs are associated with inflammatory events along the BBB

Multiple sclerosis (MS) is a *multi-component, neurodegenerative, demyelinating* disease of the CNS, characterized histopathologically by focal inflammatory infiltrates, demyelinating plaques and axonal damage [69–71]. In the most common form of the disease, relapsing/remitting MS (RRMS), patients experience discrete neurological attacks (relapses) separated by a complete or partial return to periods of normal function (remissions). Another manifestation of MS is disruption of the BBB, which is viewed both as a possible secondary effect of neuroinflammation and leukocyte transmigration, and as integral to pathogenesis [72–74]. In fact, BBB disruption is considered an early feature of the disease [75]—possibly even preceding immune cell infiltration [76]. Several observations collectively allude to the possibility EVs play a role in regulating leukocyte CNS infiltration during MS [7, 77, 78]. Key, is the increasing evidence of interactions among EVs, leukocytes, and endothelial cells in neuroinflammatory conditions. The earliest indication of this relationship is the altered appearance of endothelial EVs in the blood of MS patients. Notably, inflammation of the endothelium, which is indicated in MS brain microvasculature by up-regulation of the adhesion molecule VCAM-1 [79] and aberrant distribution of TJ proteins occludin, ZO-1 and JAM-A [80, 81] in active lesions is a potent trigger for endothelial cells, in general, to release EVs [41, 43, 82–84]. A relationship between adhesion of leukocytes to peripheral endothelial cells and release of EVs by the latter has also been described in atherosclerosis ([85]), a condition displaying evidence of peripheral vascular inflammation. Accordingly, release of EVs by endothelial cells is thought to reflect endothelial activation and/or stress [43, 86], and has been reported elevated in MS [87]—the EVs in question being designated EMPs and identified as two subtypes by their respective expression of CD31 (PECAM-1) and CD51 (vitronectin receptor). CD31+EMPs were elevated only during exacerbation, where their presence correlated positively with gadolinium-enhanced lesions, and then returned to control value at remission, while CD52+EMPs remained elevated during all phases of disease, prompting the authors to conclude the former EV subtype is a marker of acute endothelial injury, whereas the latter reflects chronic injury. Further highlighting the correlation with inflammatory state, plasma levels of CD31+EMPs were significantly reduced in MS patients treated with IFN-β1a, a standard therapy for RRMS, and declined in the same direction as clinical disability [88]. Such inflammatory responses are not limited to MS, as intracerebral injection of IL1-β into rats was also found to prompt release of endothelial cell-derived EVs, which became sequestered in the liver and mediated the acute-phase response and sickness behavior associated with CNS inflammation [64]. While it is important to keep in mind that the circulating and liver-bound EVs described in these studies were not explicitly identified as coming from the CNS microvasculature, when EVs released from IL1-β-treated BMEC cultures where injected back into rats, they elicited the same behavioral pathology.

EVs bind to/stimulate leukocytes during neuroinflammation

Once discharged from endothelial cells, circulating EVs can bind to leukocytes and influence their activity [89], though, once again, the vascular bed of origin of these EVs is uncertain. The physical closeness between endothelial cells and marginating leukocytes could conceivably allow for EVs released by endothelial cells to more effectively interact with leukocytes in a juxtacrine (i.e., contact-dependent) manner, without being diluted in the circulation or affecting off-target sites (Fig. 2a). EV:leukocyte binding was initially revealed by detection of endothelial EV:monocyte complexes in blood of MS patients [82], and formation of similar complexes in vitro. That these complexes were significantly elevated during disease relapse versus remission or compared to controls, and correlated with gadolinium enhancement on MRI, further underscore their clinical relevance as harbingers of neuroinflammation and possibly a role for endothelial EVs as key players in the inflammatory process. In keeping with this inflammatory profile, EVs obtained from the supernatant cultures of endothelial cells stimulated with the pro-inflammatory cytokine TNF-α facilitated monocyte chemotaxis [90]. EVs released by TNF-α stimulation of cultured BMECs have also been shown to interact with and stimulate proliferation of T cells [91]. A pro-inflammatory impact on T cells outside the CNS has been observed as well, with endothelial EVs (identified as $CD31^+/CD42^-$, with diameters < 1 μm) in plasma from patients with acute coronary syndrome positively correlated with IFN-γ, possibly upregulating the differentiation and function of Th1 cells through increasing the expression of T-bet mRNA and protein [92]. In contrast, endothelial EVs can additionally suppress monocyte activation via transferring anti-inflammatory miRNAs, suggesting EVs can both promote and inhibit inflammation via differential actions on leukocytes [93].

Subpopulations of EVs released from BMECs in culture [92], and into the circulation by unidentified endothelial sources in vivo [94], have also been reported to contain various adhesion proteins. Moreover, such proteins appear more prominently expressed in exosomes versus microvesicles, in EVs released from TNF-α-stimulated BMEC [23]. While the physiological significance of these particular EVs remains to be clarified by experimentation, their detection suggests possible further EV interactions with leukocytes. For example, EVs expressing TJ protein CLN-5 [44] have been isolated from both BMEC cultures and peripheral blood of mice with experimental autoimmune encephalomyelitis (EAE), an animal model of demyelinating neuroinflammation that recapitulates seminal facets of MS—including leukocyte migration across the BBB. And another TJ protein, occludin [45], likewise has been detected on EVs released from cultured BMEC, and in the circulation following TBI, a condition, like MS/EAE, associated with neuroinflammation and CNS leukocyte infiltration. As peripheral blood leukocytes from MS patients were reported to increase ectopic expression of both CLN-5 and occludin during disease relapse, and down regulate them in remission or following anti-inflammatory therapy [95], it is tempting to speculate EVs mediate transfer of TJ proteins from endothelial cells—in particular BMEC—to leukocytes during neuroinflammation. This possibility is reinforced by findings that eGFP-labeled CLN-5 expressed exclusively by endothelial cells could be transferred to leukocytes during EAE, while eGFP-CLN-5^+ EVs isolated from plasma of these mice also bound to leukocytes in vitro [44]. What purpose leukocyte-associated TJ proteins serve awaits resolution, but they have been argued to play an accessory role in leukocyte transendothelial migration (TEM) via a *zipper mechanism*, whereby inter-endothelial junctional contacts are temporarily replaced by homophilic interactions between leukocyte and endothelial junctional proteins [95, 96]

(Fig. 2b). Because basal high-level expression of TJ proteins on circulating leukocytes would be a risk for cell aggregation in blood, focal binding of endothelial-derived, TJ protein^{+} EVs to leukocytes at the BBB during neuroinflammation could, conceivably, avert this problem.

EVs are associated with enhanced TEM

That binding of endothelial EVs to leukocytes might facilitate leukocyte extravasation is lent credence by the observation endothelial EV:monocyte complexes obtained from blood of MS patients showed enhanced ability, when compared to unconjugated leukocytes, in migrating across monolayer cultures of human BMEC [36, 77]. A close, physical association among endothelial cells, EVs and leukocytes during EAE—at sites of leukocyte margination along spinal venules—was additionally demonstrated using serial electron microscopy and 3D contour-based surface reconstruction [44] and provides more suggestive evidence supporting a role for endothelial-derived EVs in regulating leukocyte behavior during neuroinflammation. However, confirmation of a direct role for these EVs in promoting leukocyte TEM, awaits demonstration that their binding to, and not merely association with, a given leukocyte population stimulates the extravasation process.

EVs and neuropathogenesis of human immunodeficiency virus (HIV)

Despite treatment of HIV infection with antiretroviral therapy (ART), the CNS is still a major target and reservoir of the virus. Recent reports indicate that even in the presence of ART, chronic neuroinflammation cannot be fully prevented, leading to the development of HIV-1-associated neurocognitive disorders (HAND) in HIV-infected patients through increased neuroinflammation and BBB/vascular disruption [97–100]. Subsets of activated monocytes that express CD16 and/or CD163 are expanded both in HIV-infected individuals and in Rhesus macaques infected with simian immunodeficiency virus (SIV) [101], an HIV-like virus that can infect monkeys and apes and causes an AIDS-like disease. In fact, CD16+monocytes serve as a continuous means of trafficking HIV from the periphery into the brain [102]. While these cells are refractory to replication, they differentiate into macrophages in the brain which can effectively sequester and replicate the virus. Although the production of EVs from various cell types are a characterized occurrence during HIV pathogenesis, not much is known about the EV response from brain endothelial cells during the course of viral infection. The only report that points to this possibility notes EVs are significantly released by cultured BMEC from the human-derived cell line, hCMEC/D3, when these cells are exposed to HIV viral particles. Although particle concentration was analyzed, the cargo from these cells was not. Figure 3 corroborates the above findings, showing generation of EVs following exposure of primary human BMECs to recombinant HIV proteins. Importantly, the EVs isolated showed the presence of p-glycoprotein (Pgp) and TJ proteins, occludin and claudin-5. These results suggest that BMECs are sensitive to HIV-1 viral proteins and respond by generating EVs that contain proteins associated with the tight junction complex and transport barrier. Moreover, using a migration assay with isolated human monocytes exposed to BMEC-derived EVs, the number of monocytes crossing BMEC monolayers significantly increased compared to monocytes not treated with EVs. These analyses are consistent with the report by Paul et al. [44], which showed endothelial-derived CLN-5 being transferred to leukocytes both in the blood and CNS of mice with EAE, as well as BMEC-derived CLN-5+EVs able to bind to leukocytes in vitro. Thus, it is possible that EV-assisted immunoinvasion by HIV infected immune cells may represent a previously unrecognized cellular mechanism in the development of NeuroAids.

Intercellular communication to brain ECs

Activated immune cells release EVs that activate ECs

Since their discovery, EVs have been envisioned as a means of communication by which one cell type can affect specific cell types in other organ systems [57]. Much of how donor cell EVs communicate with recipient cells comes from in vitro studies in which the isolated EV subtype is added to the target cell. In general, EVs can affect inter-cellular communication by presenting ligands on their surface to receptors on the target cell plasma membrane. Alternatively, internalization of EVs can occur via either direct fusion of the EV membrane with the plasma membrane of the target cell, by phagocytosis and micropinocytosis, or by clathrin-mediated endocytosis. Endothelial cells, in particular, appear to use endocytic pathways rather than fusion mechanisms to uptake exosomes from different cell types [103]. In the study by Svenson et al. barrier forming HUVECs were shown to internalize exosomes from HeLa, U87MG, CHO and MEF cells by an endocytic process that followed a time, concentration, and temperature-dependent manner [103]. Although it is clear EVs can induce a wide variety of biological responses, little is known about the molecular mechanisms that transduce EV binding/uptake into actions by the recipient cell.

In the context of the brain endothelium, recent studies point to EV-mediated intercellular communication between immune cells and the cerebral vasculature.

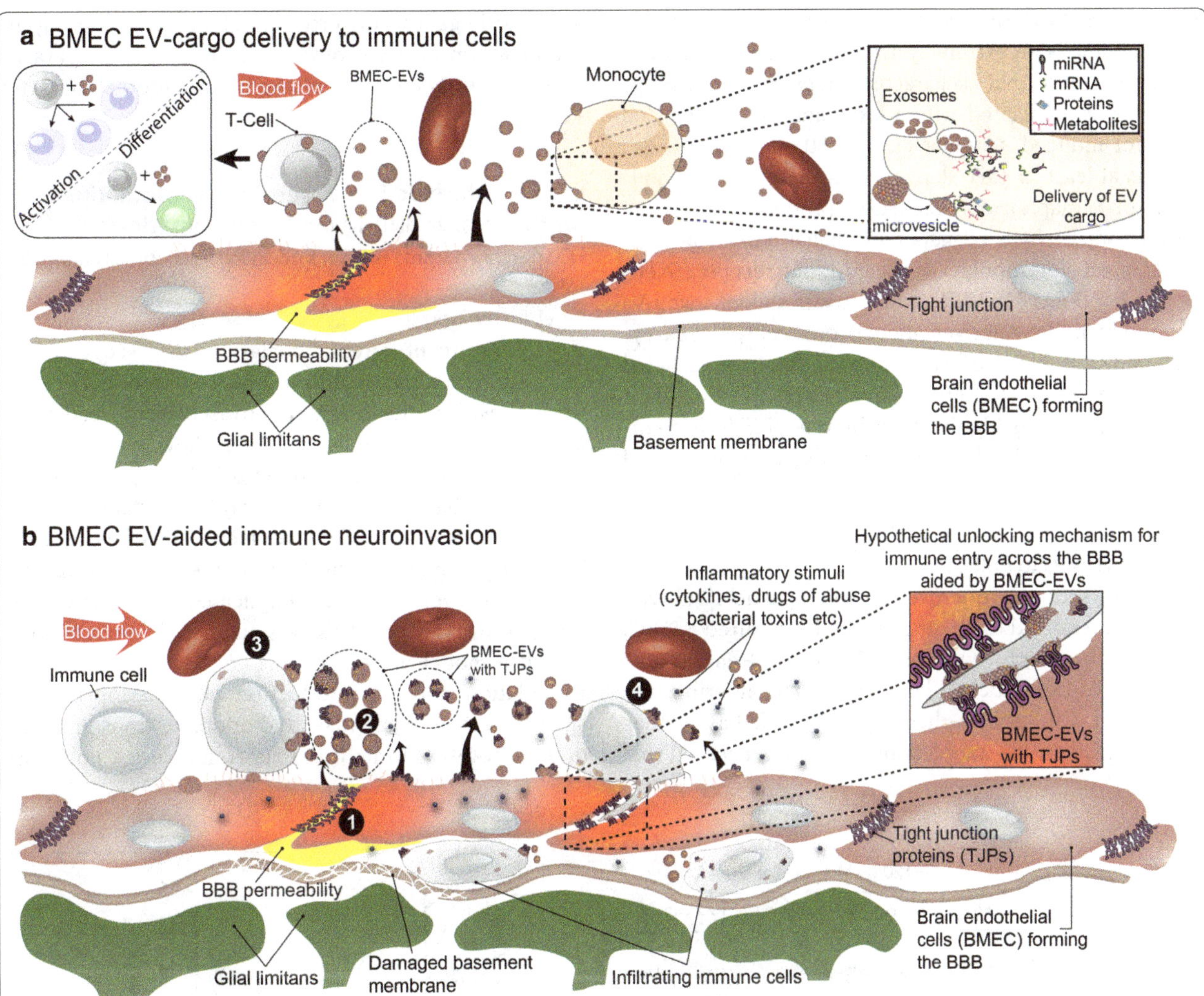

Fig. 2 Hypothetical schematic model of EV-cargo delivery to immune cells and EV-aided immune transendothelial migration. **a** Exomes produced by the BMEC, can deliver its cargo via cellular endocytic internalization. Conversely, microvesicle fusion with cell membranes of the target cell facilities emptying of their cargo. The contents in EVs can be highly heterogenous (in terms of composition and amount) although it's generally recognized that proteins, genetic material, and metabolites encompass most of its components. The biological consequences that BMEC-EVs could have on immune cells remains largely unknown. However, recent evidence suggests that EVs could affect T cell activation and differentiation status. **b** The presence of inflammatory mediators activates the brain endothelium and results in localized blood–brain barrier instability (BBB) (*1*). Subsequent hyperpermeability at the BBB may be explained by the temporal production of microvesicles and exosomes (EVs) (*2*). Importantly, brain endothelial derived EVs are known to contain tight junction proteins in their cargo [44, 45]. Although inflammatory mediators, drugs of abuse etc., induce the biogenesis of EVs from the endothelium, we propose that only activated immune cells can efficiently use these vesicles for gaining entry into the CNS. In the case illustrated, we hypothesize activated monocytes bind EVs containing TJ proteins (*3*), which then allows for direct "unzipping" of intercellular tight junction complexes at the BBB (*4*), leading to immune cell access to the perivascular space

For example, experiments revealed EVs from activated monocytes stimulated human BMEC to upregulate adhesion molecules ICAM1 and VCAM1, the chemoattractant CCL2/MCP1 and pro-inflammatory cytokines IL6 and IL1β [104]. The authors further showed monocyte derived EVs may transfer miRNAs that can modulate endothelial activation. And though it has yet to be demonstrated whether transfer of miRNA by these exosomes can also regulate BBB status, work by Chugh et al. revealed EVs could promote endothelial migration [105]. Specifically, EVs from patients positive for Kaposi's sarcoma enhanced the cellular migration of an immortalized cell line derived from HUVECs, suggesting a possible role for EVs in promoting angiogenic responses [105].

Glioblastoma EVs induce BBB permeability

Glioblastoma is an extremely aggressive, highly vascularized brain tumor that is characterized by very poor prognosis and is associated with a large amount edema due to tumor-induced, vascular leakage [106]. This vascular leakage, at least in part, derives from the pro-permeability factor Semaphorin3A (Sema3A) produced within the glioblastoma, which triggers endothelial barrier permeability most commonly via engaging its receptor Neuropilin 1 (NRP1) [107]. Recently, it was shown that EVs released by patient-derived glioblastoma cells, and carrying Sem3A on their surface, can disrupt brain endothelial barrier function in vivo and in vitro in a NRP1-dependent manner [108], thus highlighting the role of EVs in mediating communication between the BBB and parenchymal cells.

Platelet EVs/MPs to BMECs

Platelet EVs of the microvesicle/microparticle subtype have been reported to be internalized by cultured BMEC, entering both early endosome 1 antigen+endosomes and LysoTracker-labeled lysosomes, and altering the endothelial cell surface phenotype [109]. It has further been suggested such interaction(s) may play a crucial role in the pathogenesis of cerebral malaria by promoting the cytoadhesion of erythrocytes infected with the parasite *Plasmodium falciparum* to the brain endothelium [109, 110].

Brain EC-derived EVs as serological biomarkers for BBB status during neuroinflammation

EC-specific markers (CD31, Endoglin) likely on circulating EVs

Cerebral malaria

A key feature of cerebral malaria is the sequestration of *Plasmodium falciparum*-parasitized red blood cells (PRBC) within the brain microvasculature, leading to disturbances in microcirculatory flow, neuroinflammation and metabolic dysfunction [111, 112]. Consistent with inflammation and endothelial distress being signals for release of EVs from endothelial cells, EMP levels in plasma were observed to rise in Malawain children with severe malaria complicated with coma [113]. The pathogenicity of EVs was further demonstrated in a mouse model of cerebral malaria [114]. Inhibition of vesiculation and EV production conferred protection against neurologic disease, and adoptive transfer of fluorescently-labeled microparticles/microvesicles obtained

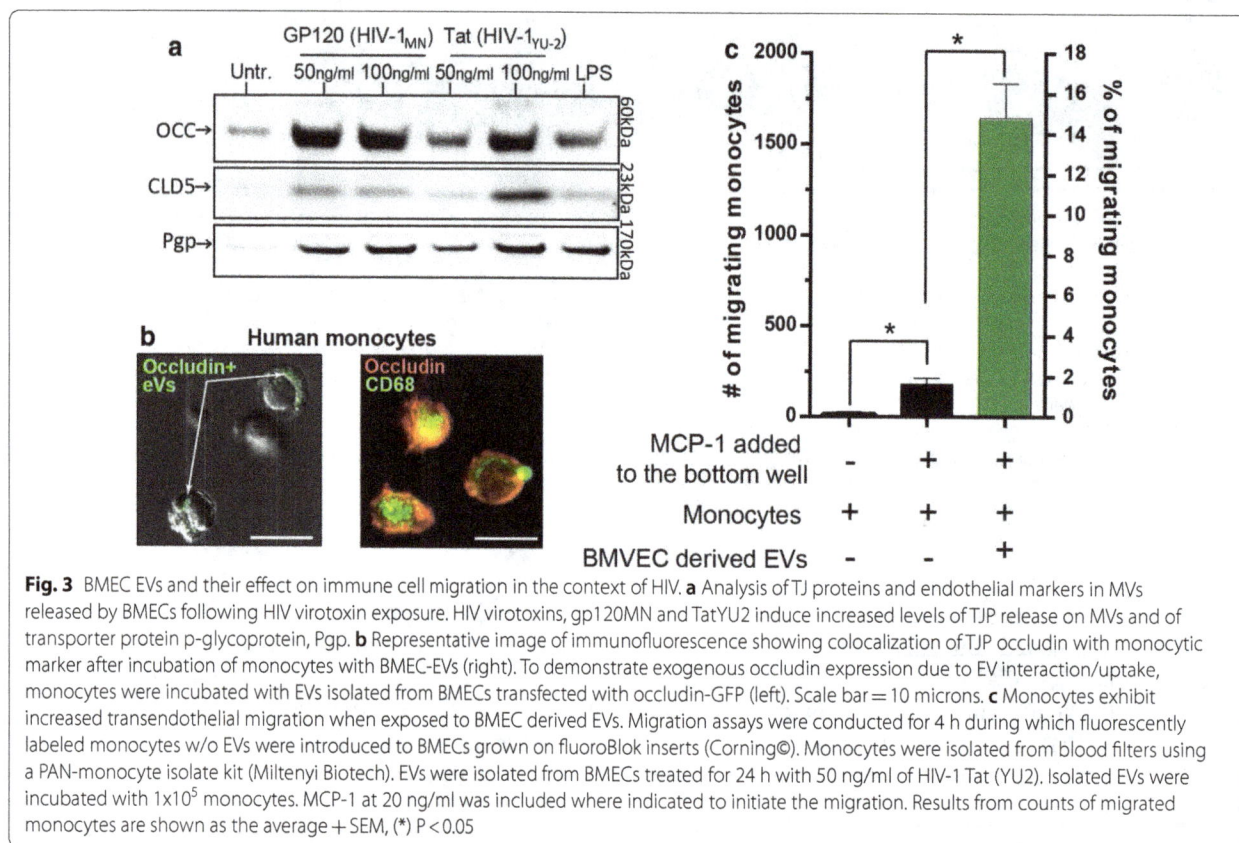

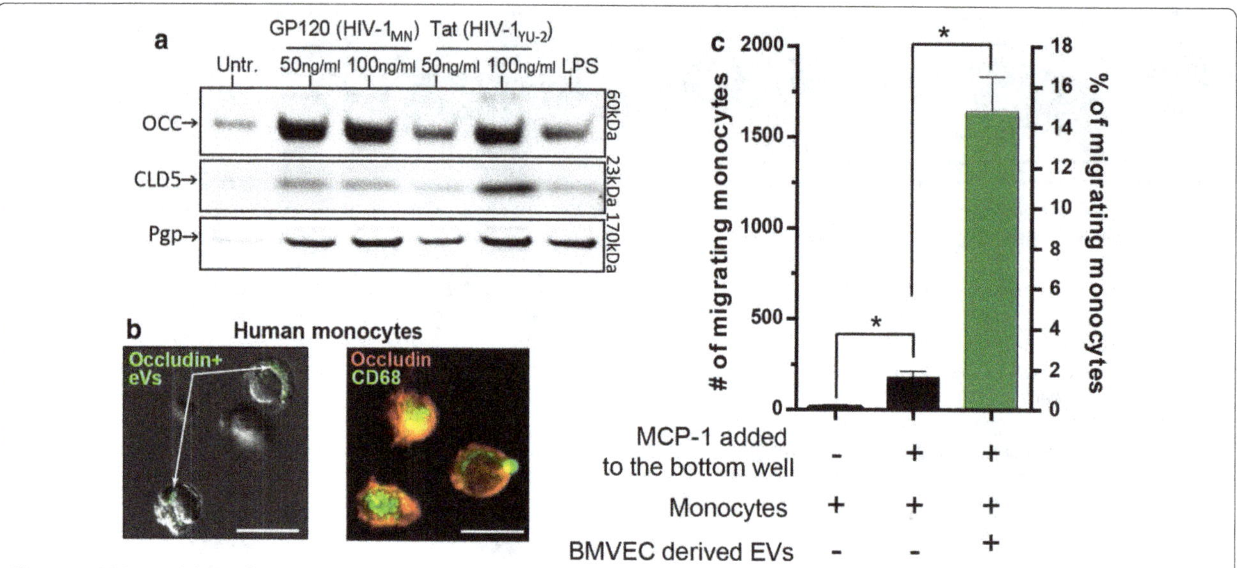

Fig. 3 BMEC EVs and their effect on immune cell migration in the context of HIV. **a** Analysis of TJ proteins and endothelial markers in MVs released by BMECs following HIV virotoxin exposure. HIV virotoxins, gp120MN and TatYU2 induce increased levels of TJP release on MVs and of transporter protein p-glycoprotein, Pgp. **b** Representative image of immunofluorescence showing colocalization of TJP occludin with monocytic marker after incubation of monocytes with BMEC-EVs (right). To demonstrate exogenous occludin expression due to EV interaction/uptake, monocytes were incubated with EVs isolated from BMECs transfected with occludin-GFP (left). Scale bar = 10 microns. **c** Monocytes exhibit increased transendothelial migration when exposed to BMEC derived EVs. Migration assays were conducted for 4 h during which fluorescently labeled monocytes w/o EVs were introduced to BMECs grown on fluoroBlok inserts (Corning©). Monocytes were isolated from blood filters using a PAN-monocyte isolate kit (Miltenyi Biotech). EVs were isolated from BMECs treated for 24 h with 50 ng/ml of HIV-1 Tat (YU2). Isolated EVs were incubated with $1x10^5$ monocytes. MCP-1 at 20 ng/ml was included where indicated to initiate the migration. Results from counts of migrated monocytes are shown as the average + SEM, (*) $P < 0.05$

from plasma of mice with CM resulted in these EVs lining the endothelium of brain microvessels of infected, but not healthy, recipient mice.

Ischemic stroke

Reflecting distress, EVs are elevated in vascular diseases in general, and in cerebrovascular accidents, like stroke, in particular [115] (for a concise review on the subject see Deng et al. [116]. Analysis of patients who suffered either a mild or moderate-severe stroke revealed higher levels of endothelial derived EVs when compared to non-stroke controls. This same study further reported the level of endothelial EVs correlated significantly with brain lesion volume, as measured by diffusion-weighted magnetic resonance imaging. In particular, EVs characterized by flow cytometry as $CD105^{+}CD54^{+}CD45^{-}$ appeared to show the strongest correlation with lesion volume. Another study provided further support that endothelial EVs could effectively be used as biomarkers in the diagnosis for ischemic injury severity [117]. In this latter case, EVs isolated from 68 patients with acute ischemic stroke were compared to those isolated from age-matched controls. The results showed the elevated presence of $CD31^{+}$ $CD41a^{-}$ EVs in patients with acute ischemic stroke. Significantly, the profile of circulating endothelial EVs may offer a way to monitor and/or risk stratify cerebrovascular disease leading to stroke [115]. For example, individuals with intracranial arterial stenosis had higher levels of both $CD31^{+}$ and $CD42b^{-}$ EVs and $CD31^{+}$ and annexin V^{+} microvesicles. No studies to date, however, have investigated whether any of these those populations of endothelial EVs contain proteins enriched at the brain endothelium. Such EVs may serve as useful surrogates for assessing the status of BBB in cerebrovascular disease and stroke.

MS

In light of release of endothelial EVs being associated with inflammation and endothelial distress, there has been considerable speculation as to whether they can serve as accessible biomarkers for MS—essentially "liquid biopsies" with potential diagnostic and prognostic value—as well as possible response indicators to treatment [7, 78, 118]. EMPs (identified by flow cytometry as < 3.0 um in diameter, and $CD31^{+}/CD42b^{-}$ or $CD62E^{+}$) in platelet poor plasma (PPP) from patients with different clinical forms of MS—RRMS, primary progressive MS, secondary progressive MS, and CSI—were all found to be elevated when compared to healthy controls [119]. Significantly, MPs prepared in batch from PPP of RRMS patients, when compared to controls, significantly disturbed the integrity and barrier properties of cultured human endothelial cells (as reflected by diminished transendothelial electrical resistance) and altered these cells' immunofluorescence staining of ZO-1 and the integral adherence junctional protein, VE-cadherin. Other reports have described changes in miRNA profiles of EVs—specifically exosomes—obtained from blood sera of MS patients [7, 120], but did not determine whether the EVs in question, in whole or in part, originated from endothelial cells.

Alzheimer's disease

Cerebrovascular dysfunction is a hallmark of Alzheimer's disease (AD) pathology. It thus stands to reason that in AD, endothelial remodeling and inflammatory responses would yield endothelial derived EVs. In fact, levels and marker profiles of endothelial EVs in the plasma of AD patients have been found to differ from those of healthy controls [121]. In the study by Xue et al. significant increases in the levels of $CD31^{+}CD42^{-}$ and $CD62e^{+}CD42^{-}$ EVs, respectively, were detected in the AD group relative to the controls. However, the elevation in EVs did not showed a difference as a function of AD severity (mild to severe) groups. In another study, a comparative endothelial EV analysis was performed in AD patients with and without vascular risk factors, such as hypertension, diabetes, dyslipidemia, stroke, coronary artery disease and smoking. Interestingly, this study did not indicate a difference in EV levels between AD patients and controls. However, a significant difference did appear between AD patients diagnosed with vascular risk factors and those without [122]. This topic clearly warrants further study, in which EV phenotyping could be expanded to include other surface markers, monitored in different forms of dementias and assessed in longitudinal studies.

Traumatic brain injury (TBI)

TBI represents a major public health concern with long lasting effects on both the patient and surrounding communities (i.e., long-term care). Currently, there are no clinically approved biomarkers to diagnose TBI or monitor the recovery [123]. However, several neuronal or astrocytic markers have been examined including S100β, neuron-specific enolase, glial fibrillary acidic protein, and Tau [124]. Consequently, the use of brain endothelial biomarkers represents a largely unexplored avenue for biomarker discovery. It is well established that TBI causes cerebral vascular damage both during the primary phase (induced by forces that are linear or rotational) and the secondary phase (a result of inflammation). These resulting changes in vascular integrity and BBB permeability, in some cases, can last for months or years following the original injury [125] and can result in delayed neuronal death and dysfunction [126]. This timeline for endothelial damage may suggest the use of brain EC-derived vesicle biomarkers over the course of both phases of TBI pathology. Some initial studies have examined the detection of endothelial-enriched markers following TBI. First, elevated levels of the TJ protein occludin were detected in patient serum following a mild TBI [127]. Around that same time, Andrews et al. sought to demonstrate that brain ECs release EVs in response to mechanical injury and that these vesicles contain TJ proteins such as occludin. Using an in vitro model, commonly used to simulate TBI on neurons, they showed that BMECs released vesicles containing PECAM-1, ICAM-1 and occludin. They further confirmed the elevated release of vesicles containing occludin in serum following TBI in vivo by flow cytometry and cryo-EM [45]. However, in both these studies, the authors did not delineate EVs released from the endothelium versus the epithelium—both of which express occludin. However, they do offer proof of principal for the detection of brain EC-enriched EV proteins as possible biomarkers. Future studies using dual or a combination of markers would be able to identify BBB specific vesicles and the potential for monitoring the recovery of the vasculature over time following TBI.

Role of EVs derived from other CNS barriers

Blood–spinal cord barrier (BSCB)

Largely analogous to the BBB in function and structure, with regard to restricting the passage of soluble and cellular elements between the blood circulation and CNS parenchyma, the BSCB nevertheless exhibits some distinguishing features compared to its brain counterpart [128, 129]. These include greater inherent permeability [130] and heightened susceptibility to stimuli that regulate endothelial integrity [131]. Such differences might at least partially stem from comparatively reduced expression of TJ proteins occludin and ZO-1 by spinal cord microvascular endothelial cells [27]. EV interactions with the spinal cord microvasculature should thus be viewed as possibly reflecting unique spinal endothelial properties. In this respect, pharmacologic inhibition of exosome production by pericytes, which lie adventitial to the endothelium and are integral to the NVU of both the BBB and BSCB, was found to preclude these cells' ability to promote angiogenesis when placed in co-culture with a spinal cord explant [132]. Insofar as cross-talk via soluble mediators between pericytes and CNS microvascular endothelial cells is critical for maintenance of barrier properties and regulation of inflammation [133, 134], pericyte-derived EVs might also be fundamental to these processes.

Blood–cerebrospinal fluid barrier (BCSFB)

The CSF space, occupied by the brain ventricles, subarachnoid spaces (SAS) of the brain and spinal cord, and central spinal canal, is separated from the blood circulation by the BCSFB. At the level of the choroid plexus (CP), which projects into the brain ventricular system and is a major producer of CSF, the BSCFB lies at the choroidal epithelium—a high resistance layer of simple columnar epithelial cells possessing tight junctions and a series of asymmetrically positioned ion transporters, enzymes and receptors that facilitate production of CSF. This epithelium encapsulates a vascular stroma comprised of fenestrated capillaries lacking typical BBB properties [135]—an arrangement establishing the BCSFB. The lateral foramina of Lushka and medial foramen of Magendie of the brain allow direct communication between the CSF in ventricles and that in the SAS. Evidence has accumulated that choroidal epithelial cells exploit EVs to shuttle specific cargo through the CSF to distant CNS regions. An example of this is the delivery of folate to the brain [136]. The folate receptor (FRα) on that basolateral surface of choroidal epithelial cells (i.e., the side facing the stromal capillaries) can pick up extravasated folate and, following endocytosis, be incorporated (complexed with folate) into MVBs. MVBs containing the FRα-folate complex can then fuse with the apical membrane of the choroidal epithelial cells, thereby releasing the FRα-folate complex as folate-bearing exosomes into the CSF. Once in the CSF, these exosomes can be delivered across the ependymal cells lining the brain ventricles and into the parenchyma. Additionally, EVs released by CP choroidal epithelial cells appear to play a role in relaying inflammatory signals from the periphery to the CNS. When peripherally injected into mice, LPS, a component of the cell wall of Gram negative bacteria, typically induces florid inflammation similar to that seen in sepsis [137]. However, it was recently shown that systemic LPS injection resulted in a large increase in nascent exosomes (in the form of intraluminal vesicles) within MVBs in CP choroidal epithelial cells [138]. Contemporaneous elevation of exosomes bearing by the CP marker, transthyretin, was detected in the CSF, suggesting the CP is an important source of EVs during system inflammation. This rise in CSF exosomes further correlated with changes in expression in both CSF and CP of miRNAs associated with inflammation: miR-1a and miR-9 were significantly down-regulated, while miR-146a and miR-155 were significantly up-regulated. And, intracerebroventricular injection of GW4869, an exosome inhibitor, reduced the amount of EVs in the CSF while causing accumulation of miRNA-146a, miRNA-155, and miR-9 in the CP. These LPS-elicited EVs were additionally observed to cross the ependymal cells and penetrate into the brain parenchyma, where they located in close proximity to GFAP+astrocytes. Studies with primary mixed cortical cultures confirmed this EV: astrocyte affinity and further identified GFAP+astrocytes and IBA1+microglia as target cells that can take up these EVs and, as a consequence, suffer downregulation of a number of genes linked to inflammatory pathways. This last series of findings offer strong support for the following scenario: EVs are produced by the BCSFB and deposited into the CSF in response to peripheral challenges, travel via the CSF to target sites, and then transmit their miRNA cargo into recipient parenchymal neural cells to effect gene regulation within the CNS [138].

Blood–retinal barrier (BRB)

The retinal pigmented epithelium (RPE) forms the outer BRB between the systemic circulation (on its basolateral side) and the retina (on its apical side) [139]. Cultured RPE cells grown in dual-chamber Transwell format were shown to release exosomes in a polarized manner; of 631 proteins identified by protein correlation profiling mass spectrometry, 299 were uniquely released apically, while 94 uniquely released basolaterally. It has further been posited that exosomes secreted by RPE cells serve as a mode of communication between the RPE and outer retina [140]. In a model system using posterior poles with retina removed from fresh human donor eyes, L-DOPA stimulation of GPR143, a G-protein couple expressed by RPE cells that contributes to pigmentation of eyes and skin, inhibited constitutive release of RPE exosomes. Concomitantly, myocilin, a protein involved in regulating intra-ocular pressure and that interacts with GPR143 in a signal transduction-dependent manner, was recruited to the endocytic compartment, indicating GPR143 and myocillin cooperate in a signal transduction pathway that regulates RPE exosome release. EVs can also act pathologically at the BRB, as EVs from mesenchymal stem cells that were cultured under diabetic-like conditions were shown to elicit features of diabetic retinopathy by elevating miR-126 expression in pericytes and causing up-regulation of angiogenic molecules VEGF and HIF-1a [141].

Use of EVs for therapeutic applications

Mediators to improve vascular pathology

The promise of EVs for therapeutic applications has sparked much interest in recent years. Much of the work thus far has focused on evaluating the therapeutic use of EVs collected from mesenchymal stem cells (MSCs) or human induced pluripotent cell–derived mesenchymal stem cells (hiPSC–MSCs) [142] (see Samsonraj et al. [143] for a recent review). EVs used as therapeutic agents have, in large, been tested in the context of tissue regeneration and wound healing. In terms of vascular injury, it is noteworthy that EVs from nearly every cell type appear to affect angiogenic responses; this includes EVs derived from cardiac progenitor cells, adipose-derived stem cells, and peripheral blood mononuclear cells to name a few. Although the positive effects of EVs on the endothelium remains unknown, it is thought that revascularization and survival factors produced by triggering the angiogenic program is a key component for recovery and tissue regeneration.

MSCs are generally recognized as adult stem cells that are able to give rise to mature mesenchymal cell types, e.g., osteoblasts, adipocytes and chondrocytes, and secrete a wide variety of bioactive molecules that display properties with considerable potential therapeutic importance: anti-apoptotic, anti-inflammatory, anti-scarring, angiogenic and chemotactic [144]. As such, there is great tendency to exploit them for their reparative capabilities in conditions where CNS barriers are disturbed [143].

MSC-derived EVs have been shown to mediate a variety of therapeutic effects [145–147], revealing their strong immunomodulatory role(s). Suggestive reparative actions of EVs at CNS barriers have also emerged as shown by examples of EV-driven remediation of vascular-associated brain injury [148, 149]. For example, multipotent human bone marrow-derived MSCs improved functional recovery after traumatic brain injury in rats, in part, by stimulating angiogenesis and neurogenesis, while also suppressing neuroinflammation [150]. In a preclinical model of hypoxic-ischemic brain injury in ovine fetuses, in utero intravenous administration of MSC-EVs reduced the total number and duration of seizures and preserved baroreceptor reflex sensitivity [151]. And, two-repetitive doses of MSV-derived EVs were found to attenuate effects of intraperitoneal injection of LPS, significantly lessening inflammation-induced neuronal cellular degeneration and microgliosis, restoring myelination and reversing long-term microstructural abnormalities of the white matter, and improving lost-lasting cognitive functions [152].

Perhaps the ability of MSC-derived EVs to execute therapeutic effects on the brain and CNS barriers stem from the capacity of EVs to intimately interact with and cross the BBB. Transwell assays employing BMECs, revealed luciferase-carrying exosomes from HEK293 cells were internalized by BMECs via endocytosis, co-localized with endosomes, and exploited the transcytotic pathway [153]. Significantly, BMEC transit only occurred when BMEC were placed under a stroke-like, inflamed condition by pre-treatment with TNF-α, suggesting EVs may remediate brain injury best under situations where the BBB is already compromised [153].

To date, there have been but a few reports on the therapeutic potential of EVs derived from BMECs. Kurachi et al. demonstrated the advantageous outcome that these EVs have on oligodendrocyte precursor cells (OPC) [63]. In this study, the investigators observed EVs derived from rat BMEC promoted proliferation and motility of cultured rat OPCs. The group additionally determined that endothelial EVs from other vascular beds or from human also shared the potential to promote OPC survival. As the authors postulated, perhaps it is via release of EVs that transplanted BMECs confer protection to OPCs in an animal model of ischemic white matter infarct [154]. These pioneering studies thus offer promise of endothelial EV based therapies for the treatment of demyelinating diseases. It is also intriguing to consider BMEC-generated EVs may represent an untapped therapeutic resource for neuroprotection, anti-inflammation and regeneration.

Drug carriers/delivery agents

A major obstacle in the treatment of CNS diseases is the high rate of failure of systemically administered drugs to effectively cross the BBB and reach therapeutic levels in the brain parenchyma [155]. Thus, there is a dire need to discover new, or modify existing, delivery vehicles that can successful encapsulate a therapeutic agent and deliver it to the CNS. Recent developments in CNS drug delivery have taken advantage of the fundamental properties of EVs to package cellular proteins and genetic material from the host cell. In this way, EVs add to the toolbox of nanomedicine, viral constructs and liposome platforms [156]. EVs make excellent delivery vehicles for various reasons. First, as reported, immunogenicity of EVs is extremely low, which helps increase bioavailability [157]. Second, cellular targeting can be controlled since ligand composition of EV membranes can be engineered or selected based on the donor cell of origin. Experiments reported by Liu et al. provide an example of how EVs are used in this manner. Employing EVs generated from human neural progenitor cells (NPC), Liu and colleagues demonstrated the addition of NPC EVs loaded with miR-210 protected human brain endothelial cells from insult [158]. Specifically, miR-210, a known mediator of antioxidant endothelial responses, when internalized by BMECs, provided endothelial protection against angiotensin II-induced ROS overproduction and EC dysfunction. In addition to mRNA, miRNA and siRNA loading of EVs, recombinant protein delivery to the CNS via EVs has also shown promising results. For example, in a model for the neurodegenerative disorder cerebral folate transport deficiency, investigators showed folate receptor-α containing EVs injected via the intraventricular route restored folate transport [136]. The therapeutic potential of including recombinant proteins in EV cargo was also displayed in a report in which recombinant catalase was captured in macrophage derived EVs and administered intranasally or intra-venously in a Parkinson's mouse model [159]. Injection of these EVs provided considerable protection to dopaminergic neurons. Drug loading of EVs, a procedure often used in the context of anti-cancer treatment, has been demonstrated using many different types of cells [160]. Also, a strategy combining liposome-containing hydrophobic compounds in EVs has been devised as a means to potentially package anti-tumor compounds [161]. The latest novel utilization of EVs as delivery vehicles includes the encapsulation of AAV gene therapy vectors (vexosomes) for the treatment of CNS diseases [162, 163]. These vexosomes not only can target the CNS, but also enable stable transgene expression by the AAV component [156–160].

Although many challenges still remain, such as loading efficiency, specific targeting, scalability and batch to batch consistency, promising results so far are clearly paving the way for the utility of EVs as CNS delivery vehicles.

Perspectives and future directions

As biomarkers

The potential for using EVs as biomarkers in diseases remains of great interest. However, key questions remain regarding how EV subtype and composition change as a function of disease or recovery. Furthermore, can a "signature" EV (i.e., panel in a vesicle biomarker) be identified with the potential to specifically identify a disease or disease severity especially between two conditions with similar pathology? Observations in a recent study found that while 4 markers were increased in both mild TBI and orthopedic patients (compared to healthy controls) only the combination of galectin-3 and occludin was able to distinguish between the two injury types [164]. It is important to note in this study that the authors did not isolate EVs; hence, these markers may be soluble or EV-associated. In some cases, it may be unnecessary to have a biomarker that can distinguish between two related diseases such as TBI and stroke, which have very defined initiation events. However, co-occurring events (i.e. TBI and orthopedic injury) may require more unique biomarkers to identify the prognosis of each injury. In addition, slowly progressing diseases may be harder to discern against the background of individual baselines or noise from multiple conditions. Many initial studies into biomarker utility are restricted and low in power, and the noted effects may become negligible when investigations are expanded. Overall, a panel approach of various biomarkers, along with large-scale multicenter longitudinal approaches will be needed to fully evaluate the utility of blood biomarkers in diagnosing and monitoring recovery following disease or injury onset [124].

In pathology

(i) Do different immune cell subtypes favor brain EVs with a particular TJ protein composition for CNS entry? And, is the act of TJ protein$^+$ EV: leukocyte binding determined by activation state of the leukocyte, or does it determine leukocyte activation state? These questions remain to be answered, and results will shed necessary light on the role(s) of these EVs during pathology. Observations that both circulating EVs and leukocytes display TJ proteins in neuroinflammatory conditions [44, 45, 95], and leukocytes receive at least some of their TJ protein from endothelial cells possibly through EV transmission [44], have prompted suggestion EV:leukocyte communication can regulate leukocyte extravasation into the CNS through a TJ protein-mediated zipper mechanism. However, it remains to be determined that such a scenario operates. As leukocyte TEM occurs both through intercellular (between cells) and transcellular (through cells) routes, EV interactions with particular leukocyte subtypes might influence which route prevails. In this regard, it's been hypothesized that different leukocyte subtypes prefer one route over the other [165], and the extent of leukocyte activation may yet be another determining factor [166]. Future studies detailing whether specific leukocyte subtypes bind EVs containing specific TJ or other adhesion proteins, how this binding may be related to leukocyte activation state, and what effect this binding has on leukocyte TEM, could provide insight into which route of TEM is preferred—and why.

(ii) Do EV interactions at the BBB regulate tumor metastasis to the brain? Given EVs released from varied cell types can impact BMEC gene expression, adhesive properties, and permeability in vitro and in vivo [108], it is reasonable to consider EVs derived from tumor cells could potentially manipulate the BBB to support brain metastasis. Indeed, EVs (comprised of exosomes and microvesicles) isolated from culture supernatants of human breast cancer cells having brain high-metastatic potential were shown to trigger the breakdown of the BBB though a miR-181c-mediated action that interferes with subcortical action dynamics in BMEC (demonstrated using a monkey-derived culture model), promote brain metastasis of breast cancer cell lines, and become preferentially incorporated into the brain of mice in vivo [167]. And it has further been demonstrated that exosomes from mouse and human brain tropic tumor cells, when injected into mice, fuse preferentially with brain endothelial cells [168]. These findings highlight the prospect that interfering with EV release may have therapeutic potential in cancer treatment by mitigating brain involvement.

(iii) Does inhibition of EV biogenesis confer BBB protection? To effectively pursue this question, it is important to recognize acknowledge that certain steps in EV biogenesis are universal for all cell types, while others are not [169]. Thus, answering how EV biogenesis in a brain ECs differ from other cell types or from ECs in other vasculature are likely to produce key insight into how this important biological process can be regulated in diseases of the CNS. Perhaps as a starting point, known pharmacological agents that appear to inhibit EV production could be tested. To date, no reports can be found in which inhibition of EV release has been tested as a therapeutic avenue in the context of neuroinflammation. Should EVs facilitate TEM, it stands to reason that interference with EV release would mitigate neuroinflammation and sustain BBB integrity. However, in support for the idea that interference of EV biogenesis can provide beneficial outcomes, is the utilization of GW4869 in experimental sepsis [170]. Specifically, in vivo inhibition of exosome biogenesis/release by injection of GW4869, was found to lower amounts of exosomes and pro-inflammatory cytokines in serum, and diminish sepsis-induced inflammation and myocardial depression following systemic LPS treatment or cecal ligation/punction surgery in mice [170]. GW4869 administration also alleviated various asthmatic features in a rodent disease model [171], and blocked exosomes from mature dendritic cells from contributing to endothelial inflammation [172], additionally arguing that suppression of EV biogenesis/release attenuates inflammatory-associated disruption to epithelial/endothelial tissues. This raises the prospect that interfering with EV:leukocyte interaction—perhaps by targeting TJ proteins shared by both these elements and BBB endothelial cells—could block formation of EV:leukocyte complexes that have enhanced TEM capability [36, 77] and, thereby, frustrate leukocyte invasion of the CNS.

Conclusions

Just as the complexity of the endothelium—once conventionally dismissed as functionally inert—has become widely recognized, so too has appreciation of the physiological and pathophysiological importance of EVs burgeoned rapidly. What might have begun as "dust" is unlikely to return to dust any time soon. With increased understanding of their association with neuroinflammatory and neurodegenerative disease, EVs are providing a window on the world of CNS barrier status in these conditions. Accessibility of biological fluids is key, as acquisition of EVs from these compartments is minimally invasive and can be performed repeatedly. While blood has most commonly been analyzed, and is a depot of EVs released from all circulating blood elements as well as the luminal surface of the endothelium, EVs present in the CSF are also considered "biomarker treasure chests" [173]. In particular, CSF EVs are likely to more accurately reflect activity of the choroidal epithelial cells of the BCSFB and leptomeningeal cells of the BLMB, as well as immune cell enterprises within the meninges [174]. Improvements in isolating EVs from small amounts of biological fluids and CNS tissues [175], and resolving EV heterogeneity by using high sensitivity/high resolution flow cytometry and cell surface markers to identify donor cell types [176, 177], will prove crucial to realizing the full impact of EVs in the physiology and pathophysiology of CNS barriers.

Abbreviations

AAV: adeno-associated virus; AD: Alzheimer's disease; ARF6: ADP-ribosylation factor 6; ART: antiretroviral therapy; BBB: blood–brain barrier; BCSFB: blood–cerebral-spinal-fluid barrier; BLMB: blood–leptomeningeal barrier; BMEC: brain microvascular endothelial cell; BRB: blood–retinal barrier; CLN-5: claudin-5; CM: cerebral malaria; CP: choroid plexus; CNS: central nervous system; CSI: clinically isolated syndrome; EAE: experimental autoimmune encephalomyelitis; EC: endothelial cell; EMPs: endothelial microparticles; EV: extracellular vesicles; FRα: folate receptor; HAND: HIV-1-associated neurocognitive disorders; hiPSC-MSCs: human induced pluripotent cell-derived mesenchymal stem cells; MP: microparticle; MS: multiple sclerosis; MRI: magnetic resonance imaging; MSC: mesenchymal stem cell; MV: microvesicle; MVB: multi-vesicular bodies; NPC: neural progenitor cells; NRP1: Neuropilin 1; NVU: neurovascular unit; OPC: oligodendrocyte precursor cells; Pgp: p-glycoprotein; PPP: platelet poor plasma; PRBC: parasitized red blood cells; ROS: reactive oxygen species; RPE: retinal pigmented epithelium; RRMS: relapsing/remitting MS; SAS: subarachnoid space; TEM: transendothelial migration; TJ: tight junctions; TBI: traumatic brain injury; vWF: von Willibrand factor.

Authors' contributions

JSP, SHR, AMA and DP wrote the manuscript. SHR and AMA performed experiments and analyzed the data. Illustrations were generated by SHR. All authors read and approved the final manuscript.

Author details

[1] Department of Pathology and Laboratory Medicine, The Lewis Katz School of Medicine at Temple University, 3500 N Broad St, Philadelphia, PA 19140, USA. [2] Shriners Hospital Pediatric Research Center, Philadelphia, PA 19140, USA. [3] Center for Substance Abuse Research, The Lewis Katz School of Medicine at Temple University, Philadelphia, PA 19140, USA. [4] Department of Immunology, Blood-Brain Barrier Laboratory & Laser Capture Microdissection Core, UConn Health, 263 Farmington Ave., Farmington, CT 06070, USA.

Acknowledgements

We would like to acknowledge Ms. Holly Dykstra for her technical contributions (shown in Fig. 2) of this manuscript.

Competing interests

The authors declare that they have no competing interests.

Funding

This work was supported in part by: NIH/NIDA P30 DA013429-16 (SHR), NIH/NINDS R01 NS086570-01 (SHR), NIH/NINDS R01 NS099855-01 (JSP), National Multiple Sclerosis Society RG-1702-27045 (JSP), F32 DA041282-02 (AMA).

References

1. Wolf P. The nature and significance of platelet products in human plasma. Br J Haematol. 1967;13:269–88.
2. van der Pol E, Boing AN, Harrison P, Sturk A, Nieuwland R. Classification, functions, and clinical relevance of extracellular vesicles. Pharmacol Rev. 2012;64:676–705.
3. Kalra H, Drummen GP, Mathivanan S. Focus on extracellular vesicles: introducing the next small big thing. Int J Mol Sci. 2016;17:170.
4. Sharma P, Schiapparelli L, Cline HT. Exosomes function in cell-cell communication during brain circuit development. Curr Opin Neurobiol. 2013;23:997–1004.
5. Morton MC, Feliciano DM. Neurovesicles in brain development. Cell Mol Neurobiol. 2016;36:409–16.
6. Gupta A, Pulliam L. Exosomes as mediators of neuroinflammation. J Neuroinflammation. 2014;11:68.
7. Selmaj I, Mycko MP, Raine CS, Selmaj KW. The role of exosomes in CNS inflammation and their involvement in multiple sclerosis. J Neuroimmunol. 2017;306:1–10.
8. Sampey GC, Meyering SS, Zadeh MA, Saifuddin M, Hakami RM, Kashanchi F. Exosomes and their role in CNS viral infections. J Neurovirol. 2014;20:199–208.
9. Hu G, Yang L, Cai Y, Niu F, Mezzacappa F, Callen S, Fox HS, Buch S. Emerging roles of extracellular vesicles in neurodegenerative disorders: focus on HIV-associated neurological complications. Cell Death Dis. 2016;7:e2481.
10. Levy E. Exosomes in the diseased brain: first insights from in vivo studies. Front Neurosci. 2017;11:142.
11. Quek C, Hill AF. The role of extracellular vesicles in neurodegenerative diseases. Biochem Biophys Res Commun. 2017;483:1178–86.
12. Ciregia F, Urbani A, Palmisano G. Extracellular vesicles in brain tumors and neurodegenerative diseases. Front Mol Neurosci. 2017;10:276.
13. Giusti I, Di Francesco M, Dolo V. Extracellular vesicles in glioblastoma: role in biological processes and in therapeutic applications. Curr Cancer Drug Targets. 2017;17:221–35.
14. Tsilioni I, Panagiotidou S, Theoharides TC. Exosomes in neurologic and psychiatric disorders. Clin Ther. 2014;36:882–8.
15. Brites D, Fernandes A. Neuroinflammation and depression: microglia activation, extracellular microvesicles and microRNA dysregulation. Front Cell Neurosci. 2015;9:476.
16. Simons M, Raposo G. Exosomes–vesicular carriers for intercellular communication. Curr Opin Cell Biol. 2009;21:575–81.
17. Camussi G, Deregibus MC, Tetta C. Paracrine/endocrine mechanism of stem cells on kidney repair: role of microvesicle-mediated transfer of genetic information. Curr Opin Nephrol Hypertens. 2010;19:7–12.
18. Ludwig AK, Giebel B. Exosomes: small vesicles participating in intercellular communication. Int J Biochem Cell Biol. 2012;44:11–5.
19. Maas SL, Breakefield XO, Weaver AM. Extracellular vesicles: unique intercellular delivery vehicles. Trends Cell Biol. 2017;27:172–88.
20. Raposo G, Stoorvogel W. Extracellular vesicles: exosomes, microvesicles, and friends. J Cell Biol. 2013;200:373–83.
21. Abels ER, Breakefield XO. Introduction to extracellular vesicles: biogenesis, RNA cargo selection, content, release, and uptake. Cell Mol Neurobiol. 2016;36:301–12.
22. Kanada M, Bachmann MH, Hardy JW, Frimannson DO, Bronsart L, Wang A, Sylvester MD, Schmidt TL, Kaspar RL, Butte MJ, et al. Differential fates of biomolecules delivered to target cells via extracellular vesicles. Proc Natl Acad Sci USA. 2015;112:E1433–42.

23. Dozio V, Sanchez JC. Characterisation of extracellular vesicle-subsets derived from brain endothelial cells and analysis of their protein cargo modulation after TNF exposure. J Extracell Vesicles. 2017;6:1302705.
24. Andreu Z, Yanez-Mo M. Tetraspanins in extracellular vesicle formation and function. Front Immunol. 2014;5:442.
25. Xu R, Greening DW, Zhu HJ, Takahashi N, Simpson RJ. Extracellular vesicle isolation and characterization: toward clinical application. J Clin Investig. 2016;126:1152–62.
26. Nuzziello N, Blonda M, Licciulli F, Liuni S, Amoruso A, Valletti A, Consiglio A, Avolio C, Liguori M. Molecular characterization of peripheral extracellular vesicles in clinically isolated syndrome: preliminary suggestions from a pilot study. Med Sci (Basel). 2017;5:19.
27. Ge S, Pachter JS. Isolation and culture of microvascular endothelial cells from murine spinal cord. J Neuroimmunol. 2006;177:209–14.
28. Ueno M, Asada K, Toda M, Nagata K, Sotozono C, Kosaka N, Ochiya T, Kinoshita S, Hamuro J. Concomitant evaluation of a panel of exosome proteins and miRs for qualification of cultured human corneal endothelial cells. Investig Ophthalmol Vis Sci. 2016;57:4393–402.
29. Engelhardt B, Ransohoff RM. Capture, crawl, cross: the T cell code to breach the blood-brain barriers. Trends Immunol. 2012;33:579–89.
30. Filippidis AS, Zarogiannis SG, Ioannou M, Gourgoulianis K, Molyvdas PA, Hatzoglou C. Permeability of the arachnoid and pia mater. The role of ion channels in the leptomeningeal physiology. Childs Nerv Syst. 2012;28:533–40.
31. Engelhardt B, Carare RO, Bechmann I, Flugel A, Laman JD, Weller RO. Vascular, glial, and lymphatic immune gateways of the central nervous system. Acta Neuropathol. 2016;132:317–38.
32. Lightman S, Rechthand E, Terubayashi H, Palestine A, Rapoport S, Kador P. Permeability changes in blood-retinal barrier of galactosemic rats are prevented by aldose reductase inhibitors. Diabetes. 1987;36:1271–5.
33. Hamilton RL, Wong JS, Guo LS, Krisans S, Havel RJ. Apolipoprotein E localization in rat hepatocytes by immunogold labeling of cryothin sections. J Lipid Res. 1990;31:1589–603.
34. Patel KD, Zimmerman GA, Prescott SM, McIntyre TM. Novel leukocyte agonists are released by endothelial cells exposed to peroxide. J Biol Chem. 1992;267:15168–75.
35. Combes V, Simon AC, Grau GE, Arnoux D, Camoin L, Sabatier F, Mutin M, Sanmarco M, Sampol J, Dignat-George F. In vitro generation of endothelial microparticles and possible prothrombotic activity in patients with lupus anticoagulant. J Clin Investig. 1999;104:93–102.
36. Jimenez JJ, Jy W, Mauro LM, Horstman LL, Bidot CJ, Ahn YS. Endothelial microparticles (EMP) as vascular disease markers. Adv Clin Chem. 2005;39:131–57.
37. Ordonez NG. Immunohistochemical endothelial markers: a review. Adv Anat Pathol. 2012;19:281–95.
38. Muller AM, Hermanns MI, Skrzynski C, Nesslinger M, Muller KM, Kirkpatrick CJ. Expression of the endothelial markers PECAM-1, vWf, and CD34 in vivo and in vitro. Exp Mol Pathol. 2002;72:221–9.
39. Kim I, Yilmaz OH, Morrison SJ. CD144 (VE-cadherin) is transiently expressed by fetal liver hematopoietic stem cells. Blood. 2005;106:903–5.
40. Yong PJ, Koh CH, Shim WS. Endothelial microparticles: missing link in endothelial dysfunction? Eur J Prev Cardiol. 2013;20:496–512.
41. Dignat-George F, Boulanger CM. The many faces of endothelial microparticles. Arterioscler Thromb Vasc Biol. 2011;31:27–33.
42. Markiewicz M, Richard E, Marks N, Ludwicka-Bradley A. Impact of endothelial microparticles on coagulation, inflammation, and angiogenesis in age-related vascular diseases. J Aging Res. 2013;2013:734509.
43. Chironi GN, Boulanger CM, Simon A, Dignat-George F, Freyssinet JM, Tedgui A. Endothelial microparticles in diseases. Cell Tissue Res. 2009;335:143–51.
44. Paul D, Baena V, Ge S, Jiang X, Jellison ER, Kiprono T, Agalliu D, Pachter JS. Appearance of claudin-5(+) leukocytes in the central nervous system during neuroinflammation: a novel role for endothelial-derived extracellular vesicles. J Neuroinflamm. 2016;13:292.
45. Andrews AM, Lutton EM, Merkel SF, Razmpour R, Ramirez SH. Mechanical injury induces brain endothelial-derived microvesicle release: implications for cerebral vascular injury during traumatic brain injury. Front Cell Neurosci. 2016;10:43.
46. Lovren F, Verma S. Evolving role of microparticles in the pathophysiology of endothelial dysfunction. Clin Chem. 2013;59:1166–74.
47. Endemann DH, Schiffrin EL. Endothelial dysfunction. J Am Soc Nephrol. 2004;15:1983–92.
48. Jaiswal JK, Andrews NW, Simon SM. Membrane proximal lysosomes are the major vesicles responsible for calcium-dependent exocytosis in nonsecretory cells. J Cell Biol. 2002;159:625–35.
49. Robbins PD, Morelli AE. Regulation of immune responses by extracellular vesicles. Nat Rev Immunol. 2014;14:195–208.
50. Hessvik NP, Llorente A. Current knowledge on exosome biogenesis and release. Cell Mol Life Sci. 2018;75:193–208.
51. Daleke DL. Regulation of transbilayer plasma membrane phospholipid asymmetry. J Lipid Res. 2003;44:233–42.
52. Hugel B, Martinez MC, Kunzelmann C, Freyssinet JM. Membrane microparticles: two sides of the coin. Physiology (Bethesda). 2005;20:22–7.
53. Tricarico C, Clancy J, D'Souza-Schorey C. Biology and biogenesis of shed microvesicles. Small GTPases. 2017;8:220–32.
54. Tkach M, Thery C. Communication by extracellular vesicles: where we are and where we need to go. Cell. 2016;164:1226–32.
55. Schiera G, Di Liegro CM, Di Liegro I. Extracellular membrane vesicles as vehicles for brain cell-to-cell interactions in physiological as well as pathological conditions. Biomed Res Int. 2015;2015:152926.
56. Chivet M, Javalet C, Laulagnier K, Blot B, Hemming FJ, Sadoul R. Exosomes secreted by cortical neurons upon glutamatergic synapse activation specifically interact with neurons. J Extracell Vesicles. 2014;3:24722.
57. Huang-Doran I, Zhang CY, Vidal-Puig A. Extracellular vesicles: novel mediators of cell communication in metabolic disease. Trends Endocrinol Metab. 2017;28:3–18.
58. Lizama CO, Zovein AC. Polarizing pathways: balancing endothelial polarity, permeability, and lumen formation. Exp Cell Res. 2013;319:1247–54.
59. Vion AC, Ramkhelawon B, Loyer X, Chironi G, Devue C, Loirand G, Tedgui A, Lehoux S, Boulanger CM. Shear stress regulates endothelial microparticle release. Circ Res. 2013;112:1323–33.
60. Andrews AM, Rizzo V. Microparticle-induced activation of the vascular endothelium requires caveolin-1/caveolae. PLoS ONE. 2016;11:e0149272.
61. Huber J, Vales A, Mitulovic G, Blumer M, Schmid R, Witztum JL, Binder BR, Leitinger N. Oxidized membrane vesicles and blebs from apoptotic cells contain biologically active oxidized phospholipids that induce monocyte-endothelial interactions. Arterioscler Thromb Vasc Biol. 2002;22:101–7.
62. Jansen F, Yang X, Franklin BS, Hoelscher M, Schmitz T, Bedorf J, Nickenig G, Werner N. High glucose condition increases NADPH oxidase activity in endothelial microparticles that promote vascular inflammation. Cardiovasc Res. 2013;98:94–106.
63. Kurachi M, Mikuni M, Ishizaki Y. Extracellular vesicles from vascular endothelial cells promote survival, proliferation and motility of oligodendrocyte precursor cells. PLoS ONE. 2016;11:e0159158.
64. Couch Y, Akbar N, Roodselaar J, Evans MC, Gardiner C, Sargent I, Romero IA, Bristow A, Buchan AM, Haughey N, Anthony DC. Circulating endothelial cell-derived extracellular vesicles mediate the acute phase response and sickness behaviour associated with CNS inflammation. Sci Rep. 2017;7:9574.
65. Hazleton I, Yates A, Dale A, Roodselaar J, Akbar N, Ruitenberg M, Anthony DC, Couch Y. Exacerbation of acute traumatic brain injury by circulating extracellular vesicles. J Neurotrauma. 2017;35:639–51.
66. Andras IE, Toborek M. Extracellular vesicles of the blood-brain barrier. Tissue Barriers. 2016;4:e1131804.
67. Yamamoto S, Niida S, Azuma E, Yanagibashi T, Muramatsu M, Huang TT, Sagara H, Higaki S, Ikutani M, Nagai Y, et al. Inflammation-induced endothelial cell-derived extracellular vesicles modulate the cellular status of pericytes. Sci Rep. 2015;5:8505.
68. Sun L, Wang X, Zhou Y, Zhou RH, Ho WZ, Li JL. Exosomes contribute to the transmission of anti-HIV activity from TLR3-activated brain microvascular endothelial cells to macrophages. Antivir Res. 2016;134:167–71.
69. Losy J. Is MS an inflammatory or primary degenerative disease? J Neural Transm (Vienna). 2013;120:1459–62.

70. Segal BM. Stage-specific immune dysregulation in multiple sclerosis. J Interf Cytokine Res. 2014;34:633–40.
71. Grigoriadis N, van Pesch V, Paradig MSG. A basic overview of multiple sclerosis immunopathology. Eur J Neurol. 2015;22(Suppl 2):3–13.
72. Correale J, Villa A. The blood-brain-barrier in multiple sclerosis: functional roles and therapeutic targeting. Autoimmunity. 2007;40:148–60.
73. Ortiz GG, Pacheco-Moises FP, Macias-Islas MA, Flores-Alvarado LJ, Mireles-Ramirez MA, Gonzalez-Renovato ED, Hernandez-Navarro VE, Sanchez-Lopez AL, Alatorre-Jimenez MA. Role of the blood-brain barrier in multiple sclerosis. Arch Med Res. 2014;45:687–97.
74. Spencer JI, Bell JS, DeLuca GC. Vascular pathology in multiple sclerosis: reframing pathogenesis around the blood-brain barrier. J Neurol Neurosurg Psychiatry. 2018;89:42–52.
75. Alvarez JI, Cayrol R, Prat A. Disruption of central nervous system barriers in multiple sclerosis. Biochim Biophys Acta. 2011;1812:252–64.
76. Alvarez JI, Saint-Laurent O, Godschalk A, Terouz S, Briels C, Larouche S, Bourbonniere L, Larochelle C, Prat A. Focal disturbances in the blood-brain barrier are associated with formation of neuroinflammatory lesions. Neurobiol Dis. 2015;74:14–24.
77. Horstman LL, Jy W, Minagar A, Bidot CJ, Jimenez JJ, Alexander JS, Ahn YS. Cell-derived microparticles and exosomes in neuroinflammatory disorders. Int Rev Neurobiol. 2007;79:227–68.
78. Saenz-Cuesta M, Irizar H, Castillo-Trivino T, Munoz-Culla M, Osorio-Querejeta I, Prada A, Sepulveda L, Lopez-Mato MP, Lopez de Munain A, Comabella M, et al. Circulating microparticles reflect treatment effects and clinical status in multiple sclerosis. Biomark Med. 2014;8:653–61.
79. Allavena R, Noy S, Andrews M, Pullen N. CNS elevation of vascular and not mucosal addressin cell adhesion molecules in patients with multiple sclerosis. Am J Pathol. 2010;176:556–62.
80. Plumb J, McQuaid S, Mirakhur M, Kirk J. Abnormal endothelial tight junctions in active lesions and normal-appearing white matter in multiple sclerosis. Brain Pathol. 2002;12:154–69.
81. Padden M, Leech S, Craig B, Kirk J, Brankin B, McQuaid S. Differences in expression of junctional adhesion molecule-A and beta-catenin in multiple sclerosis brain tissue: increasing evidence for the role of tight junction pathology. Acta Neuropathol. 2007;113:177–86.
82. Jy W, Minagar A, Jimenez JJ, Sheremata WA, Mauro LM, Horstman LL, Bidot C, Ahn YS. Endothelial microparticles (EMP) bind and activate monocytes: elevated EMP-monocyte conjugates in multiple sclerosis. Front Biosci. 2004;9:3137–44.
83. Meziani F, Tesse A, Andriantsitohaina R. Microparticles are vectors of paradoxical information in vascular cells including the endothelium: role in health and diseases. Pharmacol Rep. 2008;60:75–84.
84. Leroyer AS, Anfosso F, Lacroix R, Sabatier F, Simoncini S, Njock SM, Jourde N, Brunet P, Camoin-Jau L, Sampol J, Dignat-George F. Endothelial-derived microparticles: biological conveyors at the crossroad of inflammation, thrombosis and angiogenesis. Thromb Haemost. 2010;104:456–63.
85. Paudel KR, Panth N, Kim DW. Circulating endothelial microparticles: a key hallmark of atherosclerosis progression. Scientifica (Cairo). 2016;2016:8514056.
86. Yun JW, Xiao A, Tsunoda I, Minagar A, Alexander JS. From trash to treasure: the untapped potential of endothelial microparticles in neurovascular diseases. Pathophysiology. 2016;23:265–74.
87. Minagar A, Jy W, Jimenez JJ, Sheremata WA, Mauro LM, Mao WW, Horstman LL, Ahn YS. Elevated plasma endothelial microparticles in multiple sclerosis. Neurology. 2001;56:1319–24.
88. Sheremata WA, Jy W, Delgado S, Minagar A, McLarty J, Ahn Y. Interferon-beta1a reduces plasma CD31 + endothelial microparticles (CD31 + EMP) in multiple sclerosis. J Neuroinflamm. 2006;3:23.
89. Arteaga RB, Chirinos JA, Soriano AO, Jy W, Horstman L, Jimenez JJ, Mendez A, Ferreira A, de Marchena E, Ahn YS. Endothelial microparticles and platelet and leukocyte activation in patients with the metabolic syndrome. Am J Cardiol. 2006;98:70–4.
90. Akbar N, Digby JE, Cahill TJ, Tavare AN, Corbin AL, Saluja S, Dawkins S, Edgar L, Rawlings N, Ziberna K, et al. Endothelium-derived extracellular vesicles promote splenic monocyte mobilization in myocardial infarction. JCI Insight. 2017. https://doi.org/10.1172/jci.insight.93344.
91. Wheway J, Latham SL, Combes V, Grau GE. Endothelial microparticles interact with and support the proliferation of T cells. J Immunol. 2014;193:3378–87.
92. Lu Y, Li L, Yan H, Su Q, Huang J, Fu C. Endothelial microparticles exert differential effects on functions of Th1 in patients with acute coronary syndrome. Int J Cardiol. 2013;168:5396–404.
93. Njock MS, Cheng HS, Dang LT, Nazari-Jahantigh M, Lau AC, Boudreau E, Roufaiel M, Cybulsky MI, Schober A, Fish JE. Endothelial cells suppress monocyte activation through secretion of extracellular vesicles containing antiinflammatory microRNAs. Blood. 2015;125:3202–12.
94. Takahashi T, Kobayashi S, Fujino N, Suzuki T, Ota C, He M, Yamada M, Suzuki S, Yanai M, Kurosawa S, et al. Increased circulating endothelial microparticles in COPD patients: a potential biomarker for COPD exacerbation susceptibility. Thorax. 2012;67:1067–74.
95. Mandel I, Paperna T, Glass-Marmor L, Volkowich A, Badarny S, Schwartz I, Vardi P, Koren I, Miller A. Tight junction proteins expression and modulation in immune cells and multiple sclerosis. J Cell Mol Med. 2012;16:765–75.
96. Alexander JS, Zhu Y, Elrod JW, Alexander B, Coe L, Kalogeris TJ, Fuseler J. Reciprocal regulation of endothelial substrate adhesion and barrier function. Microcirculation. 2001;8:389–401.
97. Gannon P, Khan MZ, Kolson DL. Current understanding of HIV-associated neurocognitive disorders pathogenesis. Curr Opin Neurol. 2011;24:275–83.
98. Atluri VS, Hidalgo M, Samikkannu T, Kurapati KR, Jayant RD, Sagar V, Nair MP. Effect of human immunodeficiency virus on blood-brain barrier integrity and function: an update. Front Cell Neurosci. 2015;9:212.
99. Lescure FX, Omland LH, Engsig FN, Roed C, Gerstoft J, Pialoux G, Kronborg G, Larsen CS, Obel N. Incidence and impact on mortality of severe neurocognitive disorders in persons with and without HIV infection: a Danish nationwide cohort study. Clin Infect Dis. 2011;52:235–43.
100. Lescure FX, Moulignier A, Savatovsky J, Amiel C, Carcelain G, Molina JM, Gallien S, Pacanovski J, Pialoux G, Adle-Biassette H, Gray F. CD8 encephalitis in HIV-infected patients receiving cART: a treatable entity. Clin Infect Dis. 2013;57:101–8.
101. Fischer-Smith T, Tedaldi EM, Rappaport J. CD163/CD16 coexpression by circulating monocytes/macrophages in HIV: potential biomarkers for HIV infection and AIDS progression. AIDS Res Hum Retrovir. 2008;24:417–21.
102. Shiramizu B, Gartner S, Williams A, Shikuma C, Ratto-Kim S, Watters M, Aguon J, Valcour V. Circulating proviral HIV DNA and HIV-associated dementia. AIDS. 2005;19:45–52.
103. Svensson KJ, Christianson HC, Wittrup A, Bourseau-Guilmain E, Lindqvist E, Svensson LM, Morgelin M, Belting M. Exosome uptake depends on ERK1/2-heat shock protein 27 signaling and lipid Raft-mediated endocytosis negatively regulated by caveolin-1. J Biol Chem. 2013;288:17713–24.
104. Dalvi P, Sun B, Tang N, Pulliam L. Immune activated monocyte exosomes alter microRNAs in brain endothelial cells and initiate an inflammatory response through the TLR4/MyD88 pathway. Sci Rep. 2017;7:9954.
105. Chugh PE, Sin SH, Ozgur S, Henry DH, Menezes P, Griffith J, Eron JJ, Damania B, Dittmer DP. Systemically circulating viral and tumor-derived microRNAs in KSHV-associated malignancies. PLoS Pathog. 2013;9:e1003484.
106. Abbruzzese C, Matteoni S, Signore M, Cardone L, Nath K, Glickson JD, Paggi MG. Drug repurposing for the treatment of glioblastoma multiforme. J Exp Clin Cancer Res. 2017;36:169.
107. Roth L, Prahst C, Ruckdeschel T, Savant S, Westrom S, Fantin A, Riedel M, Heroult M, Ruhrberg C, Augustin HG. Neuropilin-1 mediates vascular permeability independently of vascular endothelial growth factor receptor-2 activation. Sci Signal. 2016;9:42.
108. Treps L, Edmond S, Harford-Wright E, Galan-Moya EM, Schmitt A, Azzi S, Citerne A, Bidere N, Ricard D, Gavard J. Extracellular vesicle-transported Semaphorin3A promotes vascular permeability in glioblastoma. Oncogene. 2016;35:2615–23.
109. Faille D, Combes V, Mitchell AJ, Fontaine A, Juhan-Vague I, Alessi MC, Chimini G, Fusai T, Grau GE. Platelet microparticles: a new player in malaria parasite cytoadherence to human brain endothelium. FASEB J. 2009;23:3449–58.

110. Rowe JA, Claessens A, Corrigan RA, Arman M. Adhesion of Plasmodium falciparum-infected erythrocytes to human cells: molecular mechanisms and therapeutic implications. Expert Rev Mol Med. 2009;11:e16.
111. Ho M, White NJ. Molecular mechanisms of cytoadherence in malaria. Am J Physiol. 1999;276:C1231–42.
112. Dunst J, Kamena F, Matuschewski K. Cytokines and chemokines in cerebral malaria pathogenesis. Front Cell Infect Microbiol. 2017;7:324.
113. van der Heyde HC, Nolan J, Combes V, Gramaglia I, Grau GE. A unified hypothesis for the genesis of cerebral malaria: sequestration, inflammation and hemostasis leading to microcirculatory dysfunction. Trends Parasitol. 2006;22:503–8.
114. El-Assaad F, Wheway J, Hunt NH, Grau GE, Combes V. Production, fate and pathogenicity of plasma microparticles in murine cerebral malaria. PLoS Pathog. 2014;10:e1003839.
115. Jung KH, Chu K, Lee ST, Park HK, Bahn JJ, Kim DH, Kim JH, Kim M, Kun Lee S, Roh JK. Circulating endothelial microparticles as a marker of cerebrovascular disease. Ann Neurol. 2009;66:191–9.
116. Deng F, Wang S, Zhang L. Endothelial microparticles act as novel diagnostic and therapeutic biomarkers of circulatory hypoxia-related diseases: a literature review. J Cell Mol Med. 2017;21:1698–710.
117. Li P, Qin C. Elevated circulating VE-cadherin + CD144 + endothelial microparticles in ischemic cerebrovascular disease. Thromb Res. 2015;135:375–81.
118. Porro C, Trotta T, Panaro MA. Microvesicles in the brain: Biomarker, messenger or mediator? J Neuroimmunol. 2015;288:70–8.
119. Marcos-Ramiro B, Oliva Nacarino P, Serrano-Pertierra E, Blanco-Gelaz MA, Weksler BB, Romero IA, Couraud PO, Tunon A, Lopez-Larrea C, Millan J, Cernuda-Morollon E. Microparticles in multiple sclerosis and clinically isolated syndrome: effect on endothelial barrier function. BMC Neurosci. 2014;15:110.
120. Ebrahimkhani S, Vafaee F, Young PE, Hur SSJ, Hawke S, Devenney E, Beadnall H, Barnett MH, Suter CM, Buckland ME. Exosomal micro-RNA signatures in multiple sclerosis reflect disease status. Sci Rep. 2017;7:14293.
121. Xue S, Cai X, Li W, Zhang Z, Dong W, Hui G. Elevated plasma endothelial microparticles in Alzheimer's disease. Dement Geriatr Cogn Disord. 2012;34:174–80.
122. Hosseinzadeh S, Noroozian M, Mortaz E, Mousavizadeh K. Plasma microparticles in Alzheimer's disease: the role of vascular dysfunction. Metab Brain Dis. 2017;33:293–9.
123. Forde CT, Karri SK, Young AM, Ogilvy CS. Predictive markers in traumatic brain injury: opportunities for a serum biosignature. Br J Neurosurg. 2014;28:8–15.
124. Kawata K, Liu CY, Merkel SF, Ramirez SH, Tierney RT, Langford D. Blood biomarkers for brain injury: What are we measuring? Neurosci Biobehav Rev. 2016;68:460–73.
125. Korn A, Golan H, Melamed I, Pascual-Marqui R, Friedman A. Focal cortical dysfunction and blood-brain barrier disruption in patients with Postconcussion syndrome. J Clin Neurophysiol. 2005;22:1–9.
126. Shlosberg D, Benifla M, Kaufer D, Friedman A. Blood-brain barrier breakdown as a therapeutic target in traumatic brain injury. Nat Rev Neurol. 2010;6:393–403.
127. Shan R, Szmydynger-Chodobska J, Warren OU, Zink BJ, Mohammad F, Chodobski A. A new panel of blood biomarkers for the diagnosis of mild traumatic brain injury/concussion in adults. J Neurotrauma. 2015;33:49–57.
128. Bartanusz V, Jezova D, Alajajian B, Digicaylioglu M. The blood-spinal cord barrier: morphology and clinical implications. Ann Neurol. 2011;70:194–206.
129. Reinhold AK, Rittner HL. Barrier function in the peripheral and central nervous system-a review. Pflug Arch. 2017;469:123–34.
130. Prockop LD, Naidu KA, Binard JE, Ransohoff J. Selective permeability of [^{3}H]-D-mannitol and [^{14}C]-carboxyl-inulin across the blood-brain barrier and blood-spinal cord barrier in the rabbit. J Spinal Cord Med. 1995;18:221–6.
131. Naidu KA, Fu ES, Prockop LD. Epinephrine increases the selective permeability of epidurally administered [^{3}H]-D-mannitol and [^{14}C]-carboxyl-inulin across the blood-spinal cord barrier. J Spinal Cord Med. 1996;19:176–82.
132. Mayo JN, Bearden SE. Driving the hypoxia-inducible pathway in human pericytes promotes vascular density in an exosome-dependent manner. Microcirculation. 2015;22:711–23.
133. Fisher M. Pericyte signaling in the neurovascular unit. Stroke. 2009;40:S13–5.
134. Hill J, Rom S, Ramirez SH, Persidsky Y. Emerging roles of pericytes in the regulation of the neurovascular unit in health and disease. J Neuroimmune Pharmacol. 2014;9:591–605.
135. Tumani H, Huss A, Bachhuber F. The cerebrospinal fluid and barriers—anatomic and physiologic considerations. Handb Clin Neurol. 2017;146:21–32.
136. Grapp M, Wrede A, Schweizer M, Huwel S, Galla HJ, Snaidero N, Simons M, Buckers J, Low PS, Urlaub H, et al. Choroid plexus transcytosis and exosome shuttling deliver folate into brain parenchyma. Nat Commun. 2013;4:2123.
137. Cavaillon JM: Exotoxins and endotoxins: Inducers of inflammatory cytokines. *Toxicon* 2017.
138. Balusu S, Brkic M, Libert C, Vandenbroucke RE. The choroid plexus-cerebrospinal fluid interface in Alzheimer's disease: more than just a barrier. Neural Regen Res. 2016;11:534–7.
139. Klingeborn M, Dismuke WM, Skiba NP, Kelly U, Stamer WD, Bowes Rickman C. Directional exosome proteomes reflect polarity-specific functions in retinal pigmented epithelium monolayers. Sci Rep. 2017;7:4901.
140. Locke CJ, Congrove NR, Dismuke WM, Bowen TJ, Stamer WD, McKay BS. Controlled exosome release from the retinal pigment epithelium in situ. Exp Eye Res. 2014;129:1–4.
141. Mazzeo A, Beltramo E, Iavello A, Carpanetto A, Porta M. Molecular mechanisms of extracellular vesicle-induced vessel destabilization in diabetic retinopathy. Acta Diabetol. 2015;52:1113–9.
142. Bruno S, Grange C, Deregibus MC, Calogero RA, Saviozzi S, Collino F, Morando L, Busca A, Falda M, Bussolati B, et al. Mesenchymal stem cell-derived microvesicles protect against acute tubular injury. J Am Soc Nephrol. 2009;20:1053–67.
143. Samsonraj RM, Raghunath M, Nurcombe V, Hui JH, van Wijnen AJ, Cool SM. Concise review: multifaceted characterization of human mesenchymal stem cells for use in regenerative medicine. Stem Cells Transl Med. 2017;6:2173–85.
144. Meirelles Lda S, Nardi NB. Methodology, biology and clinical applications of mesenchymal stem cells. Front Biosci (Landmark Ed). 2009;14:4281–98.
145. Borger V, Bremer M, Ferrer-Tur R, Gockeln L, Stambouli O, Becic A, Giebel B. Mesenchymal stem/stromal cell-derived extracellular vesicles and their potential as novel immunomodulatory therapeutic agents. Int J Mol Sci. 2017;18:1450.
146. Gimona M, Pachler K, Laner-Plamberger S, Schallmoser K, Rohde E. Manufacturing of human extracellular vesicle-based therapeutics for clinical use. Int J Mol Sci. 2017;18:1190.
147. Pistoia V, Raffaghello L. Mesenchymal stromal cells and autoimmunity. Int Immunol. 2017;29:49–58.
148. Marote A, Teixeira FG, Mendes-Pinheiro B, Salgado AJ. MSCs-derived exosomes: cell-secreted nanovesicles with regenerative potential. Front Pharmacol. 2016;7:231.
149. Yang H, Zheng Y, Zhang Y, Cao Z, Jiang Y. Mesenchymal stem cells derived from multiple myeloma patients protect against chemotherapy through autophagy-dependent activation of NF-kappaB signaling. Leuk Res. 2017;60:82–8.
150. Zhang Y, Chopp M, Liu XS, Katakowski M, Wang X, Tian X, Wu D, Zhang ZG. Exosomes derived from mesenchymal stromal cells promote axonal growth of cortical neurons. Mol Neurobiol. 2017;54:2659–73.
151. Ophelders DR, Wolfs TG, Jellema RK, Zwanenburg A, Andriessen P, Delhaas T, Ludwig AK, Radtke S, Peters V, Janssen L, et al. Mesenchymal stromal cell-derived extracellular vesicles protect the fetal brain after hypoxia-ischemia. Stem Cells Transl Med. 2016;5:754–63.
152. Drommelschmidt K, Serdar M, Bendix I, Herz J, Bertling F, Prager S, Keller M, Ludwig AK, Duhan V, Radtke S, et al. Mesenchymal stem cell-derived extracellular vesicles ameliorate inflammation-induced preterm brain injury. Brain Behav Immun. 2017;60:220–32.

153. Chen CC, Liu L, Ma F, Wong CW, Guo XE, Chacko JV, Farhoodi HP, Zhang SX, Zimak J, Segaliny A, et al. Elucidation of exosome migration across the blood-brain barrier model in vitro. Cell Mol Bioeng. 2016;9:509–29.
154. Puentes S, Kurachi M, Shibasaki K, Naruse M, Yoshimoto Y, Mikuni M, Imai H, Ishizaki Y. Brain microvascular endothelial cell transplantation ameliorates ischemic white matter damage. Brain Res. 2012;1469:43–53.
155. Upadhyay RK. Drug delivery systems, CNS protection, and the blood brain barrier. Biomed Res Int. 2014;2014:869269.
156. Kim SM, Kim HS. Engineering of extracellular vesicles as drug delivery vehicles. Stem Cell Investig. 2017;4:74.
157. Kramer-Albers EM. Ticket to ride: targeting proteins to exosomes for brain delivery. Mol Ther. 2017;25:1264–6.
158. Liu H, Wang J, Chen Y, Chen Y, Ma X, Bihl JC, Yang Y. NPC-EXs alleviate endothelial oxidative stress and dysfunction through the miR-210 downstream Nox2 and VEGFR2 pathways. Oxid Med Cell Longev. 2017;2017:9397631.
159. Haney MJ, Klyachko NL, Zhao Y, Gupta R, Plotnikova EG, He Z, Patel T, Piroyan A, Sokolsky M, Kabanov AV, Batrakova EV. Exosomes as drug delivery vehicles for Parkinson's disease therapy. J Control Release. 2015;207:18–30.
160. Pascucci L, Cocce V, Bonomi A, Ami D, Ceccarelli P, Ciusani E, Vigano L, Locatelli A, Sisto F, Doglia SM, et al. Paclitaxel is incorporated by mesenchymal stromal cells and released in exosomes that inhibit in vitro tumor growth: a new approach for drug delivery. J Control Release. 2014;192:262–70.
161. Lee J, Kim J, Jeong M, Lee H, Goh U, Kim H, Kim B, Park JH. Liposome-based engineering of cells to package hydrophobic compounds in membrane vesicles for tumor penetration. Nano Lett. 2015;15:2938–44.
162. Gyorgy B, Fitzpatrick Z, Crommentuijn MH, Mu D, Maguire CA. Naturally enveloped AAV vectors for shielding neutralizing antibodies and robust gene delivery in vivo. Biomaterials. 2014;35:7598–609.
163. Wassmer SJ, Carvalho LS, Gyorgy B, Vandenberghe LH, Maguire CA. Exosome-associated AAV2 vector mediates robust gene delivery into the murine retina upon intravitreal injection. Sci Rep. 2017;7:45329.
164. Shan R, Szmydynger-Chodobska J, Warren OU, Mohammad F, Zink BJ, Chodobski A. A new panel of blood biomarkers for the diagnosis of mild traumatic brain injury/concussion in adults. J Neurotrauma. 2016;33:49–57.
165. Weber C, Fraemohs L, Dejana E. The role of junctional adhesion molecules in vascular inflammation. Nat Rev Immunol. 2007;7:467–77.
166. Muller WA. Mechanisms of leukocyte transendothelial migration. Annu Rev Pathol. 2011;6:323–44.
167. Tominaga N, Kosaka N, Ono M, Katsuda T, Yoshioka Y, Tamura K, Lotvall J, Nakagama H, Ochiya T. Brain metastatic cancer cells release microRNA-181c-containing extracellular vesicles capable of destructing blood-brain barrier. Nat Commun. 2015;6:6716.
168. Hoshino A, Costa-Silva B, Shen TL, Rodrigues G, Hashimoto A, Tesic Mark M, Molina H, Kohsaka S, Di Giannatale A, Ceder S, et al. Tumour exosome integrins determine organotropic metastasis. Nature. 2015;527:329–35.
169. Lai RC, Tan SS, Yeo RW, Choo AB, Reiner AT, Su Y, Shen Y, Fu Z, Alexander L, Sze SK, Lim SK. MSC secretes at least 3 EV types each with a unique permutation of membrane lipid, protein and RNA. J Extracell Vesicles. 2016;5:29828.
170. Essandoh K, Yang L, Wang X, Huang W, Qin D, Hao J, Wang Y, Zingarelli B, Peng T, Fan GC. Blockade of exosome generation with GW4869 dampens the sepsis-induced inflammation and cardiac dysfunction. Biochim Biophys Acta. 2015;1852:2362–71.
171. Kulshreshtha A, Ahmad T, Agrawal A, Ghosh B. Proinflammatory role of epithelial cell-derived exosomes in allergic airway inflammation. J Allergy Clin Immunol. 2013;131:1194–203.
172. Gao W, Liu H, Yuan J, Wu C, Huang D, Ma Y, Zhu J, Ma L, Guo J, Shi H, et al. Exosomes derived from mature dendritic cells increase endothelial inflammation and atherosclerosis via membrane TNF-alpha mediated NF-kappaB pathway. J Cell Mol Med. 2016;20:2318–27.
173. Welton JL, Loveless S, Stone T, von Ruhland C, Robertson NP, Clayton A. Cerebrospinal fluid extracellular vesicle enrichment for protein biomarker discovery in neurological disease; multiple sclerosis. J Extracell Vesicles. 2017;6:1369805.
174. Bechter K, Schmitz B. Cerebrospinal fluid outflow along lumbar nerves and possible relevance for pain research: case report and review. Croat Med J. 2014;55:399–404.
175. Furi I, Momen-Heravi F, Szabo G. Extracellular vesicle isolation: present and future. Ann Transl Med. 2017;5:263.
176. Marcoux G, Duchez AC, Rousseau M, Levesque T, Boudreau LH, Thibault L, Boilard E. Microparticle and mitochondrial release during extended storage of different types of platelet concentrates. Platelets. 2017;28:272–80.
177. Morales-Kastresana A, Telford B, Musich TA, McKinnon K, Clayborne C, Braig Z, Rosner A, Demberg T, Watson DC, Karpova TS, et al. Labeling extracellular vesicles for nanoscale flow cytometry. Sci Rep. 1878;2017:7.
178. Yang T, Martin P, Fogarty B, Brown A, Schurman K, Phipps R, Yin VP, Lockman P, Bai S. Exosome delivered anticancer drugs across the blood-brain barrier for brain cancer therapy in *Danio rerio*. Pharm Res. 2015;32:2003–14.
179. Hazelton I, Yates A, Dale A, Roodselaar J, Akbar N, Ruitenberg MJ, Anthony DC, Couch Y. Exacerbation of acute traumatic brain injury by circulating extracellular vesicles. J Neurotrauma. 2018;35:639–51.
180. Haqqani AS, Delaney CE, Tremblay TL, Sodja C, Sandhu JK, Stanimirovic DB. Method for isolation and molecular characterization of extracellular microvesicles released from brain endothelial cells. Fluids Barriers CNS. 2013;10:4.
181. Jimenez JJ, Jy W, Mauro LM, Horstman LL, Ahn YS. Elevated endothelial microparticles in thrombotic thrombocytopenic purpura: findings from brain and renal microvascular cell culture and patients with active disease. Br J Haematol. 2001;112:81–90.

21

Characteristics of the cerebrospinal fluid pressure waveform and craniospinal compliance in idiopathic intracranial hypertension subjects

Monica D. Okon[1], Cynthia J. Roberts[1,2*], Ashraf M. Mahmoud[1,2], Andrew N. Springer[3], Robert H. Small[1,3], John M. McGregor[4] and Steven E. Katz[5]

Abstract

Background: Idiopathic intracranial hypertension (IIH) is a condition of abnormally high intracranial pressure with an unknown etiology. The objective of this study is to characterize craniospinal compliance and measure the cerebrospinal fluid (CSF) pressure waveform as CSF is passively drained during a diagnostic and therapeutic lumbar puncture (LP) in IIH.

Methods: Eighteen subjects who met the Modified Dandy Criteria, including papilledema and visual field loss, received an ultrasound guided LP where CSF pressure (CSFP) was recorded at each increment of CSF removal. Joinpoint regression models were used to calculate compliance from CSF pressure and the corresponding volume removed at each increment for each subject. Twelve subjects had their CSFP waveform recorded with an electronic transducer. Body mass index, mean CSFP, and cerebral perfusion pressure (CPP) were also calculated. T-tests were used to compare measurements, and correlations were performed between parameters.

Results: Cerebrospinal fluid pressure, CSFP pulse amplitude (CPA), and CPP were found to be significantly different ($p < 0.05$) before and after the LP. CSFP and CPA decreased after the LP, while CPP increased. The craniospinal compliance significantly increased ($p < 0.05$) post-LP. CPA and CSFP were significantly positively correlated.

Conclusions: Both low craniospinal compliance (at high CSFP) and high craniospinal compliance (at low CSFP) regions were determined. The CSFP waveform morphology in IIH was characterized and CPA was found to be positively correlated to the magnitude of CSFP. Future studies will investigate how craniospinal compliance may correlate to symptoms and/or response to therapy in IIH subjects.

Keywords: Idiopathic intracranial hypertension, Cerebrospinal fluid pressure waveform, Cerebrospinal fluid pressure pulse amplitude, Craniospinal compliance, Pressure–volume curves, Compliance, Cerebrospinal fluid pressure

Background

Idiopathic intracranial hypertension (IIH) is a condition of abnormally high intracranial pressure (ICP) with unknown etiology. However, factors such as obesity and stenosis of the venous sinus have been potentially linked [1, 2]. Symptoms include persistent headache, pulsatile tinnitus, diplopia, and visual disturbances such as photophobia [3, 4]. The persistent elevated pressure eventually leads to optic atrophy and vision loss [5]. The management of IIH focuses on the reduction of ICP and ultimately, the protection of vision.

Weight loss, medications, optic nerve sheath fenestrations, and neurosurgical shunting procedures are all therapeutic considerations for the control of intractable headache and the protection of visual function. None of these medical and surgical treatments are curative and they have different risk–benefit profiles. Furthermore, the response to treatment varies between individuals, and there is a lack of consensus in the literature on which

*Correspondence: roberts.8@osu.edu
[1] Department of Biomedical Engineering, The Ohio State University, 1080 Carmack Rd, Columbus, OH 43210, USA
Full list of author information is available at the end of the article

intervention is the most effective [6–8]. Aspects of the craniospinal system such as compliance may vary among individuals and thus influence the expression of the disease and response to treatment.

The purpose of this study is to develop a clinical technique to assess craniospinal compliance during the diagnostic lumbar puncture (LP) in IIH. Analysis of the CSFP waveform and the pressure–volume response in IIH will provide information that may assist in management of the disease.

Methods

Eighteen subjects who presented with signs and symptoms of IIH based on the Modified Dandy Criteria [9] were prospectively recruited under a protocol approved by The Ohio State Institutional Review Board: IRB 2012H0254: long term follow-up of subjects with IIH. Each subject received a standard ophthalmic evaluation by a neuro-ophthalmologist, including visual acuity with a Snellen chart, a slit lamp exam, fundoscopy, and Humphrey Visual Fields (Zeiss Humphrey System, Dublin, California).

Before the LP, all subjects underwent MRI and MRV to rule out structural issues such as mass lesion, infiltrative/inflammatory disease, and venous sinus thrombosis. Each subject subsequently underwent an LP with ultrasound guidance using Siemens Antares Stellar Plus with a CH4-1 transducer (Siemens Medical Solutions, Malvern, PA). An anesthesiologist conducted all of the LPs using either a 4-in. 24-gauge Pencan pencil-point needle, a 4.75-in. 24-gauge Sprotte, or 6-in. 22-gauge Sprotte pencil-point needle to confirm the diagnosis. During the LP, the CSF was passively drained to therapeutically reduce CSFP, in 2–4 ml increments, with a target closing pressure (CP) of 12 mmHg. In 12 subjects, the CSFP waveform was also recorded using an electronic transducer (Edwards LifeScience, Irvine, CA) after each increment of CSF removal.

Measured mean CSFP was plotted against volume removed at each increment for all subjects, with the change in pressure divided by the change in volume representing elastance, which is the inverse of compliance. Löfgren et al. described pressure–volume curves with two compliance regions, a low compliance region at higher CSFP (Region 1) and a high compliance region at lower CSFP (Region 2) [10]. Joinpoint (Joinpoint Regression Program, version 4.5.0.1) is open access software that identifies multiple linear regions in a general dataset, as well as the intersection point they share [11]. This software package was used to determine the two compliance regions in each subject's dataset for the current study. Based on the Bayesian Information Criterion, Joinpoint calculated a transition point from Region 1 to Region 2 in the pressure–volume curves. This transition point between linear regions was defined as the joinpoint. An example of this method is shown in Additional file 1. The craniospinal compliance in each of these regions was then calculated for all subjects as the absolute inverse of the slope of the pressure–volume regression line in each region. The CSF pressure at the joinpoint from the linear regression model was also recorded.

Calculations

From the data collected, body mass index (BMI), the mean CSFP, CSFP pulse amplitude (CPA), cerebral perfusion pressure (CPP), and the craniospinal compliance were calculated. BMI was calculated by using the standard method [12]. The mean CSFP was determined as the average between the peak and trough of the CSFP waveform. The CSFP pulse amplitude (CPA) was the difference in pressure at the peak and trough of the CSFP waveform. The cerebral perfusion pressure (CPP) for each subject was the difference between the measured CSFP and the calculated mean arterial blood pressure. The mean arterial blood pressure was calculated as $(pulse\,pressure/3) + diastolic\,pressure$.

Bivariate normal density ellipses for a probability of 0.95 and linear regression analyses were performed between Opening Pressure (OP) and compliance in both regions, between OP and the CSF pressure at the joinpoint, between compliance in Region 1 and compliance in Region 2, as well as between CPA and mean CSFP for each individual subject as well as for the overall population.

T-tests were performed comparing CSFP, CPA, and CPP before and after the LP, as well as between compliance in Region 1 and Region 2, with $p < 0.05$ as the significance threshold.

Results

All subjects were previously undiagnosed, untreated, and were undergoing an LP for diagnosis and possible therapeutic intervention. Each subject's height, BMI, and the results from the standard ophthalmic evaluation can be found in the Additional file 2. One subject had a BMI less than 25, and thus was not in the overweight or obese category [12]. The Frisén score in subject 1 was not recorded in the chart. Figure 1 shows the relationship between CSFP and CSF volume removal for all subjects. Table 1 summarizes the statistical analysis of the initial and final measurements of CSF pressure, cerebral perfusion pressure (CPP), and CPA, as well as the compliance in Region 1 and Region 2 in all subjects. CSFP, CPA, and CPP were significantly different pre and post LP. CSFP and CPA were all reduced while CPP increased post LP, as expected. The CSFP waveform was not initially studied

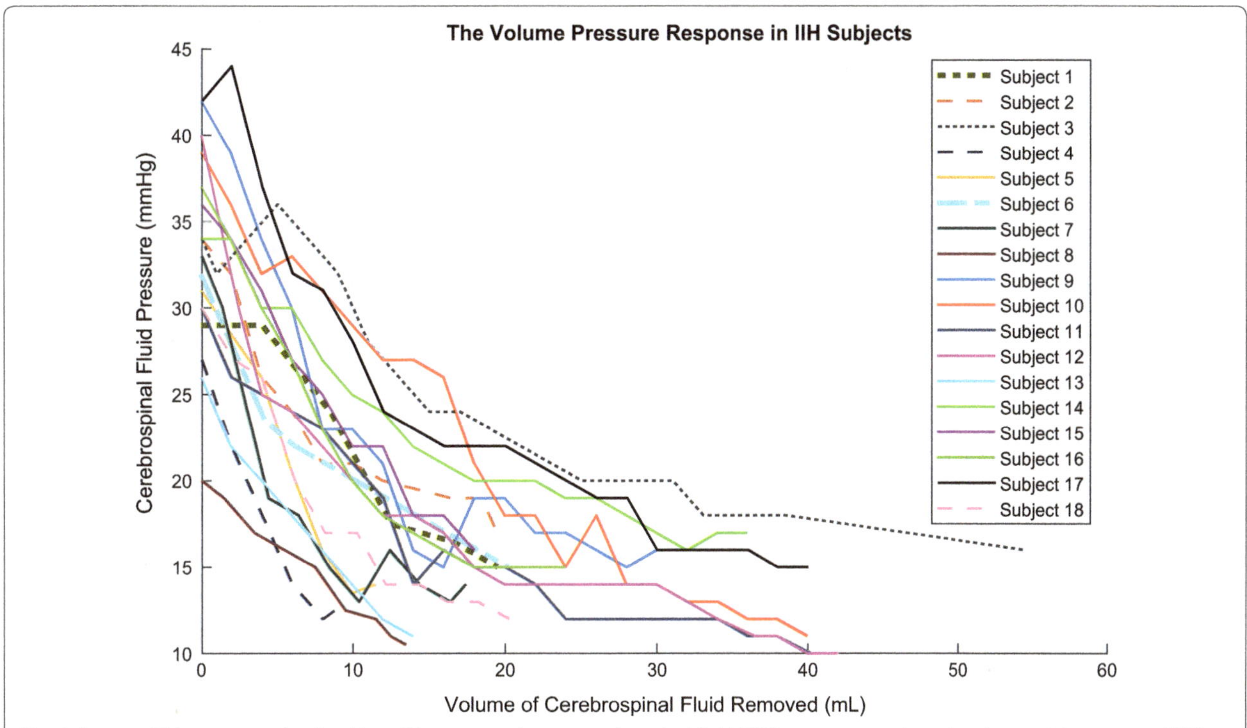

Fig. 1 Pressure-Volume curves for all subjects. The measured mean cerebrospinal fluid (CSF) pressure was plotted against each increment of CSF volume removed for all subjects

Table 1 Statistical Summary of the Pre, During, and Post LP

Measurement (during LP)	N	(R1)	(R2)	p value
Compliance[a] (mL/mmHg)	n = 15	0.70 ± 0.34 (range 0.28–1.5)	3.39 ± 1.84 (range 1.05–7.69)	< 0.0001
Measurement (pre/post LP)	**N**	**Pre-LP**	**Post-LP**	**p value**
CSFP (mmHg)	n = 18	33.11 ± 5.78 (range 20–42)	13.73 ± 2.44 (range 10–17)	< 0.0001
CPA (mmHg)	n = 12	8.08 ± 2.48 (range 4.37–13.66)	1.29 ± 0.64 (range 0.54–2.29)	< 0.0001
CPP (mmHg)	n = 18	53.22 ± 14.45 (range 30–87)	72.33 ± 10.58 (range 59–103)	< 0.0001

[a] Only subjects with two compliance regions identified by Joinpoint were used in the mean calculation

in Subjects 1–4 because the equipment was not available. Waveforms from subjects 6 and 10 were not recorded due to technical difficulties. Compliance in Region 1 and Region 2 were also found to be significantly different.

No joinpoint was identified by the software in three subjects, who were subsequently removed from compliance comparisons and any analysis requiring a joinpoint. In one of these subjects, the opening pressure was 20 mmHg, which is close to the average CSF pressure at the joinpoint of 19.40 ± 3.08 (range 13.26–23.99) mmHg. Therefore, this subject exhibited only Region 2. The other two subjects had insufficient points in either Region 1 or Region 2 for the Joinpoint program to work. The regression lines in Additional file 1 represent elastance, and the mean absolute value of the reciprocal of each, represents compliance. The mean compliance in the first region for the 15 subjects with a joinpoint was significantly lower than the mean compliance in the second region (Table 1).

The CSFP pulse amplitude showed an overall decrease with passive drainage of CSF (Table 1, Additional file 3). A sample set of recorded waveforms for a single subject is given in Additional file 3 and shows the characteristic reduction of CPA with lowering of CSFP. The CPA and CSFP for the 12 subjects with recorded waveforms were positively correlated ($p < 0.005$) for each individual linear regression analysis (Fig. 2). The mean of the slopes for the 12 subjects in Fig. 2 was 0.42 ± 0.14 (range 0.26–0.70). The mean of the R^2 values was 0.94 ± 0.07 (range

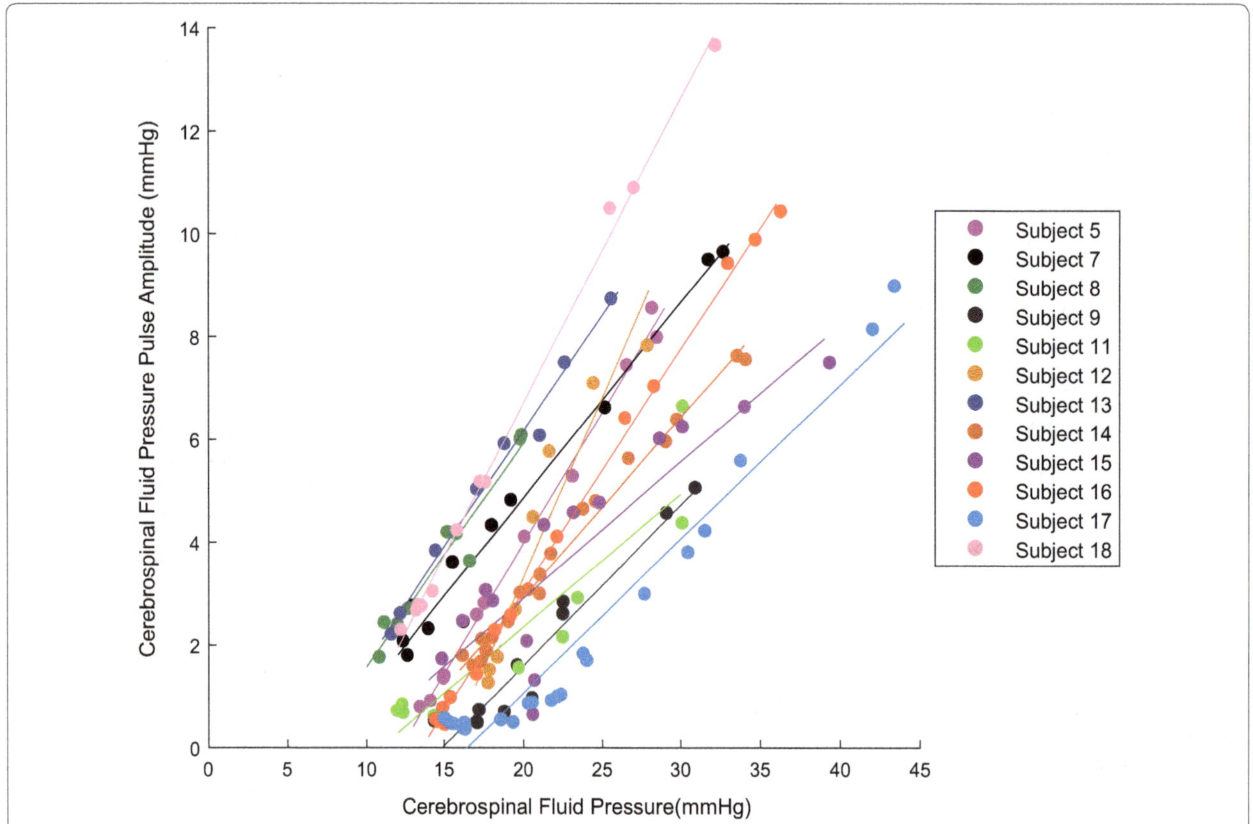

Fig. 2 Cerebrospinal fluid pressure pulse amplitude (CPA) with respect to the mean cerebrospinal fluid pressure (CSFP). The CPA and CSFP were positively correlated ($p < 0.005$) for each individual linear regression analysis of the 12 subjects with recorded waveforms. Note that the strong linear relationship was maintained through both the low compliance region and the high compliance region

0.76–0.998) whereas the overall linear regression analysis for the subjects as a whole population had an R^2 value of 0.55 with $p < 0.05$.

The regression between OP and compliance in Regions 1 and 2 was not significant. The regression between OP and the CSFP at the joinpoint was also found to be not significant. BMI and OP were found to be positively correlated (R^2 value of 0.38 with $p < 0.05$). The correlation between compliance in Region 1 and Region 2 was also not significant. However, the mean values in each region were found to be significantly different (Table 1).

Discussion

Studies have used the pressure response to induced cerebrospinal fluid (CSF) volume changes, including the associated pressure waveform, to describe craniospinal elastance and cerebral hemodynamics in multiple forms of hydrocephalus (communicating, non-communicating, and normal-tension), traumatic brain injuries, IIH and healthy subjects [1, 2, 13–17]. Most of these studies assessed the response to increase in ICP through direct bolus injection. In addition, only a few studies have examined craniospinal compliance and cerebral hemodynamics in IIH [1, 18, 19]. These reported experimental techniques do not translate well to a clinically implementable procedure that might be used to assist in the management of IIH. An LP is required to confirm diagnosis in IIH, and injection of fluid would be inappropriate in the presence of increased ICP. As a consequence, the method proposed in the current study can be used to measure the change of CSF pressure (CSFP) with the passive drainage of CSF during a diagnostic LP, which is also used therapeutically to generate a temporary reduction in ICP. The technique of fluid removal has been reported in the literature to experimentally assess compliance in normal pressure hydrocephalus subjects [20]. However, the opening pressure in these subjects was in the normal range, rather than the abnormal range for IIH.

The clinical lumbar puncture used to obtain the diagnostic opening pressure was also used to characterize craniospinal compliance and investigate the CSFP waveform in the current study. The method of passive drainage to calculate compliance was based on all subjects having an initial elevated CSFP. In Region 1, a small change in CSF volume generated a large change in measured CSFP. In Region 2, a large change in CSF volume generated a small change in measured CSFP. The target pressure of 12 mmHg was not reached in some subjects, as the Region 2 pressure stabilized at a higher level, even as CSF continued to be drained. Therefore, the LP was concluded once Region 2 was well established and CSFP did not change further. All subjects had CSFP reduced below 16 mmHg.

Analyzing the pressure volume curve with two linear regions, as discussed by Löfgren in dogs, was chosen for the current study due to the nature of the pressure–volume relationship associated with our IIH subjects [10]. Löfgren's study used a pressure range that was broader than other studies and characterized the composite pressure–volume response as a function of both cranial and spinal responses [10, 21]. In addition, Anile and Kasprowicz have shown that craniospinal response is viscoelastic [13, 22]. The shape of the pressure–volume curve would be affected by whether fluid is added or removed. Smielewski discussed how bolus manipulation, constant infusion, lumbar ventricular perfusion, and constant pressure infusion may induce a vasomotor response which can disturb a pressure reading [20]. To our knowledge, there are no current human models that measured a pressure–volume curve generated by passive drainage of CSF from an abnormally high CSFP, as in IIH. Previous studies have shown an exponential rise in CSFP with a bolus injection of fluid [17, 23]. A limitation of the current study is the lack of knowledge regarding the repeatability of this technique to calculate compliance. However, treatment is designed to lower intracranial pressure and therefore it may affect compliance, so the pressure–volume curve would be expected to be different.

Other investigators have focused their efforts on measuring compliance noninvasively through models based on MRI measurements and anatomical changes [1, 24–26]. However, these efforts to make the measurement non-invasive would be more helpful after a baseline has been established. One study found reduced compliance in IIH when compared to healthy subjects using MRI [32]. However, the reduced compliance in IIH can be expected because CSFP is presumably higher than in normal subjects. The current study utilizes the diagnostic lumbar puncture as an avenue to characterize an individual's craniospinal compliance. This method quantifies an individual's cerebrospinal system response, and may help clinicians to better tailor IIH disease management. The measurement of craniospinal compliance in IIH may provide clinical benefit by evaluating the cerebrospinal system's ability to adapt to changes [27]. The ability to respond to changes in the cerebrospinal system may lead to differences in the manifestation of symptoms or responses to treatment.

Previous studies have shown that the amplitude of pulsations in the CSFP waveform can be influenced by compliance, the magnitude of CSFP, and cerebral blood flow [15, 28–31]. Szewczykowski, Avezaat, Czosnyka, and Qvarlander found a positive relationship between the overall CPA and mean value of CSFP waveform in subjects with and without CSF disorders, which is also consistent with the data reported in the current study, and shown in Fig. 2 [32–37]. However, some previous studies have also reported a region of constant compliance below 10 mmHg [32, 35–37]. None of our subjects were evaluated in this region, since the target closing pressure for the lumbar puncture was 12 mmHg. This target was not achieved in several of our subjects where the CSFP leveled above 12 mmHg and did not reduce in this region even with passive fluid removal.

Additional file 3 shows the influence of CSF drainage on CSFP and craniospinal compliance as it inversely affects the overall amplitude of the CSFP waveform pulsations. As cerebral perfusion pressure increases, the pulse amplitude decreases, due to a change in compliance. Eide et al. reported that all of their IIH subjects who were undergoing a shunt placement had an elevated pulse amplitude (above 4 mmHg) despite having a normal ICP level [38]. The CPA in those subjects ranged from 4–8.7 mmHg [38]. Eide measured the ICP waveform in the frontal brain parenchyma while the current study measured in the lumbar region.

It is interesting to note the change in waveform morphology as CSFP is reduced and compliance is increased, as illustrated in Additional file 3. The pulsatile nature is attributed to the arterial and venous pulsations [30], and the CSFP waveform directly reflects cardiovascular events. At the highest CSFP where compliance is low, the dicrotic notch is clearly visible, similar to an arterial waveform [31]. As CSF volume was removed, the CSFP was reduced and the morphology of CSFP waveform also changed. When the CSFP was lowered to a normal range (< 20 mmHg), the distinct dicrotic notch in the waveform disappeared. Thus, the distinct features of the arterial waveform are transmitted to the CSF system when it is in a low compliance state, but not in a high compliance state.

Conclusions

The objective of the current study was to develop a clinically implementable technique for characterizing the CSFP waveform and craniospinal compliance in IIH. This objective was met using passive drainage of CSF during the diagnostic lumbar puncture, rather than bolus injection. Regions of low and high compliance were reported that corresponded to high CSFP and low CSFP, respectively, as well as a CSF pressure where a transition between the two regions occurred. CSFP magnitude, craniospinal compliance, and cerebral hemodynamics influence the CSFP waveform measured while using a technique that is clinically feasible. These parameters may predict the cerebrospinal system's ability to adjust to induced changes. The next step would be to investigate whether such parameters can be associated to severity of symptoms and response to treatment in IIH.

Abbreviations

BMI: body mass index; CP: closing pressure; CPA: CSFP pulse amplitude; CPP: cerebral perfusion pressure; CSFP: cerebrospinal fluid pressure; ICP: intracranial pressure; IIH: idiopathic intracranial hypertension; LP: lumbar puncture; OP: opening pressure.

Authors' contributions

CJR, RHS, JMM, and SEK contributed to the conception and design of the study. All authors contributed to the acquisition of data. MDO, CJR, AMM, RHS, and SEK contributed to the analysis and interpretation of data. MDO, CJR, RHS, and SEK were involved in drafting and revising the manuscript. All authors read and approved the final manuscript.

Author details

[1] Department of Biomedical Engineering, The Ohio State University, 1080 Carmack Rd, Columbus, OH 43210, USA. [2] Department of Ophthalmology & Visual Science, The Ohio State University, 915 Olentangy River Rd, Columbus, OH 43212, USA. [3] Department of Anesthesiology, The Ohio State University, 410W. 10th Avenue, Columbus, OH 43210, USA. [4] Department of Neurosurgery, The Ohio State University, 1581 Dodd Drive, Columbus, OH 43210, USA. [5] Ohio Neuro-Ophthalmology, Orbital Disease & Oculoplastics, 3545 Olentangy River Rd, Suite 200, Columbus, OH 43214, USA.

Acknowledgements

Not applicable

Competing interests

The authors declare that they have no competing interests.

References

1. Alperin N, Lam BL, Tain RW, et al. Evidence for altered spinal canal compliance and cerebral venous drainage in untreated idiopathic intracranial hypertension. Acta Neurochir Suppl. 2012;114:201–5.
2. Alperin N, Ranganathan S, Bagci AM, et al. MRI evidence of impaired CSF homeostasis in obesity-associated idiopathic intracranial hypertension. AJNR Am J Neuroradiol. 2013;34(1):29–34.
3. Yuh EL, Dillon WP. Intracranial hypotension and intracranial hypertension. Neuroimaging Clin N Am. 2010;20(4):597–617.
4. Biousse V, Bruce BB, Newman NJ. Update on the pathophysiology and management of idiopathic intracranial hypertension. J Neurol Neurosurg Psychiatry. 2012;83(5):488–94.
5. Passi N, Degnan AJ, Levy LM. MR imaging of papilledema and visual pathways: effects of increased intracranial pressure and pathophysiologic mechanisms. AJNR Am J Neuroradiol. 2013;34(5):919–24.
6. Feldon SE. Visual outcomes comparing surgical techniques for management of severe idiopathic intracranial hypertension. Neurosurg Focus. 2007;23(5):E6.
7. Wall M, Kupersmith MJ, Kieburtz KD, et al. The idiopathic intracranial hypertension treatment trial: clinical profile at baseline. JAMA Neurol. 2014;71(6):693–701.
8. Lueck C, McIlwaine G. Interventions for idiopathic intracranial hypertension. Cochrane Database Syst Rev. 2005;3(3):CD003434.
9. Wall M. Idiopathic intracranial hypertension. Neurol Clin. 2010;28(3):593–617.
10. Löfgren J, Essen CV, Zwetnow NN. The pressure-volume curve of the cerebrospinal fluid space in dogs. Acta Neurol Scand. 1973;49(4):557–74.
11. Statistical Methodology and Application Branch. Joinpoint regression program, version 4.5.0.1; 2017.
12. Calculate your body mass index. http://www.nhlbi.nih.gov/health/educational/lose_wt/BMI/bmicalc.htm. Accessed 16 June 2017.
13. Kasprowicz M, Czosnyka M, Czosnyka Z, et al. Hysteresis of the cerebrospinal pressure-volume curve in hydrocephalus. Acta Neurochir Suppl. 2003;86:529–32.
14. Maset AL, Marmarou A, Ward JD, et al. Pressure-volume index in head injury. J Neurosurg. 1987;67(6):832–40.
15. Carrera E, Kim DJ, Castellani G, et al. What shapes pulse amplitude of intracranial pressure? J Neurotrauma. 2010;27(2):317–24.
16. Czosnyka M, Czosnyka Z, Keong N, et al. Pulse pressure waveform in hydrocephalus: what it is and what it isn't. Neurosurg Focus. 2007;22(4):E2.
17. Shapiro K, Marmarou A, Shulman K. Characterization of clinical CSF dynamics and neural axis compliance using the pressure-volume index: I. the normal pressure-volume index. Ann Neurol. 1980;7(6):508–14.
18. Sklar FH, Beyer CW Jr, Clark WK. Physiological features of the pressure-volume function of brain elasticity in man. J Neurosurg. 1980;53(2):166–72.
19. Sklar FH, Diehl JT, Beyer CW Jr, Clark WK. Brain elasticity changes with ventriculomegaly. J Neurosurg. 1980;53(2):173–9.
20. Smielewski P, Czosnyka M, Roszkowski M, Walencik A. Identification of the cerebrospinal compensatory mechanisms via computer-controlled drainage of the cerebrospinal fluid. Childs Nerv Syst. 1995;11(5):297–300.
21. J Löfgren, Zwetnow NN. Cranial and spinal components of the cerebrospinal fluid pressure-volume curve. Acta Neurol Scand. 1973;49(5):575–85.
22. Anile C, Portnoy HD, Branch C. Intracranial compliance is time-dependent. Neurosurgery. 1987;20(3):389–95.
23. Marmarou A, Shulman K, LaMorgese J. Compartmental analysis of compliance and outflow resistance of the cerebrospinal fluid system. J Neurosurg. 1975;43(5):523–34.
24. Bruce BB. Noninvasive assessment of cerebrospinal fluid pressure. J Neuro Ophthalmol. 2014;34(3):288–94.
25. Eklund A, Smielewski P, Chambers I, et al. Assessment of cerebrospinal fluid outflow resistance. Med Biol Eng Comput. 2007;45(8):719–35.
26. Czosnyka M, Pickard JD. Monitoring and interpretation of intracranial pressure. J Neurol Neurosurg Psychiatry. 2004;75(6):813–21.
27. Tain R, Bagci AM, Lam BL, Sklar EM, Ertl-Wagner B, Alperin N. Determination of cranio-spinal canal compliance distribution by MRI: methodology and early application in idiopathic intracranial hypertension. J Magn Reson Imaging. 2011;34(6):1397–404.
28. Anile C, De Bonis P, Mangiola A, Mannino S, Santini P. A new method of estimating intracranial elastance. Interdiscip Neurosurg. 2014;1(2):26–30.
29. Eide PK. The correlation between pulsatile intracranial pressure and indices of intracranial pressure-volume reserve capacity: results from ventricular infusion testing. J Neurosurg. 2016;125:1493–1503.
30. Adolph R, Fukusumi H, Fowler N. Origin of cerebrospinal fluid pulsations. Am J Physiol Legacy Content. 1967;212(4):840–6.
31. Cardoso ER, Rowan JO, Galbraith S. Analysis of the cerebrospinal fluid pulse wave in intracranial pressure. J Neurosurg. 1983;59(5):817–21.
32. Szewczykowski J, liwka S, Kunicki A, Dytko P, Korsak-liwka J. A fast method of estimating the elastance of the intracranial system. J Neurosurg. 1977;47(1):19–26.
33. Avezaat CJ, van Eijndhoven JH, Wyper DJ. Cerebrospinal fluid pulse pressure and intracranial volume-pressure relationships. J Neurol Neurosurg Psychiatr. 1979;42(8):687–700.
34. Czosnyka M, Guazzo E, Whitehouse M, et al. Significance of intracranial pressure waveform analysis after head injury. Acta Neurochir. 1996;138(5):531–41 **(discussion 541-2)**.
35. Qvarlander S, Malm J, Eklund A. The pulsatility curve—the relationship between mean intracranial pressure and pulsation amplitude. Inst Phys Eng Med. 2010;31(11):1517.

22

Comparative transcriptomics of choroid plexus in Alzheimer's disease, frontotemporal dementia and Huntington's disease: implications for CSF homeostasis

Edward G. Stopa[1†], Keith Q. Tanis[2†], Miles C. Miller[1], Elena V. Nikonova[2], Alexei A. Podtelezhnikov[2], Eva M. Finney[2], David J. Stone[2], Luiz M. Camargo[2], Lisan Parker[2], Ajay Verma[3], Andrew Baird[4], John E. Donahue[1], Tara Torabi[1], Brian P. Eliceiri[4], Gerald D. Silverberg[1] and Conrad E. Johanson[1*]

Abstract

Background: In Alzheimer's disease, there are striking changes in CSF composition that relate to altered choroid plexus (CP) function. Studying CP tissue gene expression at the blood–cerebrospinal fluid barrier could provide further insight into the epithelial and stromal responses to neurodegenerative disease states.

Methods: Transcriptome-wide Affymetrix microarrays were used to determine disease-related changes in gene expression in human CP. RNA from post-mortem samples of the entire lateral ventricular choroid plexus was extracted from 6 healthy controls (Ctrl), 7 patients with advanced (Braak and Braak stage III–VI) Alzheimer's disease (AD), 4 with frontotemporal dementia (FTD) and 3 with Huntington's disease (HuD). Statistics and agglomerative clustering were accomplished with MathWorks, MatLab; and gene set annotations by comparing input sets to GeneGo (http://www.genego.com) and Ingenuity (http://www.ingenuity.com) pathway sets. Bonferroni-corrected hypergeometric p-values of <0.1 were considered a significant overlap between sets.

Results: Pronounced differences in gene expression occurred in CP of advanced AD patients vs. Ctrls. Metabolic and immune-related pathways including acute phase response, cytokine, cell adhesion, interferons, and JAK-STAT as well as mTOR were significantly enriched among the genes upregulated. Methionine degradation, claudin-5 and protein translation genes were downregulated. Many gene expression changes in AD patients were observed in FTD and HuD (e.g., claudin-5, tight junction downregulation), but there were significant differences between the disease groups. In AD and HuD (but not FTD), several neuroimmune-modulating interferons were significantly enriched (e.g., in AD: IFI-TM1, IFN-AR1, IFN-AR2, and IFN-GR2). AD-associated expression changes, but not those in HuD and FTD, were enriched for upregulation of VEGF signaling and immune response proteins, e.g., interleukins. HuD and FTD patients distinctively displayed upregulated cadherin-mediated adhesion.

Conclusions: Our transcript data for human CP tissue provides genomic and mechanistic insight for differential expression in AD vs. FTD vs. HuD for stromal as well as epithelial components. These choroidal transcriptome characterizations elucidate immune activation, tissue functional resiliency, and CSF metabolic homeostasis. The BCSFB undergoes harmful, but also important functional and adaptive changes in neurodegenerative diseases; accordingly,

*Correspondence: Conrad_Johanson@brown.edu
†Edward G. Stopa and Keith Q. Tanis contributed equally to this work
[1] Departments of Neurosurgery and Pathology (Neuropathology Division), Rhode Island Hospital, The Warren Alpert Medical School, Brown University, Providence, RI, USA
Full list of author information is available at the end of the article

the enriched JAK-STAT and mTOR pathways, respectively, likely help the CP in adaptive transcription and epithelial repair and/or replacement when harmed by neurodegeneration pathophysiology. We anticipate that these precise CP translational data will facilitate pharmacologic/transgenic therapies to alleviate dementia.

Keywords: Choroid plexus transcriptome, Neuroimmune CSF regulation, Blood–CSF barrier inflammatome, Janus kinase/signal transducers and activators of transcription (JAK-STAT), Peroxisome-proliferator-activated receptor (PPAR), Cadherin-mediated adhesion, Vascular endothelial growth factor, LRP-1, Choroid plexus methionine, CSF homocysteine, Mechanistic target of rapamycin (mTOR)

Background

The choroid plexus (CP) is a CNS secretory tissue within the cerebroventricular system consisting of a vascular stroma surrounded by epithelium [1, 2]. Although the primary function of choroidal tissue is to produce and regulate cerebrospinal fluid (CSF), it also importantly provides a permeability-regulating blood–CSF barrier (BCSFB) [3]. Other additional roles of CP relate to CNS wound repair [4], sex hormone modulation of BCSFB-CNS [5], catabolite detoxification [6], ion regulation [7], a selective leukocyte gate [8], and CSF–brain neuroimmune homeostasis, including interferon actions [9–13]. Recently, the BCSFB tissue has been examined for unique CP changes in diverse disorders: mitochondrial diseases [14], multiple sclerosis/experimental autoimmune encephalitis [15, 16], schizophrenia [17], acute response to peripheral immune challenge [18], normal pressure hydrocephalus [19], and Alzheimer's disease (AD) [20, 21].

Analyzing the transformed CP tissue composition and pathophysiologic functions in neurodegeneration elucidates specific metabolic/secretory processes underlying CSF–CNS disease pathogenesis [22]. BCSFB alterations such as choroid epithelial cell atrophy, stromal fibrosis, vascular thickening, tight junction (claudin-5) downregulation, and basement membrane thickening are associated with AD pathology [20]. These changes in the epithelial–stromal nexus likely affect secretion and transport, resulting in diminished CSF turnover and modified neuroimmune regulation. Neuroimmune phenomena in the CP and/or CSF include adjustments in the level of proteins (e.g., neurotrophins, interferons and growth factors), cytokines, and certain immune cells [12, 22]. Oxidative stressors in AD and other dementias may also differentially impact CP's ability to synthesize/transport proteins/hormones, and to regulate cellular/CSF metabolites such as methionine/homocysteine [23], Aβ/tau [24], and creatine/creatinine [25].

This investigation at the Brown University Medical School, in collaboration with Merck & Co., analyzed gene expression in CP tissues from late-stage Alzheimer patients, for comparison with control subjects (Ctrl) and two other diseases: frontotemporal dementia (FTD) and Huntington's disease (HuD). Our working hypothesis anticipated: (i) common denominators of altered CP expression in the three diseases, as well as (ii) differential expression patterns due to disease-specific alterations in neural metabolites, that by 'homeostatic feedback signaling' via volume transmission from brain to CSF to CP, could uniquely modulate gene expression at the BCSFB.

Investigating CP tissue gene expression in various CNS diseases likely informs on diverse BCSFB adjustments to neurodegeneration. Bergen et al. [26] focused on gene expression changes by CP epithelial cells in AD. In this study, we analyze CP tissue responses (epithelium plus stroma) by providing profiles of mRNA changes. The altered expression profiles in AD, FTD and HuD are discussed in relation to restorative homeostatic mechanisms, as well as to chronic BCSFB damage and disrupted CSF–brain homeostasis.

Methods

Project approval, sample collection and demographics

This research with banked specimens of human CP tissue was approved by the Institutional Review Board for Clinical Research at *Lifespan*, Rhode Island Hospital, Providence, RI. Post-mortem tissue samples from 6 healthy Ctrls of mean age 60 years, mean post-mortem interval (PMI) 22 h; and from 7 patients with advanced AD (Braak and Braak stage III–VI, 80 years, PMI 17 h), 4 FTD (72 years, PMI NA) and 3 HuD (71 years, PMI 19 h), were snap frozen in liquid N_2 and stored at − 80 °C in the Brown University Brain Tissue for Neurodegenerative Disorders Resource Center until processed. Demographic and disease data for the individual controls and patients are presented in Table 1.

Microarray design and analysis

RNA from CP was extracted using TRIzol reagent in accordance with instructions by manufacturer (ThermoFisher, Grand Island, NY). Isolated RNA samples were assayed for quality via the Agilent RNA 6000 Pico Kit on Agilent Bioanalyzer (Santa Clara, CA) and RNA yield via Quanti-iT RiboGreen RNA Assay Kit (ThermoFisher). Samples were amplified and labeled using an automated version of the NuGEN Ovation WB protocol

Table 1 Demographic and clinical data of choroid plexus samples collected

Sample ID #	Diagnosis	Age	Sex	PMI
CP_CTR_007	Control	62	M	23.9
CP_CTR_008	Control	55	F	29
CP_CTR_009	Control	37	M	18.7
CP_CTR_010	Control	64	M	25.8
CP_CTR_011	Control	69	F	12.3
CP_CTR_012	Control	70	M	N/A
CP_ALZ_015	AD (Braak III–IV)	74	F	15
CP_ALZ_017	AD (severe Braak V–VI)	84	F	N/A
CP_ALZ_018	AD (severe Braak V–VI)	84	M	N/A
CP_ALZ_019	AD (severe + Lewy body disease)	84	F	N/A
CP_ALZ_020	AD (severe Braak V–VI)	89	M	N/A
CP_ALZ_022	AD (severe Braak V–VI)	73	M	24.5
CP_ALZ_023	AD (severe Braak V–VI)	70	M	10.8
CP_FTD_024	FTD	76	M	N/A
CP_FTD_025	FTD and motor neuron disease	75	F	N/A
CP_FTD_026	FTD Pick's disease	58	M	N/A
CP_FTD_027	FTD	80	F	N/A
CP_HuD_029	HuD (grade IV)	68	M	30.1
CP_HuD_030	HuD (grade IV)	65	F	3.5
CP_HuD_031	HuD (grade IV)	80	M	24

after normalizing to 50 ng total RNA input (NuGEN Technologies, San Carlos, CA). Gene expression profiling was performed with a customized Human Affymetrix GeneChip microarray (GEO platform GPL 10379) that included 57,060 probe sets (Affymetrix, Santa Clara, CA). Hybridization (45 °C for 18 h), labeling, and scanning, using Affymetrix ovens, fluidics stations, and scanners, were conducted following the protocols recommended (NuGEN Technologies). All 20 samples passed RNA integrity and Affymetrix quality control metrics. The final sample set contained RNA from 6 Ctrl, 7 AD, 4 FTD and 3 HuD subjects (Table 1, Additional file 1: Table S1).

Data processing, statistics and annotation

Data were normalized by robust multiarray average (RMA) [27], and each sample was ratioed to the average of the Ctrl samples [28]. Statistical analysis and agglomerative clustering were performed using MathWorks MatLab (Natick, MA). In some statistical analyses, due to insufficient power, HuD and FTD data were combined into one non-AD disease grouping, as indicated by: (HuD + FTD). Gene set annotation analysis was performed by comparing input sets to GeneGo (http://www.genego.com) and Ingenuity (http://www.ingenuity.com) pathway sets. Bonferroni-corrected hypergeometric p-values (expectation (e)-values) of <0.1 were considered a significant overlap between sets.

Results

We first compared the genome-wide differences in gene expression between diseased and Ctrl CP. p-value distributions from T-test comparisons, between the Ctrl group and each of the neurodegenerative disease groups (AD, HuD, FTD), revealed significant effects on the CP transcriptome in each of the 3 diseases (Fig. 1a, Additional file 2: Table S2). The AD group had the highest number of differentially expressed probe sets likely due, at least in part, to the higher number of AD subjects compared to HuD and FTD. 3935 (7%) out of the 57,060 probe sets on the array were differentially expressed [$p < 0.01$, false discovery rate (FDR) = 14%] between AD and Ctrl subjects, while 1287 (FDR = 44%) and 2136 (FDR = 27%) probe sets were regulated with $p < 0.01$ in HuD and FTD, respectively (Fig. 1a, b, Additional file 2: Table S2). Despite the limited statistical power and resulting high false discovery rates in the HuD and FTD comparisons, there was a large degree of overlap in the genes identified in each of the comparisons (Fig. 1b, c, Additional file 2: Table S2). Almost all probe sets differentially expressed ($p < 0.01$) in the AD samples had significant or a trend toward differential expression in the same direction in the other two disease groups (Fig. 1c, Additional file 2: Table S2). In Additional file 4: Table S4 are listed the top 10 most upregulated and 10 most downregulated genes from the AD vs. Ctrl comparison; 80% of these findings were confirmed by multiple probe sets when available on the array.

In order to validate these findings with different subjects and gene expression platforms, we compared the results in whole CP to those obtained by Bergen et al. in laser-dissected CP epithelial cells from control and AD subjects [26]. We anticipated that the changes reported in CP epithelial cells would also be evident in the whole CP samples but to a lesser degree given the presence of additional cell types such as stroma and immune cells in the whole tissue samples. Indeed, the 36 genes reported as differentially expressed in AD CP epithelium by microarray, and in some cases [17] also by quantitative PCR (Bergen et al. Tables 1 and 2 in [26]), were regulated similarly in AD whole CP tissue in our study ($r^2 \sim 0.7$), but to a lesser magnitude (by ~ 35%, as indicated by linear regression in Fig. 1d). 34 of the 36 differentially expressed genes reported by Bergen et al. [26] were modulated in the same direction from Ctrl in both studies, with 20 obtaining significance ($p < 0.05$) in the current AD whole CP tissue comparison. Similarly the expression values in whole CP from FTD and HuD

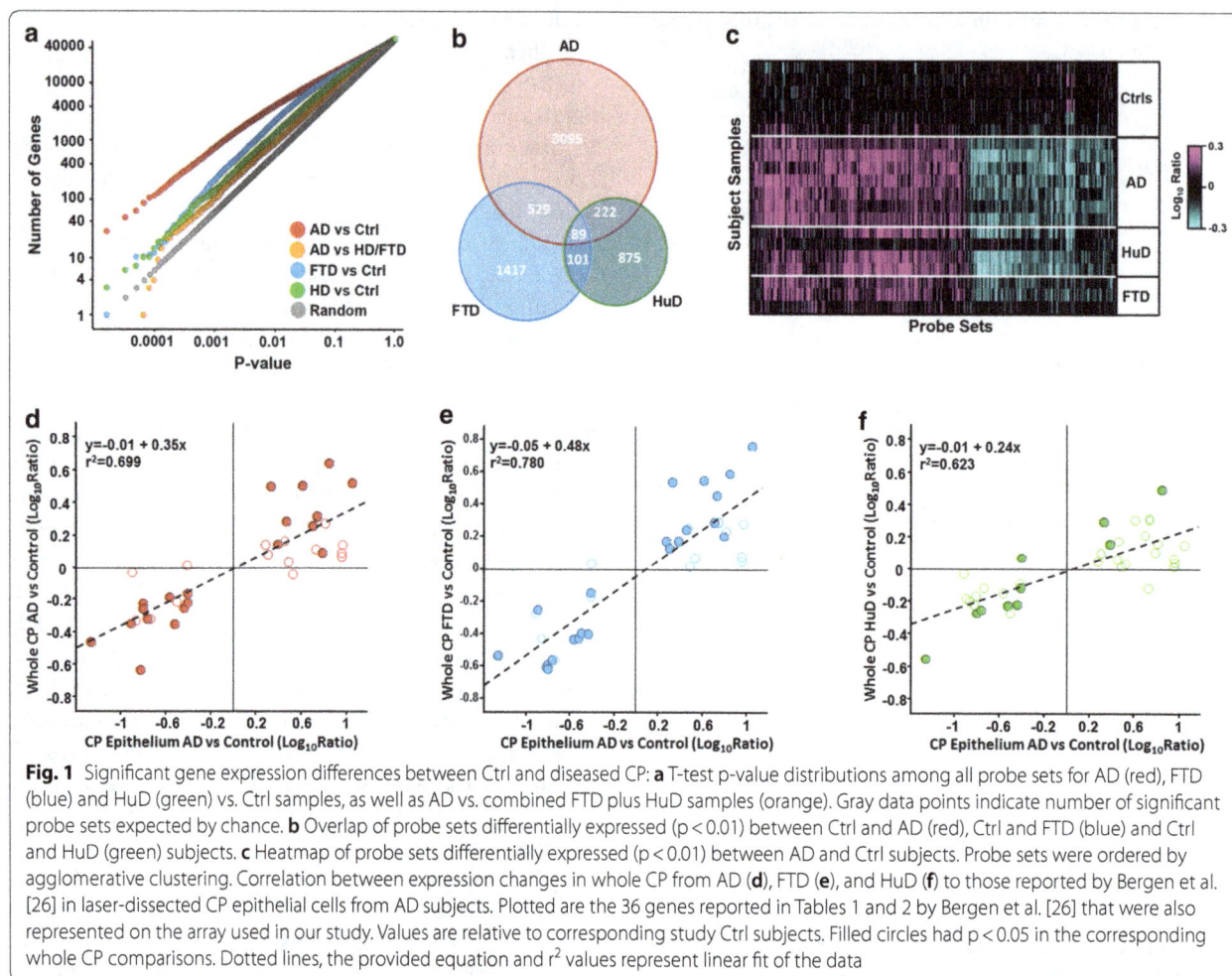

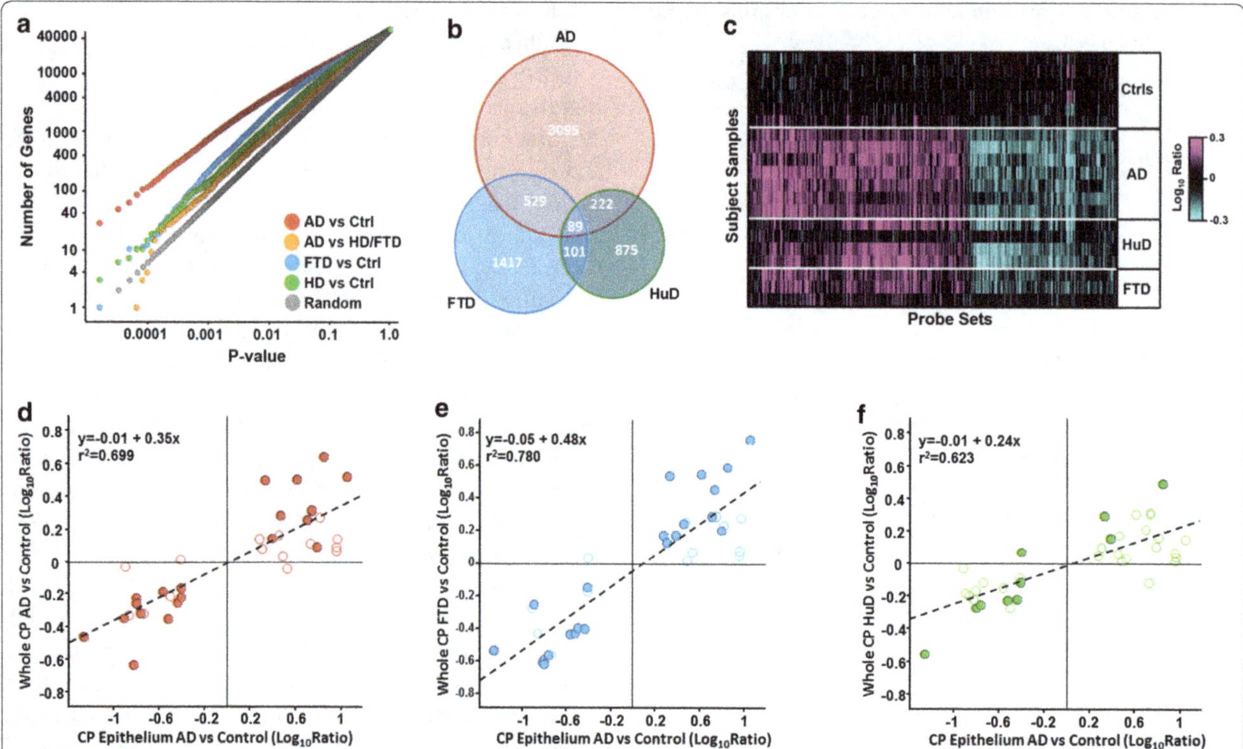

Fig. 1 Significant gene expression differences between Ctrl and diseased CP: **a** T-test p-value distributions among all probe sets for AD (red), FTD (blue) and HuD (green) vs. Ctrl samples, as well as AD vs. combined FTD plus HuD samples (orange). Gray data points indicate number of significant probe sets expected by chance. **b** Overlap of probe sets differentially expressed ($p<0.01$) between Ctrl and AD (red), Ctrl and FTD (blue) and Ctrl and HuD (green) subjects. **c** Heatmap of probe sets differentially expressed ($p<0.01$) between AD and Ctrl subjects. Probe sets were ordered by agglomerative clustering. Correlation between expression changes in whole CP from AD (**d**), FTD (**e**), and HuD (**f**) to those reported by Bergen et al. [26] in laser-dissected CP epithelial cells from AD subjects. Plotted are the 36 genes reported in Tables 1 and 2 by Bergen et al. [26] that were also represented on the array used in our study. Values are relative to corresponding study Ctrl subjects. Filled circles had $p<0.05$ in the corresponding whole CP comparisons. Dotted lines, the provided equation and r^2 values represent linear fit of the data

also correlated with those reported for AD CP epithelium in reference # [26] ($r^2=0.8$ and 0.6, respectively, Fig. 1e, f).

In this study, among the 3935 probe sets differentially expressed ($p<0.01$) in AD compared to Ctrl subjects, 2332 were upregulated and 1603 downregulated (Fig. 1b, Additional file 2: Table S2). The differentially expressed genes were examined for overlap with ~2000 GeneGo and Ingenuity pathways. Ninety-two pathways were enriched (Bonferroni corrected p-value, i.e., e-value, <0.01) among the upregulated genes. These enrichments represented primarily immune-related pathways, including acute phase response, cytokine and interferon signaling, NFkB, and cell adhesion, as well as growth factor, JAK-STAT and mTOR signaling pathways, PPAR signaling and protein/nucleic acid salvage pathways (Fig. 2, Additional file 3: Table S3a). Pathway enrichment among downregulated genes was less extensive (12 pathways with $e<0.01$), including genes involved in methionine degradation and protein translation (Fig. 2, Additional file 3: Table S3b).

Many differences between AD and Ctrl were also observed in HuD vs. FTD (Fig. 1, Additional file 2: Table S2). However, there were also some significant differences between AD vs. HuD+FTD, with 902 (1.6%) probe sets significant at $p<0.01$ (63% FDR) (Fig. 3). Figure 3a displays the genes up and down-regulated in AD more than in the combined HuD+FTD group; whereas Fig. 3b presents the opposite, i.e., genes regulated more in HuD+FTD than in AD. The 513 probe sets uniquely upregulated in AD: AD vs. Ctrl ($p<0.01$) and AD vs. HuD+FTD ($p<0.05$) were enriched ($e<0.1$) predominately in interleukin and VEGF signaling genes (Additional file 3: Table S3c). There were 272 probe sets uniquely downregulated in AD: AD vs. Ctrl ($p<0.01$) and AD vs. HuD+FTD ($p<0.05$) but were not significantly ($e<0.1$) enriched in any queried pathway. The 112 probe sets uniquely upregulated in HuD+FTD, that is, HuD+FTD vs. Ctrl ($p<0.01$), and HuD+FTD vs. AD ($p<0.05$), were enriched ($e<0.1$) in cadherin-mediated cell adhesion (Additional file 3: Table S3d). The 115 probe sets uniquely downregulated in AD vs. Ctrl ($p<0.01$),

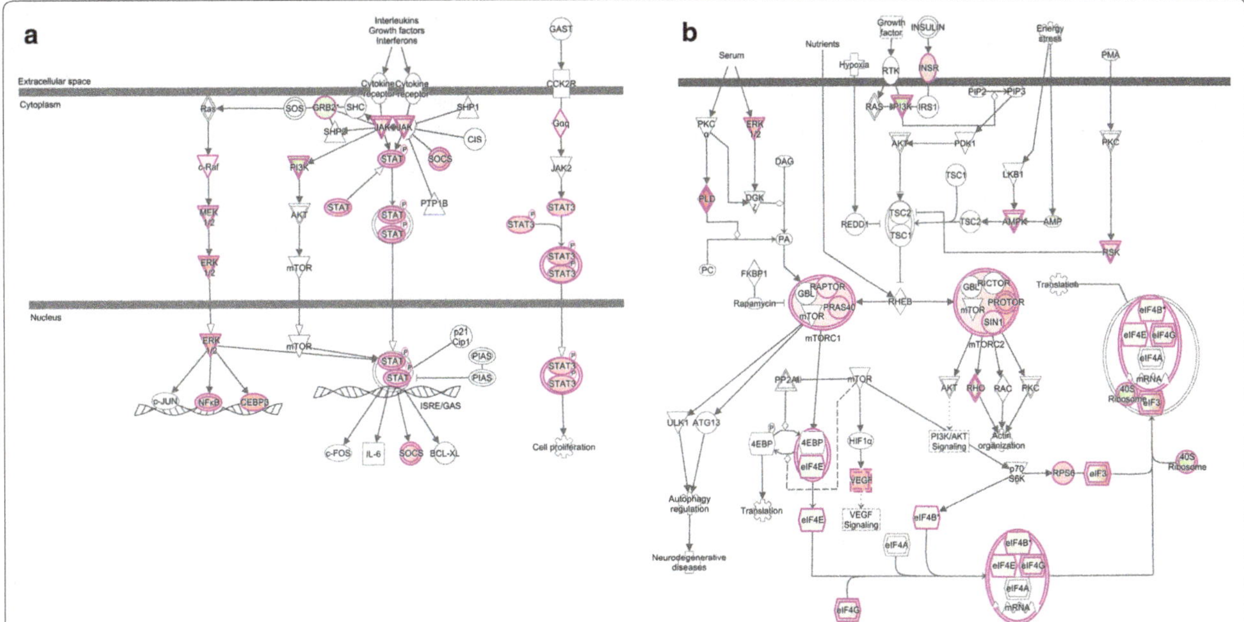

Fig. 2 Up-regulation of the JAK-STAT and mTOR pathways: Ingenuity pathway maps for **a** JAK-STAT signaling (transducing extracellular signals to transcriptional responses) and **b** mTOR signaling (a master regulator for many fundamental cellular repair processes). Genes with AD vs. Ctrl ($p < 0.01$) are outlined in red, and filled with red or green, indicating the magnitude of increased or decreased expression, respectively, in AD

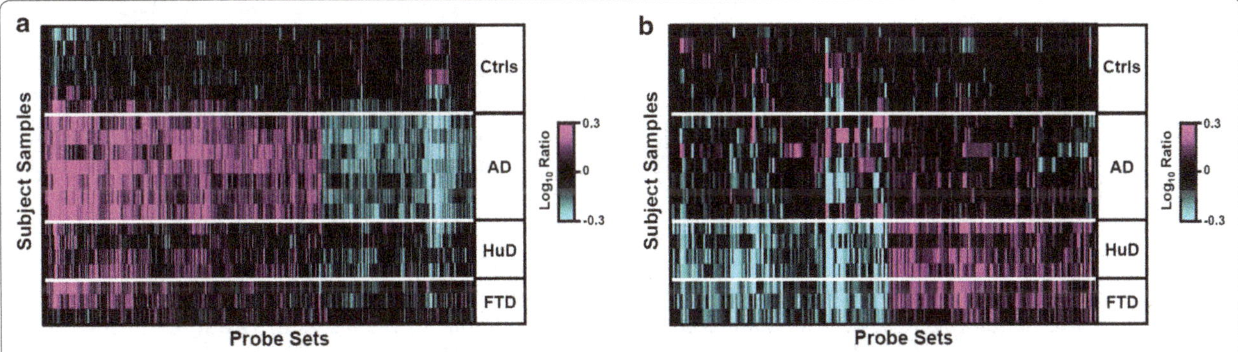

Fig. 3 Expression changes unique to AD, or to the combined HuD + FTD, non-AD 'disease control' group: **a** Heatmap of probe sets differentially expressed between AD and Ctrl subjects ($p < 0.01$), and altered more relative to the control in the AD group than in the non-AD 'disease control' group (AD/Ctrl)/(HuD + FTD/Ctrl) > 1, and AD vs. HuD + FTD, ($p < 0.05$). Probe sets are ordered by agglomerative clustering. **b** Heatmap of probe sets differentially expressed between the combined HuD + FTD group and Ctrl subjects ($p < 0.01$), and altered more relative to the combined HuD + FTD disease control group than in the AD group (HuD + FTD/Ctrl)/(AD/Ctrl) > 1, and HuD + FTD vs. AD, ($p < 0.05$). Probe sets were ordered by agglomerative clustering. Red (magenta) and green (cyan) indicate the magnitude of increased and decreased expression, respectively

and AD vs. HuD + FTD ($p < 0.05$), were not significantly ($e < 0.1$) enriched in assessed biological pathways.

The emphasis here is on gene sets and associated biological pathways. Still, it is instructive to focus on several genes/proteins currently of great interest in CP pathophysiology. Altered tight junction protein claudin-5 in CP is associated with BCSFB breaching [26], while interferon has a protein-signaling role that couples choroidal-cerebral neuroimmune interactions [13]. Claudin-5 was downregulated 1.6-, 1.9- and 2.5-fold in AD, FTD and HuD, respectively, reaching significance in FTD (respective p values of 0.071, 0.028 and 0.059). Multiple interferon signaling genes were upregulated in AD: IFI-TM1 ($p = 0.0008$), IFN-AR1 ($p = 0.006$), IFN-AR2 ($p = 0.0007$) and IFN-GR2 ($p = 0.0002$). The complete lists of differentially-expressed genes, as well as enriched biological pathways, are provided in Additional file 2: Table S2, Additional file 3: Table S3, Additional file 4: Table S4.

Discussion

Comparing gene expression in CP of AD subjects to that of Ctrls and other neurodegenerative diseases reveals important biological functions altered by dementia generation and progression. The CP as a dynamic interface between blood, CSF and brain, is able to monitor distortions and homeostatically respond, e.g., by the JAK-STAT pathway as well as cytokine and protein-signaling molecules [12, 13]. These homeostatic adjustments impact neural viability. This intimates that CP beneficial adjustments, as well as BCSFB malfunctioning, are pertinent to AD progression. The strategic role of CSF to safeguard brain is manifested by CP upregulation of many genes in response to neurodegeneration ([26] and this investigation); and by its ability to protect basic CSF composition (e.g., K, pH and vitamin homeostasis) even in advanced AD [7]. Nevertheless, the CP in AD incurs structural damage [20] and distorted epithelial metabolism and transport (e.g., Aβ, cytokine (e.g., TNFα) and methionine/homocysteine [24, 29]). The injured epithelium likely depends on enhanced mTOR expression to facilitate cellular repair and/or replacement. Accordingly, the state of CP–CSF viability in ongoing neurodegeneration is a balance between debilitating and restorative events at the BCSFB [29–31].

In this study we have shown numerous transcriptional alterations in the CP of subjects with neurodegenerative disease. Given that the BCSFB makes adjustments in CSF composition, the prolific disease-induced expression changes in CP fits previous homeostasis modeling [1, 30]. Most transcript changes were common to AD, FTD and HuD, while fewer genes were modulated differently between AD and HuD + FTD. It is instructive to compare the present observations with an earlier transcriptional investigation of the BCSFB in AD [26]. Whereas we studied homogenates of entire CP, including epithelium and stroma, Bergen et al. studied single epithelial cells captured by laser microscopy [26]. Thus, Bergen et al. provided data on epithelium-specific changes in AD (larger-fold changes, see Fig. 1d–f), while our dataset also includes potential pathophysiological interactions between CP stroma and epithelium. Indeed, robust inflammatory responses were not reported by Bergen et al. [26], suggesting deductively that the immune-reactive pathophysiology occurs primarily within CP stroma.

Some limitations of our study include the small number of patients in the HuD and FTD groups, and the lack of direct confirmation of specific genes by RT-PCR. Future studies with a larger N value for HuD and FTD will increase the statistical power for disease comparisons. For post-mortem tissue, RNA stability is challenging with autopsy specimens collected at various PMIs; however, we carefully assessed RNA integrity, using only samples passing stringent criteria. Moreover, our emphasis was on significantly-enriched pathways (affecting multiple genes within a given pathway) rather than specific gene targets, with possible individual false discoveries. Any residual blood elements in specimens would unlikely explain differences in tissue mRNA among the three disease groups. The somewhat younger Ctrl group may be advantageous in avoiding potentially confounding issues with clinically-silent early dementia in an older 'Ctrl' cohort, otherwise presumed normal.

We used GeneGo (http://www.genego.com) and Ingenuity (http://www.ingenuity.com) sets for pathway analysis. In AD compared to Ctrls, this revealed *upregulated* inflammation genes: acute phase response, cell adhesion and cytokine, interferon, JAK-STAT signaling (for translating extracellular signals into transcriptional responses). Notable *downregulated* pathways were methionine degradation and protein translation; both are implicated in AD pathology. Claudin-5 expression was downregulated, consistent with the enhanced leakiness of the BCSFB [31] encountered in neurodegenerative diseases [26] and pathophysiology models [29]. Amyloid beta peptide (Aβ) damages CP tight junctions by activating matrix metalloproteineases, thereby increasing paracellular permeability [32]. The functional significance of such altered CP pathways, for disease outcome, awaits elucidation.

Prominent in AD was *upregulated* inflammation-related signaling. These inflammation signatures differ from cortex-associated microglial infiltration [33, 34]. Key marker genes of cortical inflammation-APOE, TREM2, TYROBP-did not upregulate in AD CP. Rather, acute phase response genes dominated the upregulation: multiple cytokine and interferon receptors, JAK-STAT signaling components, MAPK, NFκB signaling and cell adhesion. Cytokines and growth factors in disease-associated reactions in BCSFB come from brain [35], blood, or CP itself. The CP responds biochemically and transcriptionally to circulating cytokines, central injury and systemic diseases [18, 36, 37]. Localized CP immunoreactions (e.g., inflammation-resolving leukocyte trafficking) may benefit brain by sensing 'injury signals' flowing from brain to CSF to CP, then feeding back to make homeostatic neural adjustments [35].

At certain stages of advancing neuroinflammation (caused by brain-residing pro-inflammatory microglial responses to Aβ loads), the CP receives plasma interferon-γ as a signal to promote homeostatic transport of anti-inflammatory monocyte-derived macrophages into CSF for resolving parenchymal inflammation [12]. Disease-induced disruption of this neuroimmune interferon adjustment at the BCSFB [38] could compromise the ability of the CSF–brain to thwart AD exacerbation. The CP competently adapts to AD stress [39] by maintaining an immunosuppressant profile of factors, e.g., VEGF and TGFβ1 in CSF, to help manage brain inflammation after neuronal injury [40].

Increased expression of LRP-1, a choroidal Aβ transporter, agrees with mouse AD modeling [24]. Upregulated LRP-1 in the apical membrane expedites Aβ removal from CSF [24]. Augmented reabsorptive clearance of Aβ at the BCSFB aids the CNS because cerebral capillaries in AD extrude less Aβ [41]. This compensatory Aβ removal by CP counters the disabled microvessels [42]. Titers of inflammatory cytokines and choroidal proteins, in CSF and blood, present in different degrees in AD [43]. Activated astrocytes and microglia congregate in Aβ plaques [44]. The manner in which CP inflammatory-signaling molecules modify AD pathogenesis is heterogeneous. Acute inflammation may beneficially promote CSF clearance of affected cells and Aβ aggregates, protecting neurons. However, persistently-elevated CP–CSF cytokines and sustained activation of microglia adversely affect neurons. An effective CP will balance the beneficial vs. detrimental effects of CSF cytokine changes in AD, FTD and HuD.

Amyloid beta induces cytokine production; and astrocytes activated by Aβ, release inflammatory factors that sustain Aβ production. Clearly the CP–CSF, using soluble signals and upregulated cellular adhesion factors, appropriately distributes certain T cell phenotypes to CSF [12]; such leukocyte penetration into CSF helps to control neuroinflammation and Aβ levels in AD brain. The dynamic relationship between pro-inflammatory and anti-inflammatory cytokines in CP–CSF impacts neuroinflammation processes and AD pathology.

Peroxisome-proliferator-activated receptor (PPAR) signaling genes, including PPARδ and its obligate heterodimer RXRα, were enriched in AD CP. PPAR/RXRs are neuroprotective in AD and Aβ therapies due to anti-inflammatory and endothelial actions [43]. PPAR activation, through endogenous or synthetic ligands, likely protects CP by increasing antioxidant capacity and improving energy supply; this maintains fuel for the Na pump [45] and CSF secretion [46], and increases expression of Aβ transporters [47]. The novel GFT1803 agent (a pan-PPAR agonist that activates all 3 PPAR isoforms) attenuates Aβ loading-induced damage and neuroinflammation [48]. PPAR thus deserves attention as a potential pathway for restoring CP–CSF integrity in AD in order to counter neurodegeneration.

Significant expression differences were also observed between AD and FTD+HuD. The VEGF signaling pathway (including VEGFA and VEGF receptors FLT1 and FLT4) displayed significant upregulation in AD but not in FTD or HuD. This agrees with our previous findings of increased VEGF within AD CP [1]. VEGF is required for maintaining endothelial cell fenestration in CP capillaries [49], an important microstructural feature for delivering plasma substances into the choroidal interstitium for epithelial processing.

Cadherin, on the other hand, was upregulated in FTD and HuD but not AD. Cadherin is a superfamily of cellular adhesion molecules (CAM), that maintain tissue structure and boundaries between cells and organelles. CAM binding also modifies gene expression. Cell–cell adhesions mediate specific immune actions [50], of which there is a plethora in CP of FTD and HuD patient specimens. A cadherin family member prominent in CP is γ-protocadherin (γ-Pcdh), expressed at the apical membrane [51]. Mutation of γ-Pcdh causes ventricular collapse. Keep et al. proposed an immune and CSF dynamics role for CP γ-Pcdh [52], that co-expresses with the NaBCN2 Na transporter supporting CSF secretion. This gene may function in CP ion transport-CSF formation by way of apical–microskeletal membrane interactions with NaBCN2 that regulate ion trafficking [32]. Moreover, Kolmer immune cells, attached to CP apical surface [53], may have an altered function in neurodegenerative diseases when cadherin is upregulated.

We hypothesize that the downregulated expression observed in this study reflects failing metabolic pathways involved in choroid cell and CSF homeostasis. Reduction in methionine-degradation genes is intriguing given that excessive homocysteine, a product of methionine metabolism, is a risk factor for AD [54–57]. Methionine loading increases brain homocysteine, Aβ and phospho-tau in mouse models [58]. Decreased expression in AD CP of the methionine-degrading gene may relate to elevated homocysteine levels in CSF [59]. The impact of augmented CSF homocysteine on raising brain Aβ and tau hints that additional methionine gene studies on CP transcription factors and metabolism in neurodegenerative diseases are needed.

We also determined a decreased expression of protein translation genes, including multiple eukaryotic translation initiation factors (EIF genes) and ribosomal proteins. CP has a major role in producing and secreting CSF proteins, e.g., transthyretin that stabilizes Aβ conformation. In AD there is decreased choroidal synthesis of transthyretin [24], lowering its CSF concentration [60]. Moreover, the heat stress glucose regulatory proteins 78 and 94 in human AD CP are diminished [39], implicating suboptimal glucose or calcium homeostasis. Altered heat stress proteins at the AD BCSFB deserve examination for impact on cerebral metabolism.

Expression of mTOR associates with controlling cell growth and proliferation [61], possibly a factor as damaged choroid epithelial cells need replacement. Our finding of increased fatty acid oxidation and upstream mTOR signaling (Fig. 2), with juxtaposed downregulated protein translation, fits existing concepts suggesting altered energy metabolism in AD onset and progression. While increased PPAR activity downstream of mTOR fits the compensatory adaptation to retain CP resiliency, there is a disconnect between upregulated mTOR and the downregulated protein translation machinery typically induced by mTOR. This suggests a break in normal mTOR signaling (see Fig. 2) that could undermine CP function or resiliency when challenged with neurodegeneration. This is significant because of CP's pivotal role in providing brain with supportive factors and immune cells that migrate across BCSFB into CSF–brain. Studies need to assess the role of the dynamic CP transcriptome in providing resiliency to the BCSFB, in order to retain CSF homeostatic reserve for staving off neurodegeneration.

Conclusions

The AD transcript findings reported herein for bulk CP tissue compare favorably with and expand prior analysis in laser-captured epithelial cells [26]. Such concurrence is remarkable given the different tissue sampling, measurement platforms and patient cohorts. Highlights of our investigation include *upregulated* genes linked to inflammation and interferon neuroimmune homeostasis, as well as to JAK-STAT and mTOR; and *downregulated* genes for methionine degradation, protein translation and claudin-5 (tight junction). CP is a complex homeostatic tissue. The BCSFB undergoes deleterious, but sometimes functional and adaptive, changes in dementia-related pathophysiology. The enriched JAK-STAT and mTOR pathways (Fig. 2), respectively, are likely instrumental in promoting adaptive transcriptional responses and epithelial repair/replacement when CP is harmed by injuries associating with neurodegeneration. Analyzing biological pathway mechanisms expedites specific pharmacologic targeting.

Future transcriptome work with larger cohorts should delineate gene expression by demographic endpoints, Braak staging, Aβ plaque score, disease duration, ApoE genotype, co-morbidity, and other disease characteristics. The transcriptome distinctions here precisely describe CP–CSF function in, and response to, certain neuropathologies: AD vs. FTD vs. HuD. This categorical approach provides crucial knowledge on the BCSFB role in pathogenesis; and hopefully should improve prophylaxis of various neural diseases. The goal: To identify exact CP targets to exploit when implementing pharmacologic/genetic therapies to alleviate CSF–brain metabolic distortions in dementia.

Abbreviations

Aβ: amyloid beta; AD: Alzheimer's disease; APOE: apolipoprotein; BCSFB: blood–CSF barrier; CP: choroid plexus; CSF: cerebrospinal; EIF: eukaryotic translation initiation factors; FDR: false discovery rate; FTD: frontotemporal dementia; HuD: Huntington's disease; JAK-STAT: Janus kinase/signal transducers and activators of transcription; LRP1: low density lipoprotein receptor-related protein 1; mTOR: mechanistic target of rapamycin; PMI: post-mortem interval; PPAR: peroxisome-proliferator-activate receptor; RAGE: receptor for advanced glycation end product; TGFβ: transforming growth factor beta; VEGF: vascular endothelial growth factor.

Authors' contributions

ES conceived the original research design, wrote/edited a significant part of the paper, and coordinated the manuscript input from various authors. KT conducted the bioinformatics/statistical analyses, constructed figures/tables, and wrote/edited part of the manuscript. MM processed the choroid plexus specimens, contributed to research design, and organized datasets for uploading to the Gene Expression Omnibus (GEO). EN, AP, EF, DS, LC, LP, AV, AB, JD, TT, BE, and GS participated in tissue collection/processing, discussed aspects of experimental design/execution, or helped with manuscript preparation. CJ participated in the project planning, wrote/edited a large part of the paper, and integrated manuscript input from all authors. All authors read and approved the final manuscript.

Author details

[1] Departments of Neurosurgery and Pathology (Neuropathology Division), Rhode Island Hospital, The Warren Alpert Medical School, Brown University, Providence, RI, USA. [2] Genetics and Pharmacogenomics, Merck & Co., Inc., West Point, PA, USA. [3] United Neuroscience, Dublin, Ireland. [4] Department of Surgery, University of California San Diego Medical Center, Hillcrest, 212 Dickinson Street, San Diego, CA, USA.

Acknowledgements

The authors would like to thank the families of patients with AD, referred from the Department of Neurology at Rhode Island Hospital, for donating patient brains to the Brown University Brain Tissue for Neurodegenerative Disorders Resource Center.

Funding

This study was supported by funds provided by Merck & Co. (for CP tissue transcript analyses and bioinformatical/statistical work), and by the Division of Neuropathology at Rhode Island Hospital (for CP tissue storage/processing and manuscript costs).

References

1. Stopa EG, Berzin TM, Kim S, Song P, Kuo-LeBlanc V, Rodriguez-Wolf M, Baird A, Johanson CE. Human choroid plexus growth factors: what are the implications for CSF dynamics in Alzheimer's disease? Exp Neurol. 2001;167(1):40–7.
2. Davson H, Segal M. Physiology of the CSF and blood–brain barriers. Boca Raton: CRC; 1996. p. 822.
3. Johanson CE, Stopa E, McMillan PN. The blood–cerebrospinal fluid barrier: structure and functional significance. In: Nag S, editor. The blood–brain and other neural barriers, vol. 686. New York: Springer; 2011. p. 475.

4. Walter HJ, Berry M, Hill DJ, Cwyfan-Hughes S, Holly JM, Logan A. Distinct sites of insulin-like growth factor (IGF)-II expression and localization in lesioned rat brain: possible roles of IGF binding proteins (IGFBPs) in the mediation of IGF-II activity. Endocrinology. 1999;140(1):520–32.
5. Marques F, Sousa JC, Brito MA, Pahnke J, Santos C, Correia-Neves M, Palha JA. The choroid plexus in health and in disease: dialogues into and out of the brain. Neurobiol Dis. 2017;107:32–40.
6. Strazielle N, Khuth ST, Ghersi-Egea JF. Detoxification systems, passive and specific transport for drugs at the blood–CSF barrier in normal and pathological situations. Adv Drug Deliv Rev. 2004;56(12):1717–40.
7. Spector R, Johanson CE. Sustained choroid plexus function in human elderly and Alzheimer's disease patients. Fluids Barriers CNS. 2013;10(1):28.
8. Balusu S, Brkic M, Libert C, Vandenbroucke RE. The choroid plexus-cerebrospinal fluid interface in Alzheimer's disease: more than just a barrier. Neural Regen Res. 2016;11(4):534–7.
9. Engelhardt B, Sorokin L. The blood–brain and the blood–cerebrospinal fluid barriers: function and dysfunction. Semin Immunopathol. 2009;31(4):497–511.
10. Reboldi A, Coisne C, Baumjohann D, Benvenuto F, Bottinelli D, Lira S, Uccelli A, Lanzavecchia A, Engelhardt B, Sallusto F. C–C chemokine receptor 6-regulated entry of TH-17 cells into the CNS through the choroid plexus is required for the initiation of EAE. Nat Immunol. 2009;10(5):514–23.
11. Lauer AN, Tenenbaum T, Schroten H, Schwerk C. The diverse cellular responses of the choroid plexus during infection of the central nervous system. Am J Physiol. 2017. https://doi.org/10.1152/ajpcell.00137.2017.
12. Schwartz M, Baruch K. The resolution of neuroinflammation in neurodegeneration: leukocyte recruitment via the choroid plexus. EMBO J. 2014;33(1):7–22.
13. Schwartz M, Deczkowska A. Neurological disease as a failure of brain-immune crosstalk: the multiple faces of neuroinflammation. Trends Immunol. 2016;37(10):668–79.
14. Spector R, Johanson CE. Choroid plexus failure in the Kearns-Sayre syndrome. Cerebrospinal Fluid Res. 2010;7(1):14.
15. Vercellino M, Votta B, Condello C, Piacentino C, Romagnolo A, Merola A, Capello E, Mancardi GL, Mutani R, Giordana MT, et al. Involvement of the choroid plexus in multiple sclerosis autoimmune inflammation: a neuropathological study. J Neuroimmunol. 2008;199(1–2):133–41.
16. Millward JM, Ariza de Schellenberger A, Berndt D, Hanke-Vela L, Schellenberger E, Waiczies S, Taupitz M, Kobayashi Y, Wagner S, Infante-Duarte C. Application of europium-doped very small iron oxide nanoparticles to visualize neuroinflammation with MRI and fluorescence microscopy. Neuroscience. 2017. https://doi.org/10.1016/j.neuroscience.2017.12.014.
17. Kim S, Hwang Y, Lee D, Webster MJ. Transcriptome sequencing of the choroid plexus in schizophrenia. Transl Psychiatry. 2016;6(11):e964.
18. Marques F, Sousa JC, Coppola G, Falcao AM, Rodrigues AJ, Geschwind DH, Sousa N, Correia-Neves M, Palha JA. Kinetic profile of the transcriptome changes induced in the choroid plexus by peripheral inflammation. J Cereb Blood Flow Metab. 2009;29(5):921–32.
19. Silverberg GD, Huhn S, Jaffe RA, Chang SD, Saul T, Heit G, Von Essen A, Rubenstein E. Downregulation of cerebrospinal fluid production in patients with chronic hydrocephalus. J Neurosurg. 2002;97(6):1271–5.
20. Serot JM, Bene MC, Faure GC. Choroid plexus, aging of the brain, and Alzheimer's disease. Front Biosci. 2003;8:s515–21.
21. Gorlé N, Van Cauwenberghe C, Libert C, Vandenbroucke RE. The effect of aging on brain barriers and the consequences for Alzheimer's disease development. Mamm Genome. 2016;27(7–8):407–20.
22. Johanson C, McMillan P, Tavares R, Spangenberger A, Duncan J, Silverberg G, Stopa E. Homeostatic capabilities of the choroid plexus epithelium in Alzheimer's disease. Cerebrospinal Fluid Res. 2004;1(1):3.
23. Oikonomidi A, Lewczuk P, Kornhuber J, Smulders Y, Linnebank M, Semmler A, Popp J. Homocysteine metabolism is associated with cerebrospinal fluid levels of soluble amyloid precursor protein and amyloid beta. J Neurochem. 2016;139(2):324–32.
24. González-Marrero I, Giménez-Llort L, Johanson CE, Carmona-Calero EM, Castañeyra-Ruiz L, Brito-Armas JM, Castañeyra-Perdomo A, Castro-Fuentes R. Choroid plexus dysfunction impairs beta-amyloid clearance in a triple transgenic mouse model of Alzheimer's disease. Front Cell Neurosci. 2015;9:17.
25. Johanson CE, Stopa EG, Daiello L, de la Monte S, Ott B. Disrupted blood-CSF barrier to urea and creatinine in mild cognitive impairment and Alzheimer's disease. J Alzheimer's Dis Parkinsonism 2018;8:2. https://doi.org/10.4172/2161-0460.1000435
26. Bergen AA, Kaing S, ten Brink JB, Gorgels TG, Janssen SF, Bank NB. Gene expression and functional annotation of human choroid plexus epithelium failure in Alzheimer's disease. BMC Genomics. 2015;16:956.
27. López-Romero P, González MA, Callejas S, Dopazo A, Irizarry RA. Processing of Agilent microRNA array data. BMC Res Notes. 2010;3:18.
28. Irizarry RA, Hobbs B, Collin F, Beazer-Barclay YD, Antonellis KJ, Scherf U, Speed TP. Exploration, normalization, and summaries of high density oligonucleotide array probe level data. Biostatistics. 2003;4(2):249–64.
29. Steeland S, Gorlé N, Vandendriessche C, Balusu S, Brkic M, Van Cauwenberghe C, Van Imschoot G, Van Wonterghem E, De Rycke R, Kremer A, et al. Counteracting the effects of TNF receptor-1 has therapeutic potential in Alzheimer's disease. EMBO Mol Med. 2018. https://doi.org/10.15252/emmm.201708300.
30. Johanson C, Silverberg G, Donahue J, Duncan J, Stopa E. Choroid plexus and CSF in Alzheimer's disease: altered expression and transport of proteins and peptides. London: CRC Press LLC; 2005. p. 307–39.
31. Chalbot S, Zetterberg H, Blennow K, Fladby T, Andreasen N, Grundke-Iqbal I, Iqbal K. Blood-cerebrospinal fluid barrier permeability in Alzheimer's disease. J Alzheimers Dis. 2011;25(3):505–15.
32. Brkic M, Balusu S, Van Wonterghem E, Gorlé N, Benilova I, Kremer A, Van Hove I, Moons L, De Strooper B, Kanazir S, et al. Amyloid β oligomers disrupt blood–CSF barrier integrity by activating matrix metalloproteinases. J Neurosci. 2015;35(37):12766–78.
33. Podtelezhnikov AA, Tanis KQ, Nebozhyn M, Ray WJ, Stone DJ, Loboda AP. Molecular insights into the pathogenesis of Alzheimer's disease and its relationship to normal aging. PLoS ONE. 2011;6(12):e29610.
34. Keren-Shaul H, Spinrad A, Weiner A, Matcovitch-Natan O, Dvir-Szternfeld R, Ulland TK, David E, Baruch K, Lara-Astaiso D, Toth B, et al. A unique microglia type associated with restricting development of Alzheimer's disease. Cell. 2017;169(7):1276–90.
35. Kunis G, Baruch K, Rosenzweig N, Kertser A, Miller O, Berkutzki T, Schwartz M. IFN-gamma-dependent activation of the brain's choroid plexus for CNS immune surveillance and repair. Brain. 2013;136(Pt 11):3427–40.
36. Johanson CE, Duncan JA, Stopa EG, Baird A. Enhanced prospects for drug delivery and brain targeting by the choroid plexus-CSF route. Pharm Res. 2005;22(7):1011–37.
37. Vallieres L, Rivest S. Regulation of the genes encoding interleukin-6, its receptor, and gp130 in the rat brain in response to the immune activator lipopolysaccharide and the proinflammatory cytokine interleukin-1beta. J Neurochem. 1997;69(4):1668–83.
38. Mesquita SD, Ferreira AC, Gao F, Coppola G, Geschwind DH, Sousa JC, Correia-Neves M, Sousa N, Palha JA, Marques F. The choroid plexus transcriptome reveals changes in type I and II interferon responses in a mouse model of Alzheimer's disease. Brain Behav Immun. 2015;49:280–92.
39. Anthony SG, Schipper HM, Tavares R, Hovanesian V, Cortez SC, Stopa EG, Johanson CE. Stress protein expression in the Alzheimer-diseased choroid plexus. J Alzheimers Dis. 2003;5(3):171–7.
40. Knuckey NW, Finch P, Palm DE, Primiano MJ, Johanson CE, Flanders KC, Thompson NL. Differential neuronal and astrocytic expression of transforming growth factor beta isoforms in rat hippocampus following transient forebrain ischemia. Brain Res Mol Brain Res. 1996;40(1):1–14.
41. Deane R, Wu Z, Zlokovic BV. RAGE (yin) versus LRP (yang) balance regulates alzheimer amyloid beta-peptide clearance through transport across the blood–brain barrier. Stroke J Cereb Circulation. 2004;35(11 Suppl 1):2628–31.
42. Silverberg G, Flaherty-Slone S, Messier A, Soltman S, Miller M, Szmydynger-Chodobska J, Chodobski A, Johanson C. Amyloid transporter expression is altered by aging at the blood–brain barrier and choroid plexus. In: Gordon Research Conference. Tilton: New Hampshire; 2006.
43. Brosseron F, Krauthausen M, Kummer M, Heneka MT. Body fluid cytokine levels in mild cognitive impairment and Alzheimer's disease: a comparative overview. Mol Neurobiol. 2014;50(2):534–44.
44. McDonald CL, Hennessy E, Rubio-Araiz A, Keogh B, McCormack W, McGuirk P, Reilly M, Lynch MA. Inhibiting TLR2 activation attenuates amyloid accumulation and glial activation in a mouse model of Alzheimer's disease. Brain Behav Immun. 2016;58:191–200.

45. Vates TS Jr, Bonting SL, Oppelt WW. Na–K activated adenosine triphosphatase formation of cerebrospinal fluid in the cat. Am J Physiol. 1964;206:1165–72.
46. Johanson CE, Duncan JA 3rd, Klinge PM, Brinker T, Stopa EG, Silverberg GD. Multiplicity of cerebrospinal fluid functions: new challenges in health and disease. Cerebrospinal Fluid Res. 2008;5:10.
47. Pascale CL, Miller MC, Chiu C, Boylan M, Caralopoulos IN, Gonzalez L, Johanson CE, Silverberg GD. Amyloid-beta transporter expression at the blood–CSF barrier is age-dependent. Fluids Barriers CNS. 2011;8:21.
48. Kummer MP, Schwarzenberger R, Sayah-Jeanne S, Dubernet M, Walczak R, Hum DW, Schwartz S, Axt D, Heneka MT. Pan-PPAR modulation effectively protects APP/PS1 mice from amyloid deposition and cognitive deficits. Mol Neurobiol. 2014;51(2):661–71.
49. Maharaj AS, Walshe TE, Saint-Geniez M, Venkatesha S, Maldonado AE, Himes NC, Matharu KS, Karumanchi SA, D'Amore PA. VEGF and TGF-beta are required for the maintenance of the choroid plexus and ependyma. J Exp Med. 2008;205(2):491–501.
50. Turner ML. Cell adhesion molecules: a unifying approach to topographic biology. Biol Rev Camb Philos Soc. 1992;67(3):359–77.
51. Lobas MA, Helsper L, Vernon CG, Schreiner D, Zhang Y, Holtzman MJ, Thedens DR, Weiner JA. Molecular heterogeneity in the choroid plexus epithelium: the 22-member γ-protocadherin family is differentially expressed, apically localized, and implicated in CSF regulation. J Neurochem. 2012;120(6):913–27.
52. Keep RF, Xiang J, Andjelkovic AV. Where did the ventricles go? J Neurochem. 2012;120(6):851–2.
53. Singhrao SK, Neal JW, Rushmere NK, Morgan BP, Gasque P. Differential expression of individual complement regulators in the brain and choroid plexus. Lab Invest J Tech Methods Pathol. 1999;79(10):1247–59.
54. Clarke R, Smith AD, Jobst KA, Refsum H, Sutton L, Ueland PM. Folate, vitamin B12, and serum total homocysteine levels in confirmed Alzheimer disease. Arch Neurol. 1998;55(11):1449–55.
55. McCaddon A, Davies G, Hudson P, Tandy S, Cattell H. Total serum homocysteine in senile dementia of Alzheimer type. Int J Geriatr Psychiatry. 1998;13(4):235–9.
56. Seshadri S, Beiser A, Selhub J, Jacques PF, Rosenberg IH, D'Agostino RB, Wilson PW, Wolf PA. Plasma homocysteine as a risk factor for dementia and Alzheimer's disease. N Engl J Med. 2002;346(7):476–83.
57. Van Dam F, Van Gool WA. Hyperhomocysteinemia and Alzheimer's disease: a systematic review. Arch Gerontol Geriatr. 2009;48(3):425–30.
58. McCampbell A, Wessner K, Marlatt MW, Wolffe C, Toolan D, Podtelezhnikov A, Yeh S, Zhang R, Szczerba P, Tanis KQ, et al. Induction of Alzheimer's-like changes in brain of mice expressing mutant APP fed excess methionine. J Neurochem. 2011;116(1):82–92.
59. van Wijk N, Slot RER, Duits FH, Strik M, Biesheuvel E, Sijben JWC, Blankenstein MA, Bierau J, van der Flier WM, Scheltens P, et al. Nutrients required for phospholipid synthesis are lower in blood and cerebrospinal fluid in mild cognitive impairment and Alzheimer's disease dementia. Alzheimers Dement (Amst). 2017;8:139–46.
60. Hansson SF, Andréasson U, Wall M, Skoog I, Andreasen N, Wallin A, Zetterberg H, Blennow K. Reduced levels of amyloid-beta-binding proteins in cerebrospinal fluid from Alzheimer's disease patients. J Alzheimers Dis. 2009;16(2):389–97.
61. Lee H. Phosphorylated mTOR expression profiles in human normal and carcinoma tissues. Dis Markers. 2017;2017:1397063.

Cerebral influx of Na^+ and Cl^- as the osmotherapy-mediated rebound response in rats

Eva Kjer Oernbo[1], Kasper Lykke[1,5], Annette Buur Steffensen[1], Kathrin Töllner[2,3], Christina Kruuse[4], Martin Fredensborg Rath[1], Wolfgang Löscher[2,3] and Nanna MacAulay[1,6*]

Abstract

Background: Cerebral edema can cause life-threatening increase in intracranial pressure. Besides surgical craniectomy performed in severe cases, osmotherapy may be employed to lower the intracranial pressure by osmotic extraction of cerebral fluid upon intravenous infusion of mannitol or NaCl. A so-called rebound effect can, however, hinder continuous reduction in cerebral fluid by yet unresolved mechanisms.

Methods: We determined the brain water and electrolyte content in healthy rats treated with osmotherapy. Osmotherapy (elevated plasma osmolarity) was mediated by intraperitoneal injection of NaCl or mannitol with inclusion of pharmacological inhibitors of selected ion-transporters present at the capillary lumen or choroidal membranes. Brain barrier integrity was determined by fluorescence detection following intravenous delivery of Na^+-fluorescein.

Results: NaCl was slightly more efficient than mannitol as an osmotic agent. The brain water loss was only ~60% of that predicted from ideal osmotic behavior, which could be accounted for by cerebral Na^+ and Cl^- accumulation. This electrolyte accumulation represented the majority of the rebound response, which was unaffected by the employed pharmacological agents. The brain barriers remained intact during the elevated plasma osmolarity.

Conclusions: A brain volume regulatory response occurs during osmotherapy, leading to the rebound response. This response involves brain accumulation of Na^+ and Cl^- and takes place by unresolved molecular mechanisms that do not include the common ion-transporting mechanisms located in the capillary endothelium at the blood–brain barrier and in the choroid plexus epithelium at the blood–CSF barrier. Future identification of these ion-transporting routes could provide a pharmacological target to prevent the rebound effect associated with the widely used osmotherapy.

Keywords: Osmotherapy, Rebound effect, Brain edema, Brain barriers, Ion-transporting mechanisms

Background

The ion and fluid homeostasis in the mammalian brain is tightly controlled to preserve the intracranial pressure (ICP) within a normal range. Cerebral edema, as occurring in pathologies such as traumatic brain injury and stroke, can cause the ICP to rise to life-threateningly high levels [1]. In severe cases, a decompressive craniectomy can be initiated to lower the ICP [2]. Alternatively, osmotherapy can be used to osmotically extract cerebral fluid into the blood circulation by intravenous (i.v.) infusion of mannitol or NaCl [3], although it remains disputed which of these osmotic agents is most efficient for brain water extraction. The initial target when applying osmotherapy is a plasma osmolarity up to 320 mOsm but depending on the clinical circumstances, this recommended value may be exceeded [1]. Osmotherapy induces an immediate loss of brain fluid, which can, however, be reduced or even reversed due to yet incompletely understood mechanisms; a phenomenon referred to as the rebound

*Correspondence: macaulay@sund.ku.dk
[6] Department of Neuroscience, Faculty of Health and Medical Sciences, University of Copenhagen, Blegdamsvej 3, 2200 Copenhagen, Denmark
Full list of author information is available at the end of the article

effect [4, 5]. The rebound effect has been suggested to arise from a compensatory accumulation of cerebral osmolytes, generating an osmotic gradient favoring fluid movement back into the brain particularly upon dilution of the plasma osmolarity by renal excretion and/or withdrawal of the osmotic agent [4, 5]. It remains uncertain to what extent brain ion accumulation participates in the rebound response, and if so, which molecular transporting mechanisms contribute to this volume regulatory response. The secretion of ions may take place at one or both of the two major interfaces between the brain and blood: the capillary endothelium forming the blood–brain barrier (BBB) and/or the cerebrospinal fluid (CSF)-secreting choroid plexus epithelium, which forms the blood–CSF barrier (BCSFB) [6, 7]. The capillary endothelium and the choroid plexus epithelium express several ion-transporting mechanisms, i.e. the Na^+–K^+–$2Cl^-$ co-transporter 1 (NKCC1), the Na^+–H^+ anti-porter 1 (NHE1), Na^+-coupled bicarbonate transporters (NBCs), and the amiloride-sensitive Na^+ channel (ENaC) [8–10]. These transport mechanisms may be potential candidates for brain ion and water regulation, and could, as such, participate in electrolyte translocation from blood to brain during the elevated blood osmolarity resulting from osmotherapy treatment. Inhibition of a subset of these ion transporters has been associated with improved outcome in an experimental animal model of stroke [11, 12], which may indicate involvement of such transport mechanisms in brain ion and water dynamics. Here, we employed in vivo investigations of healthy non-edematous rats to obtain the brain volume regulatory response to increased plasma osmolarity in the absence of pathological events, such as stroke/haemorrhage, and investigate a putative role of a range of transport mechanisms in the brain volume regulatory gain of ions.

Methods

Animals

This study was performed in accordance with the European Community guidelines for the use of experimental animals using protocols approved either by the Lower Saxony State Office for Consumer Protection and Food Safety (Niedersachsen, Germany) or Supervisory Authority on Animal Testing (Danish Veterinary and Food Administration, Denmark). To avoid variation due to mixed gender, only female Sprague–Dawley rats were employed, aged 9–13 weeks (Taconic A/S, Lille Skensved, Denmark or Janvier Labs, Le Genest-Saint-Isle, France). Whether the present findings hold for male rats as well will require further studies in the future. Rats were housed in groups of 2–5 per cage (Tp III cages, 22 °C, 12:12 h light/dark cycle) with access to unlimited water and standard altromin rodent diet. The allocation of rats into the treatment groups was randomized, and all experiments were reported in compliance with the ARRIVE guidelines (Animal Research: Reporting in Vivo Experiments) [13].

Brain water extraction by elevated plasma osmolarity

Rats were anesthetized using isoflurane inhalation mixed in O_2 (1.5–5%, 1 l/min) and anaesthesia was maintained throughout the entire experiment. The body temperature was controlled to 37 °C using an electric heating pad (Harvard Apparatus, Holliston, MA, US) and monitored by a rectal probe during the entire procedure. To avoid systemic regulation of blood osmolytes upon hyperosmotic treatment, a functional nephrectomy was performed immediately prior to the initiation of the experiment in all animals except for naïve animals, which were not exposed to isosmolar- or hyperosmolar treatment but underwent anaesthesia induction shortly before decapitation, see Table 1 for grouping of experimental animals. In brief, laparotomy incision areas were treated with local analgesia [2–4 drops 2% tetracaine (Sigma-Aldrich, Brøndbyvester, Denmark, T7508) or xylocaine (1 mg/ml, AstraZeneca A/S, Copenhagen, Denmark, N01BB02)/bupivacaine (0.5 mg/ml, Amgros I/S, Copenhagen, Denmark, N01BB01) (both in 0.9% w/v NaCl)] prior to opening of the abdominal cavity either from the dorsal or the ventral side in the fully anesthetized animals. The renal artery and vein were ligated using non-absorbable suture. For rats given ventral incision, a catheter (for i.p. delivery, see below) was placed during suturing of the incision, while for rats with dorsal incisions, the smaller openings were closed with metal wound clamps immediately after i.p. delivery. The rats received a single i.p. bolus of a physiological NaCl solution (0.9% w/v NaCl) as an isosmolar control treatment, while an equiosmolar bolus of NaCl (1.17 g/kg, 1 M [14]) or mannitol (7.29 g/kg, dissolved in 0.9% w/v NaCl; 2 M) was given to elevate the plasma osmolarity to a similar extent. All solutions were heated to 37 °C and delivered as 2 ml/100 g body weight. We employed i.p. delivery of the osmotic agent as this delivery route gives similar plasma osmolarities as i.v. delivery [14]. For i.v. inhibitor experiments, a catheter was inserted into the tail vein and an inhibitor mixture containing bumetanide (10 mg/kg [11], Sigma-Aldrich, B3023), amiloride (6 mg/kg [15], Sigma-Aldrich, A7410), and methazolamide (20 mg/kg [16], Sigma-Aldrich, SML0720) or vehicle (specified below) was injected 5 min prior to i.p. treatment with isosmolar- or hyperosmolar NaCl, see Table 1 for grouping of experimental animals. Inhibitors were given in a mixture to minimize the number of rats used for experiments. While drug concentrations in the blood are difficult to assess due to unspecific binding to tissue

Table 1 Overview of experimental animal groups

Experiment	Label	Osmotic agent	Treatment	Delivery route	# rats
Brain water and ion quantification	Control	–	Vehicle	i.v.	9
		–	Inhibitors	i.v.	7
		–	Vehicle	i.c.v.	6
		–	Inhibitors	i.c.v.	6
	Osmotherapy	NaCl (i.p.)	Vehicle	i.v.	9
		NaCl (i.p.)	Inhibitors	i.v.	8
		NaCl (i.p.)	3× vehicle	i.v.	4
		NaCl (i.p.)	3× inhibitors	i.v.	4
		NaCl (i.p.)	Vehicle	i.c.v.	6
		NaCl (i.p.)	Inhibitors	i.c.v.	6
		Mannitol (i.p.)	–	–	6
	Naïve	–	–	–	3
Brain barrier permeability	Control	–	NaFl	i.v.	3
	Osmotherapy	NaCl (i.p.)	NaFl	i.v.	3
	Naïve	–	–	–	3
Monitoring of ICP		–	Evans blue	i.c.v.	3
Blood pressure measurement		–	Vehicle	i.v.	3
		–	Inhibitors	i.v.	3

i.p., intraperitoneal; i.v., intravenous; i.c.v., intra(cerebro)ventricular; 3×, triple doses; NaFl, Na^+-fluorescein

and blood proteins, we estimate maximal blood concentrations of 0.4 mM for bumetanide and amiloride, and 1.2 mM for methazolamide based on estimated blood volume of 7% of the rat body weight (average: 233 g). In a few experiments, rats were given a triple inhibitor or vehicle dose into the tail vein. In this case, a bolus injection of inhibitors or vehicle was given 20 min and 5 min before and 15 min after delivery of isosmolar or hyperosmolar NaCl. In other experiments, rats were positioned in a stereotactic frame (Stoelting, Wood Dale, IL, US, 51500) and a micro drill (CircuitMedic, Haverhill, MA, US, 110-4102) employed to induce a burr hole in the skull (coordinates from bregma: 1.4 mm lateral, 0.8 mm posterior). A Hamilton syringe (G27, Agntho's AB, Lidingö, Sweden, 2100521) filled with inhibitor mixture (bumetanide: 33 µM, amiloride and methazolamide: 167 µM, final ventricular concentrations estimated to be 20 and 100 µM [17–22]) or vehicle dissolved in equilibrated (95% O_2/5% CO_2) artificial CSF (aCSF) (120 mM NaCl, 2.5 mM KCl, 1.3 mM $MgSO_4 \times 7\ H_2O$, 1 mM NaH_2PO_4, 25 mM $NaHCO_3$, 10 mM glucose × H_2O, 2.5 mM $CaCl_2$, pH 7.4 at 37 °C) was fastened to the stereotactic apparatus and introduced into the right lateral ventricle (4.7 mm ventral). Two min prior to isosmolar or hyperosmolar i.p. treatment, 6 µl inhibitor or vehicle solution was injected in 2 s (volume and rate adjusted to hit both lateral ventricles), see Table 1 for grouping of experimental animals. To maintain an optimal intraventricular inhibitor dose, inhibitor or vehicle solution was injected into the ventricular system every 15 min. All the experiments were terminated by decapitation of the animal 1 h after i.p. injection of osmotic agent or physiological saline. A 1 h treatment period was chosen according to the reported near stabilization of plasma osmolarity and brain volume within 30 min after a hyperosmolar challenge [14]. All inhibitor solutions were made freshly each day (some from frozen stock solutions). Bumetanide and methazolamide were dissolved in 0.1 M NaOH (pH adjusted with 0.1 M HCl to pH 11 and 9, respectively) and diluted to 10 mg/ml for injection into the tail vein, while amiloride was dissolved in heated water at 10 mg/ml. Inhibitors, which were introduced into the ventricular system, were dissolved in DMSO (final concentration of 0.2% in aCSF).

Brain water and electrolyte quantification

The brain was removed immediately after decapitation. The olfactory bulbs and medulla oblongata were discarded and the remaining brain tissue was placed in a pre-weighed porcelain evaporation beaker and weighed within minutes after isolation to reduce loss of brain water. Brain tissue was homogenized in the pre-weighed evaporation beaker using a steel pestle and dried at 100 °C for 3–4 days to a constant mass for determination of the brain water content. The dried brain tissue (75–130 mg) was extracted in 1 ml 0.75 M HNO_3 on a horizontal shaker table for 3 days at room temperature (RT). The Cl^- content in the brain extracts was quantified by a colorimetric method using a QuantiChrom™ Chloride Assay Kit (MEDIBENA Life Science & Diagnostic Solution, Vienna, Austria), while the Na^+ and K^+ content was quantified using flame photometry (Instrument Laboratory 943, Bedford, MA, US).

Plasma osmolarity and ion quantification

A heparin-coated tube (Jørgen Kruuse A/S, Langeskov, Denmark) was filled with pooled blood (venous and arterial) from the neck region upon decapitation of the rats. Blood samples were kept cold for maximal 4 h until centrifugation at 1300*g* for 10 min at RT. The plasma layer was collected and stored at − 20 °C. The plasma osmolarity was determined by a freezing point depression osmometer (Löser, Berlin, Germany), while the content of Na^+, Cl^-, urea and creatinine was measured using a RAPIDLab® blood gas analyzer (Siemens, Münich, Germany) or flame photometer (Instrument Laboratory 943).

Analysis of data

If assuming that the barriers between blood and brain behave as semipermeable membranes, i.e. permeable only to water but not to solutes, a new steady state in brain water content V_h (h; hyperosmolar, in ml/g dry weight) mediated by an elevated plasma osmolarity C^h_{osm} (mOsm) can be given by Eq. 1 as described in [14], where V_i is brain water content (i; isosmolar, in ml/g dry weight) in rats with isosmolar plasma osmolarity C^i_{osm} (mOsm).

$$V_h = V_i \cdot \frac{C^i_{osm}}{C^h_{osm}} \tag{1}$$

If the brain water loss is less than predicted by Eq. 1, this will imply that the brain gains osmotically active solutes given that the plasma and brain water is in osmotic equilibrium. The predicted gain of electrolytes, ΔQ (mmol/kg dry weight), can then be given by

$$\Delta Q = V_h \cdot C^h_{osm} - V_i \cdot C^i_{osm} \tag{2}$$

Brain barrier permeability

To assess the paracellular permeability of the brain barriers, anaesthetized rats were subjected to a functional nephrectomy. The experiments were initiated as above, after which a 4% Na^+-fluorescein (Sigma-Aldrich, F63772) solution (2 ml/kg, 0.25 ml/min, dissolved in 0.9% w/v NaCl) was infused into the femoral vein through a catheter; Na^+-fluorescein is a marker of paracellular permeability and has been used to identify paracellular BBB disruption by osmotic shock [23]. Five min hereafter, isosmolar or hyperosmolar NaCl was injected into the abdominal cavity as described above, see Table 1 for grouping of experimental animals. Rats were decapitated after 1 h, and the brains were removed immediately and frozen on crushed solid CO_2. Coronal sections (12 μm) were cut in a cryostat and mounted on slides. Na^+-fluorescein was visualized using an Axioplan 2 epifluoresence microscope (Carl Zeiss Vision, München-Halbergmoos, Germany) equipped with a Plan Neofluar and an AxioCam MR digital camera by use of the AxioVision 4.4 software (Carl Zeiss Vision, Birkerød, Denmark). Image acquisition was performed in a blinded fashion. Representative images were captured of brain regions comprising the neocortex, hippocampus, thalamus, and the lateral ventricle. The pineal gland was used as an internal positive control due to its lack of BBB [24]. Phase contrast images were included to visualize brain structures in transmitted light. Image processing (brightness and contrast) was performed using Adobe Photoshop (San Jose, CA, US).

Monitoring of ICP

In order to monitor the ICP of the anaesthetized rats, a micro drill (1 mm bit) was applied to manually induce a burr hole into the skull until transparency was observed. The thin skull layer was gently ruptured using a 0.6 mm bit (without disruption of dura mater) after which a tweezer was employed to remove skull flakes. An epidural probe (Plastics One, Roanoke, VA, US, C313GS-5-3UP, 0 mm below pedestal) was gently placed onto dura mater, and fastened to the skull by cement (GC, Kortrijk, Belgium, Fuji I, 000136). ICP fluctuations were detected by PicoLog Recorder software (Pico Technology, Cambridgeshire, UK). To ensure proper probe insertion in the epidural space, the jugular vein was compressed before the beginning of each experiment and a raised ICP detected as a positive control. An Evans blue (Sigma-Aldrich, E2129) solution (0.003% w/v in 0.9% w/v NaCl) was infused into the right lateral ventricle (6 μl in total, 3 μl/s) using a Hamilton syringe, while ICP recordings were collected, see Table 1 for grouping of experimental animals. 10 min after intraventricular injections, rats were euthanized by decapitation. The brains were isolated and cerebral hemispheres separated to confirm intraventricular Evans blue staining.

Blood pressure measurement

Female Sprague–Dawley rats (22–28 weeks) were anaesthetized with chloral hydrate (400 mg/kg, i.p.), see Table 1 for grouping of experimental animals. A catheter was inserted into the left femoral artery to measure the intra-arterial blood pressure (BioSys software, TSE Systems, Bad Homburg, Germany). The intra-arterial blood pressure was monitored until 1 h after i.v. injection of inhibitors (10 mg/kg bumetanide, 6 mg/kg amiloride and

20 mg/kg methazolamide) or vehicle, and experiments were terminated by decapitation of the rats.

Statistical analysis

All data are given as mean values ± standard error of mean (SEM). To evaluate statistically significant differences between mean values of two groups, an unpaired two-tailed Student's t-test was applied, while a one-way analysis of variance (ANOVA) followed by Dunnett's or Tukey's multiple comparisons post hoc test was applied to compare mean values of multiple groups. Comparison of two factors was evaluated by a two-way ANOVA followed by Tukey's multiple comparisons post hoc test. $p < 0.05$ was considered statistically significant. All statistical analyses were performed in GraphPad Prism 7.0 (GraphPad Software, Inc., La Jolla, CA, US) and indicated in the respective figure legend.

Results

Osmotherapy caused cerebral water loss and influx of Na^+ and Cl^-

To determine the effect of osmotherapy on the brain water and electrolyte content, we employed a rat in vivo model in which the plasma osmolarity was elevated by i.p. injection of NaCl (1.17 g/kg, 2 ml/100 g body weight). To isolate the effect of brain volume regulation, rats were functionally nephrectomized prior to the procedure, the success of which was evident from the increased plasma content of creatinine and urea in these animals compared to naïve rats, which had not undergone nephrectomy (Fig. 1a, b, see figure legend for values). The plasma osmolarity in the nephrectomized rats treated with isosmolar NaCl (303 ± 1 mOsm, n = 9, termed 'control' henceforward) was not significantly different from that of the naïve rats (298 ± 1 mOsm, n = 3, Fig. 1c), indicating that the extended experimental protocol in itself did not interfere with plasma osmolarity. Following a single bolus injection with hyperosmotic NaCl (termed 'osmotherapy' henceforward), the plasma osmolarity was increased to 355 ± 1 mOsm after 1 h (n = 9, $p < 0.001$, Fig. 1c), with an associated increase in the plasma content of Na^+ and Cl^- (n = 9, $p < 0.001$, Fig. 1d, e, see figure legend for values).

The brain water content of the naïve rats, which were not exposed to isosmolar or hyperosmolar treatment, (3.72 ± 0.03 ml/g dry weight, n = 3) was slightly lower than that of the control rats exposed to the isosmolar NaCl treatment (3.79 ± 0.01 ml/g dry weight, n = 9, $p < 0.05$, Fig. 2a), while osmotherapy caused a 9% reduction in the brain water content (to 3.46 ± 0.01, n = 9, $p < 0.001$, Fig. 2a). However, this reduction in brain water content amounted to only ~60% of that predicted from ideal osmotic behavior (calculated according to Eq. 1 and illustrated as a dashed red line in Fig. 2a), which indicates that volume regulation takes place. The osmotherapy-mediated reduction in the brain water loss was associated with an increase in brain electrolyte content, with a 15% increase in brain Na^+ ($p < 0.001$, Fig. 2b) and a 31% increase in brain Cl^- ($p < 0.001$, Fig. 2c) (see figure legend for values). There was a minor 2% increase in the brain K^+ content (control: 463 ± 2 mmol/kg dry weight vs. osmotherapy: 471 ± 2 mmol/kg dry weight, n = 9, $p < 0.05$). The brain Na^+ and Cl^- content in control rats was not significantly different from that obtained in naïve rats, Fig. 2b, c, see figure legend for values. The total increase in osmolyte content represented by Na^+, Cl^-, and K^+, $\Delta Q_{observed}$, amounted to 79 mmol/kg dry weight, which represents 104% of the predicted osmolyte gain, $\Delta Q_{predicted} = 76$ mmol/kg dry weight (Eq. 2). The osmotherapy-mediated gain of brain Na^+ and Cl^-, and to a minor extent K^+, can thereby account for the reduction in brain water loss observed 1 h after administration of the hyperosmolar challenge.

NaCl is slightly more potent than mannitol in osmotherapy

To determine the potency of osmotherapy conducted with NaCl vs. mannitol, we performed a parallel experimental series with mannitol as the osmotic agent. The increased Na^+ and Cl^- plasma concentration observed with NaCl infusion (as above, $p < 0.001$), was absent, and even slightly reversed compared to control rats upon i.p. delivery of mannitol (7.29 g/kg, 2 ml/100 g body weight) ($p < 0.001$ for Na^+ and $p < 0.05$ for Cl^-, Fig. 2d, e, see figure legend for values). Mannitol treatment yielded a plasma osmolarity (356 ± 3 mOsm, n = 6) similar to that obtained in rats treated with NaCl (355 ± 1 mOsm, n = 9, Fig. 1c, p = 0.71). Mannitol efficiently reduced the brain water content (to 3.51 ± 0.02 ml/g dry weight, $p < 0.001$), although slightly less effectively than NaCl ($p < 0.05$), Fig. 2a. Osmotherapy performed with mannitol increased the brain Na^+ content by 6% ($p < 0.001$), which was less than with NaCl as the osmotic agent (15%, $p < 0.001$), Fig. 2b. The brain Cl^- content, in contrast, increased to a similar extent upon treatment with either of the osmolytes (31% with NaCl, $p < 0.001$ and 38% with mannitol, $p < 0.001$, Fig. 2c), which was also evident for the brain K^+ content (p = 0.23; 2% with NaCl, n = 9, $p < 0.01$, and 3% with mannitol, n = 6, $p < 0.001$). Osmotherapy thus reduced the brain water content, but promoted brain electrolyte accumulation (predominantly in the form of Na^+ and Cl^-) irrespective of the osmotic agent employed, with NaCl being slightly more effective than mannitol for brain water extraction under our experimental conditions.

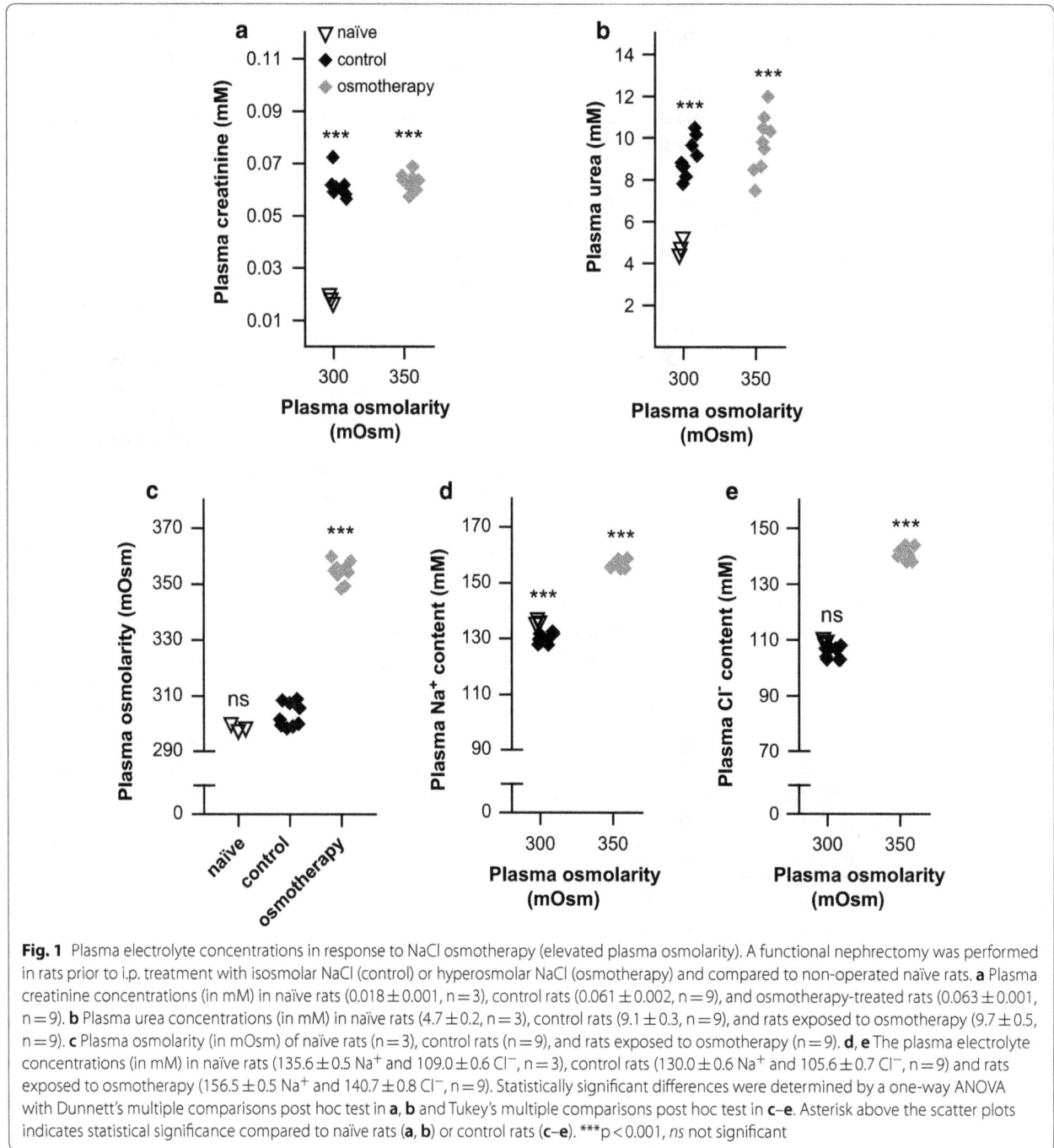

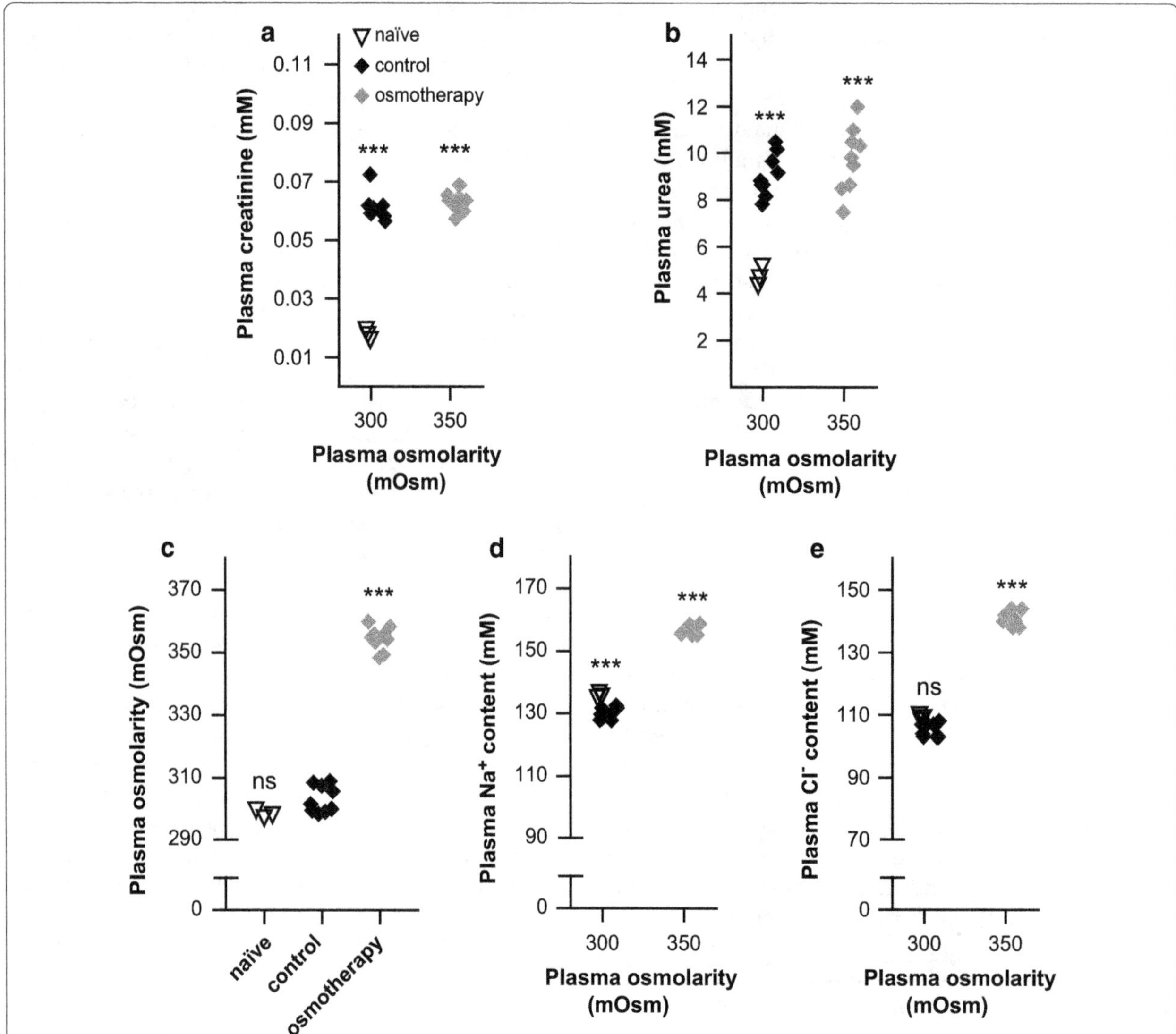

Fig. 1 Plasma electrolyte concentrations in response to NaCl osmotherapy (elevated plasma osmolarity). A functional nephrectomy was performed in rats prior to i.p. treatment with isosmolar NaCl (control) or hyperosmolar NaCl (osmotherapy) and compared to non-operated naïve rats. **a** Plasma creatinine concentrations (in mM) in naïve rats (0.018 ± 0.001, n = 3), control rats (0.061 ± 0.002, n = 9), and osmotherapy-treated rats (0.063 ± 0.001, n = 9). **b** Plasma urea concentrations (in mM) in naïve rats (4.7 ± 0.2, n = 3), control rats (9.1 ± 0.3, n = 9), and rats exposed to osmotherapy (9.7 ± 0.5, n = 9). **c** Plasma osmolarity (in mOsm) of naïve rats (n = 3), control rats (n = 9), and rats exposed to osmotherapy (n = 9). **d**, **e** The plasma electrolyte concentrations (in mM) in naïve rats (135.6 ± 0.5 Na^+ and 109.0 ± 0.6 Cl^-, n = 3), control rats (130.0 ± 0.6 Na^+ and 105.6 ± 0.7 Cl^-, n = 9) and rats exposed to osmotherapy (156.5 ± 0.5 Na^+ and 140.7 ± 0.8 Cl^-, n = 9). Statistically significant differences were determined by a one-way ANOVA with Dunnett's multiple comparisons post hoc test in **a**, **b** and Tukey's multiple comparisons post hoc test in **c**–**e**. Asterisk above the scatter plots indicates statistical significance compared to naïve rats (**a**, **b**) or control rats (**c**–**e**). ***$p < 0.001$, *ns* not significant

Inhibitors of ion-transporting mechanisms at the blood-side membranes of the BBB capillary endothelium and choroid plexus had no effect on the brain water loss or electrolyte gain upon osmotherapy

To identify the molecular mechanisms governing the hyperosmotic-induced brain ion accumulation and resulting volume regulation, the experimental regime from above (with NaCl as the osmotic agent) was repeated in rats during i.v. exposure to a mixture of inhibitors targeting a selection of ion-transporting mechanisms expressed in the BBB capillary endothelium and the blood-facing side of the choroid plexus. The diuretic compound bumetanide was applied for NKCC1 inhibition [25], amiloride to target NHE1 and ENaC [19], while the carbonic anhydrase inhibitor methazolamide [16] was applied to indirectly inhibit the NBCs. Importantly,

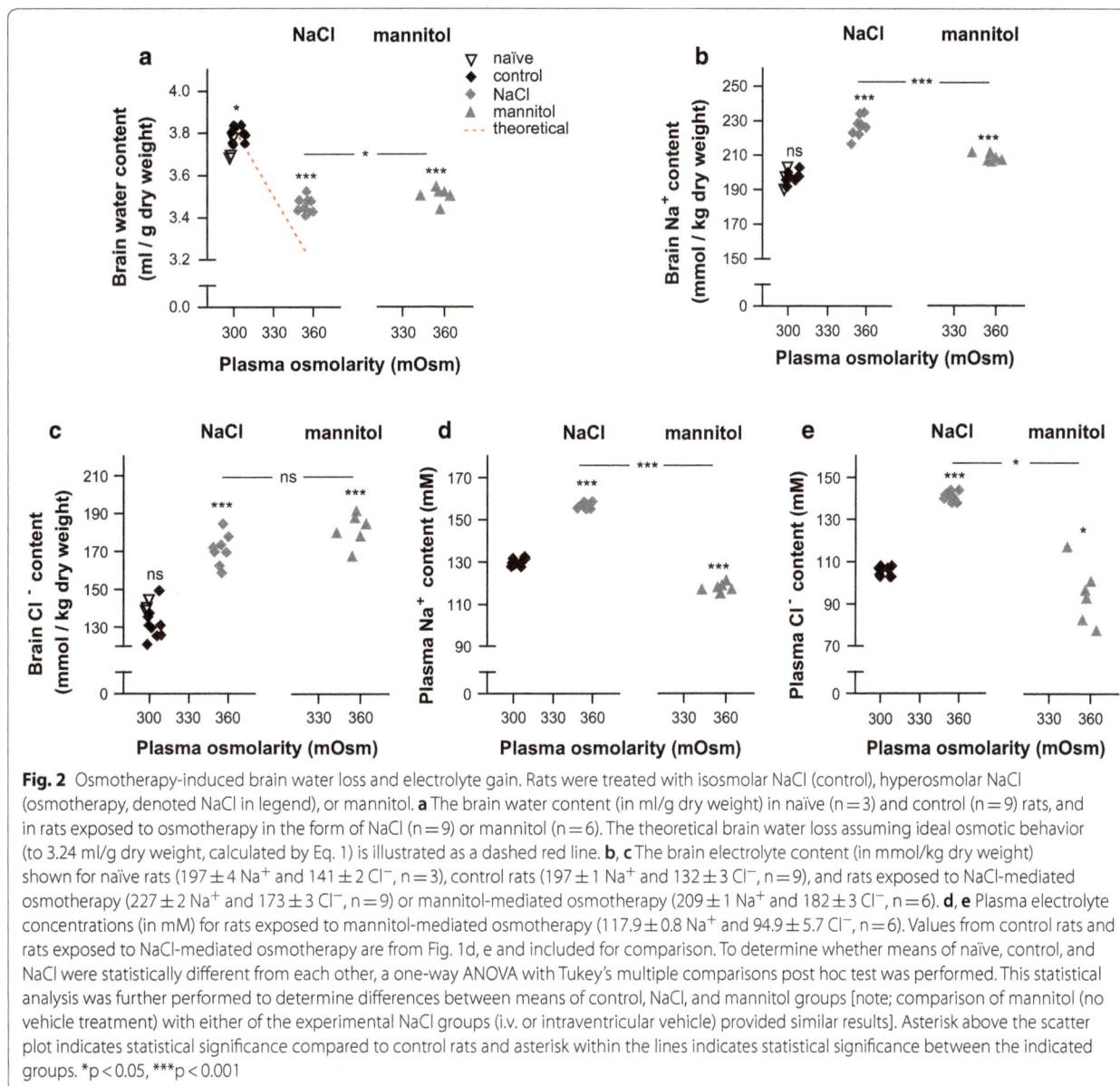

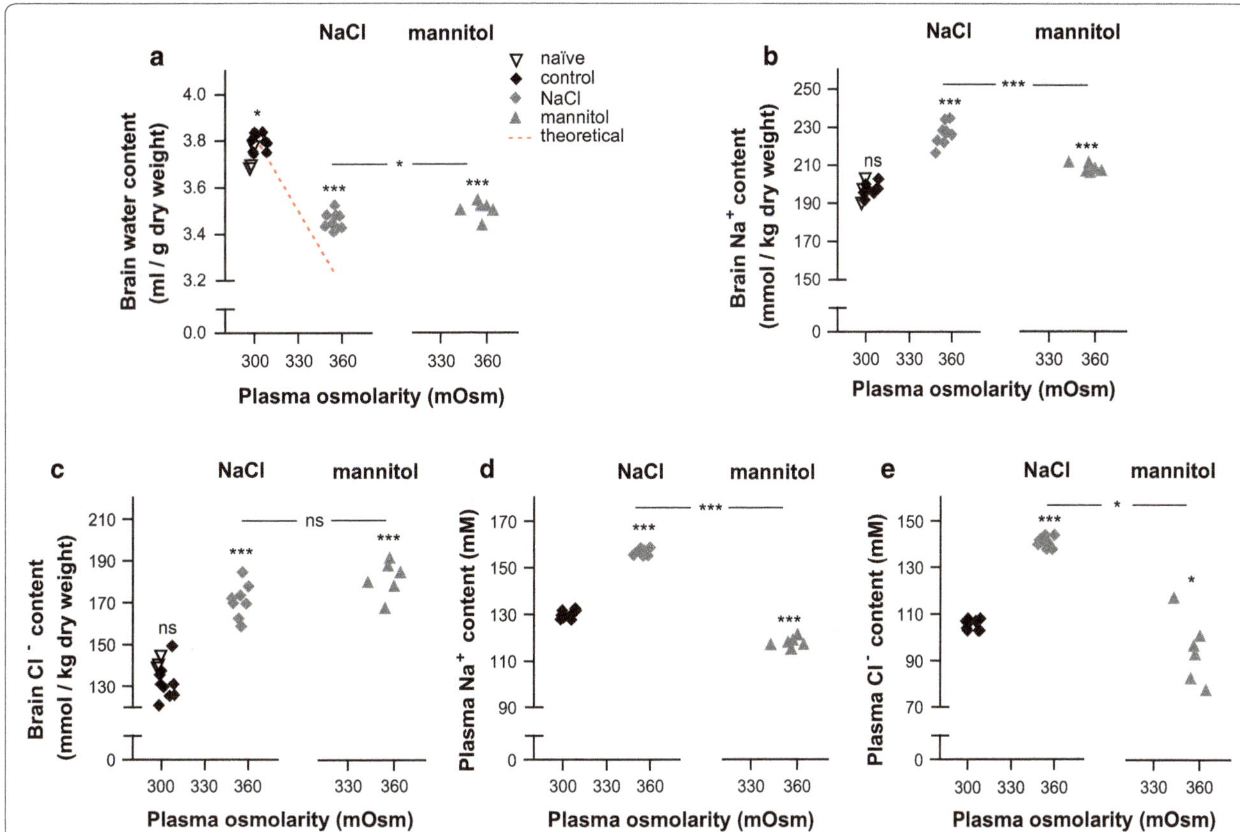

Fig. 2 Osmotherapy-induced brain water loss and electrolyte gain. Rats were treated with isosmolar NaCl (control), hyperosmolar NaCl (osmotherapy, denoted NaCl in legend), or mannitol. **a** The brain water content (in ml/g dry weight) in naïve (n = 3) and control (n = 9) rats, and in rats exposed to osmotherapy in the form of NaCl (n = 9) or mannitol (n = 6). The theoretical brain water loss assuming ideal osmotic behavior (to 3.24 ml/g dry weight, calculated by Eq. 1) is illustrated as a dashed red line. **b, c** The brain electrolyte content (in mmol/kg dry weight) shown for naïve rats (197 ± 4 Na^+ and 141 ± 2 Cl^-, n = 3), control rats (197 ± 1 Na^+ and 132 ± 3 Cl^-, n = 9), and rats exposed to NaCl-mediated osmotherapy (227 ± 2 Na^+ and 173 ± 3 Cl^-, n = 9) or mannitol-mediated osmotherapy (209 ± 1 Na^+ and 182 ± 3 Cl^-, n = 6). **d, e** Plasma electrolyte concentrations (in mM) for rats exposed to mannitol-mediated osmotherapy (117.9 ± 0.8 Na^+ and 94.9 ± 5.7 Cl^-, n = 6). Values from control rats and rats exposed to NaCl-mediated osmotherapy are from Fig. 1d, e and included for comparison. To determine whether means of naïve, control, and NaCl were statistically different from each other, a one-way ANOVA with Tukey's multiple comparisons post hoc test was performed. This statistical analysis was further performed to determine differences between means of control, NaCl, and mannitol groups [note; comparison of mannitol (no vehicle treatment) with either of the experimental NaCl groups (i.v. or intraventricular vehicle) provided similar results]. Asterisk above the scatter plot indicates statistical significance compared to control rats and asterisk within the lines indicates statistical significance between the indicated groups. *$p < 0.05$, ***$p < 0.001$

these inhibitors did not demonstrate an effect on the arterial blood pressure of anaesthetized rats compared with vehicle (at 1 h endpoint, n = 3, Fig. 3a).

A single i.v. dose of inhibitors did not alter the plasma osmolarity compared to vehicle treatment in either control rats (vehicle: 303 ± 1 mOsm vs. inhibitors: 303 ± 2 mOsm, n = 7–9, p = 0.76) or osmotherapy-treated rats (vehicle: 355 ± 1 mOsm vs. inhibitors: 357 ± 2 mOsm, n = 8–9, p = 0.35). Delivery of inhibitors did not affect the brain water, Na^+, and Cl^- content in control rats and failed to modulate the osmotherapy-induced changes in brain water, Na^+, and Cl^- content, Fig. 3b–d. The K^+ content was also unaffected by i.v. inhibitor application (in mmol/kg dry weight: control; vehicle: 463 ± 2 vs. inhibitors: 460 ± 2, osmotherapy; vehicle: 471 ± 2 vs. inhibitors: 474 ± 2, n = 7–9, p > 0.80). To increase the probability for the inhibitors to reach their targets in sufficient concentrations, we performed an additional experimental series with triple inhibitor application (20 min and 5 min prior to initiation of hyperosmotic treatment and 15 min after). These increased inhibitor doses did not affect the brain water content (Fig. 3b, inset). The unchanged electrolyte contents following inhibitor exposure aligns with the stable brain water content. These results suggest that NKCC1,

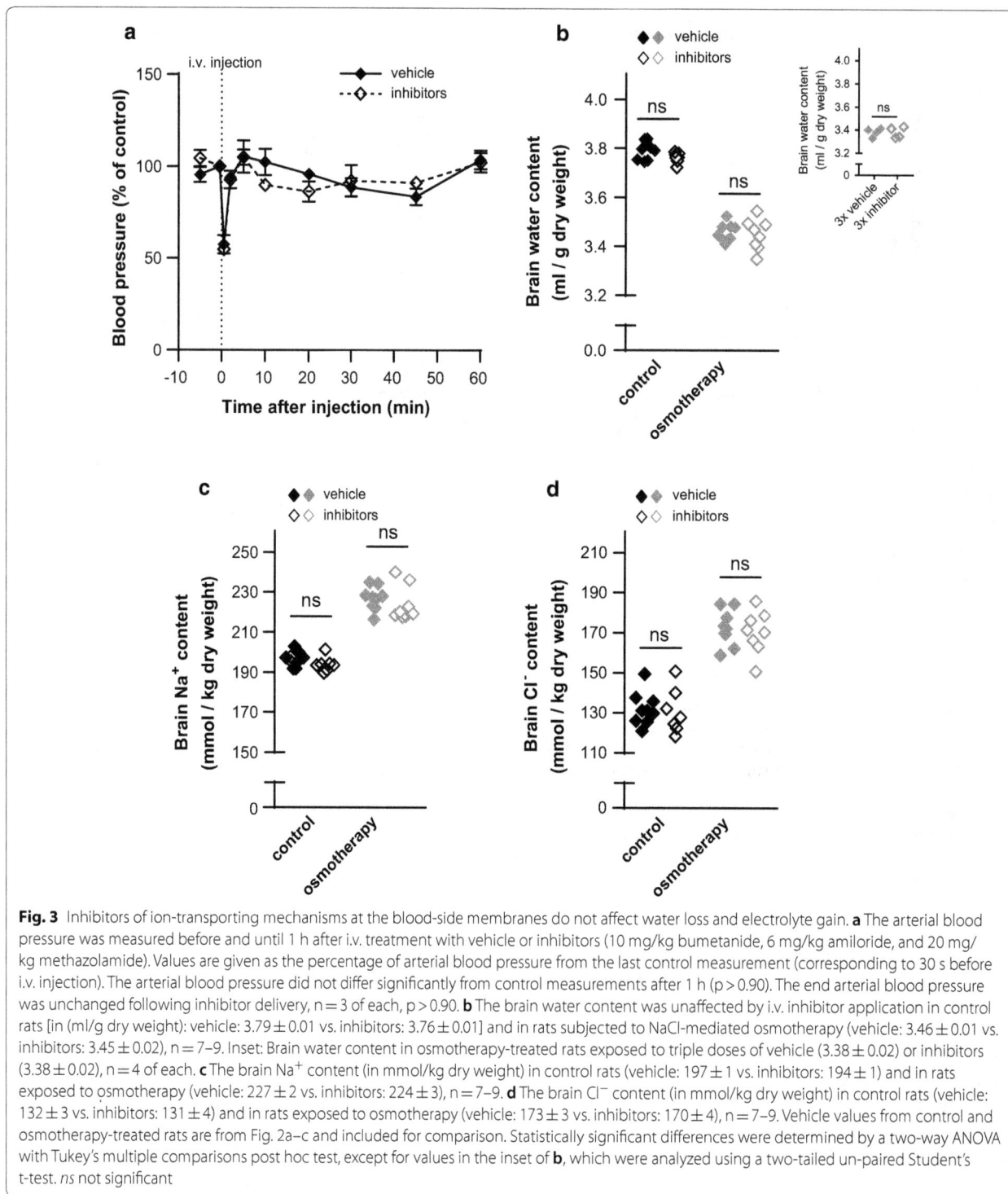

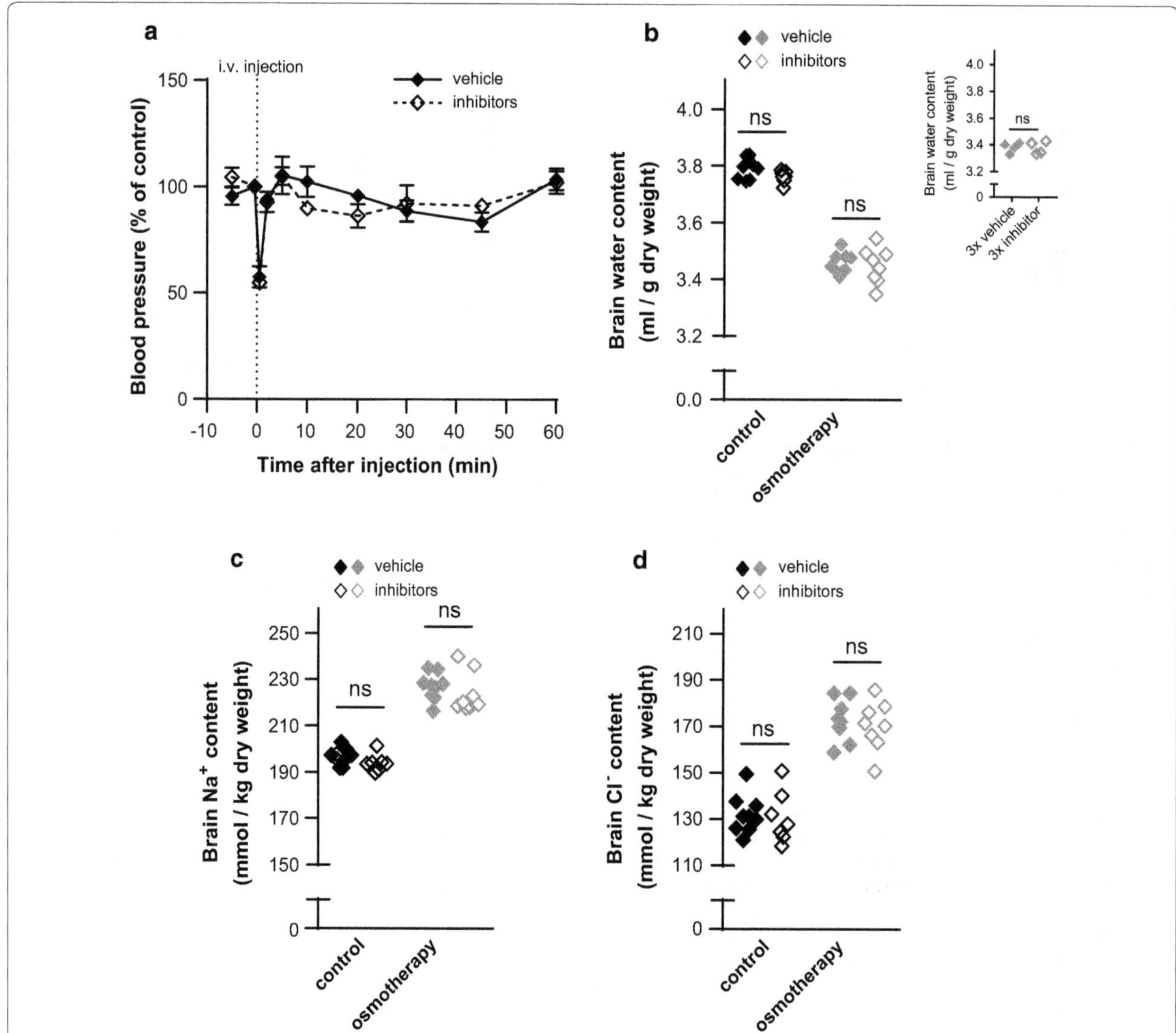

Fig. 3 Inhibitors of ion-transporting mechanisms at the blood-side membranes do not affect water loss and electrolyte gain. **a** The arterial blood pressure was measured before and until 1 h after i.v. treatment with vehicle or inhibitors (10 mg/kg bumetanide, 6 mg/kg amiloride, and 20 mg/kg methazolamide). Values are given as the percentage of arterial blood pressure from the last control measurement (corresponding to 30 s before i.v. injection). The arterial blood pressure did not differ significantly from control measurements after 1 h ($p > 0.90$). The end arterial blood pressure was unchanged following inhibitor delivery, $n = 3$ of each, $p > 0.90$. **b** The brain water content was unaffected by i.v. inhibitor application in control rats [in (ml/g dry weight): vehicle: 3.79 ± 0.01 vs. inhibitors: 3.76 ± 0.01] and in rats subjected to NaCl-mediated osmotherapy (vehicle: 3.46 ± 0.01 vs. inhibitors: 3.45 ± 0.02), $n = 7$–9. Inset: Brain water content in osmotherapy-treated rats exposed to triple doses of vehicle (3.38 ± 0.02) or inhibitors (3.38 ± 0.02), $n = 4$ of each. **c** The brain Na^+ content (in mmol/kg dry weight) in control rats (vehicle: 197 ± 1 vs. inhibitors: 194 ± 1) and in rats exposed to osmotherapy (vehicle: 227 ± 2 vs. inhibitors: 224 ± 3), $n = 7$–9. **d** The brain Cl^- content (in mmol/kg dry weight) in control rats (vehicle: 132 ± 3 vs. inhibitors: 131 ± 4) and in rats exposed to osmotherapy (vehicle: 173 ± 3 vs. inhibitors: 170 ± 4), $n = 7$–9. Vehicle values from control and osmotherapy-treated rats are from Fig. 2a–c and included for comparison. Statistically significant differences were determined by a two-way ANOVA with Tukey's multiple comparisons post hoc test, except for values in the inset of **b**, which were analyzed using a two-tailed un-paired Student's t-test. *ns* not significant

NHE1, ENaC, and NBCs localized at the blood-facing side of the BBB capillary endothelium and the choroidal membrane are not the primary access routes for brain electrolyte entry during osmotherapy and therefore not the molecular mechanisms underlying brain volume regulation under these conditions.

Osmotherapy-induced brain water loss and ion accumulation were unaffected by inhibitors of ion-transporting mechanisms at the CSF-facing choroidal membrane

Ion-transporting mechanisms localized at the other major interface; the ventricular side of the choroid plexus, may instead contribute to the volume regulatory gain of cerebral electrolytes upon administration of osmotherapy in the form of a hyperosmotic NaCl challenge. The select ion-transporting mechanisms expressed at the luminal membrane of the choroid plexus epithelium were targeted by injection of the inhibitor mixture (estimated ventricular concentrations of 20 μM bumetanide, 100 μM amiloride, and 100 μM methazolamide) directly into one of the lateral ventricles. Initially, the maximal inhibitor volume and infusion rate were chosen from two criteria: (1) both lateral ventricles should be exposed to inhibitors even though injections were given into only one of the lateral ventricles (verified with Evans blue, see Fig. 4a for a representative image) and (2) the ICP should remain fairly stable upon intraventricular inhibitor infusion (the ICP increased briefly to only a minor extent; 2.6 ± 0.7 mmHg, n = 3, Fig. 4b, with a brief compression of the jugular vein illustrated as a positive control).

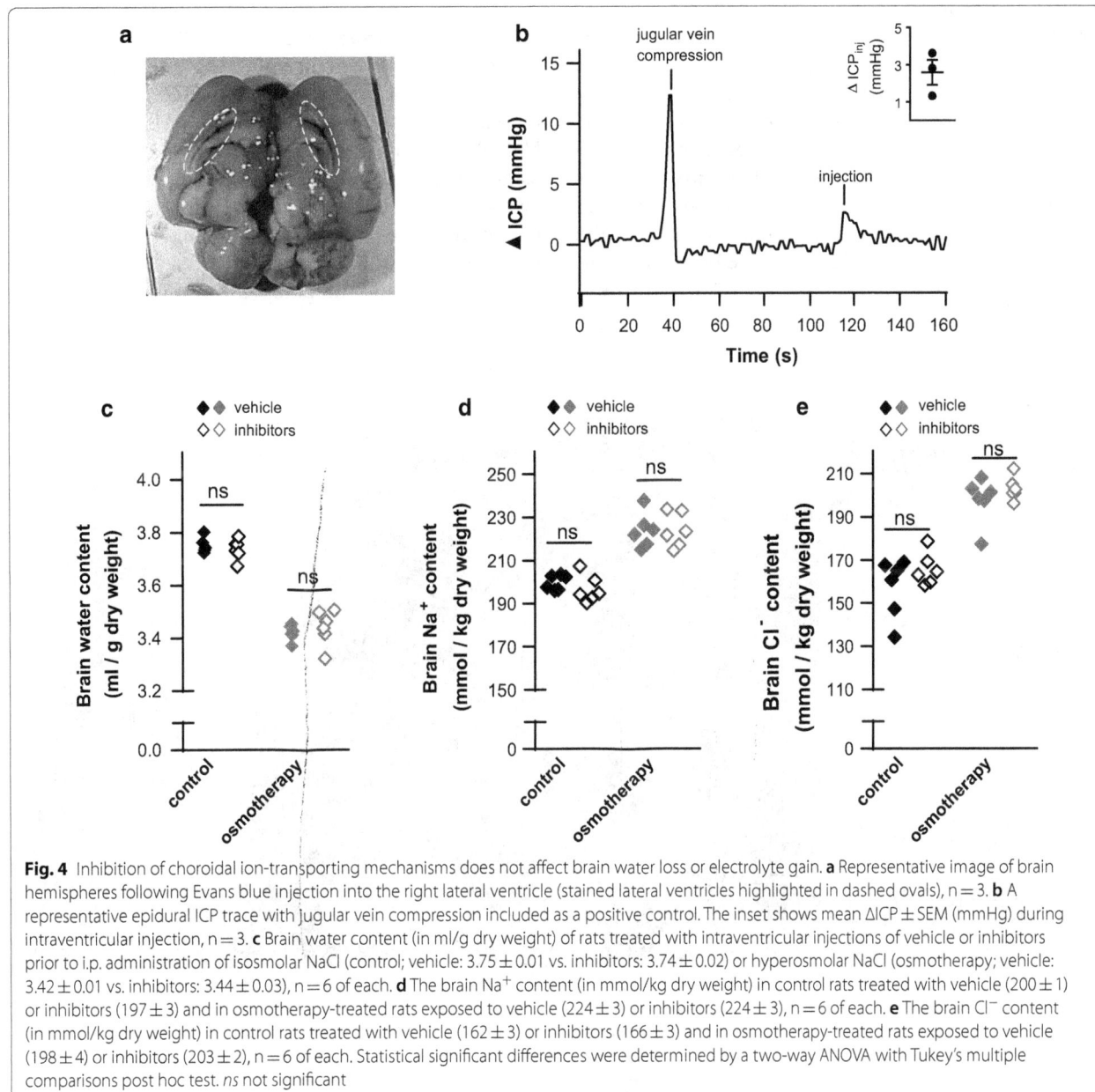

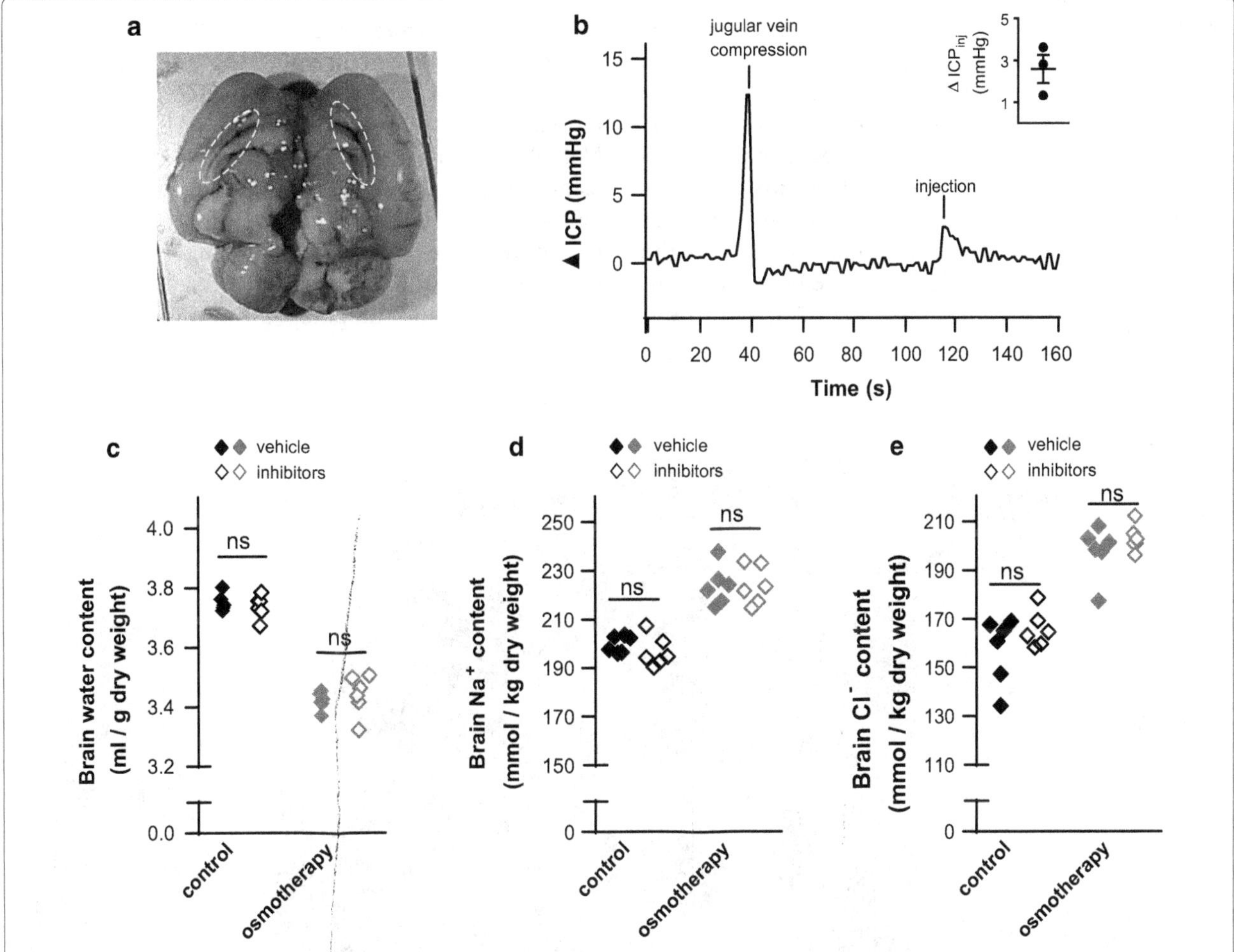

Fig. 4 Inhibition of choroidal ion-transporting mechanisms does not affect brain water loss or electrolyte gain. **a** Representative image of brain hemispheres following Evans blue injection into the right lateral ventricle (stained lateral ventricles highlighted in dashed ovals), n = 3. **b** A representative epidural ICP trace with jugular vein compression included as a positive control. The inset shows mean ΔICP ± SEM (mmHg) during intraventricular injection, n = 3. **c** Brain water content (in ml/g dry weight) of rats treated with intraventricular injections of vehicle or inhibitors prior to i.p. administration of isosmolar NaCl (control; vehicle: 3.75 ± 0.01 vs. inhibitors: 3.74 ± 0.02) or hyperosmolar NaCl (osmotherapy; vehicle: 3.42 ± 0.01 vs. inhibitors: 3.44 ± 0.03), n = 6 of each. **d** The brain Na^+ content (in mmol/kg dry weight) in control rats treated with vehicle (200 ± 1) or inhibitors (197 ± 3) and in osmotherapy-treated rats exposed to vehicle (224 ± 3) or inhibitors (224 ± 3), n = 6 of each. **e** The brain Cl^- content (in mmol/kg dry weight) in control rats treated with vehicle (162 ± 3) or inhibitors (166 ± 3) and in osmotherapy-treated rats exposed to vehicle (198 ± 4) or inhibitors (203 ± 2), n = 6 of each. Statistical significant differences were determined by a two-way ANOVA with Tukey's multiple comparisons post hoc test. *ns* not significant

Vehicle or inhibitors were thus injected into the ventricular system of anesthetized rats prior to osmotherapy followed by another drug application every 15 min during the 1 h experimental time period to maintain a maximal targeting effect despite risk of wash-out by the high ventricular CSF flow rate [26]. The plasma osmolarity was similar in vehicle- and inhibitor-treated rats exposed to isosmolar NaCl solution (vehicle: 297 ± 2 mOsm vs. inhibitors: 298 ± 2 mOsm, n = 6, p = 0.94) and in rats subjected to osmotherapy (vehicle: 347 ± 1 mOsm vs. inhibitors: 347 ± 2 mOsm, n = 6, p = 0.87). Osmotherapy led to a reduction in the brain water content and to an increased Na^+ (12%) and Cl^- (22%) content in the brain of vehicle-treated rats (n = 6, p < 0.001 for both, Fig. 4c–e), with an unaltered brain K^+ content (in mmol/kg dry weight: control: 472 ± 3 vs. osmotherapy: 471 ± 4, n = 6, p > 0.90). Intraventricular inhibitor application had no effect on the brain water content in control rats or in osmotherapy-treated rats, Fig. 4c. The brain Na^+ and Cl^- content in control- or osmotherapy-treated rats was, likewise, unaffected by inhibitor application into the lateral ventricles (n = 6, for all conditions, Fig. 4d, e), which was also seen for brain K^+ content (in mmol/kg dry weight: control; vehicle: 472 ± 3 vs. inhibitors: 469 ± 4, osmotherapy; vehicle: 471 ± 4 vs. inhibitors: 472 ± 2, n = 6, p > 0.90 for both). These results suggest that osmotherapy-mediated brain electrolyte influx does not originate from increased activity of choroidal transporters (NKCC1, NHE1, NBCs, or ENaC) expressed at the luminal CSF-facing side of the membrane.

The integrity of the brain barriers was preserved after osmotherapy treatment

To assess whether Na^+ and Cl^- entered the brain through a possible breach in the brain barriers in response to osmotherapy, we delivered Na^+-fluorescein i.v. 5 min prior to osmotherapy treatment (as above). Histological analysis of coronal brain sections (Fig. 5a) from the control rats revealed a weak background fluorescent signal in the brain parenchyma, as illustrated before [23], near-absence of Na^+-fluorescein in the neocortex, hippocampus, and thalamus, and minor staining in the lateral ventricle [23] (from choroid plexus with fenestrated blood capillaries), n = 3, Fig. 5c. Notably, the observed staining pattern was unaltered by osmotherapy treatment as illustrated in representative images of the neocortex, hippocampus, thalamus, and lateral ventricle, while no fluorescence was detected in naïve rats, which did not receive Na^+-fluorescein (n = 3, Fig. 5b–d). The pineal gland (Fig. 5e) served as

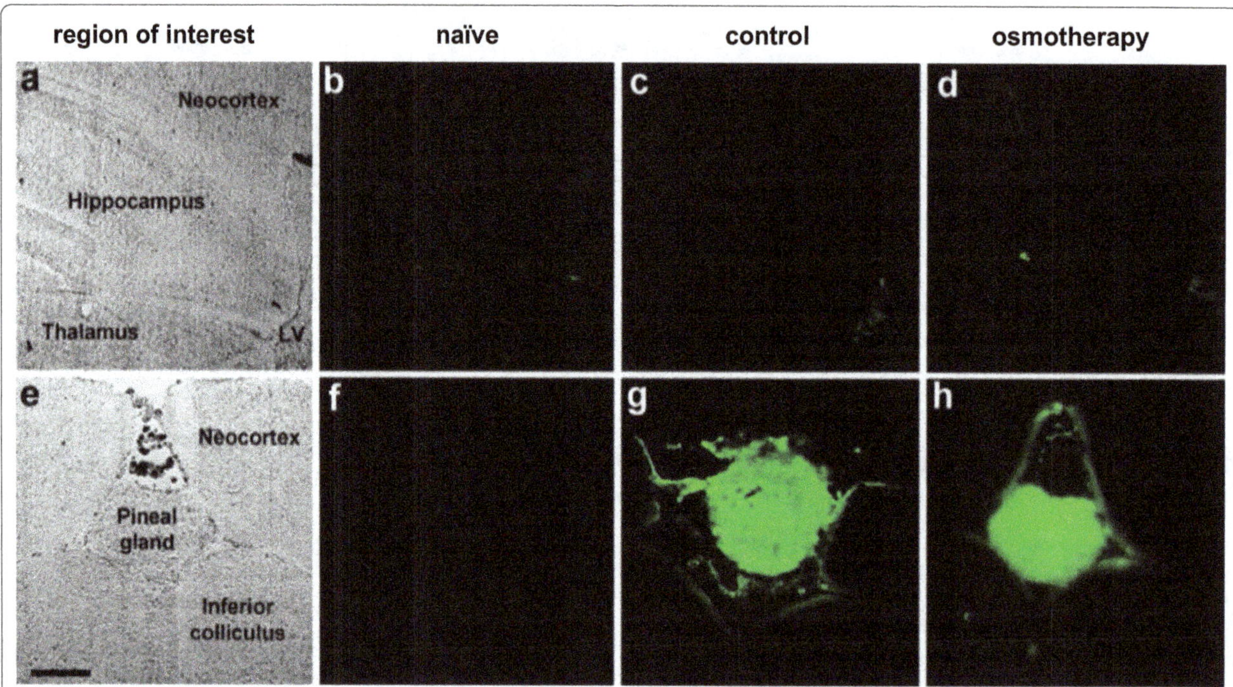

Fig. 5 Osmotherapy does not alter the brain barrier permeability. Na^+-fluorescein (green fluorescence) was injected into the blood circulation of rats prior to i.p. exposure of isosmolar NaCl (control) or hyperosmolar NaCl (osmotherapy). Naïve rats did not receive Na^+-fluorescein and were euthanized immediately after anaesthesia induction. **a, e** Phase contrast images illustrate structures of the brain regions of interest in transmitted white light. Representative images of Na^+-fluorescein in **b–d** hippocampus, thalamus, neocortex, and the lateral ventricle (LV) and **f–h** pineal gland (positive control) of naïve rats, control rats, and osmotherapy-treated rats, n = 3. Scale bar = 500 μm

a positive control due to the lack of BBB in this brain structure. Hence, Na^+-fluorescein was detected in the pineal gland of control rats and osmotherapy-treated rats, while no fluorescence was observed in the pineal gland of naïve rats, which did not receive Na^+-fluorescein (n = 3, Fig. 5f–h). The absence of osmotherapy-induced penetration of Na^+-fluorescein into the brain indicates that the integrity of the BBB and BCSFB remained intact during the applied osmotherapy treatment.

Discussion

We have demonstrated in rats that following osmotherapy (~ 50 mOsm increase in plasma osmolarity), water is osmotically extracted from the brain, although to a lesser extent than can be predicted from theoretical calculations. The reduced osmotic extraction was assigned predominantly to brain Na^+ and Cl^- accumulation (6–15% for Na^+ and 22–38% for Cl^-) and to a minor extent, if any, brain K^+ accumulation (up to 3% increase) as a function of increased plasma osmolarity, in agreement with an earlier report [14]. Notably, it is not simply the ion *concentration* that increases with the systemic hyperosmolarity but the actual ion *content*. These findings indicate that specific volume regulatory transporting mechanisms are activated in response to and/or as a consequence of increased plasma osmolarity. Employment of NaCl as the osmotic agent contributed to an increased Na^+ and Cl^- concentration in the plasma, which, in itself, could affect the brain electrolyte content. However, we observed that mannitol-mediated osmotherapy of identical magnitude and delivered volume led to similar effects on the brain electrolyte/water content [14], indicating that plasma hyperosmolarity, and not the increased plasma Na^+ and Cl^- concentrations, causes the brain electrolyte accumulation. Osmotic extraction of cerebral fluid was slightly more effective with NaCl as the osmotic agent, rather than mannitol, even though the cerebral accumulation of Na^+ was significantly higher in rats treated with NaCl. The reduced osmotic fluid extraction (and thus osmolyte increase) observed with mannitol as the osmotic agent may instead be explained by an unknown but substantial influx of other osmolytes, e.g. mannitol itself, which has previously been detected in the rat brain following mannitol-induced elevation in the plasma osmolarity [14]. With the similar Cl^- accumulation obtained with both NaCl and mannitol as the osmotic agent, one may, however, from the principle of electroneutrality, expect accumulation of another cationic electrolyte (or reduced retention of a different anion). Taken together, our findings indicate that the osmotherapy-induced rebound response may be regulated differently depending on the osmotic agent applied, although overlapping mechanisms, such as the observed gain of brain Na^+ and Cl^-, clearly exist.

According to theoretical considerations based on reflection coefficients of both osmotic agents, i.e. the relative impermeability across the BBB, NaCl treatment has been predicted to induce a larger osmotic response than mannitol [27], as confirmed by our findings. While previous findings demonstrated that NaCl was superior with regard to initial reduction of the ICP, maintenance of a lowered ICP [28, 29], and an increased cerebral water loss [29] in experimental animal models of brain injuries, other researchers observed an equal efficiency of NaCl or mannitol as the osmotic agent [30, 31], or a higher efficiency with mannitol in healthy animals [32]. Two of the latter observations may, however, be influenced by the unequal end plasma osmolarity induced by either osmotic agent [30, 32], which essentially prevents a comparative analysis. A line of clinical trials, mainly performed on patients with traumatic brain injury, reported that osmotherapy using NaCl solutions with additives (e.g. dextran, lactate, or hydroxyethyl starch solutions) [33–35] or NaCl alone [36] more effectively lowered the ICP compared with mannitol. While these reports support the findings from our animal experiments, two other clinical trials found an equal efficacy of the two osmotic agents on the ICP [37, 38]. However, a direct comparison between the few head-to-head studies carried out is challenged by the varying treatment strategies; (i) continuous or bolus injections, (ii) different doses/volumes of the osmotic agent, and (iii) different time windows, which altogether resulted in variable plasma osmolarities. In addition, diverse patient populations and outcome measurements [39] further hamper the comparison between clinical trials. It is, therefore, still questionable which osmotic agent is superior [1, 40] and animal/clinical studies, which allow direct comparison, are warranted. Mannitol remains the recommended standard osmotic agent for treatment of patients with severe head injury (Level II evidence), whereas hyperosmolar NaCl is recommended for children (Level III evidence) [41]. The choice of osmotic agent may, however, rather be based on side-effect profiles of the osmotic agents and how those will affect the clinical situation (comorbidities, age) [1].

Neither the signaling cascades, nor the molecular transport mechanisms, that couple systemic plasma hyperosmolarity to brain electrolyte accumulation have been identified. In the present study, we therefore introduced a mixture of inhibitors targeting ion-transporting proteins expressed in the BBB capillary endothelium and/or the choroid plexus epithelium, and determined their effect on osmotherapy-induced brain ion accumulation. While amiloride and methazolamide may target abluminal ion-transporting mechanisms [21, 42], we expect insignificant bumetanide interaction at the abluminal membrane of the capillaries forming the BBB because of its poor BBB permeability [43, 44]. We failed to detect evidence in favor of NKCC1, NHE1, ENaC or carbonic anhydrase (indirectly targeting the bicarbonate transporters) located at the BBB endothelium or in choroid plexus participating in this brain volume regulation. Hence, we were unable to reproduce a previously reported reduction of hyperosmotic plasma-induced brain water extraction by methazolamide [14]. The reasons for this discrepancy are unclear, although the previous study employed a very high dose of methazolamide, which was delivered i.p. instead of i.v. as in the present study. We cannot rule out that the inhibitor concentrations applied in this study were not sufficient for effective blockage of the target proteins, even though a procedure with triple doses was incorporated to enhance inhibitor efficiency. The free unbound inhibitor concentration may, however, be significantly reduced by potential binding of inhibitors to plasma proteins, as shown for bumetanide [45]. We recently found that hyperosmotic conditions enhanced the activity of abluminal Na^+/K^+-ATPase in endothelial cells, which were co-cultured with astrocytes in an in vitro BBB model [46], indicating that this transport mechanism may counteract osmotic extraction from the brain by cerebral accumulation of Na^+ in response to a hyperosmotic challenge. With the damaging effect of pump inhibition, it is, however, not simple to verify this finding by currently available techniques in animal models in vivo: a direct effect of Na^+/K^+-ATPase inhibition is difficult to deduce, due to disruption of electrochemical gradients controlling secondary active and passive transporting mechanisms. The Na^+/K^+-ATPase expressed at the CSF-facing membrane of the choroid plexus could also be a potential candidate in brain volume regulation upon osmotherapy, since the Na^+/K^+-ATPase may contribute to CSF production [47], in addition to the recently reported significant contribution of NKCC1 in murine CSF production [48]. To this end, it is important to note that the wet-dry technique, employed to determine brain water content, favors parenchymal water content over CSF, as the major part of CSF is lost in the brain isolation process. If the ion-transporting mechanisms were to regulate the CSF production per se, and the equilibrium rate between CSF and brain interstitial fluid is slow, such regulatory functions could well be missed by this experimental design.

While the ion-transporting mechanisms (NKCC1, NHE1, NBCs, and ENaC) at the BBB capillary endothelium and choroid plexus epithelium were shown not to be involved in the osmotherapy-mediated translocation of Na^+ and Cl^- from the blood into the rat brain under our experimental conditions, Na^+ and Cl^- could instead enter the brain via paracellular transport routes, which may become available with hyperosmolar plasma. However, we demonstrated that the two major brain barriers, i.e. the BBB and BCSFB, appeared to remain intact upon osmotherapy, as we detected no changes in cerebral Na^+-fluorescein accumulation whether or not the animals had been exposed to osmotherapy. Notably, we cannot exclude that Na^+ and Cl^-, which are of a smaller molecular weight (22.99 Da and 35.45 Da) than Na^+-fluorescein (376.27 Da), can cross the brain barriers via a paracellular route *provided* that the given hyperosmotic challenge promoted an increase in the permeability of the brain barriers towards smaller permeants, while excluding the fluorescent dye. However, a previous study showed that a change in barrier function, corresponding to BBB opening towards mannitol and Na^+, occurred only with hyperosmotic challenges rendering the plasma osmolarity >385 mOsm [49]. An alternative manner of accumulating brain electrolytes during conditions of elevated plasma osmolarity could be via increased bulk flow of CSF into the brain interstitial fluid [50] or via a potential regulation of fluid drainage at arachnoid granulations [51], dural lymphatic vessels [52, 53], and/or at glymphatic paravascular drainage routes [54]. Parenchymal cell volume regulation may, in addition, indirectly affect electrolyte movement across the brain barriers.

The present experimental protocol was designed to quantitatively resolve the *direct* consequences of increased plasma osmolarity (mimicked osmotherapy) on brain water and ion accumulation (hence the choice of nephrectomized animals, in which the inflicted change in plasma osmolarity could be tightly controlled). In various severities of stroke-induced brain edema in animal models, one may well expect altered BBB integrity (in the afflicted area) and potentially even altered expression/activity of membrane transporters in the BBB capillary endothelium. Such stroke-induced membrane transport responses could potentially affect ion and water accumulation during osmotherapy, and may serve to explain the observed beneficial effect of bumetanide treatment in an animal stroke model [11]. Future studies should therefore address whether the osmotherapy-mediated influx of cerebral Na^+ and Cl^- likewise contribute to the rebound response in animal models of stroke-induced cerebral edema.

Conclusions

While osmotherapy immediately lowers the ICP of patients with cerebral edema, a delayed rebound response can limit or even reverse the otherwise effective drainage. We here demonstrated that the mammalian brain loses less water than predicted from osmotically obliged water extraction when exposed to hyperosmolar plasma; osmotherapy. This volume regulatory mechanism, the rebound effect, hinges on initiation of brain ion accumulation predominantly in the form of Na^+ and Cl^-. We propose that the brain ion accumulation occurs via transcellular pathways, one of which may well be hyperosmolar-induced abluminal Na^+/K^+-ATPase activity [46], rather than due to a hyperosmolar-induced breach in the brain barriers. In the absence of identified luminal transport mechanisms, altered bulk flow (CSF-to-parenchyma flow) or drainage ((g)lymphatic pathways) may well contribute to osmolarity-induced brain electrolyte accumulation. The transport mechanisms proposed to promote osmotherapy-induced brain ion accumulation remain unresolved, since we found no evidence of NKCC1, NHE1, ENaC, and NBCs appearing amongst these under our experimental conditions in healthy non-edematous rats. Future identification of such ion-transporting mechanisms might provide a useful therapeutic target for pharmacological prevention of the rebound effect during osmotherapy in patients experiencing brain edema.

Abbreviations

aCSF: artificial CSF; ANOVA: analysis of variance; BBB: blood–brain barrier; BCSFB: blood–CSF barrier; CSF: cerebrospinal fluid; ENaC: amiloride-sensitive Na^+ channel; ICP: intracranial pressure; i.p.: intraperitoneal; i.v.: intravenous; NBCs: Na^+-coupled bicarbonate transporters; NHE1: Na^+–H^+ anti-porter 1; NKCC1: Na^+–K^+–$2Cl^-$ co-transporter 1; RT: room temperature; SEM: standard error of mean.

Authors' contributions

EKO, KL, ABS, KT, MFR, WL, and NM contributed substantially to the design/concept of experiments, experimental performance, data analysis, or interpretation. EKO, KL, ABS, KT, CK MFR, WL, and NM drafted or critically revised the manuscript, and approved the version to be published. All authors read and approved the final manuscript.

Author details

[1] Department of Neuroscience, University of Copenhagen, Copenhagen, Denmark. [2] Department of Pharmacology, Toxicology, and Pharmacy, University of Veterinary Medicine Hannover, Hannover, Germany. [3] Center for Systems Neuroscience, Hannover, Germany. [4] Neurovascular Research Unit, Department of Neurology, Herlev Gentofte Hospital, University of Copenhagen, Herlev, Copenhagen, Denmark. [5] Present Address: AJVaccines, Copenhagen, Denmark. [6] Department of Neuroscience, Faculty of Health and Medical Sciences, University of Copenhagen, Blegdamsvej 3, 2200 Copenhagen, Denmark.

Acknowledgements

We thank Edith Kaczmarek, Kristoffer Racz, Rikke Lundorf, and Charlotte Mehlin for technical and surgical assistance and Prof. Dr. Andrea Tipold for measuring plasma electrolyte concentrations.

Funding

This study was funded by the Independent Research Fund Denmark (Sapere Aude, 0602-02344B FSS, to NM) and the Deutsche Forschungsgemeinschaft (Bonn, Germany, Lo 274/15-1, to WL).

References

1. Ropper AH. Management of raised intracranial pressure and hyperosmolar therapy. Pract Neurol. 2014;14:152–8.
2. Ucar T, Akyuz M, Kazan S, Tuncer R. Role of decompressive surgery in the management of severe head injuries: prognostic factors and patient selection. J Neurotrauma. 2005;22:1311–8.
3. McManus ML, Churchwell KB, Strange K. Regulation of cell volume in health and disease. N Engl J Med. 1995;333:1260–6.
4. Todd MM. Hyperosmolar therapy and the brain: a hundred years of hard-earned lessons. Anesthesiology. 2013;118:777–9.
5. Paczynski RP. Osmotherapy. Basic concepts and controversies. Crit Care Clin. 1997;13:105–29.
6. Abbott NJ, Ronnback L, Hansson E. Astrocyte–endothelial interactions at the blood–brain barrier. Nat Rev Neurosci. 2006;7:41–53.
7. Brown PD, Davies SL, Speake T, Millar ID. Molecular mechanisms of cerebrospinal fluid production. Neuroscience. 2004;129:957–70.
8. Hladky SB, Barrand MA. Fluid and ion transfer across the blood–brain and blood–cerebrospinal fluid barriers; a comparative account of mechanisms and roles. Fluids Barriers CNS. 2016;13:19.
9. Damkier HH, Brown PD, Praetorius J. Cerebrospinal fluid secretion by the choroid plexus. Physiol Rev. 2013;93:1847–92.
10. Kusche-Vihrog K, Jeggle P, Oberleithner H. The role of ENaC in vascular endothelium. Pflugers Arch. 2014;466:851–9.
11. O'Donnell ME, Tran L, Lam TI, Liu XB, Anderson SE. Bumetanide inhibition of the blood–brain barrier Na–K–Cl cotransporter reduces edema formation in the rat middle cerebral artery occlusion model of stroke. J Cereb Blood Flow Metab. 2004;24:1046–56.
12. O'Donnell ME, Chen YJ, Lam TI, Taylor KC, Walton JH, Anderson SE. Intravenous HOE-642 reduces brain edema and Na uptake in the rat permanent middle cerebral artery occlusion model of stroke: evidence for participation of the blood–brain barrier Na/H exchanger. J Cereb Blood Flow Metab. 2013;33:225–34.
13. Kilkenny C, Browne WJ, Cuthill IC, Emerson M, Altman DG. Improving bioscience research reporting: the ARRIVE guidelines for reporting animal research. J Pharmacol Pharmacother. 2010;1:94–9.
14. Cserr HF, DePasquale M, Patlak CS. Regulation of brain water and electrolytes during acute hyperosmolality in rats. Am J Physiol. 1987;253:F522–9.
15. Nordquist L, Isaksson B, Sjoquist M. The effect of amiloride during infusion of oxytocin in male sprague-dawley rats: a study of a possible intrarenal target site for oxytocin. Clin Exp Hypertens. 2008;30:151–8.
16. Gray WD, Rauh CE, Osterberg AC, Lipchuck LM. The anticonvulsant actions of methazolamide (a carbonic anhydrase inhibitor) and diphenylhydantoin. J Pharmacol Exp Ther. 1958;124:149–60.
17. Lykke K, Tollner K, Feit PW, Erker T, MacAulay N, Loscher W. The search for NKCC1-selective drugs for the treatment of epilepsy: structure–function relationship of bumetanide and various bumetanide derivatives in inhibiting the human cation-chloride cotransporter NKCC1A. Epilepsy Behav. 2016;59:42–9.
18. Bairamian D, Johanson CE, Parmelee JT, Epstein MH. Potassium cotransport with sodium and chloride in the choroid plexus. J Neurochem. 1991;56:1623–9.
19. Teiwes J, Toto RD. Epithelial sodium channel inhibition in cardiovascular disease. A potential role for amiloride. Am J Hypertens. 2007;20:109–17.
20. Nakamura K, Kamouchi M, Kitazono T, Kuroda J, Shono Y, Hagiwara N, Ago T, Ooboshi H, Ibayashi S, Iida M. Amiloride inhibits hydrogen peroxide-induced Ca^{2+} responses in human CNS pericytes. Microvasc Res. 2009;77:327–34.
21. Li M, Wang W, Mai H, Zhang X, Wang J, Gao Y, Wang Y, Deng G, Gao L, Zhou S, et al. Methazolamide improves neurological behavior by inhibition of neuron apoptosis in subarachnoid hemorrhage mice. Sci Rep. 2016;6:35055.
22. Sugrue MF, Gautheron P, Mallorga P, Nolan TE, Graham SL, Schwam H, Shepard KL, Smith RL. L-662,583 is a topically effective ocular hypotensive carbonic anhydrase inhibitor in experimental animals. Br J Pharmacol. 1990;99:59–64.
23. Hawkins BT, Egleton RD. Fluorescence imaging of blood–brain barrier disruption. J Neurosci Methods. 2006;151:262–7.
24. Moller M, van Deurs B, Westergaard E. Vascular permeability to proteins and peptides in the mouse pineal gland. Cell Tissue Res. 1978;195:1–15.
25. Russell JM. Sodium–potassium–chloride cotransport. Physiol Rev. 2000;80:211–76.

26. Karimy JK, Kahle KT, Kurland DB, Yu E, Gerzanich V, Simard JM. A novel method to study cerebrospinal fluid dynamics in rats. J Neurosci Methods. 2015;241:78–84.
27. Bhardwaj A, Ulatowski JA. Hypertonic saline solutions in brain injury. Curr Opin Crit Care. 2004;10:126–31.
28. Mirski AM, Denchev ID, Schnitzer SM, Hanley FD. Comparison between hypertonic saline and mannitol in the reduction of elevated intracranial pressure in a rodent model of acute cerebral injury. J Neurosurg Anesthesiol. 2000;12:334–44.
29. Qureshi AI, Wilson DA, Traystman RJ. Treatment of elevated intracranial pressure in experimental intracerebral hemorrhage: comparison between mannitol and hypertonic saline. Neurosurgery. 1999;44:1055–63.
30. Freshman SP, Battistella FD, Matteucci M, Wisner DH. Hypertonic saline (7.5%) versus mannitol: a comparison for treatment of acute head injuries. J Trauma. 1993;35:344–8.
31. Scheller MS, Zornow MH, Seok Y. A comparison of the cerebral and hemodynamic effects of mannitol and hypertonic saline in a rabbit model of acute cryogenic brain injury. J Neurosurg Anesthesiol. 1991;3:291–6.
32. Wang LC, Papangelou A, Lin C, Mirski MA, Gottschalk A, Toung TJ. Comparison of equivolume, equiosmolar solutions of mannitol and hypertonic saline with or without furosemide on brain water content in normal rats. Anesthesiology. 2013;118:903–13.
33. Battison C, Andrews PJ, Graham C, Petty T. Randomized, controlled trial on the effect of a 20% mannitol solution and a 7.5% saline/6% dextran solution on increased intracranial pressure after brain injury. Crit Care Med. 2005;33:196–202 **(discussion 257-198)**.
34. Harutjunyan L, Holz C, Rieger A, Menzel M, Grond S, Soukup J. Efficiency of 7.2% hypertonic saline hydroxyethyl starch 200/0.5 versus mannitol 15% in the treatment of increased intracranial pressure in neurosurgical patients—a randomized clinical trial [ISRCTN62699180]. Crit Care. 2005;9:R530–40.
35. Ichai C, Armando G, Orban JC, Berthier F, Rami L, Samat-Long C, Grimaud D, Leverve X. Sodium lactate versus mannitol in the treatment of intracranial hypertensive episodes in severe traumatic brain-injured patients. Intensive Care Med. 2009;35:471–9.
36. Oddo M, Levine JM, Frangos S, Carrera E, Maloney-Wilensky E, Pascual JL, Kofke WA, Mayer SA, LeRoux PD. Effect of mannitol and hypertonic saline on cerebral oxygenation in patients with severe traumatic brain injury and refractory intracranial hypertension. J Neurol Neurosurg Psychiatry. 2009;80:916–20.
37. Sakellaridis N, Pavlou E, Karatzas S, Chroni D, Vlachos K, Chatzopoulos K, Dimopoulou E, Kelesis C, Karaouli V. Comparison of mannitol and hypertonic saline in the treatment of severe brain injuries. J Neurosurg. 2011;114:545–8.
38. Cottenceau V, Masson F, Mahamid E, Petit L, Shik V, Sztark F, Zaaroor M, Soustiel JF. Comparison of effects of equiosmolar doses of mannitol and hypertonic saline on cerebral blood flow and metabolism in traumatic brain injury. J Neurotrauma. 2011;28:2003–12.
39. Asehnoune K, Lasocki S, Seguin P, Geeraerts T, Perrigault PF, Dahyot-Fizelier C, Paugam Burtz C, Cook F, Demeure Dit Latte D, Cinotti R, et al. Association between continuous hyperosmolar therapy and survival in patients with traumatic brain injury—a multicentre prospective cohort study and systematic review. Crit Care. 2017;21:328.
40. Burgess S, Abu-Laban RB, Slavik RS, Vu EN, Zed PJ. A systematic review of randomized controlled trials comparing hypertonic sodium solutions and mannitol for traumatic brain injury: implications for emergency department management. Ann Pharmacother. 2016;50:291–300.
41. Adelson PD, Bratton SL, Carney NA, Chesnut RM, du Coudray HE, Goldstein B, Kochanek PM, Miller HC, Partington MD, Selden NR, et al. Guidelines for the acute medical management of severe traumatic brain injury in infants, children, and adolescents. Chapter 11. Use of hyperosmolar therapy in the management of severe pediatric traumatic brain injury. Pediatr Crit Care Med. 2003;4:S40–4.
42. Durham-Lee JC, Mokkapati VU, Johnson KM, Nesic O. Amiloride improves locomotor recovery after spinal cord injury. J Neurotrauma. 2011;28:1319–26.
43. Brandt C, Nozadze M, Heuchert N, Rattka M, Loscher W. Disease-modifying effects of phenobarbital and the NKCC1 inhibitor bumetanide in the pilocarpine model of temporal lobe epilepsy. J Neurosci. 2010;30:8602–12.
44. Li Y, Cleary R, Kellogg M, Soul JS, Berry GT, Jensen FE. Sensitive isotope dilution liquid chromatography/tandem mass spectrometry method for quantitative analysis of bumetanide in serum and brain tissue. J Chromatogr B Analyt Technol Biomed Life Sci. 2011;879:998–1002.
45. Walker PC, Berry NS, Edwards DJ. Protein binding characteristics of bumetanide. Dev Pharmacol Ther. 1989;12:13–8.
46. Lykke K, Assentoft M, Horlyck S, Helms HC, Stoica A, Toft-Bertelsen TL, Tritsaris K, Vilhardt F, Brodin B, MacAulay N. Evaluating the involvement of cerebral microvascular endothelial Na(+)/K(+)-ATPase and Na(+)-K(+)-2Cl(−) co-transporter in electrolyte fluxes in an in vitro blood–brain barrier model of dehydration. J Cereb Blood Flow Metab. 2017. https://doi.org/10.1177/0271678X17736715.
47. Pollay M, Hisey B, Reynolds E, Tomkins P, Stevens FA, Smith R. Choroid plexus Na+/K+-activated adenosine triphosphatase and cerebrospinal fluid formation. Neurosurgery. 1985;17:768–72.
48. Steffensen AB, Oernbo EK, Stoica A, Gerkau NJ, Barbuskaite D, Tritsaris K, Rose CR, MacAulay N. Cotransporter-mediated water transport underlying cerebrospinal fluid formation. Nat Commun. 2018;9:2167.
49. Cserr HF, DePasquale M, Patlak CS. Volume regulatory influx of electrolytes from plasma to brain during acute hyperosmolality. Am J Physiol. 1987;253:F530–7.
50. Pullen RG, DePasquale M, Cserr HF. Bulk flow of cerebrospinal fluid into brain in response to acute hyperosmolality. Am J Physiol. 1987;253:F538–45.
51. Pollay M. The function and structure of the cerebrospinal fluid outflow system. Cerebrospinal Fluid Res. 2010;7:9.
52. Aspelund A, Antila S, Proulx ST, Karlsen TV, Karaman S, Detmar M, Wiig H, Alitalo K. A dural lymphatic vascular system that drains brain interstitial fluid and macromolecules. J Exp Med. 2015;212:991–9.
53. Louveau A, Smirnov I, Keyes TJ, Eccles JD, Rouhani SJ, Peske JD, Derecki NC, Castle D, Mandell JW, Lee KS, et al. Structural and functional features of central nervous system lymphatic vessels. Nature. 2015;523:337–41.
54. Iliff JJ, Wang M, Liao Y, Plogg BA, Peng W, Gundersen GA, Benveniste H, Vates GE, Deane R, Goldman SA, et al. A paravascular pathway facilitates CSF flow through the brain parenchyma and the clearance of interstitial solutes, including amyloid beta. Sci Transl Med. 2012;4:147ra111.

Permissions

All chapters in this book were first published in FBOC, by BioMed Central; hereby published with permission under the Creative Commons Attribution License or equivalent. Every chapter published in this book has been scrutinized by our experts. Their significance has been extensively debated. The topics covered herein carry significant findings which will fuel the growth of the discipline. They may even be implemented as practical applications or may be referred to as a beginning point for another development.

The contributors of this book come from diverse backgrounds, making this book a truly international effort. This book will bring forth new frontiers with its revolutionizing research information and detailed analysis of the nascent developments around the world.

We would like to thank all the contributing authors for lending their expertise to make the book truly unique. They have played a crucial role in the development of this book. Without their invaluable contributions this book wouldn't have been possible. They have made vital efforts to compile up to date information on the varied aspects of this subject to make this book a valuable addition to the collection of many professionals and students.

This book was conceptualized with the vision of imparting up-to-date information and advanced data in this field. To ensure the same, a matchless editorial board was set up. Every individual on the board went through rigorous rounds of assessment to prove their worth. After which they invested a large part of their time researching and compiling the most relevant data for our readers.

The editorial board has been involved in producing this book since its inception. They have spent rigorous hours researching and exploring the diverse topics which have resulted in the successful publishing of this book. They have passed on their knowledge of decades through this book. To expedite this challenging task, the publisher supported the team at every step. A small team of assistant editors was also appointed to further simplify the editing procedure and attain best results for the readers.

Apart from the editorial board, the designing team has also invested a significant amount of their time in understanding the subject and creating the most relevant covers. They scrutinized every image to scout for the most suitable representation of the subject and create an appropriate cover for the book.

The publishing team has been an ardent support to the editorial, designing and production team. Their endless efforts to recruit the best for this project, has resulted in the accomplishment of this book. They are a veteran in the field of academics and their pool of knowledge is as vast as their experience in printing. Their expertise and guidance has proved useful at every step. Their uncompromising quality standards have made this book an exceptional effort. Their encouragement from time to time has been an inspiration for everyone.

The publisher and the editorial board hope that this book will prove to be a valuable piece of knowledge for researchers, students, practitioners and scholars across the globe.

List of Contributors

Ivana Lazarevic and Britta Engelhardt
Theodor Kocher Institute, University of Bern, Freiestrasse 1, 3012 Bern, Switzerland

Edit Dósa, Krisztina Heltai, Tamás Radovits, Gabriella Molnár and Béla Merkely
Heart and Vascular Center, Semmelweis University, 68 Városmajor Street, Budapest 1122, Hungary

Judit Kapocsi
Department of Internal Medicine, Semmelweis University, 26 Üllői Street, Budapest 1085, Hungary

Rongwei Fu
Public Health and Preventive Medicine, Oregon Health and Science University, 3184 S.W. Sam Jackson Park Rd, CB669, Portland, OR 97329, USA

Nancy D. Doolittle, Gerda B. Tóth and Zachary Urdang
Department of Neurology, Oregon Health and Science University, 3184 S.W. Sam Jackson Park Rd, L603, Portland, OR 97329, USA

Edward A. Neuwelt
Department of Neurology, Oregon Health and Science University, 3184 S.W. Sam Jackson Park Rd, L603, Portland, OR 97329, USA
Department of Neurosurgery, Oregon Health and Science University, 3184 S.W. Sam Jackson Park Rd, L603, Portland, OR 97329, USA
Portland Veterans Affairs Medical Center, 3710 S.W. US Veterans Hospital Rd, Portland, OR 97239, USA
Blood–Brain Barrier and Neuro-Oncology Program, Oregon Health and Science University, 3181 S.W. Sam Jackson Park Road, L603, Portland, OR 97239, USA

Joao Prola Netto
Department of Neurology, Oregon Health and Science University, 3181 SW Sam Jackson Park Road, Portland, OR 97239, USA
Department of Neuroradiology, Oregon Health and Science University, 3181 SW Sam Jackson Park Road, Portland, OR 97239, USA

Daniel Schwartz
Department of Neurology, Oregon Health and Science University, 3181 SW Sam Jackson Park Road, Portland, OR 97239, USA
Advanced Imaging Research Center, Oregon Health and Science University, 3181 SW Sam Jackson Park Road, Portland, OR 97239, USA

Csanad Varallyay
Department of Neurology, Oregon Health and Science University, 3181 SW Sam Jackson Park Road, Portland, OR 97239, USA

Rongwei Fu
School of Public Health, Oregon Health and Science University, 3181 SW Sam Jackson Park Road, Portland, OR 97239, USA
Emergency Medicine, Oregon Health and Science University, 3181 SW Sam Jackson Park Road, Portland, OR 97239, USA

Bronwyn Hamilton
Department of Neuroradiology, Oregon Health and Science University, 3181 SW Sam Jackson Park Road, Portland, OR 97239, USA

Edward A. Neuwelt
Department of Neurology, Oregon Health and Science University, 3181 SW Sam Jackson Park Road, Portland, OR 97239, USA
Department of Veterans Affairs Medical Center, 3710 SW U.S. Veterans Hospital Road, Portland, OR 97239, USA
Department of Neurosurgery, Oregon Health and Science University, 3181 SW Sam Jackson Park Road, L603, Portland, OR 97239, USA

Zhongyun Chen, Chunyan Liu, Jie Zhang and Yan Xing
Department of Neurology, Aviation General Hospital of China Medical University and Beijing Institute of Translational Medicine, Chinese Academy of Sciences, No. 3 Anwai Beiyuan Road, Chaoyang District, Beijing 100012, China

Norman Relkin
Department of Neurology and Neuroscience, Weill Medical College of Cornell University, Cornell Memory Disorders Program, 428 East 72 Street, Suite 500, New York, NY 10021, USA

Yanfeng Li
Department of Neurology, Peking Union Medical College Hospital, Beijing, China

Catharina Conrad
Department of Neurology, Philipps University Marburg, Baldingerstr, 35033 Marburg, Germany
Department of Anesthesiology and Intensive Care Medicine, University Hospital, Albert-Schweitzer Campus 1, 48149 Münster, Germany

Kristina Dorzweiler and Jörg W. Bartsch
Department of Neurosurgery, Philipps University Marburg, Baldingerstr, 35033 Marburg, Germany

Miles A. Miller
Department of Biological Engineering, Massachusetts Institute of Technology, Cambridge, MA 02139, USA
Center for Systems Biology, Massachusetts General Hospital, Harvard Medical School, Boston, MA 02114, USA

Douglas A. Lauffenburger
Department of Biological Engineering, Massachusetts Institute of Technology, Cambridge, MA 02139, USA

Herwig Strik
Department of Neurology, Philipps University Marburg, Baldingerstr, 35033 Marburg, Germany

Grant A. Bateman
Department of Medical Imaging, John Hunter Hospital, Locked Bag 1, Newcastle Region Mail Center, Newcastle 2310, Australia
Newcastle University Faculty of Health, Callaghan Campus Newcastle, Newcastle, Australia

Jeannette Lechner-Scott
Newcastle University Faculty of Health, Callaghan Campus Newcastle, Newcastle, Australia
Department of Neurology, John Hunter Hospital, Newcastle, Australia
Hunter Medical Research Institute, Newcastle, Australia

Rodney A. Lea
Institute of Health and Biomedical Innovation, Queensland University of Technology, Brisbane, Australia

John Greenwood
Institute of Ophthalmology, University College London, London EC1V 9EL, UK

Margareta Hammarlund-Udenaes
Department of Pharmaceutical Biosciences, Uppsala University, 751 24 Uppsala, Sweden

Hazel C. Jones
Gagle Brook House, Chesterton, Bicester OX26 1UF, UK

Alan W. Stitt
Centre for Experimental Medicine, Queen's University Belfast, Belfast, Northern Ireland, UK

Roosmarijn E. Vandenbroucke
Department of Biomedical Molecular Biology, Ghent University, Ghent, Belgium
VIB-UGent Center for Inflammation Research, VIB, Ghent, Belgium

Ignacio A. Romero
School of Life, Health and Chemical Sciences, Open University, Milton Keynes, UK

Matthew Campbell
Smurfit Institute of Genetics, Lincoln Place Gate, Trinity College Dublin, Dublin 2, Ireland

Gert Fricker
Institute of Pharmacy and Molecular Biotechnology, Ruprecht-Karls University, Heidelberg, Germany

Birger Brodin
Department of Pharmacy, Faculty of Health and Medical Sciences, University of Copenhagen, Copenhagen, Denmark

Heiko Manninga
NEUWAY Pharma GmbH, Ludwig-Erhard-Allee 2, 53175 Bonn, Germany

Pieter J. Gaillard
2-BBB Medicines BV, Leiden, Netherlands

Markus Schwaninger
Institute of Experimental and Clinical Pharmacology and Toxicology, University of Lübeck, Lübeck, Germany

Carl Webster
Antibody Discovery and Protein Engineering, MedImmune, Cambridge, UK

Krzysztof B. Wicher
Ossianix Inc., Stevenage, UK

Michel Khrestchatisky
CNRS, NICN, Aix Marseille Univ, Marseille, France
Vect-Horus, Faculte de Medecine Nord, 51 Boulevard Pierre Dramard, Marseille, France

M. Guerra and E. M. Rodríguez
Instituto de Anatomía, Histología y Patología, Facultad de Medicina, Universidad Austral de Chile, Valdivia, Chile

J. L. Blázquez
Departamento de Anatomía e Histología Humana, Facultad de Medicina, Universidad de Salamanca, Salamanca, Spain

Lucas R. Sass, Mohammadreza Khani and Gabryel Connely Natividad
Neurophysiological Imaging and Modeling Laboratory, University of Idaho, 875 Perimeter Dr. MC1122, Moscow, ID 83844-1122, USA

R. Shane Tubbs
Seattle Science Foundation, 200 2nd Ave N, Seattle, WA 98109, USA

Olivier Baledent
Bioflow Image, Service de Biophysique et de Traitement de l'Image médicale, Bâtiment desécoles, CHU Nord Amiens-Picardie, Place Victor Pauchet, 80054 Amiens Cedex 1, France

Bryn A. Martin
Neurophysiological Imaging and Modeling Laboratory, University of Idaho, 875 Perimeter Dr. MC1122, Moscow, ID 83844-1122, USA
Department of Biological Engineering, University of Idaho, 875 Perimeter Dr. MC0904, Moscow, ID 83844-0904, USA

Shigenori Kanno
Department of Neurology, Southmiyagi Medical Center, 38-1, Aza-nishi, Shibata, Miyagi 989-1253, Japan
Department of Behavioural Neurology and Cognitive Neuroscience, Tohoku University Graduate School of Medicine, Sendai, Japan

Makoto Saito, Tomohito Kashinoura, Yoshiyuki Nishio, Osamu Iizuka, Hirokazu Kikuchi, Masahito Takagi and Etsuro Mori
Department of Behavioural Neurology and Cognitive Neuroscience, Tohoku University Graduate School of Medicine, Sendai, Japan

Masaki Iwasaki
Department of Neurosurgery, Tohoku University Graduate School of Medicine, Sendai, Japan

Shoki Takahashi
Department of Diagnostic Radiology, Tohoku University Graduate School of Medicine, Sendai, Japan

Erin Gallagher and Peter C. Searson
Institute for Nanobiotechnology Johns Hopkins University, 3400 North Charles Street, Baltimore, MD 21218, USA
Department of Materials Science and Engineering, Johns Hopkins University, 3400 North Charles Street, Baltimore, MD 21218, USA

Il Minn
Department of Radiology and Radiological Science, Johns Hopkins University, 3400 North Charles Street, Baltimore, MD 21231, USA

Janice E. Chambers
College of Veterinary Medicine, Mississippi State University, Mississippi State, MS 39762-6100, USA

Sadhana Jackson
Brain Cancer Program, Johns Hopkins University, David H. Koch Cancer Research Building II, 1550 Orleans Street, Room 1M16, Baltimore, MD 21287, USA
Neuro-Oncology Branch, NCI/NIH, 9030 Old Georgetown Rd, Building 82, Bethesda, MD 20892, USA

Jon Weingart and Xiaobu Ye
School of Medicine, Department of Neurosurgery, Johns Hopkins University, Baltimore, MD 21287, USA

Edjah K. Nduom
Surgical Neurology Branch, NINDS/NIH, 10 Center Drive, 3D20, Bethesda, MD 20814, USA

Thura T. Harfi
David Heart and Lung Research Institute, The Ohio State University, 374 12th Avenue, Suite 200, Columbus, OH 43210, USA

Richard T. George
Heart and Vascular Institute, Johns Hopkins University, 600 N. Wolfe Street, Sheikh Zayed Tower, Baltimore, MD 21287, USA

Dorothea McAreavey
Critical Care Medicine Department, Nuclear Cardiology Section, NIH Clinical Center, 10 Center Drive, Bethesda, MD 20892, USA

Nicole M. Anders and Michelle A. Rudek
Cancer Chemical and Structural Biology and Analytical Pharmacology Core Laboratory, Johns Hopkins University, Bunting-Blaustein Cancer Research Building I, 1650 Orleans Street, CRB1 Room 1M52, Baltimore, MD 21231, USA

Cody Peer and William D. Figg
Clinical Pharmacology, NCI/NIH, 10 Center Drive, 5A01, Bethesda, MD 20814, USA

Mark Gilbert
Neuro-Oncology Branch, NCI/NIH, 9030 Old Georgetown Rd, Building 82, Bethesda, MD 20892, USA

Stuart A. Grossman
Brain Cancer Program, Johns Hopkins University, David H. Koch Cancer Research Building II, 1550 Orleans Street, Room 1M16, Baltimore, MD 21287, USA

Tori B. Terrell-Hall, Jessica I. G. Griffith and Paul R. Lockman
Department of Basic Pharmaceutical Sciences, School of Pharmacy, West Virginia University HSC, 1 Medical Center Dr., Morgantown, WV 26506, USA

Amanda G. Ammer
WVU Cancer Institute Research Laboratories, West Virginia University HSC, Morgantown, WV 26506, USA

Masatsune Ishikawa
Rakuwa Villa Ilios, 186 Jyrakumawari-nishimachi, Nakagyouku, Kyoto 604-8402, Japan
Normal Pressure Hydrocephalus Center, Rakuwakai Otowa Hospital, 2 Chinjicho, Yamashinaku, Otowa, Kyoto 607-8062, Japan

Shigeki Yamada
Normal Pressure Hydrocephalus Center, Rakuwakai Otowa Hospital, 2 Chinjicho, Yamashinaku, Otowa, Kyoto 607-8062, Japan
Department of Neurosurgery, Rakuwakai Otowa Hospital, 2 Chinjicho, Yamashinaku, Otowa, Kyoto 607-8062, Japan

Kazuo Yamamoto
Department of Neurosurgery, Rakuwakai Otowa Hospital, 2 Chinjicho, Yamashinaku, Otowa, Kyoto 607-8062, Japan

Ken Takizawa and Mitsunori Matsumae
Department of Neurosurgery, Tokai University School of Medicine, 143 Shimokasuya, Isehara, Kanagawa 2591193, Japan

Saeko Sunohara, Satoshi Yatsushiro and Kagayaki Kuroda
Course of Science and Technology, Graduate School of Science and Technology, Tokai University, 4-1-1 Kitakaname, Hiratsuka, Kanagawa 2591292, Japan

Naoko H. Tomioka and Makoto Hosoyamada
Department of Human Physiology and Pathology, Faculty of Pharma-Sciences, Teikyo University, 2-11-1 Kaga, Itabashi-ku, Tokyo 173-8605, Japan

Yoshifuru Tamura, Shigeru Shibata and Shunya Uchida
Department of Internal Medicine, Teikyo University School of Medicine, Teikyo University, 2-11-1 Kaga, Itabashi-ku, Tokyo 173-8605, Japan

Tappei Takada and Hiroshi Suzuki
Department of Pharmacy, The University of Tokyo Hospital, Faculty of Medicine, The University of Tokyo, 7-3-1 Hongo, Bunkyo-ku, Tokyo 113-8655, Japan

Catherine A. A. Lee
Department of Genetics and Cell Development, University of Minnesota, Minneapolis, MN 55455, USA

Hannah S. Seo, Frank S. Bates and Samira M. Azarin
Department of Chemical Engineering and Materials Science, University of Minnesota, Minneapolis, MN 55455, USA

Anibal G. Armien
Ultrastructural Pathology Unit, Veterinary Diagnostic Laboratory, College of Veterinary Medicine, University of Minnesota, St. Paul, MN 55108, USA

Jakub Tolar
Department of Pediatrics, University of Minnesota, Minneapolis, MN 55455, USA

Nienke R. Wevers
Mimetas BV, J.H. Oortweg 19, 2333 CH Leiden, The Netherlands
Department of Cell and Chemical Biology, Leiden University Medical Centre, Einthovenweg 20, 2333 ZC Leiden, The Netherlands

Dhanesh G. Kasi, Karlijn J. Wilschut, Remko van Vught, Sebastiaan J. Trietsch, Paul Vulto and Henriëtte L. Lanz
Mimetas BV, J.H. Oortweg 19, 2333 CH Leiden, The Netherlands

Taylor Gray, Benjamin Smith, Graham Marsh and Birgit Obermeier
Biogen, 225 Binney Street, Cambridge, MA 02142, USA

Fumitaka Shimizu, Yasuteru Sano and Takashi Kanda
Yamaguchi University Graduate School of Medicine, Minamikogushi, Ube, Yamaguchi 7558505, Japan

Mohammad M. Faghih and M. Keith Sharp
Biofluid Mechanics Laboratory, Department of Mechanical Engineering, University of Louisville, Louisville, KY 40292, USA

Servio H. Ramirez
Department of Pathology and Laboratory Medicine, The Lewis Katz School of Medicine at Temple University, 3500 N Broad St, Philadelphia, PA 19140, USA
Shriners Hospital Pediatric Research Center, Philadelphia, PA 19140, USA
Center for Substance Abuse Research, The Lewis Katz School of Medicine at Temple University, Philadelphia, PA 19140, USA

Allison M. Andrews
Department of Pathology and Laboratory Medicine, The Lewis Katz School of Medicine at Temple University, 3500 N Broad St, Philadelphia, PA 19140, USA

Center for Substance Abuse Research, The Lewis Katz School of Medicine at Temple University, Philadelphia, PA 19140, USA

Debayon Paul and Joel S. Pachter
Department of Immunology, Blood-Brain Barrier Laboratory and Laser Capture Microdissection Core, UConn Health, 263 Farmington Ave., Farmington, CT 06070, USA

Monica D. Okon
Department of Biomedical Engineering, The Ohio State University, 1080 Carmack Rd, Columbus, OH 43210, USA

Cynthia J. Roberts and Ashraf M. Mahmoud
Department of Biomedical Engineering, The Ohio State University, 1080 Carmack Rd, Columbus, OH 43210, USA
Department of Ophthalmology and Visual Science, The Ohio State University, 915 Olentangy River Rd, Columbus, OH 43212, USA

Andrew N. Springer
Department of Anesthesiology, The Ohio State University, 410W, 10th Avenue, Columbus, OH 43210, USA

Robert H. Small
Department of Biomedical Engineering, The Ohio State University, 1080 Carmack Rd, Columbus, OH 43210, USA
Department of Anesthesiology, The Ohio State University, 410W, 10th Avenue, Columbus, OH 43210, USA

John M. McGregor
Department of Neurosurgery, The Ohio State University, 1581 Dodd Drive, Columbus, OH 43210, USA

Steven E. Katz
Ohio Neuro-Ophthalmology, Orbital Disease and Oculoplastics, 3545 Olentangy River Rd, Suite 200, Columbus, OH 43214, USA

Edward G. Stopa, Miles C. Miller, John E. Donahue, Tara Torabi, Gerald D. Silverberg and Conrad E. Johanson
Departments of Neurosurgery and Pathology (Neuropathology Division), Rhode Island Hospital, The Warren Alpert Medical School, Brown University, Providence, RI, USA

Keith Q. Tanis, Elena V. Nikonova, Alexei A. Podtelezhnikov, Eva M. Finney, David J. Stone, Luiz M. Camargo and Lisan Parker
Genetics and Pharmacogenomics, Merck and Co., Inc., West Point, PA, USA

Ajay Verma
United Neuroscience, Dublin, Ireland

Andrew Baird and Brian P. Eliceiri
Department of Surgery, University of California San Diego Medical Center, Hillcrest, 212 Dickinson Street, San Diego, CA, USA

Eva Kjer Oernbo, Annette Buur Steffensen and Martin Fredensborg Rath
Department of Neuroscience, University of Copenhagen, Copenhagen, Denmark

Kasper Lykke
Department of Neuroscience, University of Copenhagen, Copenhagen, Denmark
AJVaccines, Copenhagen, Denmark

Kathrin Töllner and Wolfgang Löscher
Department of Pharmacology, Toxicology, and Pharmacy, University of Veterinary Medicine Hannover, Hannover, Germany
Center for Systems Neuroscience, Hannover, Germany

Christina Kruuse
Neurovascular Research Unit, Department of Neurology, Herlev Gentofte Hospital, University of Copenhagen, Herlev, Copenhagen, Denmark

Nanna MacAulay
Department of Neuroscience, University of Copenhagen, Copenhagen, Denmark
Department of Neuroscience, Faculty of Health and Medical Sciences, University of Copenhagen, Blegdamsvej 3, 2200 Copenhagen, Denmark

Index